Breast Cancer: A Growing Concern

Breast Cancer: A Growing Concern

Editor: Brianna Peralta

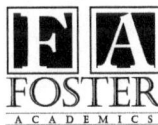

FOSTER
ACADEMICS

www.fosteracademics.com

www.fosteracademics.com

FA FOSTER
ACADEMICS

Cataloging-in-Publication Data

Breast cancer : a growing concern / edited by Brianna Peralta.
      p. cm.
Includes bibliographical references and index.
ISBN 978-1-63242-749-6
1. Breast--Cancer. 2. Breast--Tumors. 3. Breast--Cancer--Treatment. 4. Cancer in women.
I. Peralta, Brianna.
RC280.B8 B74 2019
616.994 49--dc23

Foster Academics,
118-35 Queens Blvd., Suite 400,
Forest Hills, NY 11375, USA

ISBN 978-1-63242-749-6 (Hardback)

Contents

Preface

The world is advancing at a fast pace like never before. Therefore, the need is to keep up with the latest developments. This book was an idea that came to fruition when the specialists in the area realized the need to coordinate together and document essential themes in the subject. That's when I was requested to be the editor. Editing this book has been an honour as it brings together diverse authors researching on different streams of the field. The book collates essential materials contributed by veterans in the area which can be utilized by students and researchers alike.

Breast cancer is the most common invasive cancer, affecting 12% of women worldwide. Some of the risk factors contributing to the incidence of this disease are obesity, alcohol consumption, hormone replacement therapy, lack of physical exercise, etc. Between 5-10% of breast cancer cases are attributed to genetics. Breast cancers are easy to diagnose through a biopsy or a microscopic analysis of the affected area of the breast. Its treatment can be a multidisciplinary procedure involving surgical and non-surgical modalities. The tumor is removed surgically along with the surrounding tissue, and one or more lymph nodes may also be biopsied. For someone with high risk factors, medications such as raloxifene or tamoxifen may be used to prevent this disease. The topics covered in this extensive book deal with the clinical aspects of breast cancer. The aim of this book is to present researches that have transformed this domain and aided its treatment and management. The readers would gain knowledge that would broaden their perspective about breast cancer.

Each chapter is a sole-standing publication that reflects each author's interpretation. Thus, the book displays a multi-facetted picture of our current understanding of application, resources and aspects of the field. I would like to thank the contributors of this book and my family for their endless support.

Editor

Nogo-B receptor increases the resistance to tamoxifen in estrogen receptor-positive breast cancer cells

Pin Gao[1,2,3], Xiang Wang[2,3,4], Ying Jin[1,2,3], Wenquan Hu[2,3], Yajun Duan[2,3,4], Aiping Shi[1], Ye Du[1], Dong Song[1], Ming Yang[1], Sijie Li[1], Bing Han[1], Gang Zhao[1], Hongquan Zhang[4,5*], Zhimin Fan[1,5*] and Qing Robert Miao[2,3,5*] 🅘

Abstract

Backgrounds: Tamoxifen is typically used to treat patients with estrogen receptor alpha (ERα)-positive breast cancer. However, 30% of these patients gain acquired resistance to tamoxifen during or after tamoxifen treatment. As a Ras modulator, Nogo-B receptor (NgBR) is required for tumorigenesis through the signaling crosstalk with epidermal growth factor (EGF) receptor (EGFR)-mediated pathways. NgBR is highly expressed in many types of cancer cells and regulates the sensitivity of hepatocellular carcinoma to chemotherapy. In this study, we found the expression of NgBR is increased in tamoxifen-resistant ERα-positive breast cancer cells.

Methods: Tamoxifen-resistant ERα-positive MCF-7 and T47D breast cancer cell lines were established by culturing with gradually increased concentration of 4-hydroxytamoxifen (4-OHT). The effects of NgBR on tamoxifen resistance was determined by depleting NgBR in these cell lines using previously validated small interfering RNA (siRNA). The effects of 4-OHT on cell viability and apoptosis were determined using well-accepted methods such as clonogenic survival assay and Annexin V/propidium iodide staining. The alteration of EGF-stimulated signaling and gene expression was determined by western blot analysis and real-time PCR, respectively.

Results: NgBR knockdown with siRNA attenuates EGF-induced phosphorylation of ERα and restores the sensitivity to tamoxifen in ERα-positive breast cancer cells. Mechanistically, our data demonstrated that NgBR knockdown increases the protein levels of p53 and decreases survivin, which is an apoptosis inhibitor.

Conclusions: These results suggested that NgBR is a potential therapeutic target for increasing the sensitivity of ERα-positive breast cancer to tamoxifen.

Keywords: Nogo-B receptor, Survivin, Tamoxifen, Estrogen receptor, Breast cancer

Background

Breast cancer is the most common cancer in women around the world [1, 2]. About 75% of the cases are estrogen receptor alpha (ERα)-positive breast cancer [3]. These patients undergo adjuvant endocrine therapy to increase

disease-free survival (DFS) and overall survival (OS) [4]. According to the National Comprehensive Cancer Network (NCCN) guideline, patients with invasive breast cancer who are ERα-positive or progesterone receptor (PR)-positive are eligible for tamoxifen, the selective estrogen receptor modulator (SERM) [5]. Tamoxifen, or its active metabolite 4-hydroxytamoxifen (4-OHT), are reported to induce breast cancer cell apoptosis [6]. However, recurrence within 15 years occurs in one third of patients treated with tamoxifen for 5 years [4].

The underlying mechanisms of developing resistance, especially acquired resistance, to tamoxifen are complex and numerous, including ligand-independent activation

* Correspondence: hongquan.zhang@bjmu.edu.cn; fanzhimn@163.com; qmiao@mcw.edu
[4]Department of Human Anatomy, Histology, and Embryology, Key Laboratory of Carcinogenesis and Translational Research (Ministry of Education) and State Key Laboratory of Natural and Biomimetic Drugs, Peking University Health Science Center, Beijing 100191, China
[1]Department of Breast Surgery, The First Hospital of Jilin University, 71 Xinmin street, Changchun 130021, Jilin Province, China
[2]Division of Pediatric Surgery, Department of Surgery, Children's Research Institute, Medical College of Wisconsin, 8701 W Watertown Plank Rd, Milwaukee, WI 53226, USA
Full list of author information is available at the end of the article

of ERα or its co-activators through phosphorylation, and the inhibition of apoptosis through constitutive activation of survival signaling [7]. Clinical evidence shows that patients with human epidermal growth factor receptor 2 (HER2) overexpression and lower ERα levels are more likely to become tamoxifen-resistant [8]. Preclinical studies implicate the contribution of growth factor receptor signaling pathways, such as EGFR and HER2, to tamoxifen resistance [9, 10].

Nogo isoforms, including Nogo-A, Nogo-B and Nogo-C, are members of a reticulon protein superfamily. Nogo-B is mainly expressed in peripheral tissues [11]. NgBR was identified as a Nogo-B receptor specific for the amino terminus of Nogo-B (AmNogo-B). NgBR is necessary for angiogenesis by mediating chemotaxis of endothelial cells [12], and is essential for vasculature development [13, 14]. Our recent findings demonstrated that NgBR binds farnesylated Ras and recruits Ras to the plasma membrane, which is a critical step required for receptor tyrosine kinase (RTK)-mediated activation of Ras signaling in human breast cancer cells and tumorigenesis [15]. Greater expression of NgBR in ERα-positive breast tumor tissues is significantly correlated with expression of survivin [16], which is an apoptosis inhibitor [17]. A proteomic study also showed that NgBR is essential for promoting epithelial-mesenchymal transition (EMT) in breast cancer cells [18]. However, the involvement of NgBR in tamoxifen resistance of ERα-positive breast cancer is still unknown. In this study, we showed that NgBR knockdown attenuates tamoxifen resistance in MCF-7 and T47D breast cancer cells by inhibiting EGF-stimulated phosphorylation of ERα. Also, NgBR knockdown restored the sensitivity of ERα-positive breast cancer cells to tamoxifen through decreasing p53-mediated expression of survivin. Our results suggest that NgBR is a potential therapeutic target for increasing the efficacy of tamoxifen and overcoming the resistance to tamoxifen in ERα-positive patients with breast cancer.

Methods

Antibodies, reagents and plasmids

A peptide (AHHRMRWRADGRSLEK, residues from 81 to 96 of NgBR) was used to immunize rabbits (Epitomics, Burlingame, CA, USA). Antiserum was purified using the same peptide-conjugated SulfoLink Coupling Gel (Pierce, Rockford, IL, USA). Purified NgBR rabbit polyclonal antibody was used for immunostaining. The peptide recognizing epitope 14–30 of human Nogo-B was used to immunize rabbits (IMG-5346A, Imgenex, San Diego, CA, USA). Antibodies for NgBR (#ab168351) and phosphorylated ERα (phos-S118) (#ab32396) were purchased from Abcam (Cambridge, MA, USA). Antibodies for phos-EGFR (#3777), phos-Akt (#S473), phos-p42/44 extracellular signal-related kinase (ERK)

(#9101), total Akt (#4691), total ERK (#4595), ERα (#8644), HER2 (#4290) and survivin (#2808) were purchased from Cell Signaling Technology (Beverly, MA, USA). We also used antibodies for p53 (#10442–1-AP), β-actin (#60008–1) and Hsp90 (13171–1-AP) from Proteintech (Rosement, IL, USA). EGF (#E5036) was purchased from Sigma-Aldrich (St. Louis, MO, USA). HER2 plasmid DNA was a gift from Mien-Chie Hung (Addgene plasmid # 16257).

Cell culture

Human breast cancer cell lines MCF-7 and T-47D were obtained from the American Type Culture Collection. The cells were grown in DMEM with L-Glutamine (MCF-7 Gibco) or RPMI-1640 with L-Glutamine (T47D, Gibco) supplemented with 10% FBS (Sigma, St. Louis, MO, USA) and 1% penicillin streptomycin glutamine (Gibco). The tamoxifen-resistant cell lines (MCF-7-TamR and T47D-TamR) were derived from the parental cell lines by continuous gradual exposure to 4-OHT (Sigma, St. Louis, MO, USA) to reach the final concentration of 1 μM in methanol in 6 months [19]. Culture medium was replaced every 2–3 days. Cells were incubated at 37 °C in a humidified atmosphere containing 5% CO_2. The cell lots used in this study were authenticated prior to in vitro experiments.

Small interfering RNA (siRNA) and plasmid transfection

NgBR siRNA (forward, GGAAAUACAUAGACCUACA; reverse, UGUAGGUCUAUGUAUUUCC) oligonucleotides with 3′ dTdT overhangs were synthesized by QIAGEN (Valencia, CA, USA). The specificity of NgBR siRNA has been validated in our previous publication [12]. Control siRNA in experiments refers to a non-silencing (NS) siRNA (NSF, UUCUCCGAACGUGUCACGU; NSR, ACGUGACACGUUCGG AGAA) designed and synthesized by QIAGEN. P53 siRNA (sc44218) and survivin siRNA (sc-29,499) were purchased from Santa Cruz (Dallas, TX, USA). Cells were transfected with siRNA using Lipofectamine RNAiMAX reagent (ThermoFisher Scientific). For transient NgBR overexpression experiments, MCF-7 cells were transfected with pIRES-NgBR-HA plasmid DNA using Lipofectamine 2000 reagent (ThermoFisher Scientific).

Quantitative real-time polymerase chain reaction

Total RNA was extracted from cells by using TRIzol reagent according to the manual (ThermoFisher Scientific) and complementary DNA (cDNA) was reverse-transcribed using the iScript cDNA Synthesis Kit (Bio-Rad, Hercules, CA, USA) according to the manufacturer's instructions. Real-time PCR was performed using iTaq Universal SYBR Green Supermix (Bio-Rad, USA) and was run on MyiQ Single Color Real-Time PCR Detection System (Bio-Rad). The relative messenger RNA (mRNA) expression of each gene was normalized to glyceraldehyde-3-phosphate dehydrogenase (GAPDH) RNA levels. The primers were synthesized by Integrated DNA Technologies (Coralville, IA, USA). The forward and reverse primers for NgBR are 5′-tgccagttagtagcccagaagcaa-3′ and 5′-tgatgtgccagggaa-gaaagccta-3′, respectively. The forward and reverse primers for p53 are 5′-cctttctatcagccccagaggata-3′ and 5′-GGGA CATCCTTAATTATCTGGGGT-3′, respectively. The forward and reverse primers for GAPDH are 5′-aacctgccaag-tatgatgac-3′ and 5′-tctcttgctcagtgtccttg-3′, respectively. The forward and reverse primers for EGFR are 5′-aagcca-tatgacggaatccc-3′ and 5′-ggaactttgggcgactatctg-3′, respectively. The forward and reverse primers for ERα are 5′-cgactatatgtgtccagccac-3′ and 5′-cctcttcggtctttcgtatcc-3′, respectively. The forward and reverse primers for survivin are 5′-caaggagctggaaggctg-3′ and 5′-ttcttggctctttctctgtcc-3′, respectively.

Clonogenic survival assay
Cells were seeded in triplicate into cell culture dishes (1000 cells/well). MCF-7-TamR or T47D-TamR cells were transfected with NgBR siRNA or non-silencing siRNA. At 12 h after transfection, cells were treated with or without 4-OHT. After 14 days, cells were washed with PBS, fixed with methanol for 15 min and stained with 0.1% crystal violet for 15 min. Colonies containing 50 or more cells were counted [20].

Cell viability assay
Cell viability was determined using the CCK-8 assay. Cells were seeded at the density of 5000 cells/well into 96-well plates; 10 μL of CCK-8 (Sigma) was added to each well. Then cells were incubated at 37 °C for 1–3 h. The absorbance of the reaction was measured using a plate reader (Molecular Devices, Sunnyvale, CA, USA). Another cell viability assay used in this study was trypan blue staining. Cells were seeded into 96-well plates (5000/well). Then, the cells were incubated for 24 h before transfection with NgBR siRNA. The treatment time with 4-OHT was 3 days. Before staining, cells were washed with PBS and dislodged with trypsin. Then cell suspension and trypan blue were mixed (1:1) for 3 min. The number of viable and dead cells on the hemocytometer were counted under a microscope.

Apoptosis assay by FITC Annexin V/propidium iodide (PI) staining
An FITC Annexin V Apoptosis Detection kit (# 556547) was purchased from BD Biosciences (San Jose, CA, USA). Cells cultured in 6-well plates were transfected with siRNA of NgBR, p53 or survivin, and then treated with 4-OHT for 48 h. Cells were then stained with 5 μL Annexin V-FITC and 5 μL PI in 500 uL of apoptosis reaction solution at room temperature in the dark for

15 min following the manufacture's instruction. The BD LSR II flow cytometer was used to detect apoptotic cells.

Western blot
Cells were harvested and washed with PBS, and then lysed with lysis buffer supplemented with Pierce Protease and Phosphatase Inhibitor Mini Tablets (ThermoFisher Scientific) for 10 min on ice. The whole cell lysate was scraped from the plates and then centrifuged at 12000 rpm for 10 min at 4 °C. The concentrations of protein were determined by BCA Protein Assay Kit (Bio-Rad). Cell lysates were subjected to SDS-PAGE, transferred to nitrocellulose blotting membrane (GE Healthcare Life Sciences, Pittsburgh, PA, USA), then incubated with primary specific antibodies at 4 °C overnight. The membranes were incubated with secondary antibodies (Jackson ImmunoResearch, West Grove, PA, USA) at 1:10000 dilution for 2 h at room temperature. The protein band intensities were evaluated using Amersham ECL Western Blotting Detection System (GE Healthcare Life Sciences) and were normalized to housekeeping genes, either β-actin or HSP90. All western blot experiments were performed at least three times.

Raf-pull-down assay
Ras activity was assessed using GST-Raf-1 RBD beads (RF02, Cytoskeleton, Denver, CO, USA) according to the manufacturer's protocol: 500μg total cell lysate was incubated with 10 μL GST-Raf1-RBD beads overnight at 4 °C with gentle rocking. Samples were washed five times, then dissolved in 20 μL 2X SDS sample buffer. Activated H-Ras and K-Ras was determined by western blot using specific H-Ras (GTX116041, GeneTex, San Antonio, TX, USA) or K-Ras (12063–1-AP, Proteintech, Rosemont, IL, USA) antibodies, respectively.

Tissue microarray slides
Breast cancer tissue was collected from 22 patients at the First Hospital of Jilin University (Changchun, China).

We had consent from all patients for participating in this study. All of the patients received modified radical mastectomy and were diagnosed with infiltrating ductal carcinoma via pathological diagnosis. Immunohistochemistry was performed to examine NgBR, Nogo-B, and survivin expression levels following standard methodology described in our previous publication [16]. All of these breast cancer cases were histopathologically re-evaluated on hematoxylin and eosin-stained slides by two pathologists. The breast tissue specimens are anonymous. The study was approved by the ethical committee of the First Hospital of Jilin University.

Association between NgBR or survivin expression and survival in patients with breast cancer

All data were collected from a public online clinical database (http://kmplot.com). We analyzed the association between mRNA level of NgBR (NUS1, 225071_x at from Kaplan–Meier Plot database) or survivin (BIRC5, 202094_x at from Kaplan–Meier Plot database) and survival in patients with breast cancer. Kaplan-Meier survival curves according to NgBR expression status were used to analyze the relapse-free survival (RFS) and log-rank p values (SPSS 23.0 USA).

Statistical analysis

Data were analyzed from at least three independent experiments. The results were reported as the mean ± SD. Values of $p < 0.05$ were considered statistically significant. Student's t test or analysis of variance (ANOVA) were performed as appropriate. Correlation between NgBR and survivin expression was analyzed using Fisher's test. Statistical analyses were performed using Prism 6.0 software (GraphPad software, USA).

Results

NgBR expression is increased in tamoxifen-resistant breast cancer cells

Tamoxifen resistant MCF-7 (MCF-7-TamR) and T47D (T47D-TamR) ERα-positive breast cancer cells were established following the previously described method [19]. To validate tamoxifen resistance in established MCF-7-TamR and T47D-TamR cells, both normal and tamoxifen-resistant cells were treated with 0–5 μM 4-OHT. As shown in Fig. 1a–d, 5 μM 4-OHT cannot attenuate the colony formation capability of MCF-7-TamR and T47D-TamR cells. However, parental cells cannot survive treatment with 5 μM 4-OHT. CCK-8 cell viability assay was also used for determining the response of these breast cancer cells to tamoxifen (Additional file 1: Figure S1A and B). Similarly, both MCF-7-TamR and T47D-TamR can survive treatment with 5 μM 4-OHT. The levels of NgBR transcript and protein were determined by real-time PCR (Fig. 1e and f) and western blot analysis (Fig. 1g and h). The expression of NgBR was increased in both MCF-7-TamR (Fig. 1e, g and h) and T47D-TamR cells (Fig. 1f; Additional file 2: Figure S2) as compared to that in their parental cells. The alteration of other gene expression between MCF-7 and MCF-7-TamR cells is shown in Fig. 1g and h. Consistent with many previous studies [19, 21, 22], we also noted increased expression of EGFR, HER2, and survivin, and decreased expression of p53 and ERα in MCF-7-TamR (Fig. 1g and h).

NgBR knockdown attenuates the tamoxifen resistance

To determine the contribution of increased NgBR expression to tamoxifen resistance, we knocked down the expression of NgBR with specific NgBR siRNA (siNgBR),

which has been validated in our previous reports [18]. The effects of NgBR knockdown on cell apoptosis and necrosis of MCF-7-TamR (Fig. 2a and b) and T47D-TamR (Additional file 3: Figure S3A and B) were determined by Annexin V/PI staining and flow cytometry. The results showed that NgBR knockdown increases the sensitivity of both MCF-7-TamR and T47D-TamR cells to 4-OHT. Compared to the non-treatment group, 4-OHT treatment alone did not induce significant death of tamoxifen-resistant cells. However, NgBR knockdown along with 4-OHT treatment significantly increased the percentage of cell death. Cell viability was determined by counting the number of negative trypan blue stained cells using a hemocytometer. Consistently, MCF-7-TamR and T47D-TamR cells were resistant to 4-OHT treatment. However, NgBR knockdown restored the sensitivity of MCF-7-TamR (Fig. 2c) and T47D-TamR (Additional file 3: Figure S3C) to tamoxifen. The clonogenic survival assay further demonstrated that NgBR knockdown attenuates the colony formation capability of MCF-7-TamR (Fig. 2d and e) and T47D-TamR cells (Additional file 3: Figure S3D and E) under the condition of 5 μM 4-OHT treatment. These results demonstrated that NgBR knockdown increases the sensitivity of tamoxifen-resistant ERα-positive breast cancer cells to tamoxifen.

As in our previous report [15], overexpression of NgBR in MCF-7 cells increased the membrane-associated H-Ras and K-Ras (Fig. 3a). Consequently, if we transfected plasmid DNA expressing human influenza hemagglutinin (HA) tagged NgBR (NgBR-HA) to MCF-7 cells, we appreciated that the overexpression of exogenous NgBR-HA increased the viability of MCF-7 cells treated with 4-OHT (Fig. 3b). Similarly, overexpression of HER2-HA also increased the resistance of MCF-7 cells to 4-OHT (Fig. 3b). However, NgBR knockdown attenuated the resistance of MCF-7 cells overexpressing HER2-HA (Fig. 3b). In MCF-7-TamR cells, overexpression of NgBR-HA restored the resistance of NgBR knockdown MCF-7-TamR cells to tamoxifen (Fig. 3c). As shown in Fig. 3d, transfection of NgBR-HA plasmid DNA restored the expression of NgBR in MCF-7-TamR cells transfected with NgBR siRNA (siNgBR), which targets the 3′-untranslated region (UTR) of NgBR as described in our previous publication [12]. It suggests that NgBR is one of driving forces for tamoxifen resistance. However, knockdown of Nogo-B does not affect the sensitivity of MCF-7-TamR to tamoxifen (Fig. 3c). The efficacy of Nogo-B siRNA was confirmed by western blot analysis (Fig. 3d).

NgBR knockdown promotes apoptosis by regulating the expression of p53 and survivin

Our previous study showed that NgBR deficiency in ERα-positive breast cancer cells decreases the resistance to chemotherapy by increasing p53 and decreasing

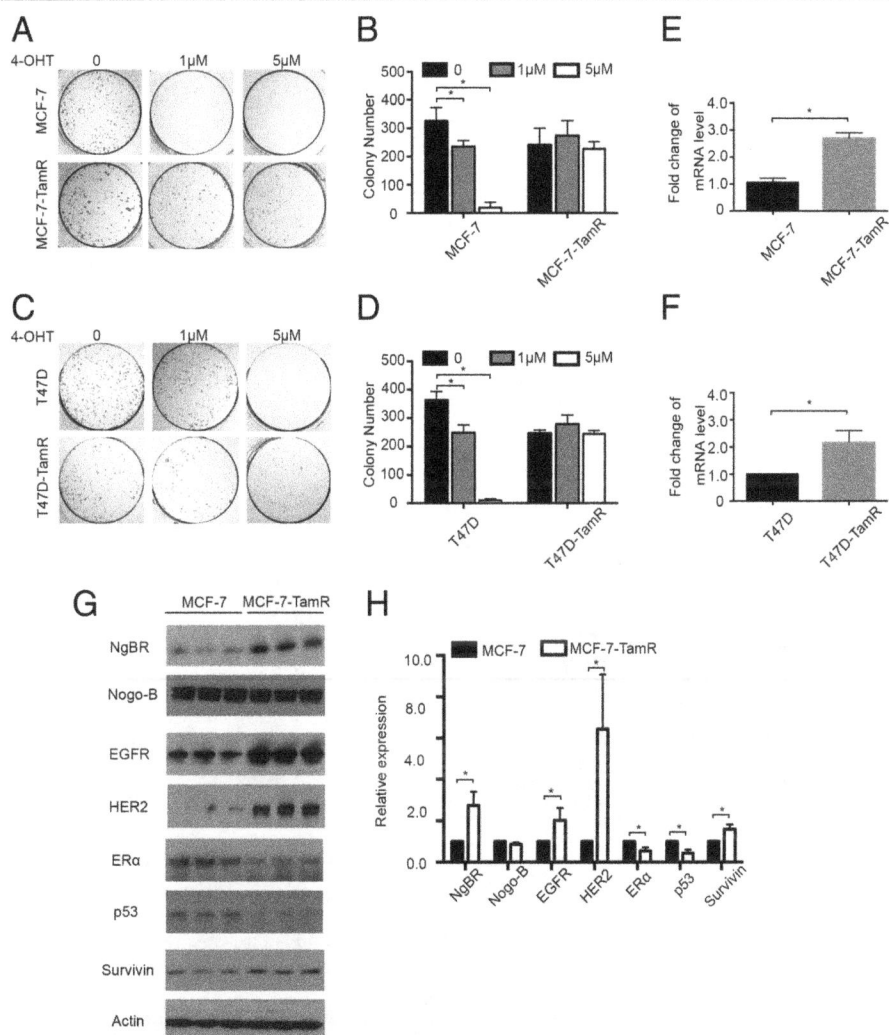

Fig. 1 Nogo-B receptor (NgBR) is highly expressed in the tamoxifen resistant MCF-7-TamR and T47D-TamR cells. **a** Colony formation assay was performed as described in "Methods". Wild-type MCF-7 and tamoxifen-resistant MCF-7-TamR cells were treated with different concentrations of 4-OHT (0, 1 and 5 μM). **b** Quantification of colony number presented in colony formation assays of MCF-7 and MCF-7-TamR cells. **c** Colony formation assay of wild-type T47D and tamoxifen-resistant T47D-TamR cells treated with different concentrations of 4-OHT (0, 1 and 5 μM). **d** Quantification of colony number in colony formation assays of T47D and T47D-TamR cells. **e, f** mRNA level of NgBR was increased in MCF-7-TamR and T47D-TamR cells as compared to wild-type MCF-7 and T47D cells, respectively. The relative amount of NgBR mRNA level was normalized to glyceraldehyde-3-phosphate dehydrogenase (GAPDH). **g** NgBR protein level was increased in MCF-7-TamR cells. Protein levels of Nogo-B, epidermal growth factor receptor (EGFR), human epidermal growth factor receptor 2 (HER2), estrogen receptor alpha (ERα), p53 and survivin in MCF-7 and MCF-7-TamR cells were determined using western blot analysis. **h** Quantitative analysis of protein levels using ImageJ and normalized to the housekeeping gene β-actin. Data are presented as fold changes in MCF-7-TamR cells compared to MCF-7 cells. The data are from three separate repeat experiments, and are presented as the mean ± SD (*$p < 0.05$, $n = 3$)

survivin [23]. To determine if and the extent to which NgBR is dependent on p53-mediated survivin expression to promote the resistance to tamoxifen, we examined the alteration of p53 and survivin expression in tamoxifen-resistant ERα-positive breast cancer cells before and after NgBR depletion. As shown in Fig. 4a and b, NgBR depletion in MCF-7-TamR cells increased the expression of p53 but decreased the amount of survivin at the protein levels. Overexpression of NgBR-HA restored the expression pattern of p53 and survivin in MCF-7-TamR cells transfected with siNgBR to levels similar to that in MCF-7-TamR cells transfected with control siRNA (Fig. 3d). When p53 was knocked down by siRNA, survivin was increased in MCF-7 cells (Fig. 4c and d). To determine if either p53 or survivin is involved in regulating the apoptosis of NgBR-deficient cells, we knocked down either p53 in MCF-7 cells or survivin in MCF-7-TamR cells using siRNA either targeting p53 (si-p53) or targeting survivin (si-survivin), respectively. As shown in Fig. 4e and f, knockdown of p53 increased

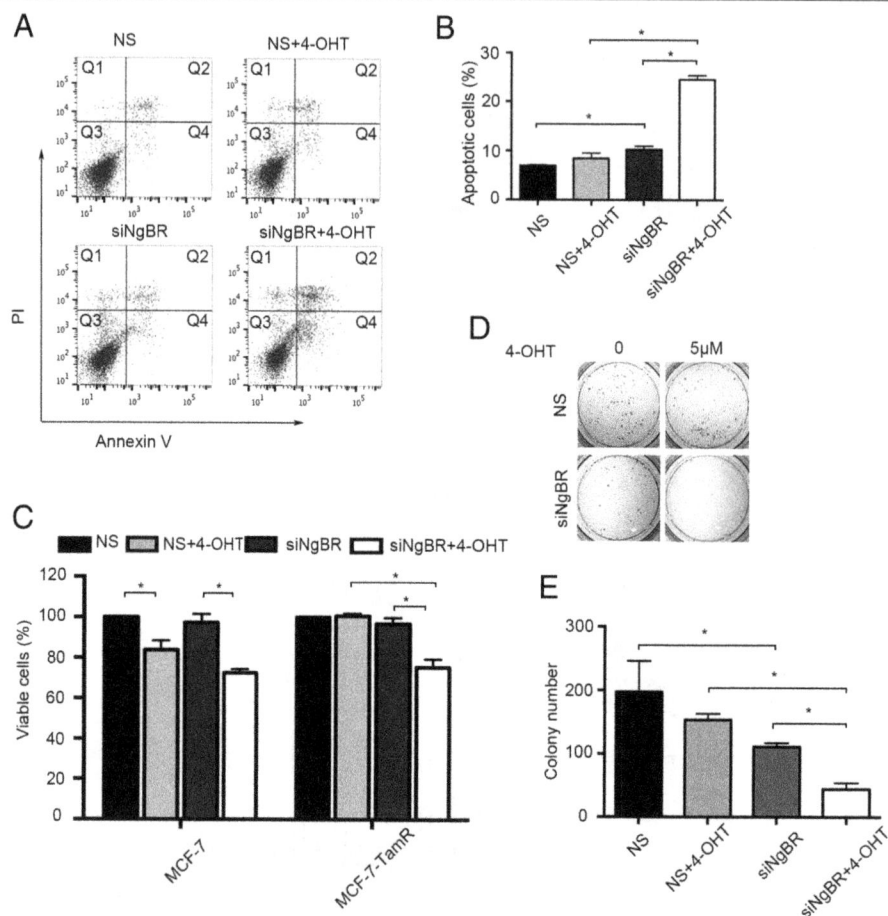

Fig. 2 Nogo-B receptor (NgBR) knockdown decreases the resistance of MCF-7-TamR cells to tamoxifen. **a** NgBR knockdown increases 4-OHT-induced apoptosis of MCF-7-TamR cells; 4-OHT, 5 μM. The apoptotic cells were detected by Annexin V-PI staining as described in "Methods". The total number of cells in the Q2 and Q4 quadrant were counted as apoptotic cells. **b** Percentages of apoptotic MCF-7-TamR cells are presented in the bar graph. **c** NgBR knockdown decreases cell viability of MCF-7-TamR cells treated with 4-OHT. Cell viability was determined using trypan blue staining. MCF-7-TamR cells were treated with 4-OHT (5 μM) for 48 h. The viable cell number in the non-silencing (NS) group is set as 100%. **d** NgBR knockdown decreases the clonogenenicity of MCF-7-TamR cells treated with 4-OHT (5 μM). Clonogenic survival assay was performed as described in "Methods". **e** Quantification of colony number in colony formation assays as described in Fig. 2d. The data were repeated in three separate experiments, and are presented as the mean ± SD (*$p < 0.05$, $n = 3$)

the resistance of MCF-7 cells to 4-OHT, while survivin knockdown restored the sensitivity of MCF-7-TamR cells to 4-OHT (Fig. 4g and h). Similar results were also observed in p53 knockdown T47D cells (Additional file 4: Figure S4A–D) and survivin knockdown T47D-TamR cells (Additional file 4: Figure S4E–F). These results demonstrated the contribution of increased p53 expression and decreased survivin expression that occurs in NgBR knockdown cells for restoring the sensitivity of ERα-positive breast cancer cells to tamoxifen. The clonogenic survival assay further demonstrated that loss of p53 in NgBR knockdown MCF-7 cells attenuated the effects of NgBR deficiency on increased sensitivity of MCF-7 cells to tamoxifen (Fig. 4i and j). In addition, knockdown of both H-Ras and K-Ras in MCF-7-TamR cells also resulted in the increased amount of p53 and

decreased amount of survivin (Fig. 5a). Overexpression of either NgBR-HA or HER2-HA in MCF-7 cells decreased the protein levels of p53 and ERα but increased the protein level of survivin (Fig. 5b). Interestingly, knockdown of NgBR in MCF-7 cells overexpressing HER2-HA restored the protein levels of p53, ERα and survivin levels to those occurring in control MCF-7 cells transfected with empty vector (Fig. 5b).

NgBR knockdown diminished EGF-stimulated phosphorylation of ERα

Phosphorylation of ERα serine 118 (S118) residue has been reported to be involved in resistance to tamoxifen [24, 25]. To examine the involvement of NgBR in regulating EGF-stimulated phosphorylation of ERα S118, we treated MCF-7-TamR cells with 100 ng/mL EGF for

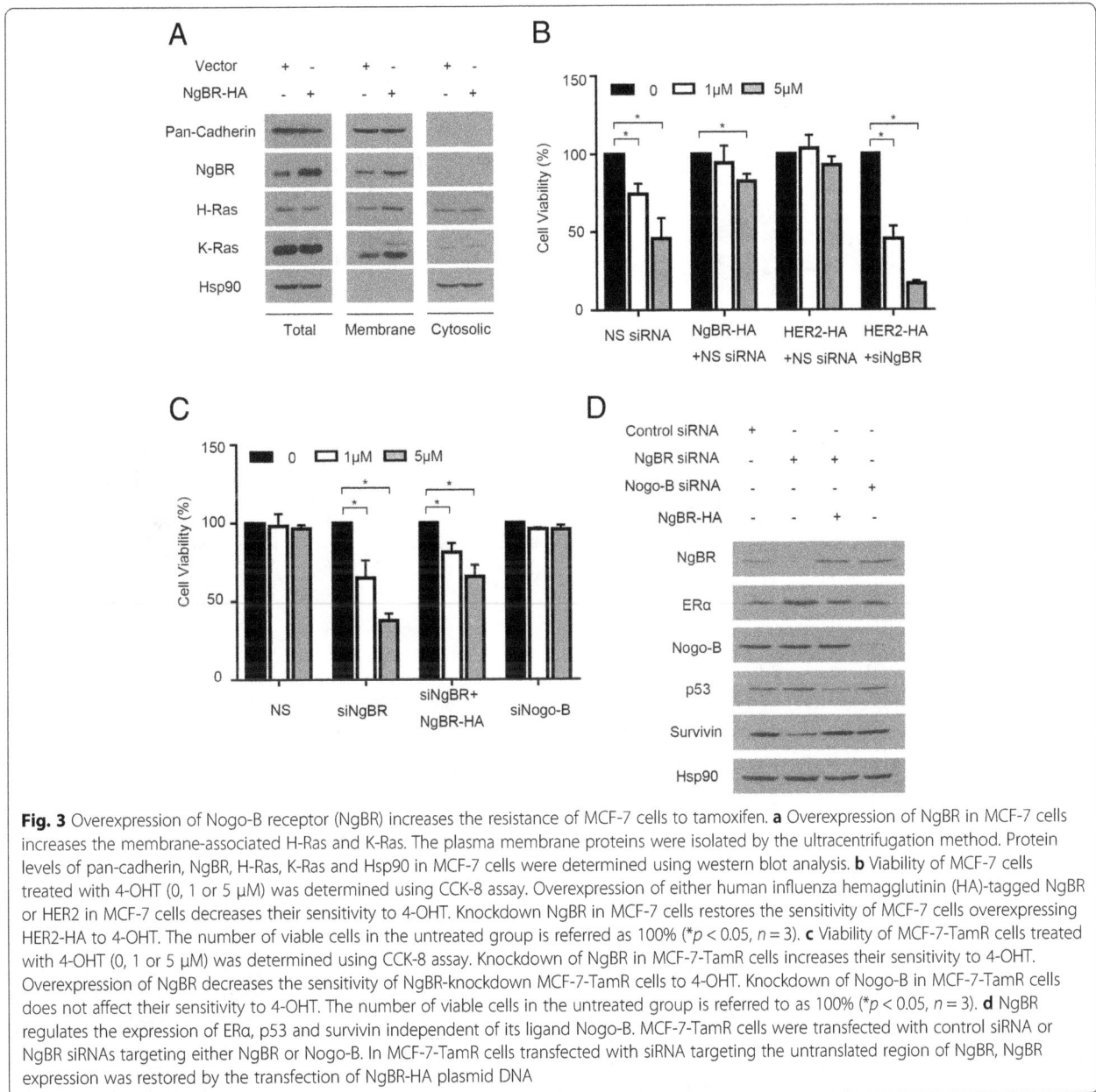

Fig. 3 Overexpression of Nogo-B receptor (NgBR) increases the resistance of MCF-7 cells to tamoxifen. **a** Overexpression of NgBR in MCF-7 cells increases the membrane-associated H-Ras and K-Ras. The plasma membrane proteins were isolated by the ultracentrifugation method. Protein levels of pan-cadherin, NgBR, H-Ras, K-Ras and Hsp90 in MCF-7 cells were determined using western blot analysis. **b** Viability of MCF-7 cells treated with 4-OHT (0, 1 or 5 μM) was determined using CCK-8 assay. Overexpression of either human influenza hemagglutinin (HA)-tagged NgBR or HER2 in MCF-7 cells decreases their sensitivity to 4-OHT. Knockdown NgBR in MCF-7 cells restores the sensitivity of MCF-7 cells overexpressing HER2-HA to 4-OHT. The number of viable cells in the untreated group is referred as 100% (*$p < 0.05$, $n = 3$). **c** Viability of MCF-7-TamR cells treated with 4-OHT (0, 1 or 5 μM) was determined using CCK-8 assay. Knockdown of NgBR in MCF-7-TamR cells to 4-OHT. Overexpression of NgBR decreases the sensitivity of NgBR-knockdown MCF-7-TamR cells to 4-OHT. Knockdown of Nogo-B in MCF-7-TamR cells does not affect their sensitivity to 4-OHT. The number of viable cells in the untreated group is referred to as 100% (*$p < 0.05$, $n = 3$). **d** NgBR regulates the expression of ERα, p53 and survivin independent of its ligand Nogo-B. MCF-7-TamR cells were transfected with control siRNA or NgBR siRNAs targeting either NgBR or Nogo-B. In MCF-7-TamR cells transfected with siRNA targeting the untranslated region of NgBR, NgBR expression was restored by the transfection of NgBR-HA plasmid DNA

5 min, which is the peak of the phosphorylation signal in response to EGF stimulation. As shown in Fig. 6a and b, EGF treatment increased the phosphorylation of AKT, ERK and MDM2 in MCF-7-TamR cells treated with control non-silencing (NS) siRNA. NgBR knockdown attenuated EGF-stimulated phosphorylation of AKT, ERK and MDM2. But NgBR knockdown did not affect the total protein levels of AKT, ERK and MDM2 or the phosphorylation of EGFR (Fig. 6a). EGF treatment not only activated the downstream signaling of the EGF pathway, but also increased the phosphorylation of ERα (S118), which is in accordance with previous studies [10, 26]. NgBR knockdown attenuated EGF-stimulated phosphorylation of ERα. The inhibitory effects of NgBR

knockdown on EGF-stimulated phosphorylation of ERα were also noted in T47D-TamR cells (Additional file 5: Figure S5).

To further investigate the underlying mechanism by which NgBR regulates the expression of p53 and survivin, we stimulated MCF-7-TamR cells with EGF (100 ng/mL) for 12 h. EGF treatment increased the protein level of survivin, and NgBR knockdown attenuated the protein level of survivin in EGF-treated cells (Fig. 6c and d). To elucidate the roles of NgBR in regulating the EGF-mediated pathway, we used glutathione (GST)-tagged Ras-binding domain of Raf (RBD) to pull down activated Ras as described in our previous publication [15]. As shown in Fig. 6e, EGF stimulation for 5 min not only induced the

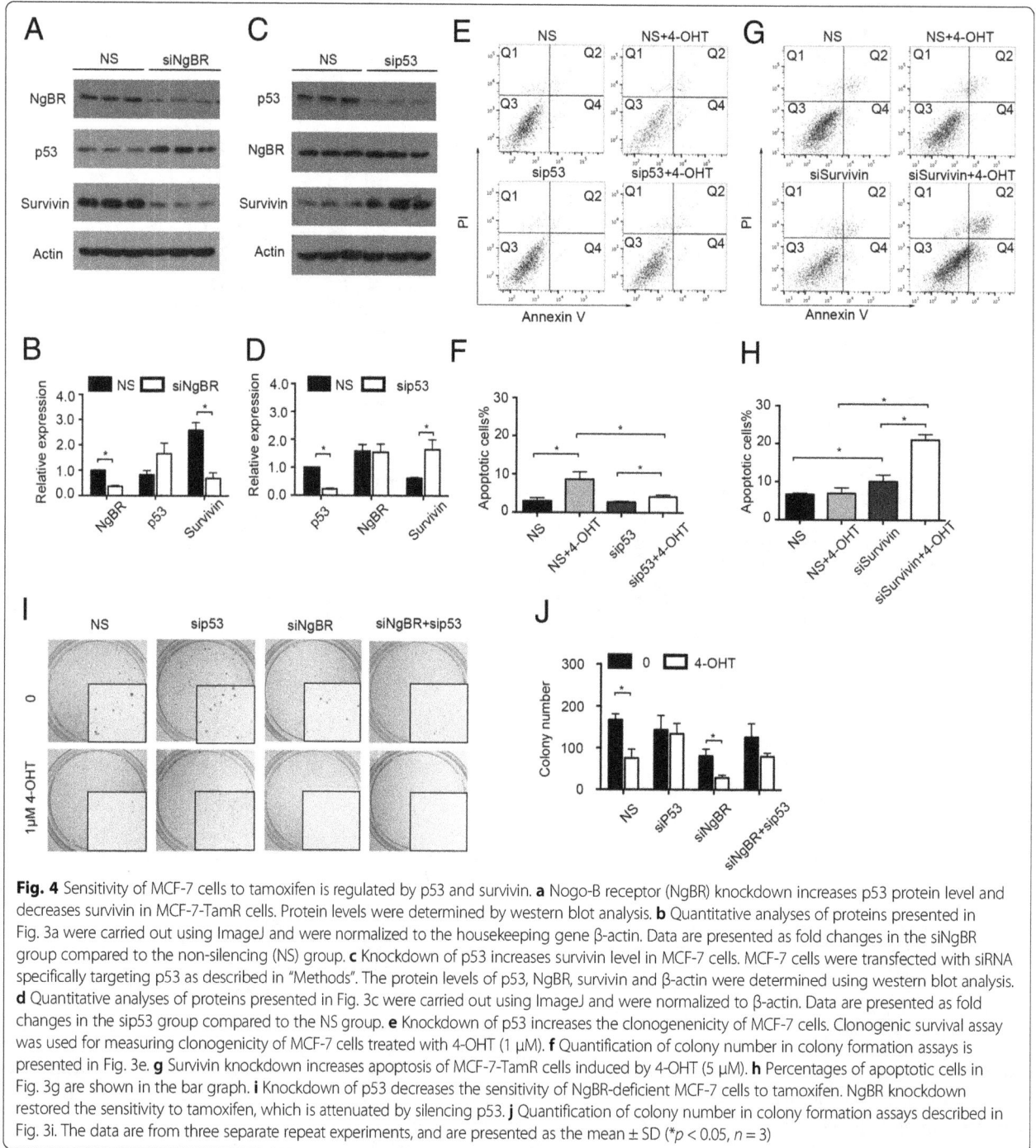

Fig. 4 Sensitivity of MCF-7 cells to tamoxifen is regulated by p53 and survivin. **a** Nogo-B receptor (NgBR) knockdown increases p53 protein level and decreases survivin in MCF-7-TamR cells. Protein levels were determined by western blot analysis. **b** Quantitative analyses of proteins presented in Fig. 3a were carried out using ImageJ and were normalized to the housekeeping gene β-actin. Data are presented as fold changes in the siNgBR group compared to the non-silencing (NS) group. **c** Knockdown of p53 increases survivin level in MCF-7 cells. MCF-7 cells were transfected with siRNA specifically targeting p53 as described in "Methods". The protein levels of p53, NgBR, survivin and β-actin were determined using western blot analysis. **d** Quantitative analyses of proteins presented in Fig. 3c were carried out using ImageJ and were normalized to β-actin. Data are presented as fold changes in the sip53 group compared to the NS group. **e** Knockdown of p53 increases the clonogenenicity of MCF-7 cells. Clonogenic survival assay was used for measuring clonogenicity of MCF-7 cells treated with 4-OHT (1 μM). **f** Quantification of colony number in colony formation assays is presented in Fig. 3e. **g** Survivin knockdown increases apoptosis of MCF-7-TamR cells induced by 4-OHT (5 μM). **h** Percentages of apoptotic cells in Fig. 3g are shown in the bar graph. **i** Knockdown of p53 decreases the sensitivity of NgBR-deficient MCF-7 cells to tamoxifen. NgBR knockdown restored the sensitivity to tamoxifen, which is attenuated by silencing p53. **j** Quantification of colony number in colony formation assays described in Fig. 3i. The data are from three separate repeat experiments, and are presented as the mean ± SD (*$p < 0.05$, $n = 3$)

activation of H-Ras and K-Ras in MCF-7-TamR cells, but also increased the amount of NgBR in the complex of activated K-Ras and H-Ras. It indicates that EGF stimulation increases the association between NgBR and activated Ras. Consistent with our previous reports [15], NgBR knockdown also attenuated the EGF-stimulated Ras activation in MCF-7-TamR cells. These results (Fig. 6) suggest that NgBR-mediated Ras activation may contribute to EGF-stimulated phosphorylation of ERα.

NgBR expression is associated with survivin and poor survival in patients with breast cancer

Our previous publication showed that expression of NgBR is much higher in ERα-positive breast cancer tissues than in normal breast tissues, and that NgBR is also highly associated with survivin expression [16]. To further confirm the relationship between survivin and NgBR, we performed immunohistochemistry (IHC) staining to examine expression in 22 samples of breast

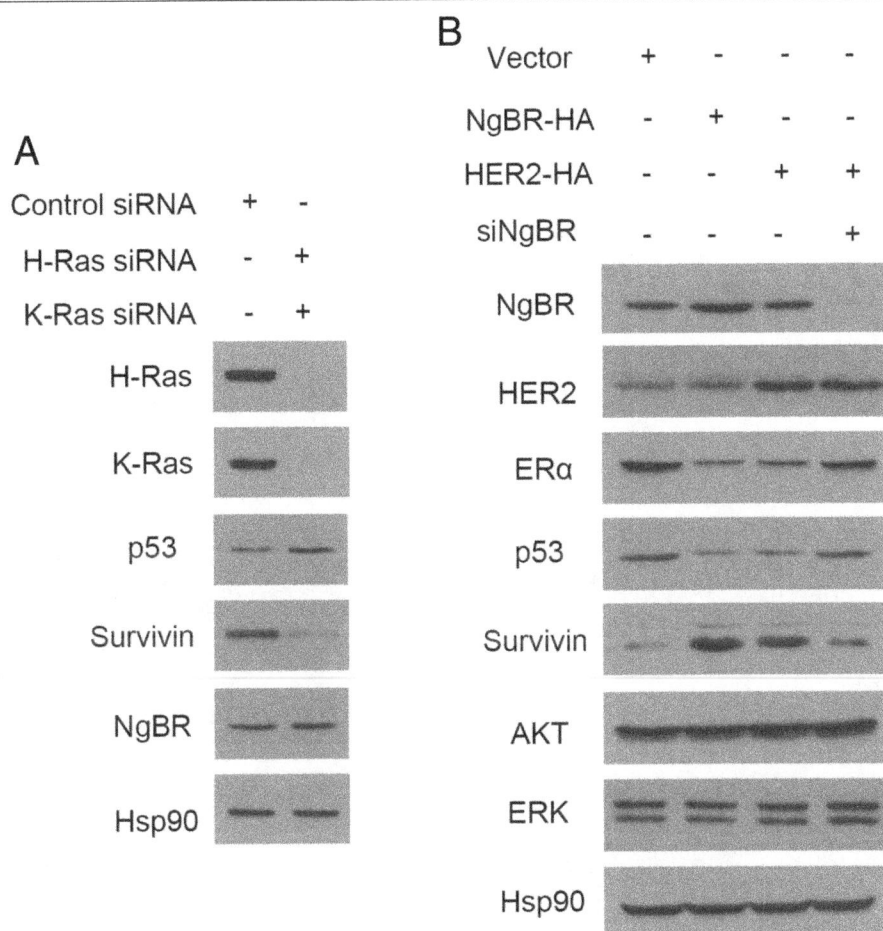

Fig. 5 Nogo-B receptor (NgBR) regulates protein levels of p53 and survivin through Ras-mediated pathways. **a** Knockdown of both H-Ras and K-Ras increases the protein levels of p53 and decreases the protein level of survivin. Control siRNA and siRNAs targeting either H-Ras or K-Ras siRNA were transfected into MCF-7-TamR cells. **b** Overexpression of either NgBR-HA or HER2-HA in MCF-7 cells decreases the protein levels of p53, ERα, and increases the protein level of survivin. Knockdown NgBR in MCF-7 cells overexpressing HER2-HA restores the protein levels of p53, ERα and survivin to levels similar to those in control MCF-7 cells transfected with empty plasmid DNA vector. Change in NgBR or human epidermal growth factor receptor 2 (HER2) has no effects on the total protein levels of AKT and extracellular signal-related kinase (ERK)

cancer tissue. The basic characteristics of the tissue samples are shown in Table 1, and the results of the quantitative analysis of IHC staining was shown in Table 2. As shown in Fig. 7a, patients with high expression of NgBR also have high expression of survivin. In patients with negative or weak expression of NgBR, the expression of survivin was also low. The association between NgBR and survivin was statistically significant (Table 2). The association between NgBR and clinical outcomes in patients with breast cancer was determined using the public Kaplan–Meier Plot database. Kaplan–Meier analysis revealed that high expression of NgBR was associated with poor RFS in patients with ERα-positive breast cancer ($n = 755$) and in patients receiving endocrine therapy ($n = 335$) (Fig. 7b; Additional files 6, 7, 8 and 9). Consistently, high expression of survivin was also associated with poor RFS in patients with ERα-positive breast

cancer ($n = 2046$) and in patients receiving endocrine therapy ($n = 928$) (Fig. 7c). The association between higher NgBR expression and poor RFS was further confirmed in the GSE6532 dataset ($n = 343$) (Additional file 10: Figure S6; Additional file 11).

Discussion

As previously confirmed, NgBR is highly expressed in ERα-positive breast cancer [16], and promotes epithelial-mesenchymal transition of breast tumor cells [18]. However, the underlying mechanism by which NgBR enhances the acquired resistance of ERα-positive breast cancer to tamoxifen has not been elucidated. In this study, we found that NgBR expression is increased in tamoxifen-resistant breast cancer cell lines (Fig. 1). High expression of NgBR was associated with poor RFS in patients with ERα-positive breast cancer and in patients

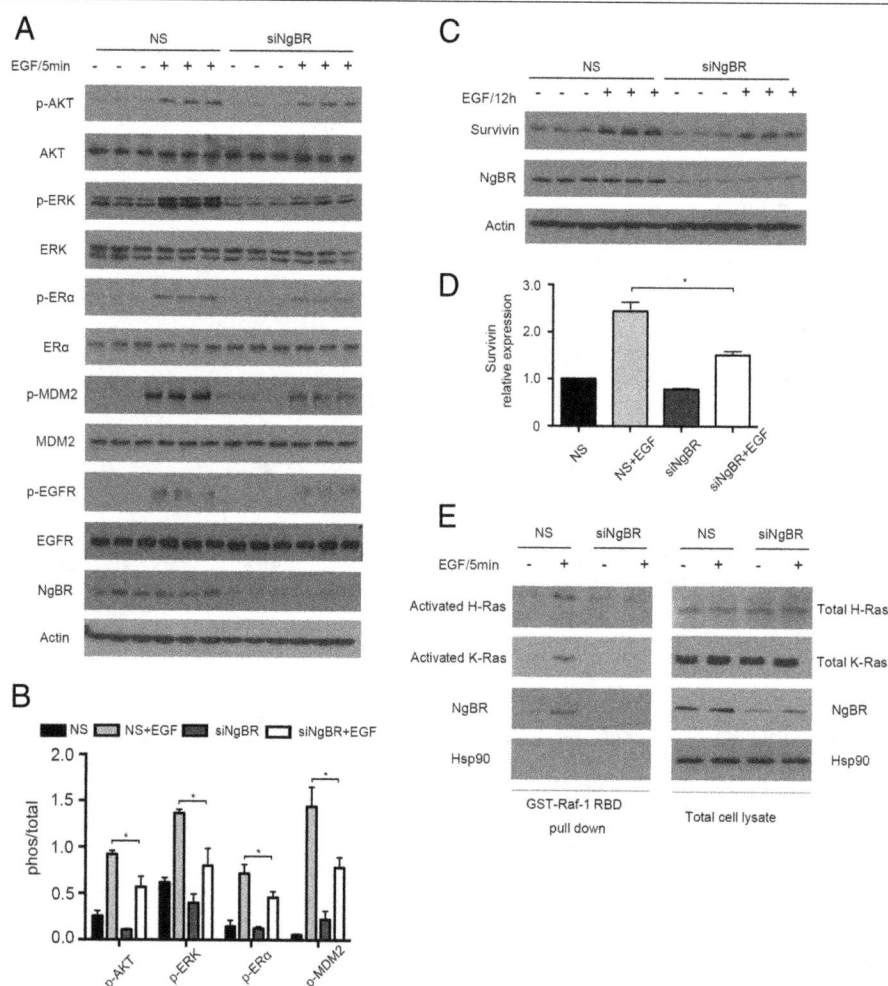

Fig. 6 Nogo-B receptor (NgBR) knockdown attenuates epidermal growth factor receptor (EGF)-stimulated signaling and estrogen receptor alpha (ERα) phosphorylation in MCF-7-TamR cells. **a** MCF-7-TamR cells were transfected with siNgBR and treated with EGF (100 ng/mL) for 5 min. Downstream signaling of the EGF pathway was determined using western blot assay. **b** Quantitative analysis of phosphorylated proteins presented in Fig. 4b were carried out using ImageJ and were normalized to total proteins. **c** MCF-7-TamR cells were transfected with siNgBR and treated with 100 ng/mL EGF for 12 h. Survivin protein levels were determined using western blot analysis. **d** Quantitative analysis of survivin protein levels presented in Fig. 4c were carried out using ImageJ and were normalized to β-actin. **e** NgBR is required for the EGF-stimulated activation of H-Ras and K-Ras in MCF-7-TamR cells. MCF-7-TamR cells were transfected with siNgBR and stimulated with 100 ng/mL EGF for 5 min. The complex of activated Ras (GTP-loaded Ras) was precipitated from total cell lysates using GST-RBD beads. Protein levels were detected by western blotting. Both Ras and NgBR were detected in the complexes precipitated by the Raf-pull-down method. The data are from three separate repeat experiments and are presented as the mean ± SD (*$p < 0.05$, $n = 3$)

receiving endocrine therapy (Fig. 5b). NgBR knockdown decreased EGF-induced expression of survivin (Fig. 4c and d) and phosphorylation of ERα (Fig. 4a). Consequently, the results of cell viability and apoptosis assays clearly demonstrate that NgBR knockdown attenuates resistance to tamoxifen (Fig. 2). Our study elucidated the important roles of NgBR in promoting the acquired resistance of ERα-positive breast cancer to tamoxifen.

For patients with ERα positive breast cancer, treatment mainly focuses on reducing estrogen levels or blocking the ERα signaling pathway. Aromatase inhibitors (AIs), such as anastrozole [27], are estrogen synthesis inhibitors. Fulvestrant is a selective ERα downregulator [28]. Tamoxifen, also

known as a selective estrogen receptor modulator, blocks the activity of estrogen by binding to ERα [29] and suppressing the classical ERE regulated genes [30]. However, 30% of patients still gain resistance to tamoxifen [31]. Many studies have elucidated potential mechanisms of tamoxifen resistance, but these are still unclear due to many unidentified factors [32]. In this study, we demonstrated that NgBR, which is upregulated in tamoxifen-resistant breast cancer cells, is a potential factor contributing to tamoxifen resistance. Our data demonstrated that NgBR knockdown restores the sensitivity of tamoxifen-resistant breast cancer cells to tamoxifen (Fig. 2). Our result indicates NgBR is a potential therapeutic target for

Table 1 Demographic and clinical characteristics of study population

	Variables	Value
ER	1+	1 (0.05)
	2+	9 (0.41)
	3+	12 (0.54)
PR	1+	4 (0.18)
	2+	5 (0.23)
	3+	13 (0.59)
HER2	–	17 (0.77)
	1+	2 (0.09)
	2+	2 (0.09)
	3+	1 (0.05)

Abbreviations: ER estrogen receptor, *PR* progesterone receptor, *HER2* human epidermal growth factor receptor 2

attenuating tamoxifen resistance. Unlike NgBR, Nogo-B protein levels do not increase in either MCF-7-TamR cells (Fig. 1g) or T47D-TamR cells (Additional file 2: Figure S2). Although NgBR was identified as a specific receptor for ligand Nogo-B, knockdown of Nogo-B does not affect the sensitivity of MCF-7-TamR cells to tamoxifen (Fig. 3c). If and the extent to which Nogo-B facilitates the NgBR-mediated Ras-signaling pathway needs further investigation.

According to previous studies, increased EGFR expression in tamoxifen-resistant cells contributes to the acquired resistance to tamoxifen [10, 21]. Consistent with previous reports, EGF stimulation also activated the phosphorylation of ERα [33]. Our recent report demonstrated that NgBR binds the farnesylated Ras and promotes Ras plasma membrane translocation [15]. NgBR-mediated accumulation of plasma membrane-associated Ras enhances EGF signaling [15]. As shown in Fig. 3a, NgBR overexpression in MCF-7 cells also increased membrane-associated H-Ras and K-Ras and resulted in increased resistance to tamoxifen (Fig. 3b). Similarly, increased expression of NgBR in tamoxifen-resistant breast cancer cells also enhances EGF-stimulated Ras activation and phosphorylation of AKT and ERK. NgBR knockdown diminishes the EGF-stimulated Ras activation and EGFR-mediated signaling (Fig. 6). Activation of these pathways leads to Akt-dependent phosphorylation of MDM2 [34], which downregulates cellular levels of p53 and decreases

Table 2 Correlation analysis of survivin and NgBR

	Survivin		Number	p
	Low	High		
NgBR				
Low	5 (71.4%)	2 (28.6%)	7 (100%)	0.014
High	2 (13.3%)	13 (86.7%)	15 (100%)	
n	7 (31.8%)	15 (68.2%)	22 (100%)	

NgBR Nogo-B receptor

p53 transcriptional activity [35]. Our previous report also demonstrated that NgBR promotes the ubiquitination of p53 in human hepatocellular carcinoma via Akt and MDM2 phosphorylation signaling [36]. Here, our data demonstrated the inverse expression patterns between p53 and NgBR in breast cancer cells (Fig. 4). The protein levels of p53 decrease in tamoxifen-resistant breast cancer cells along with increased expression of survivin and NgBR (Fig. 1g; Additional file 2: Figure S2A). Knockdown of either NgBR (Fig. 3d) or H-Ras/K-Ras (Fig. 5a) in MCF-7-TamR cells increased p53 and deceased survivin protein levels. As a tumor repressor gene, p53 is found to be mutated in many cancers [37] and promotes apoptosis in breast cancers [38]. It has been shown that p53 represses survivin expression at the transcriptional level [39]. Our data (Fig. 4c and d; Additional file 4: Figure S4A and B) also demonstrated that knockdown of p53 in breast cancer cells can induce the expression of survivin, which predicts a poor response to endocrine therapy [40]. In this study, we confirmed the effects of p53 on inducing tamoxifen resistance in parental MCF-7 and T47D cells, and survivin knockdown restored the sensitivity to 4-OHT in MCF-7-TamR (Fig. 4) and T47D-TamR cells (Additional file 4: Figure S4).

Ras is a well-known oncogene that has been shown to cause tumorigenesis and drug resistance by activating downstream kinases such as phosphatidylinositol-3-OH kinase (PI-3 K)/Akt and Raf-1 kinase/ERK [41–45]. Although Ras mutations rarely occur in breast cancer (less than 10%) [46], oncogenic Ras can contribute to the tumorigenic and invasive potential of breast epithelial cells [46]. Therefore, upregulation of normal Ras activity by RTKs, such as the EGFR and insulin growth factor receptor (IGF1-R), has been shown in ERα positive breast cancer [47–49]. The classic mechanism of E2 action is mediated by the nuclear ERα that regulates transcription of target genes containing the consensus ERE in their promoter region [47–49]. In addition, E2 can also exert its action through membrane ERα (mERα) in conjugation with the signaling complex including EGFR, IGF-1R, adaptor protein Shc/Grb2 and RasGEFs (such as SOS1 and RasGEF3) to activate Src/Ras-dependent activation of the Raf1-MARK/PI3K-Akt pathways [47–49]. This pathway promotes estrogen-dependent tumor resistance [50]. Our recent publication demonstrated that NgBR binds farnesylated Ras and is required for keeping Ras at the plasma membrane [15]. Therefore, NgBR is essential for the Ras-mediated signaling pathway [15]. Previous reports have shown that EGF induces the phosphorylation of ERα at the serine 118 residue [51], which is the confirmed signal involved in ERα-mediated resistance to endocrine therapy [25]. In this study, we demonstrated that NgBR knockdown impairs EGF-stimulated phosphorylation of ERα (Fig. 4a; Additional file 10: Figure S6A) but also

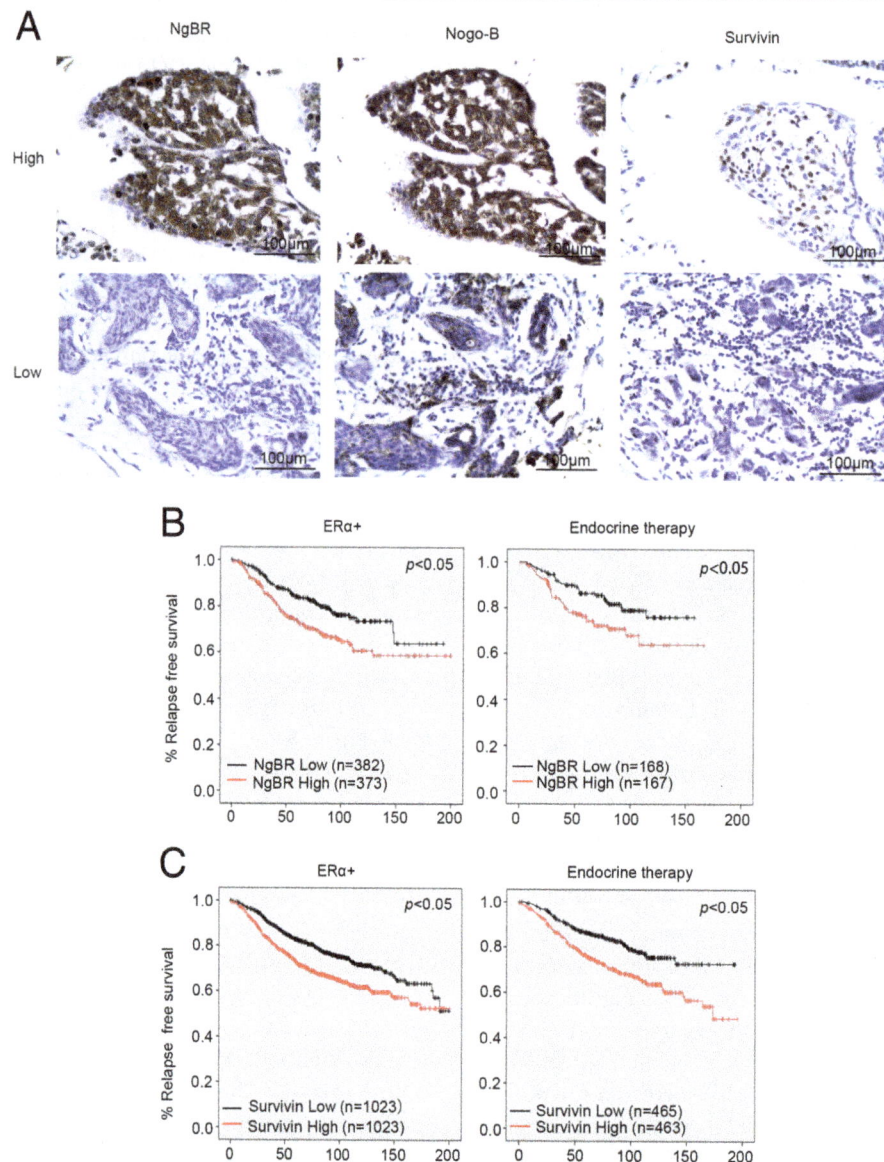

Fig. 7 Higher expression of Nogo-B receptor (NgBR) is associated with poor outcome in patients with estrogen receptor alpha (ERα) positive breast cancer. **a** Immunohistocheical (IHC) staining of NgBR, Nogo-B and survivin in 22 samples of breast cancer tissue. Images were taken using an Olympus microscope with ×20 lens. Scale bar 100 μm. **b** Relapse-free survival (RFS) in patients with ERα-positive breast cancer or endocrine therapy-treated patients. NgBR (NUS1) mRNA expression data were retrieved from a gene-expression profiling dataset (225071_x from Kaplan–Meier Plot database) of 755 cases of ERα-positive breast cancer and 335 patients with ERα-positive breast cancer treated with endocrine therapy. Kaplan–Meier analysis revealed significantly reduced RFS ($p < 0.05$) in 373 patients with ERα-positive breast cancer with high NgBR expression in tumors as compared to 382 patients with low NgBR expression in tumors. Similarly, RFS in patients with ERα-positive breast cancer treated with endocrine therapy is significantly decreased in 167 patients with high NgBR expression in tumors as compared to 168 patients with low NgBR expression in tumors ($p < 0.05$). **c** RFS in patients with ERα-positive breast cancer or endocrine therapy-treated patients. Survivin (BIRC5) mRNA expression data were retrieved from a gene-expression profiling dataset (202094_x from Kaplan–Meier Plot database) of 2046 cases of ERα-positive breast cancer and 928 patients with ERα-positive breast cancer treated with endocrine therapy. Kaplan–Meier analysis revealed significantly reduced RFS ($p < 0.05$) in 1023 patients with ERα-positive breast cancer with high survivin expression in tumors as compared to 1023 patients with low survivin expression in tumors. Similarly, RFS in patients with ERα-positive breast cancer treated with endocrine therapy is significantly decreased in 463 patients with high survivin expression in tumors as compared to 465 patients with low NgBR expression in tumors ($p < 0.05$)

attenuates resistance to tamoxifen (Fig. 2; Additional file 3: Figure S3). This finding indicates that NgBR is a potential therapeutic target for blocking concurrent endocrine-resistant signaling. However, we need further investigation to determine synergetic roles of NgBR in coordinating with other growth factor receptors, such as insulin-like growth factor 1 receptor (IGF1-R) and mERα, to promote the acquired resistance to tamoxifen.

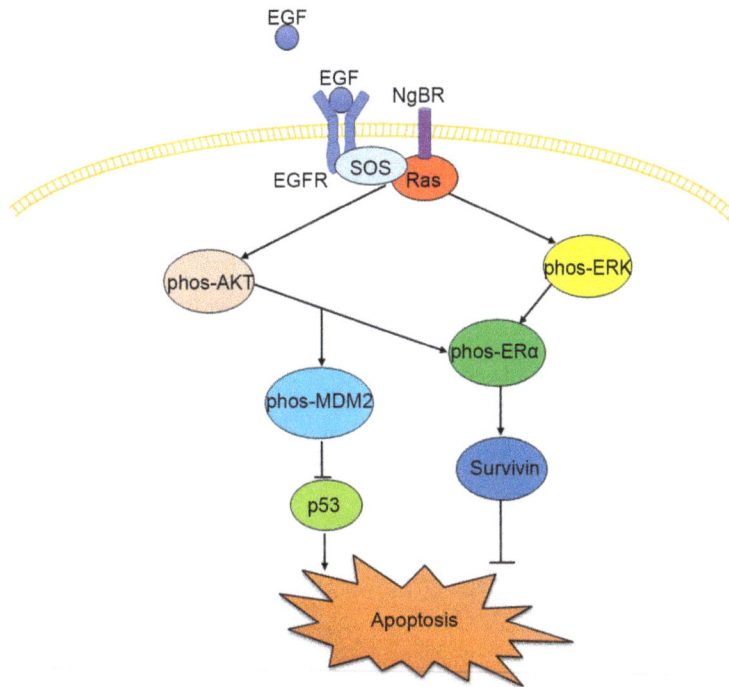

Fig. 8 Nogo-B receptor (NgBR) is required for epidermal growth factor (EGF)-acquired resistance to tamoxifen in patients with estrogen receptor alpha (ERα)-positive breast cancer. EGF binds to EGF receptor (EGFR) and recruits SOS1, an activator for Ras, to the plasma membrane. NgBR promotes the translocation of Ras to the plasma membrane and enhances EGF signaling, such as phosphorylation of Akt and extracellular signal-related kinase (ERK). Phosphorylated Akt further induces the phosphorylation of MDM2, which promotes p53 ubiquitination leading to its degradation and attenuates p53-mediated apoptosis. Phosphorylation of Akt and ERK also induce the phosphorylation of ERα, which induces the expression of survivin, an apoptosis inhibitor

Except for the contribution of growth factor receptor signaling pathways to tamoxifen resistance [9, 10], decreased ERα expression [7, 52] and increased human epidermal growth factor receptor 2 (HER2) [8, 53] are more likely to be attributed to tamoxifen resistance. Previous studies by others showed that hyperactivation of Raf kinase induces the loss of ERα in ERα-positive breast cancer cells [54] and inhibition of mitogen-activated protein kinase (MAPK) activity induced the expression of ERα in ERα-negative breast cancer cells [55]. As shown in Fig. 1g, ERα decreased and HER2 increased in MCF-7-TamR cells as compared to parental MCF-7 cells. Overexpression of either NgBR-HA or HER2-HA in MCF-7 cells decreased the protein level of ERα (Fig. 5b). Interestingly, NgBR knockdown in either MCF-7-TamR cells (Fig. 3d and c) or MCF-7 cells overexpressing HER2-HA (Figs. 5b and 3b) restored the protein level of ERα to a level similar to that in control cells as well as sensitivity to tamoxifen. The contribution of NgBR-regulated ERα expression to tamoxifen resistance needs further investigation in our future studies.

Conclusions

In summary, our results demonstrate that increased expression of NgBR in tamoxifen-resistant breast cancer cells promotes EGF signaling by increasing phosphorylation of AKT/ERK and MDM2, which attenuates the expression of p53 and increases the expression of survivin, which may lead to acquired resistance to tamoxifen as shown in Fig. 8. Higher levels of NgBR in patients with ERα-positive breast cancer are associated with poor RFS outcomes in patients with breast cancer because they lead to easier acquisition of tamoxifen resistance. Our data suggest that NgBR is a potential therapeutic target for restoring the sensitivity of tamoxifen-resistant breast cancer cells to conventional endocrine therapy.

Additional files

Additional file 1: Figure S1. MCF-7-TamR and T47D-TamR cells are resistant to 4-OHT. The 4-OHT resistant phenotype was confirmed using the CCK8 cell viability assay. (A) Cell viability was analyzed in MCF-7 and MCF-7-TamR cells treated with 1 μM 4OHT for different time periods (0, 1 day, 3 days and 5 days). (B) Cell viability was analyzed in T47D and T47D-TamR cells treated with 1 μM 4OHT for different time periods (0, 1 day, 3 days and 5 days). The OD value of untreated cells is referred to as 100%. The results show the average percentage of OD value as compared to untreated cells. The data are from in three separate repeated experiments, and are presented as the mean ± SD (*p < 0.05, n = 3). (PDF 153 kb)

Additional file 2: Figure S2. NgBR is highly expressed in the tamoxifen-resistant T47D-TamR cells. (A) NgBR level was increased in T47D-TamR cells. Protein levels of Nogo-B, ERα, p53 and survivin in T47D and T47D-TamR cells were determined using western blot analysis. (B) Quantitative analysis of proteins presented in Additional file 2: Figure S2A was carried out using ImageJ and normalized to β-actin. Data are presented as fold changes of T47D-TamR compared to the T47D cells. The data are from three separate repeated experiments and are presented as the mean ± SD (*$p < 0.05$, n = 3). (PDF 155 kb)

Additional file 3: Figure S3. NgBR decreases the resistance of T47D-TamR to tamoxifen. (A) NgBR knockdown increases apoptosis of T47D-TamR cells induced by 4-OHT (5 μM). The apoptotic cells were detected by Annexin V-PI staining. The total number of cells in the Q2 and Q4 quadrant was regarded as apoptotic cells. (B) Percentages of apoptotic cells are shown in the bar graph. (C) NgBR knockdown decreases the viability of T47D-TamR cells. Cell viability was determined using trypan blue staining of T47D-TamR cells treated with 5 μM 4-OHT for 48 h. The viable cell number of the NS group is referred to as 100%. (D) NgBR knockdown decreases the clonogenenicity of T47D-TamR cells. The clonogenic survival assay was used for measuring clonogenicity of T47D-TamR cells treated with 4-OHT (5 μM). (E) Quantification of colony number in colony formation assays presented in Additional file 3: Figure S3D. The data are from three separate repeated experiments and are presented as the mean ± SD (*$p < 0.05$, n = 3). (PDF 296 kb)

Additional file 4: Figure S4. Sensitivity of T47D cells to tamoxifen is regulated by p53 and survivin (A) Knockdown of p53 increases survivin level in T47D cells. T47D cells were transfected with siRNA specifically targeting p53 as described in "Methods". The protein levels of p53, NgBR, survivin and β-actin were determined using western blot analysis. (B) Quantitative analysis of proteins presented in Additional file 5: Figure S5A were carried out using ImageJ and were normalized to β-actin. Data are presented as fold changes in the si-p53 group compared to the NS group. (C) Knockdown of p53 decreases apoptosis of T47D cells induced by 4-OHT (1 μM). (D) Percentages of apoptotic cells in Additional file 5: Figure S5C are shown in the bar graph. (E) Survivin knockdown increases apoptosis of T47D-TamR cells induced by 4-OHT (5 μM). (F) Percentages of apoptotic cells in Additional file 5: Figure S5E are shown in the bar graph. (PDF 292 kb)

Additional file 5: Figure S5. NgBR knockdown attenuated EGF-stimulated signaling and ERα phosphorylation in T47D-TamR cells. (A) T47D-TamR cells were transfected with siNgBR and treated with EGF (100 ng/mL) for 5 min. Downstream signaling of the EGF pathway was determined using western blot assay. (B) Quantitative analysis of phosphorylated proteins presented in Additional file 10: Figure S6A were carried out using ImageJ and were normalized to total proteins. The data are from three separate repeated experiments and are presented as the mean ± SD (*$p < 0.05$, n = 3). (PDF 310 kb)

Additional file 6: NgBR (NUS1) mRNA expression data were retrieved from a gene-expression profiling dataset (225071_x from Kaplan–Meier Plot database) of 755 patients with ERα-positive breast cancer and 335 patients with ERα-positive breast cancer treated with endocrine therapy. Kaplan–Meier analysis revealed significantly reduced relapse-free survival (RFS) ($p < 0.05$) in 373 patients with ERα positive breast cancer with high NgBR expression in tumors as compared to 382 patients with low NgBR expression in tumors. (XLSX 42 kb)

Additional file 7: NgBR (NUS1) mRNA expression data were retrieved from a gene-expression profiling dataset (225071_x from Kaplan–Meier Plot database) of 755 patients with ERα-positive breast cancer and 335 patients with ERα-positive breast cancer treated with endocrine therapy. Kaplan–Meier analysis revealed that the RFS in patients with ERα-positive breast cancer treated with endocrine therapy is significantly decreased in 167 patients with high NgBR expression in tumors as compared to 168 patients with low NgBR expression in tumors ($p < 0.05$). (XLSX 32 kb)

Additional file 8: Survivin (BIRC5) mRNA expression data were retrieved from a gene-expression profiling dataset (202094_x from Kaplan–Meier Plot database) of 2046 patients with ERα-positive breast cancer and 928 patients with ERα-positive breast cancer treated with endocrine therapy. Kaplan–Meier analysis revealed significantly reduced relapse-free survival (RFS) ($p < 0.05$) in 1023 patients with ERα-positive breast cancer with high survivin expression in tumors as compared to 1023 patients with low survivin expression in tumors. (XLSX 70 kb)

Additional file 9: Survivin (BIRC5) mRNA expression data were retrieved from a gene-expression profiling dataset (202094_x from Kaplan–Meier Plot database) of 2046 patients with ERα-positive breast cancer and 928 patients with ERα-positive breast cancer treated with endocrine therapy. Kaplan–Meier analysis revealed that RFS in patients with ERα-positive breast cancer treated with endocrine therapy is significantly decreased in 463 patients with high survivin expression in tumors as compared to 465 patients with low NgBR expression in tumors ($p < 0.05$). (XLSX 60 kb)

Additional file 10: Figure S6. Relapse-free survival (RFS) in patients with ERα-positive breast cancer (n = 343). NgBR (NUS1) mRNA expression data were retrieved from the GSE6532 database. Kaplan–Meier analysis revealed significantly reduced RFS ($p < 0.05$) in patients with high NgBR expression in tumors (n = 189) as compared to patients with low NgBR expression in tumors (n = 154). (PDF 109 kb)

Additional file 11: NgBR (NUS1) mRNA expression data were retrieved from GSE6532 database. Kaplan–Meier analysis revealed significantly reduced relapse-free survival (RFS) ($p < 0.05$) in patients with high NgBR expression in tumors (n = 189) as compared to patients with low NgBR expression in tumors (n = 154). (XLS 67 kb)

Abbreviations
4-OHT: 4-Hydroxytamoxifen; AIs: Aromatase inhibitors; AmNogo-B: Amino terminus of Nogo-B; DFS: Disease-free survival; DMEM: Dulbecco's modified Eagle's medium; EGF: Epidermal growth factor; EGFR: Epidermal growth factor receptor; EMT: Epithelial-mesenchymal transition; ERα: Estrogen receptor alpha; ERK: Extracellular signal-related kinase; FBS: Fetal bovine serum; GST: Glutathione; HA: Human influenza hemagglutinin; HER2: Human epidermal growth factor receptor 2; IHC: Immunohistochemistry; MAPK: Mitogen-activated protein kinase; MCF-7-TamR: Tamoxifen resistant MCF-7 cells; mERα: Membrane ERα; mRNA: Messenger RNA; NCCN: National Comprehensive Cancer Network; NgBR: Nogo-B receptor; NgBR-HA: Human influenza hemagglutinin (HA) tagged NgBR; NS: Non-silencing small interfering RNA; OS: Overall survival; PBS: Phosphate-buffered saline; PR: progesterone receptor; RBD: Ras-binding domain of Raf; RFS: Relapse-free survival; RTKs: Receptor tyrosine kinases; SERM: Selective estrogen receptor modulator; siNgBR: Nogo-B receptor small interfering RNA; siRNA: small interfering RNA; T47D-TamR: Tamoxifen-resistant T47D cells

Acknowledgements
We thank Meghann Sytsma at the Medical College of Wisconsin (MCW) for editing the manuscript and administrative support for this study.

Funding
This work is supported in part by start-up funds from the Division of Pediatric Surgery and Division of Pediatric Pathology, MCW and Advancing a Healthier Wisconsin endowment to MCW, NIH R01HL108938, NIH R01DK112971, Wisconsin Breast Cancer Showhouse (WBCS), Institutional Research Grant # 86–004-26 from the American Cancer Society, Kathy Duffey Fogarty Award for breast cancer research, Rock River Research Foundation, State of Wisconsin Tax Check-off program for breast & prostate cancer research, We Care Fund and Children's Hospital of Wisconsin Research Institute Pilot Innovative Research Grant to QRM; the National Natural Science Foundation of China (grant no. 81041098) and Bethune Program B of Jilin University (grant no. 2012217) to ZF; the National Natural Science Foundation of China (grant No. 81472734 and 81730071) to HZ.

Authors' contributions
PG, XW, YJ, WH and YD conducted the experiments and data analysis; AS and YD collected tissue samples and performed histology analysis; PG and QRM designed the experiments and wrote the paper; ZF, HZ, AS, DS, MY, SL,

Nogo-B receptor increases the resistance to tamoxifen in estrogen receptor-positive breast...

15

BH and GZ provided reagents and edited the paper; QRM was responsible for overall integration and execution of the scientific approaches. All authors read and approved the final manuscript.

Competing interests

The authors declare that they have no competing interests.

Author details

[1]Department of Breast Surgery, The First Hospital of Jilin University, 71 Xinmin street, Changchun 130021, Jilin Province, China. [2]Division of Pediatric Surgery, Department of Surgery, Children's Research Institute, Medical College of Wisconsin, 8701 W Watertown Plank Rd, Milwaukee, WI 53226, USA. [3]Division of Pediatric Pathology, Department of Pathology, Children's Research Institute, Medical College of Wisconsin, 8701 W Watertown Plank Rd, Milwaukee, WI 53226, USA. [4]Department of Human Anatomy, Histology, and Embryology, Key Laboratory of Carcinogenesis and Translational Research (Ministry of Education) and State Key Laboratory of Natural and Biomimetic Drugs, Peking University Health Science Center, Beijing 100191, China. [5]College of Life Sciences, Nankai University, 94 Weijin Road, Tianjin 300071, China.

References

1. Jemal A, Bray F, Center MM, Ferlay J, Ward E, Forman D. Global cancer statistics. CA Cancer J Clin. 2011;61(2):69–90.
2. Siegel RL, Miller KD, Jemal A. Cancer statistics, 2017. CA Cancer J Clin. 2017;67(1):7–30.
3. Harvey JM, Clark GM, Osborne CK, Allred DC. Estrogen receptor status by immunohistochemistry is superior to the ligand-binding assay for predicting response to adjuvant endocrine therapy in breast cancer. J Clin Oncol. 1999;17(5):1474–81.
4. Early Breast Cancer Trialists' Collaborative G. Effects of chemotherapy and hormonal therapy for early breast cancer on recurrence and 15-year survival: an overview of the randomised trials. Lancet. 2005;365(9472):1687–717.
5. Gradishar WJ, Anderson BO, Blair SL, Burstein HJ, Cyr A, Elias AD, Farrar WB, Forero A, Giordano SH, Goldstein LJ, et al. Breast cancer version 3.2014. J Natl Compr Cancer Netw. 2014;12(4):542–90.
6. Obrero M, Yu DV, Shapiro DJ. Estrogen receptor-dependent and estrogen receptor-independent pathways for tamoxifen and 4-hydroxytamoxifen-induced programmed cell death. J Biol Chem. 2002;277(47):45695–703.
7. Musgrove EA, Sutherland RL. Biological determinants of endocrine resistance in breast cancer. Nat Rev. 2009;9(9):631–43.
8. Arpino G, Green SJ, Allred DC, Lew D, Martino S, Osborne CK, Elledge RM. HER-2 amplification, HER-1 expression, and tamoxifen response in estrogen receptor-positive metastatic breast cancer: a southwest oncology group study. Clin Cancer Res. 2004;10(17):5670–6.
9. Zhen LL, Zhu X, Zheng W, Wang XY, Wu ZY. Involvement of epidermal growth factor receptor signaling pathway In tamoxifen resistance of MCF 7 cells. Ai Zheng. 2006;25(7):839–43.
10. Turner N, Pearson A, Sharpe R, Lambros M, Geyer F, Lopez-Garcia MA, Natrajan R, Marchio C, Iorns E, Mackay A, et al. FGFR1 amplification drives endocrine therapy resistance and is a therapeutic target in breast cancer. Cancer Res. 2010;70(5):2085–94.
11. Huber AB, Weinmann O, Brosamle C, Oertle T, Schwab ME. Patterns of Nogo mRNA and protein expression in the developing and adult rat and after CNS lesions. J Neurosci. 2002;22(9):3553–67.
12. Miao RQ, Gao Y, Harrison KD, Prendergast J, Acevedo LM, Yu J, Hu F, Strittmatter SM, Sessa WC. Identification of a receptor necessary for Nogo-B stimulated chemotaxis and morphogenesis of endothelial cells. Proc Natl Acad Sci U S A. 2006;103(29):10997–1002.
13. Rana U, Liu Z, Kumar SN, Zhao B, Hu W, Bordas M, Cossette S, Szabo S, Foeckler J, Weiler H, et al. Nogo-B receptor deficiency causes cerebral vasculature defects during embryonic development in mice. Dev Biol. 2016;410(2):190–201.
14. Park EJ, Grabinska KA, Guan Z, Sessa WC. NgBR is essential for endothelial cell glycosylation and vascular development. EMBO Rep. 2016;17(2):167–77.
15. Zhao B, Hu W, Kumar S, Gonyo P, Rana U, Liu Z, Wang B, Duong WQ, Yang Z, Williams CL, et al. The Nogo-B receptor promotes Ras plasma membrane localization and activation. Oncogene. 2017;36(24):3406–16.
16. Wang B, Zhao B, North P, Kong A, Huang J, Miao QR. Expression of NgBR is highly associated with estrogen receptor alpha and survivin in breast cancer. PLoS One. 2013;8(11):e78083.
17. Tamm I, Wang Y, Sausville E, Scudiero DA, Vigna N, Oltersdorf T, Reed JC. IAP-family protein survivin inhibits caspase activity and apoptosis induced by Fas (CD95), Bax, caspases, and anticancer drugs. Cancer Res. 1998;58(23):5315–20.
18. Zhao B, Xu B, Hu W, Song C, Wang F, Liu Z, Ye M, Zou H, Miao QR. Comprehensive proteome quantification reveals NgBR as a new regulator for epithelial-mesenchymal transition of breast tumor cells. J Proteome. 2015;112:38–52.
19. Wang L, Zhang X, Wang ZY. The Wilms' tumor suppressor WT1 regulates expression of members of the epidermal growth factor receptor (EGFR) and estrogen receptor in acquired tamoxifen resistance. Anticancer Res. 2010;30(9):3637–42.
20. Luo J, Wang W, Tang Y, Zhou D, Gao Y, Zhang Q, Zhou X, Zhu H, Xing L, Yu J. mRNA and methylation profiling of radioresistant esophageal cancer cells: the involvement of Sall2 in acquired aggressive phenotypes. J Cancer. 2017;8(4):646–56.
21. Yuan J, Liu M, Yang L, Tu G, Zhu Q, Chen M, Cheng H, Luo H, Fu W, Li Z, et al. Acquisition of epithelial-mesenchymal transition phenotype in the tamoxifen-resistant breast cancer cell: a new role for G protein-coupled estrogen receptor in mediating tamoxifen resistance through cancer-associated fibroblast-derived fibronectin and beta1-integrin signaling pathway in tumor cells. Breast Cancer Res. 2015;17:69.
22. Thewes V, Simon R, Schroeter P, Schlotter M, Anzeneder T, Buttner R, Benes V, Sauter G, Burwinkel B, Nicholson RI, et al. Reprogramming of the ERRalpha and ERalpha target gene landscape triggers tamoxifen resistance in breast cancer. Cancer Res. 2015;75(4):720–31.
23. Jin Y, Hu W, Liu T, Rana U, Aguilera-Barrantes I, Kong A, Kumar SN, Wang B, Gao P, Wang X, et al. Nogo-B receptor increases the resistance of estrogen receptor positive breast cancer to paclitaxel. Cancer Lett. 2018;419:233–44.
24. de Leeuw R, Neefjes J, Michalides R. A role for estrogen receptor phosphorylation in the resistance to tamoxifen. Int J Breast Cancer. 2011;2011:232435.
25. Anbalagan M, Rowan BG. Estrogen receptor alpha phosphorylation and its functional impact in human breast cancer. Mol Cell Endocrinol. 2015;418(Pt 3):264–72.
26. Dai X, Cai C, Xiao F, Xiong Y, Huang Y, Zhang Q, Xiang Q, Lou G, Lian M, Su Z, et al. Identification of a novel aFGF-binding peptide with anti-tumor effect on breast cancer from phage display library. Biochem Biophys Res Commun. 2014;445(4):795–801.
27. Higuchi T, Endo M, Hanamura T, Gohno T, Niwa T, Yamaguchi Y, Horiguchi J, Hayashi S. Contribution of Estrone sulfate to cell proliferation in aromatase inhibitor (AI) -resistant, Hormone Receptor-Positive Breast Cancer. PLoS One. 2016;11(5):e0155844.
28. Paoletti C, Larios JM, Muniz MC, Aung K, Cannell EM, Darga EP, Kidwell KM, Thomas DG, Tokudome N, Brown ME, et al. Heterogeneous estrogen receptor expression in circulating tumor cells suggests diverse mechanisms of fulvestrant resistance. Mol Oncol. 2016;10(7):1078–85.
29. Kim J, Lee J, Jang SY, Kim C, Choi Y, Kim A. Anticancer effect of metformin on estrogen receptor-positive and tamoxifen-resistant breast cancer cell lines. Oncol Rep. 2016;35(5):2553–60.
30. Fan P, Agboke FA, Cunliffe HE, Ramos P, Jordan VC. A molecular model for the mechanism of acquired tamoxifen resistance in breast cancer. Eur J Cancer. 2014;50(16):2866–76.
31. Fan W, Chang J, Fu P. Endocrine therapy resistance in breast cancer: current status, possible mechanisms and overcoming strategies. Future Med Chem. 2015;7(12):1511–9.
32. Clarke R, Tyson JJ, Dixon JM. Endocrine resistance in breast cancer–an overview and update. Mol Cell Endocrinol. 2015;418(Pt 3):220–34.
33. Schiff R, Massarweh SA, Shou J, Bharwani L, Mohsin SK, Osborne CK. Cross-talk between estrogen receptor and growth factor pathways as a molecular target for overcoming endocrine resistance. Clin Cancer Res. 2004;10(1 Pt 2):331S–6S.

34. Xiong J, Su T, Qu Z, Yang Q, Wang Y, Li J, Zhou S. Triptolide has anticancer and chemosensitization effects by down-regulating Akt activation through the MDM2/REST pathway in human breast cancer. Oncotarget. 2016;7(17):23933–46.

35. Mayo LD, Donner DB. A phosphatidylinositol 3-kinase/Akt pathway promotes translocation of Mdm2 from the cytoplasm to the nucleus. Proc Natl Acad Sci U S A. 2001;98(20):11598–603.

36. Dong C, Zhao B, Long F, Liu Y, Liu Z, Li S, Yang X, Sun D, Wang H, Liu Q, et al. Nogo-B receptor promotes the chemoresistance of human hepatocellular carcinoma via the ubiquitination of p53 protein. Oncotarget. 2016;7(8):8850–65.

37. Muller PA, Vousden KH. Mutant p53 in cancer: new functions and therapeutic opportunities. Cancer Cell. 2014;25(3):304–17.

38. Bailey ST, Shin H, Westerling T, Liu XS, Brown M. Estrogen receptor prevents p53-dependent apoptosis in breast cancer. Proc Natl Acad Sci U S A. 2012; 109(44):18060–5.

39. Mirza A, McGuirk M, Hockenberry TN, Wu Q, Ashar H, Black S, Wen SF, Wang L, Kirschmeier P, Bishop WR, et al. Human survivin is negatively regulated by wild-type p53 and participates in p53-dependent apoptotic pathway. Oncogene. 2002;21(17):2613–22.

40. Span PN, Tjan-Heijnen VC, Manders P, van Tienoven D, Lehr J, Sweep FC. High survivin predicts a poor response to endocrine therapy, but a good response to chemotherapy in advanced breast cancer. Breast Cancer Res Treat. 2006;98(2):223–30.

41. Omerovic J, Laude AJ, Prior IA. Ras proteins: paradigms for compartmentalised and isoform-specific signalling. Cell Mol Life Sci. 2007; 64(19–20):2575–89.

42. Hancock JF. Ras proteins: different signals from different locations. Nat Rev Mol Cell Biol. 2003;4(5):373–84.

43. Buday L, Downward J. Many faces of Ras activation. Biochim Biophys Acta. 2008;1786(2):178–87.

44. McCubrey JA, Steelman LS, Abrams SL, Lee JT, Chang F, Bertrand FE, Navolanic PM, Terrian DM, Franklin RA, D'Assoro AB, et al. Roles of the RAF/ MEK/ERK and PI3K/PTEN/AKT pathways in malignant transformation and drug resistance. Adv Enzym Regul. 2006;46:249–79.

45. McCubrey JA, Steelman LS, Chappell WH, Abrams SL, Wong EW, Chang F, Lehmann B, Terrian DM, Milella M, Tafuri A, et al. Roles of the Raf/MEK/ERK pathway in cell growth, malignant transformation and drug resistance. Biochim Biophys Acta. 2007;1773(8):1263–84.

46. Karnoub AE, Weinberg RA. Ras oncogenes: split personalities. Nat Rev Mol Cell Biol. 2008;9(7):517–31.

47. Acconcia F, Kumar R. Signaling regulation of genomic and nongenomic functions of estrogen receptors. Cancer Lett. 2006;238(1):1–14.

48. Zhang D, Trudeau VL. Integration of membrane and nuclear estrogen receptor signaling. Comp Biochem Physiol A Mol Integr Physiol. 2006;144(3):306–15.

49. Soltysik K, Czekaj P. Membrane estrogen receptors - is it an alternative way of estrogen action? J Physiol Pharmacol. 2013;64(2):129–42.

50. Pritchard JE, Dillon PM, Conaway MR, Silva CM, Parsons SJ. A mechanistic study of the effect of doxorubicin/adriamycin on the estrogen response in a breast cancer model. Oncology. 2012;83(6):305–20.

51. Bunone G, Briand PA, Miksicek RJ, Picard D. Activation of the unliganded estrogen receptor by EGF involves the MAP kinase pathway and direct phosphorylation. EMBO J. 1996;15(9):2174–83.

52. Guo S, Li Y, Tong Q, Gu F, Zhu T, Fu L, Yang S. deltaEF1 down-regulates ER-alpha expression and confers tamoxifen resistance in breast cancer. PLoS One. 2012;7(12):e52380.

53. Knowlden JM, Hutcheson IR, Jones HE, Madden T, Gee JM, Harper ME, Barrow D, Wakeling AE, Nicholson RI. Elevated levels of epidermal growth factor receptor/c-erbB2 heterodimers mediate an autocrine growth regulatory pathway in tamoxifen-resistant MCF-7 cells. Endocrinology. 2003;144(3):1032–44.

54. Oh AS, Lorant LA, Holloway JN, Miller DL, Kern FG, El-Ashry D. Hyperactivation of MAPK induces loss of ERalpha expression in breast cancer cells. Mol Endocrinol. 2001;15(8):1344–59.

55. Bayliss J, Hilger A, Vishnu P, Diehl K, El-Ashry D. Reversal of the estrogen receptor negative phenotype in breast cancer and restoration of antiestrogen response. Clin Cancer Res. 2007;13(23):7029–36.

2

Epigenomics of mammary gland development

Holly Holliday[1,2], Laura A. Baker[1,2], Simon R. Junankar[1,2], Susan J. Clark[2,3] and Alexander Swarbrick[1,2*]

Abstract

Differentiation of stem cells into highly specialised cells requires gene expression changes brought about by remodelling of the chromatin architecture. During this lineage-commitment process, the majority of DNA needs to be packaged into inactive heterochromatin, allowing only a subset of regulatory elements to remain open and functionally required genes to be expressed. Epigenetic mechanisms such as DNA methylation, post-translational modifications to histone tails, and nucleosome positioning all potentially contribute to the changes in higher order chromatin structure during differentiation. The mammary gland is a particularly useful model to study these complex epigenetic processes since the majority of its development is postnatal, the gland is easily accessible, and development occurs in a highly reproducible manner. Inappropriate epigenetic remodelling can also drive tumourigenesis; thus, insights into epigenetic remodelling during mammary gland development advance our understanding of breast cancer aetiology. We review the current literature surrounding DNA methylation and histone modifications in the developing mammary gland and its implications for breast cancer.

Keywords: Mammary development, Breast cancer, Stem cell, Differentiation, Epithelial, Epigenetics, Chromatin, Methylation, Histone

Background

Lineage commitment in the mammary gland

The mammary gland is a dynamic tissue with rapid changes in tissue architecture occurring throughout the lifetime of the mammal in response to hormonal cues (reviewed in [1, 2]). The gland is comprised of an epithelial ductal tree embedded within a stromal fat pad comprised of a variety of cell types including adipocytes, fibroblasts, immune cells, lymphatic cells, and vascular cells that interact with each other to maintain a functional organ [2]. At birth, the gland contains a rudimentary ductal structure. The presence of oestrogen at puberty causes the ducts to undergo branching morphogenesis, generating a ductal tree that invades the stromal fat pad. Ductal elongation is driven by proliferation of cap cells located at the tips of the terminal end buds (TEBs) [1, 2]. During pregnancy and lactation, progesterone and prolactin cause extensive secondary and tertiary side branching and the formation of alveolar units that produce and secrete milk. Weaning of the offspring initiates the process

of involution, which essentially remodels the mammary gland back to the virgin state [1, 2].

The mammary ductal epithelium is comprised of two main cell lineages: the inner luminal population containing ductal and alveolar cells, and the outer basal population containing myoepithelial cells (Fig. 1). The basal population is enriched for cells capable of self-renewal and multi-lineage differentiation upon serial transplantation into cleared mammary fat pads. These cells, known as mammary stem cells (MaSCs) [3, 4], lack unique cell surface markers, complicating their purification from the bulk basal cell population (referred to as 'basal'). The luminal compartment contains proliferative luminal progenitor and mature luminal cells. During pregnancy and lactation, luminal progenitors differentiate into alveolar cells via alveolar progenitors. Transplantation experiments support a model whereby a bipotent MaSC at the apex of a differentiation hierarchy gives rise to both myoepithelial and luminal lineages [1]. The existence of bipotent MaSCs under physiological conditions is debated, with various lineage-tracing experiments yielding irreconcilable results. Some groups have found that adult basal cells give rise to both mature luminal and basal cells [5, 6]. Other groups have found that bipotent MaSCs only exist during embryonic development and that basal and luminal lineages of

* Correspondence: a.swarbrick@garvan.org.au
[1]The Kinghorn Cancer Centre, Cancer Research Division, Garvan Institute of Medical Research, Darlinghurst, NSW 2010, Australia
[2]St Vincent's Clinical School, Faculty of Medicine, UNSW, Darlinghurst, NSW 2010, Australia
Full list of author information is available at the end of the article

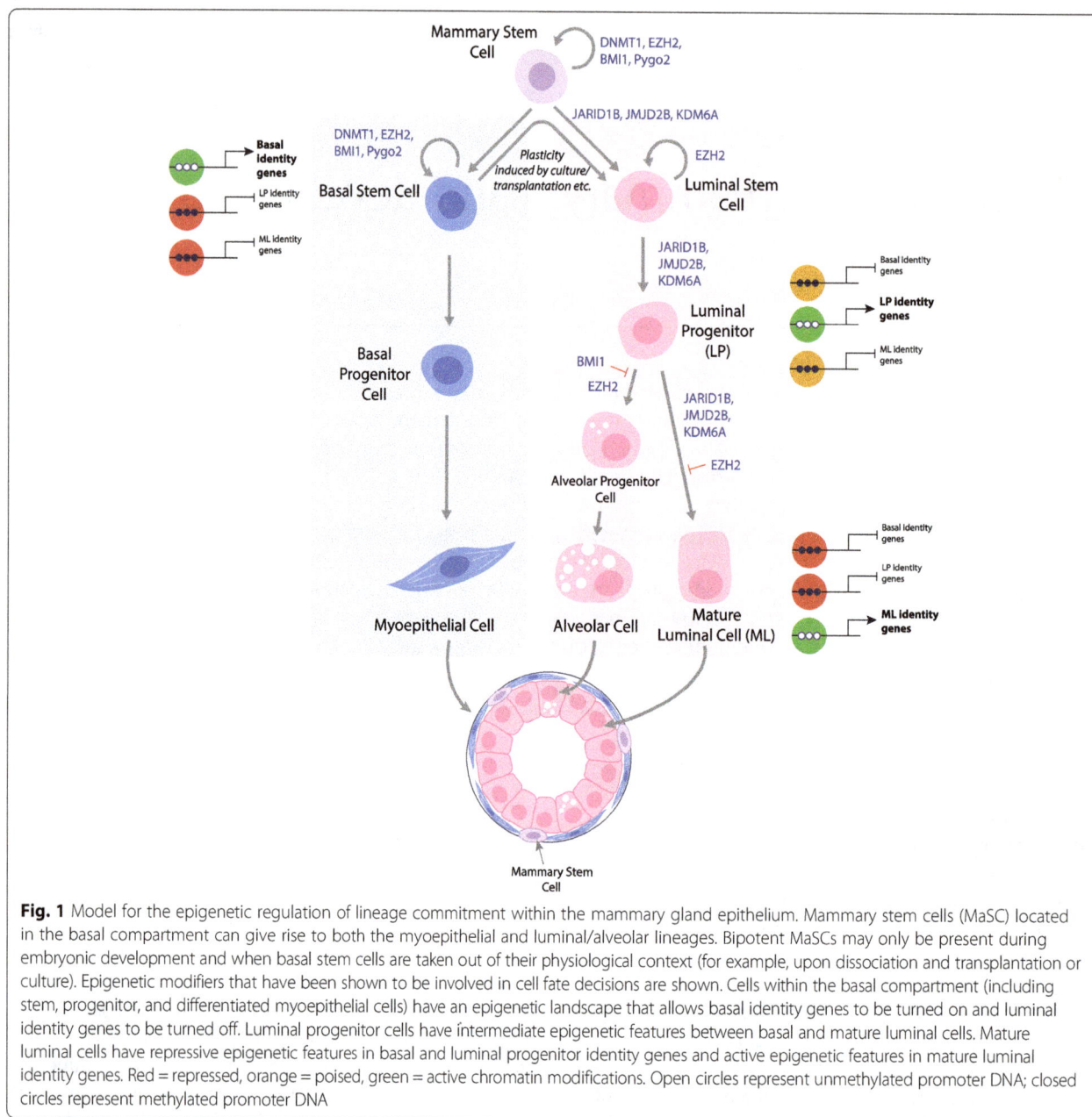

Fig. 1 Model for the epigenetic regulation of lineage commitment within the mammary gland epithelium. Mammary stem cells (MaSC) located in the basal compartment can give rise to both the myoepithelial and luminal/alveolar lineages. Bipotent MaSCs may only be present during embryonic development and when basal stem cells are taken out of their physiological context (for example, upon dissociation and transplantation or culture). Epigenetic modifiers that have been shown to be involved in cell fate decisions are shown. Cells within the basal compartment (including stem, progenitor, and differentiated myoepithelial cells) have an epigenetic landscape that allows basal identity genes to be turned on and luminal identity genes to be turned off. Luminal progenitor cells have intermediate epigenetic features between basal and mature luminal cells. Mature luminal cells have repressive epigenetic features in basal and luminal progenitor identity genes and active epigenetic features in mature luminal identity genes. Red = repressed, orange = poised, green = active chromatin modifications. Open circles represent unmethylated promoter DNA; closed circles represent methylated promoter DNA

the adult gland are maintained by distinct pools of unipotent stem cells [7–10] (Fig. 1). The different conclusions may be due to reliance on different genetic reporters that mark distinct cell populations with discrete differentiation potentials.

It is increasingly accepted that cellular differentiation is not unidirectional and that 'terminally differentiated' cells may exhibit plasticity under certain conditions of stress, injury, or experimental stimuli [11]. Indeed, differentiated myoepithelial and luminal cells have been shown to adopt stem-like properties when cultured ex vivo [12]. The molecular mechanisms underlying this cellular plasticity are largely unknown.

Epigenetics and development

Extensive changes in gene expression are required for a stem cell to undergo lineage commitment and functional differentiation during development. Changes in gene expression are associated with heritable epigenetic modifications to DNA and chromatin without changes to the DNA sequence. There are several layers of epigenetic regulation involved in the moderation of gene expression, including DNA methylation, post-translational modification to histone tails, chromatin remodelling, and higher order chromosome organisation (Fig. 2). DNA methylation is central to transcriptional repression,

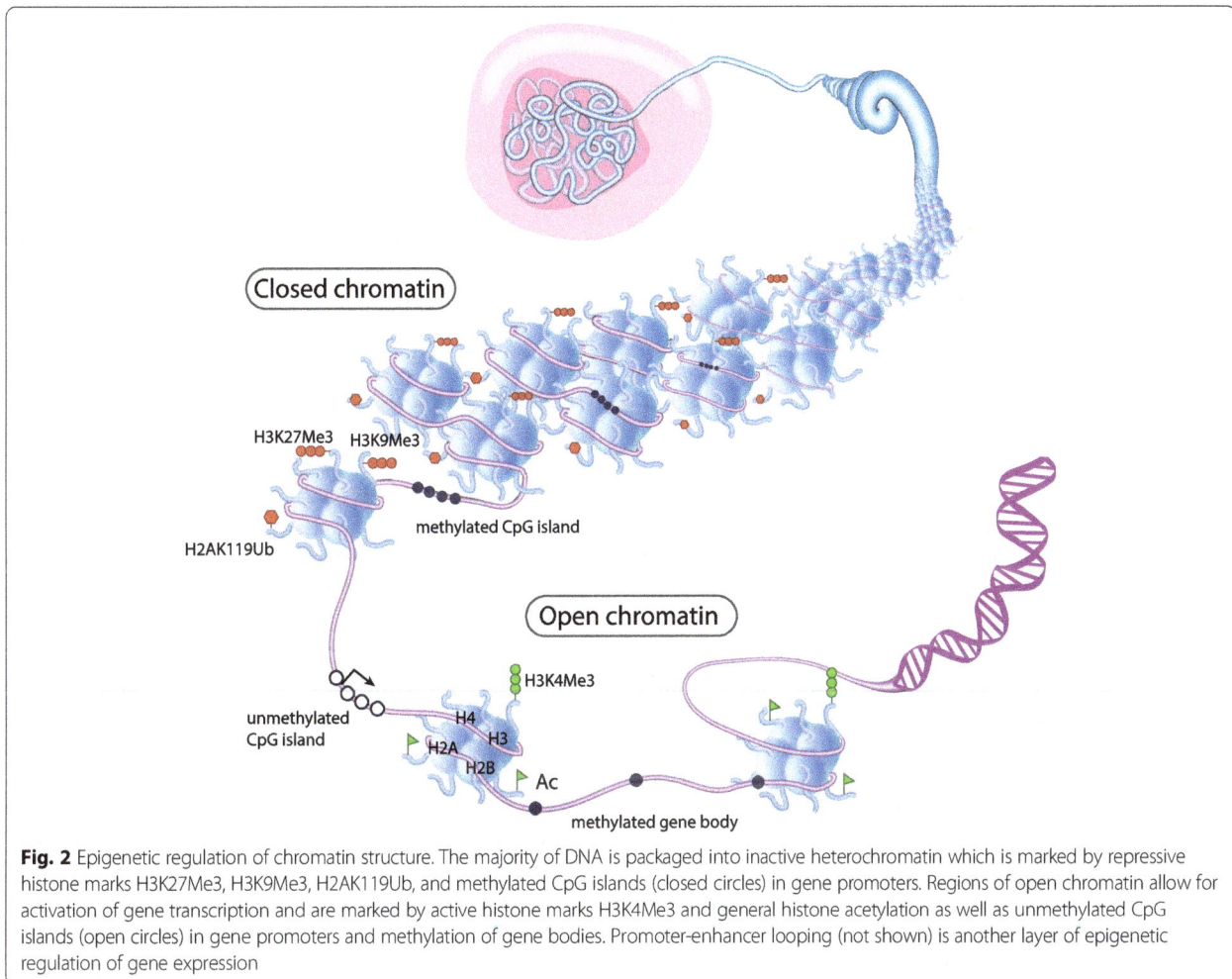

Fig. 2 Epigenetic regulation of chromatin structure. The majority of DNA is packaged into inactive heterochromatin which is marked by repressive histone marks H3K27Me3, H3K9Me3, H2AK119Ub, and methylated CpG islands (closed circles) in gene promoters. Regions of open chromatin allow for activation of gene transcription and are marked by active histone marks H3K4Me3 and general histone acetylation as well as unmethylated CpG islands (open circles) in gene promoters and methylation of gene bodies. Promoter-enhancer looping (not shown) is another layer of epigenetic regulation of gene expression

genomic imprinting, X-chromosome inactivation, and suppression of repetitive genomic elements [13, 14]. The basic chromatin subunit is the nucleosome, which is made up of ~ 147 nucleotides of DNA wrapped around a core histone octamer made up of two of each of the histone proteins H2A, H2B, H3, and H4 [15] (Fig. 2). Protruding N-terminal histone tails are subject to covalent post-translational modifications including acetylation, phosphorylation, ubiquitination, and methylation. The resulting 'histone code' ultimately influences gene transcription through multiple mechanisms (reviewed in [16]). The organisation and positioning of nucleosomes also determines which regions of the genome are active or inactive. Chromatin remodellers use ATP hydrolysis to move, destabilise, eject, or restructure nucleosomes to change chromatin accessibility and gene transcription [17].

Epigenetic regulation of differentiation in embryonic stem (ES) cells and the haematopoietic system is well characterised [18, 19]; however, far less is known about the epigenetic mechanisms underlying self-renewal and differentiation of tissue-specific epithelial stem and progenitor cells. Lineage-specific epigenetic programmes

can become deregulated and result in oncogenesis [20]. Understanding these processes under physiological circumstances provides insights into how these complex programmes are altered during carcinogenesis.

DNA methylation

The majority of CpG dinucleotides in the mammalian genome are methylated with the exception of CG-dense regions located around transcriptional start sites, known as CpG islands. These occur in approximately 70% of annotated gene promoters [14]. During development, DNA methyltransferase enzymes (DNMT1, DNMT3A, and DNMT3B) deposit and maintain methylation in a small subset of CpG island promoters causing transcriptional repression [21]. Conversely, methylation in gene bodies correlates with transcriptional activation [22] (Fig. 2). Cellular differentiation is accompanied by progressive gain of CpG island methylation resulting in silencing of developmental and non-related lineage-specific genes [23]. Demethylation of tissue-specific genes also defines cellular identity and is mediated by ten-eleven translocation (Tet) methylcytosine dioxygenases (Tet1, Tet2, Tet3) [23, 24].

DNA methylation patterns define mammary epithelial cell identity

Mammary epithelial identity is, in part, shaped by the DNA methylation landscape, which varies between cell types [25, 26]. For example, methylation profiles from mammary epithelial cells are more similar to skin cells than blood cells, in keeping with the ectodermal origin of mammary and skin epithelial cells [25].

There have been numerous efforts to analyse DNA methylation patterns of stem/progenitor cells and differentiated luminal and myoepithelial cells in mice and humans [26–30]. Stem/progenitor cells isolated from human mammary glands are hypomethylated compared with differentiated luminal and myoepithelial cell types. This suggests that DNA methylation increases as the cells undergo lineage restriction, complementing work in other stem cell populations [31]. Genes that are hypomethylated and highly expressed in stem/progenitor cells include transcription factors with known roles in stem cell maintenance (e.g. HOXA1 and TCF7L1) [27]. Conversely, genes with promoter methylation (silenced) in stem/progenitor cells and gene body methylation (activated) in mature luminal cells include luminal-driving transcription factors (e.g. GATA3). This implies that DNA methylation is important in regulating the expression of lineage-specific transcription factors [28]. Comprehensive DNA methylation profiling of mouse mammary epithelial subpopulations has revealed similar patterns; when compared to basal cells, luminal cells have hypermethylation and silencing of stem and basal cell-related genes (e.g. *Angptl2* and *Krt5*) and hypomethylation and activation of epithelial differentiation genes (e.g. *Elf5*, *Cldn4*, and *Krt8*) [25, 26, 30]. Thus, DNA methylation is important for controlling expression of transcription factors that define basal cells and luminal populations.

Murine studies have been particularly useful in determining the effects of ageing and pregnancy on DNA methylation in mammary epithelial cells [25, 26]. Pregnancy induces changes to the DNA methylome of both basal and luminal populations that persist throughout life [25, 26]. Genes involved in lactation and involution become hypomethylated in response to the pregnancy and are primed to respond robustly to subsequent pregnancies [26]. An epigenetic memory of pregnancy may explain the protective effect of early pregnancy on breast cancer risk in humans later in life [32].

DNMT1 maintains mammary stem/progenitor cells

DNMT1 has high affinity for hemimethylated DNA and is responsible for restoring the original methylation pattern present before DNA replication [21]. Its activity is required for the maintenance of adult stem cells including MaSCs [33] (Table 1). Expression of DNMT1 is similar in basal and luminal cells and increases during pregnancy [33]. Mammary-specific deletion of DNMT1 in mice severely effects TEB development and ductal elongation, results in fewer proliferative Ki67[+] mammary epithelial cells, and mammary cells have reduced mammosphere-forming capacity when cultured ex vivo [33]. Correspondingly, inhibition of DNMT activity by administering 5-azacitidine (5-AzaC) to mice decreases Cyclin D1 expression and an overall reduction in mammary cell numbers [25]. Taken together, DNMT1-mediated DNA methylation is essential for maintenance of stem/progenitor cells in the mammary gland.

Histone modifications

Histone modifications occur on lysine and arginine residues and regulate DNA accessibility, or act as protein docking sites for the initiation of downstream biological processes, including chromatin compaction, transcriptional regulation, and DNA repair [16]. Histone acetylation is associated with transcriptional activation [34], while histone methylation can either activate (trimethylation of lysine 4 on histone 3; designated as H3K4Me3) or repress (H3K27Me3 or H3K9Me3) transcription [35, 36]. Bivalent promoters, containing both active H3K4Me3 and inactive H3K27Me3 marks, are often found at the promoters of key developmental genes and signal a repressed yet poised state, which allows for rapid activation or silencing of genes during differentiation [37]. These were originally discovered in ES cells and have since been identified in adult stem cells. Histones flanking active enhancer regions are marked by H3K4Me1 and H3K27ac modifications [38]. Histone modifications are most effectively mapped using chromatin immunoprecipitation followed by DNA sequencing (ChIP-Seq).

Rewriting the histone code through mammary gland development

Mammary subpopulations and regulatory elements governing transcription have been defined through the integration of ChIP-Seq data with transcriptional signatures [28, 39–42]. The diverse chromatin states that distinguish between mammary epithelial subpopulations are as extensive as those that distinguish epithelial subpopulations from developmentally unrelated stromal cells [40]. The largest variations in chromatin state occurred in enhancer regions, although there were also significant variations in promoter regions [40]. This shows that the chromatin state of cell-specific regulatory elements is a key determinant of cell type, even within the same epithelial lineage.

Histone methylation changes correlate with gene expression changes during lineage restriction. In the mouse mammary gland, luminal progenitor-defining genes [43] have higher H3K4Me3 coverage and lower H3K27Me3 coverage in luminal progenitor cells

Table 1 Summary of epigenetic modulating proteins with known roles in mammary gland development

Protein complex or family	Members	Modification	Activating/repressive	Role in MG development	Reference
DNA methyltransferase	DNMT1, DNMT3a, DNMT3b	DNA methylation	Repressive at promoters, activating in gene bodies	DNMT1 maintains stem/progenitor cells	[33]
Polycomb repressive complex 2 (PRC2)	SUZ2, EED, RBBP4 or RBBP7 and EZH2 or EZH1	H3K27 trimethylation	Repressive	EZH2 maintains stem/progenitor cells, restricts mature luminal differentiation, and promotes alveolar differentiation.	[39, 50, 51]
Polycomb repressive complex 1 (PRC1)	PCGF BMI1 or MEL18	H2AK119 mono-ubiquitylation	Repressive	BMI1 maintains stem/progenitor cells and restricts alveolar differentiation	[52]
	CBX CBX2, CBX4, CBX6, CBX7, or CBX8				
	PHC PHC1, PHC2, or PHC3				
	SCML SCMH1 or SCML2				
	RING RING2 or RING1				
Lysine demethylase (KDM) proteins	JARID1B/KDM5B/PLU-1	H3K4Me3 demethylation	Repressive and activating	GATA3 cofactor, promotes luminal differentiation	[55, 57–59]
	JMJD2B/KDM4B	H3K9Me3 demethylation	Activating	ERα cofactor, promotes luminal differentiation	[61]
	KDM6A/UTX	H3K27Me3 demethylation	Activating	Luminal transcription factor co-factor, promotes luminal differentiation	[62]
Plant homeodomain (PHD)-containing proteins	Pygo2	Binds to H3K4Me3	Not applicable	β-catenin co-factor, maintains stem/progenitor cells by restricting Notch-mediated luminal differentiation	[65]
Bromodomain and extra-terminal domain (BET) proteins	BRD4	Binds to acetylated lysines on histones	Activating	FOXO1 cofactor, maintains basal epithelial phenotype	[76]

compared with basal cells [39]. Genes within the mature luminal signature [43] show the same pattern when comparing mature luminal cells with luminal progenitors [39]. Histone modifications are also altered upon pregnancy. Luminal cells differentiate into milk-secreting alveolar cells in preparation for lactation, which results in decreased repressive marks and increased active marks in key luminal differentiation and milk-production genes. Similar results were found in sorted human mammary epithelial populations [28, 40]. Interestingly, the genes repressed in luminal and basal subsets are often present in large regions enriched for H3K27Me3 marks (K27 blocs), which may allow for cell-type specific co-ordinated gene silencing [28]. These studies demonstrate that distinct histone methylation profiles influence gene expression changes that direct basal to luminal progenitor differentiation and the maturation of luminal progenitors to luminal and alveolar cells (Fig. 1). Histone modifications also regulate gene expression within the heterogeneous basal population. A small population of quiescent MaSCs, marked by co-expression of LGR5 and TSPAN8, have recently been purified from the mouse mammary epithelium [44]. These cells share similarities with quiescent stem cells in other tissues and have distinct H3K4Me3 and H3K27Me3 landscapes compared with the other basal cells [44].

Analysis of bivalent promoters in the mammary epithelial subpopulations has led to some interesting discoveries. Luminal progenitor cells have intermediate promoter features between basal and mature luminal cells. For example, promoters of genes involved in basal functions (such as extracellular matrix organisation) are marked by H3K4Me3 in basal cells, are bivalent in luminal progenitors, and are marked with H3K27Me3 in mature luminal cells [40]. This corresponds with a decrease in gene expression [40]. This is consistent with the model that luminal progenitors are derived from basal cells. However, it is not possible to discern whether luminal commitment of basal cells happens in the adult gland or if it occurs during embryonic development and is maintained in the adult gland. While each subset contains bivalent domains, the highest number occurs in the terminally differentiated mature luminal subset [39, 40]. This challenges the dogma that bivalent domains operate predominantly in stem cells to restrict lineage-specific gene expression [37]. Instead, bivalent domains may be a more general phenomenon in cells of all differentiation states. Key developmental transcription factors within basal and luminal cells contain bivalent promoters; this may keep these genes poised, enabling rapid response to environmental stimuli [28, 40]. For example, in differentiated myoepithelial cells, the epithelial-mesenchymal transition (EMT) transcription factor ZEB1 is held in a bivalent state. Stimulation with transforming growth factor (TGF)β results in the removal of the repressive H3K27Me3 mark while maintaining the active H3K4Me3 mark. This leads to rapid transcription of ZEB1 and de-differentiation of the myoepithelial cells into stem-like cells in culture [12].

The following section will summarise the current literature surrounding the effector proteins mediating the epigenetic changes to the histone code.

Polycomb group proteins maintain stem/progenitor cells

Polycomb group (PcG) proteins are epigenetic repressors that participate in the establishment and maintenance of cell identity. PcG proteins bind and repress genes that drive differentiation in embryonic and somatic stem cells. Differentiation is accompanied by loss of PcG binding and increased activation of PcG target genes [45]. In mammals there are two PcG chromatin-modifying complexes, Polycomb repressive complexes 1 and 2 (PRC1 and PRC2). These complexes work in a co-ordinated fashion to mediate repression [45]. The PRC2 complex is comprised of SUZ12, EED, RBBP4 or RBBP7, and EZH2 or EZH1 (Table 1). Initial recruitment of PRC2 to the chromatin depends on the DNA methylation state, pre-existing histone modifications, and recruitment by sequence-specific transcription factors [46]. EZH2 catalyses trimethylation of H3K27, which leads PRC1 recruitment. PRC1 is comprised of one member from each of the following paralog groups: PCGF, CBX, PHC, SCML, and RING [47] (Table 1). PRC1 ubiquitinates H2AK119, which represses transcription by condensing the chromatin and pausing RNA polymerase II [48].

PcG proteins are important for mammary gland development. As discussed above, H3K27 methylation is associated with gene expression changes that accompany mammary lineage commitment. EZH2, the catalytic subunit of PRC2, has been implicated in co-ordinating histone methylation changes during differentiation. Changes in EZH2 activity are regulated by progesterone during pregnancy and are mirrored by changes in global H3K27Me3 levels, coupling hormonal cues to changes in the epigenetic landscape [39]. Over-expression of EZH2 leads to multi-layered ducts and luminal cell hyperplasia, suggesting that EZH2 drives luminal expansion [49]. Conversely, EZH2 knock-out mice have delayed ductal elongation, and cells derived from these mice have a lower re-populating capacity in vivo and lower clonogenic activity in vitro. Doxycycline-inducible knock-out of EZH2 depletes the luminal progenitor pool, strengthening the role for EZH2 in maintaining luminal progenitors [50]. EZH2 supresses cell cycle inhibitors (e.g. *Ink4a* and *Cdkn1a*) and genes involved in epidermal differentiation, suggesting that EZH2 plays a critical role in progenitor cell proliferation and preventing activation of extraneous differentiation programmes [39]. Paradoxically, loss of EZH2 in the mammary epithelium did not alter H3K27Me3 ChIP-Seq profiles. However, because this was conducted on unsorted mammary tissue it is possible that stromal cells with intact EZH2 expression masked the true epigenetic modifications in the mammary epithelial cells. Another possibility is that EZH1, a weaker histone methyltransferase, compensates for EZH2 [51]. EZH2-deficient mice produce milk yet cannot support their pups. This is likely due to a combination of impaired progenitor proliferation leading to reduced alveolar unit density and impaired alveolar differentiation [39, 50].

BMI1, a member of the PCGF paralog group of the PRC1 complex, has also been implicated in mammary gland development. Like EZH2 knock-out mice, BMI1 knock-out mice have severely stunted ductal trees during pubertal development. Mammary epithelial cells from these mice have a 14-fold reduction in re-populating capacity upon serial transplantation, demonstrating the role of BMI1 in MaSC self-renewal [52]. BMI1 is also important for human MaSC self-renewal, where over-expression and knock-down of BMI1 increases and decreases mammosphere-forming capacity, respectively [53]. BMI1 also restricts alveolar differentiation; over-expression of BMI1 blocks alveolar differentiation and loss of BMI1 causes premature alveolar development [52]. The opposing roles of PcG proteins EZH2 and BMI1 in promoting and restricting alveolar differentiation, respectively, is an unexpected result that warrants further investigation.

Lysine demethylases JARID1B, JMJ2B, and KDM6A drive luminal fate commitment

While histone methylation is well studied, enzymes that remove these marks, histone demethylases (known as KDMs), have only been identified more recently. Before their discovery, it was thought that histone methylation was an irreversible modification. It is now evident that histone demethylases play pivotal roles in modifying histones to determine whether a cell maintains multipotency or differentiates. As well as modifying the histone tails directly, certain family members can recruit PcG proteins to further modify chromatin [45]. There are six families of histone demethylase proteins, KDM1–6, each with multiple members that have distinct substrate specificity [54]. Members of the KDM2–6 families contain a Jumonji (or JmjC) domain, which uses a demethylation mechanism distinct from KDM1. So far, three JmjC domain-containing proteins have been identified as important regulators of mammary gland development: JARID1B (KDM5B, PLU-1), JMJ2B (KDM4B), and KDM6A (UTX) (Table 1).

JARID1B removes tri- and di-methylation of H3K4 and is thought to repress transcription [55, 56]. Complete and functional JARID1B knock-out mice have defects in pubertal mammary gland development, including a reduced number of TEBs, less side branching, and impaired ductal elongation [57, 58]. JARID1B mRNA is expressed in both murine basal and luminal lineages (Holliday et al., unpublished data) and seems to be important for rapid epithelial cell proliferation during puberty but not in alveolar development during pregnancy since JARID1B knock-out mice are able to produce milk [58]. The mammary developmental defects in these mice are partially due to a deficiency in systemic oestrogen levels; however, JARID1B also has a mammary cell-intrinsic function [58]. Gene expression analysis on primary mammary epithelial cells and cell lines with perturbed JARID1B expression revealed that JARID1B promotes luminal lineage-specific gene expression and represses basal-specific genes [56, 58, 59]. Key luminal lineage commitment genes (*Elf5*, *Esr1*, *Pgr*, *Prlr*, and *Stat5a*) are downregulated in the JARID1B-deficient mammary epithelial cells and breast cancer cell lines [58, 59]. In some but not all cases, increased gene expression was a consequence of JARID1B binding directly to chromatin, overlapping with active H3K4Me2/3 modifications. This is counter-intuitive given its histone demethylase activity on H3K4. It has been suggested that the PHD domain of JARID1B mediates recognition and binding to H3K4Me3 marks, leading to fine-tuning of H3K4 methylation [59, 60]. Zou et al. [58] observed co-binding of JARID1B and the luminal transcription factor GATA3 at the *Foxa1* and *Stat5a* promoters and loss of GATA3 binding in JARID1B knock-out mammary epithelial cells, arguing that JARID1B and GATA3 can act co-operatively to mediate transcription. JARID1B has also been shown to interact with oestrogen receptor (ER)α in the COS-7 cell line [57]. However, this has not been validated in mammary epithelial cells.

Trimethylation of H3K9 and H3K27 is associated with an inactive chromatin state. JMJD3B and KDM6A demethylate H3K9 and H3K27, respectively, and are therefore transcriptional activators [54]. Knock-out of either of these proteins results in defects in pubertal mammary gland development [61, 62]. JMJD2B interacts with ERα and oestrogen stimulation causes JMJD2B and ERα to localise to chromatin and demethylate H3K9 at ERα target genes [61]. KDM6A knock-out luminal mammary epithelial cells have a gene expression signature more similar to wild-type basal cells than wild-type luminal cells [62]. Like JMJD2B, KDM6A may also be a co-factor for luminal transcription factors since ChIP-Seq analysis on whole mammary glands reveals that KDM6A could bind to promoters and enhancers of ERα, progesterone receptor (PR), and ELF5 target genes [62]. Paradoxically, H3K27Me3 marks were unchanged upon KDM6A knock-out, suggesting that KDM6A has histone demethylase-independent functions, or that KDM6B can compensate for KDM6A loss [62].

Pygo2 maintains mammary stem cells

The chromatin binding protein Pygo2 is part of the Pygopus family of proteins, which contain a highly conserved PHD domain. Pygo2 is an essential component of the Wnt/β-catenin signalling pathway [63], fundamental for maintaining stem cell self-renewal in many tissues including the mammary gland [8]. Unlike the PcG and the KDM proteins, Pygo2 does not directly modify chromatin; instead it recognises and binds active H3K4Me3 modifications via its PHD domain. Basal-specific deletion of Pygo2 results in a two-fold reduction of the basal population, decreased the re-populating capacity, and a basal cell gene expression profile which more closely resembles a luminal signature than a MaSC/basal signature [64, 65]. Components of the Notch signalling pathway, a key driver of luminal cell differentiation [66], are upregulated in Pygo2-deficient basal cells suggesting that Pygo2 normally acts to repress Notch signalling. Pygo2 is required for recruiting β-catenin to the Notch3 locus and maintaining the Notch3 gene in a bivalent state, such that loss of Pygo2 permits Notch-mediated luminal differentiation [65]. Taken together, these studies highlight the role of Pygo2 as a Wnt/β-catenin co-factor that maintains the basal fate by suppression of Notch signalling.

Relevance to breast cancer

There is increasing evidence that different breast cancer subtypes arise from distinct developmental stages along the differentiation hierarchy and retain characteristics of their cell of origin [67]. The epigenetic processes that determine cell fate in normal cells are often hijacked by cancer cells [20, 68]. A comprehensive review of epigenetic perturbation in breast cancer is beyond the scope of this review, although several key examples of developmental epigenetic mechanisms gone awry in breast cancer are discussed below.

The genomes of cancer cells are globally hypomethylated compared with normal cells, resulting in genomic instability [69]. Cancer cells also harbour selective hypermethylation of promoter CpG islands in tumour suppressor genes [69, 70]. Consistent with the role of DNMT1 in maintaining MaSCs, it is also required for cancer stem cell (CSC) maintenance in the MMTV-Neu-Tg mouse mammary tumour model of HER2+ breast cancer [33, 71]. DNMT1 is highly expressed in breast CSCs where it methylates and silences several tumour suppressor genes including Isl1, whose gene product inhibits ERα-mediated transcription [33]. Treatment of mice with the clinical DNMT inhibitor 5-AzaC reduces the CSC pool and significantly improves survival,

especially when combined with a histone deacetylase (HDAC) inhibitor [71].

In addition to DNA methylation, cancer cells also display perturbation of histone modifiers [20]. For example, in non-malignant cells, the core PRC2 component, EZH2, is required for the proliferation of progenitor cells [39, 51]. EZH2 is over-expressed in high-grade basal-like breast cancer where it likely plays a similar role [72]. Similarly, the PRC1 protein BMI1, whose role is to sustain self-renewal of normal mammary stem cells [52, 53], also has proto-oncogenic functions in breast cancer. BMI1 is over-expressed in aggressive basal-like breast cancers where it promotes EMT and self-renewal and is thought to confer drug resistance [73, 74]. JARID1B normally promotes luminal differentiation [58] and is frequently amplified and over-expressed in luminal breast cancer [59]. In this context, JARID1B is a highly active luminal lineage-specific proto-oncogene that correlates with poor patient outcome [59]. These examples highlight the need to understand the context-dependent regulation of these epigenetic factors in normal development.

Unlike genetic aberrations, epigenetic modifications are reversible, making epigenetic therapy an attractive avenue for treatment. Bromodomain and extra-terminal (BET) domain inhibitors are currently under clinical trial for the treatment of various cancers [75]. These drugs target proteins with a bromodomain, which recognises acetylated histone marks. Bromodomain-containing protein 4 (BRD4) co-operates with FOXO1 to promote the expression of basal genes in MCF10A normal mammary epithelial cells [76]. BET domain inhibitors are generally more efficacious in triple-negative breast cancer (TNBC) cell lines compared with luminal and HER2+ breast cancer cell lines [77]. Interestingly, these drugs seem to push the TNBC cells to a more differentiated luminal state [77].

Breast tumours are not only made up of epithelial cells, but also contain a heterogeneous microenvironment encompassing multiple different cell types including cancer-associated fibroblasts, dendritic cells, macrophages, and lymphocytes [78]. Epigenetic drugs do not only target the epithelial cells intrinsically but can also target the cross-talk between the epithelial cells and stromal cells. It has recently been shown that epigenetic therapies can sensitise cancer cells to the host immune system and boost the effects of immunotherapies such as check-point inhibitors (reviewed in [79]). This is particularly relevant to breast cancer, where treatment with check-point inhibitors has been shown to have limited efficacy compared with other cancer types [80].

Studying the context-dependent role of epigenetic modifiers in development has shaped our understanding of their role in different breast cancer subtypes. This research has uncovered exciting potential novel therapeutic targets and this list is continuing to grow.

Conclusions

In response to microenvironmental cues, multiple layers of epigenetic regulation work in concert to maintain the undifferentiated MaSC state, or to direct the differentiation into specialised myoepithelial, luminal, and alveolar cells (Fig. 1). This review has focused on DNA methylation and the histone code but did not include nucleosome positioning and the three-dimensional organisation of chromatin within the nucleus. Systematic studies of genome-wide chromatin remodelling through mammary gland development and cell fate decisions are lacking and present an exciting area for further investigation.

Perturbation of epigenetic mechanisms can lead to the onset of different subtypes of cancer in a highly lineage-specific manner. A rigorous understanding of the epigenetic processes governing normal mammary development is central to our understanding of breast cancer aetiology and also for employing epigenetic therapies, which are becoming more commonly used in cancer treatment.

There is an increasing appreciation that differentiation occurs as a continuous spectrum, rather than proceeding through stable populations of cells with discrete identities [81]. This presents a challenge when studying bulk cell populations, as do the majority of studies described in this review. Technical advancement in this space has made it possible to perform single-cell ChIP-Seq, RNA-Seq, and the newly developed ATAC-Seq to decipher regions of open and closed chromatin [82]. Future studies will employ these cutting-edge technologies to generate chromatin maps and gene expression profiles to better understand the epigenomic and transcriptomic events that accompany lineage commitment at cellular resolution.

Abbreviations

5-AzaC: 5-Azacitidine; ATAC: Assay for transposase-accessible chromatin; BET: Bromodomain and extra-terminal; ChIP: Chromatin immunoprecipitation; CSC: Cancer stem cell; DNMT: DNA methyltransferase; EMT: Epithelial-mesenchymal transition; ER: Oestrogen receptor; ES: Embryonic stem; HDAC: Histone deacetylase; KDM: Lysine demethylase; MaSC: Mammary stem cell; PcG: Polycomb group; PR: Progesterone receptor; PRC: Polycomb repressive complex; TEB: Terminal end bud; Tet: Ten-eleven translocation; TNBC: Triple-negative breast cancer

Acknowledgements

The author would like to thank Dr. Kate Patterson for illustrating the template for Fig. 2.

Funding

This work was supported by funding from the NHMRC in the form of Australian Postgraduate Awards (to HH and LAB) and a Project Grant (to AS). The McMurtrie Family and the estate of the late R.T. Hall also provided support for this work.

Authors' contributions

HH conducted the literature search and wrote the draft of this manuscript. LAB, SRJ, and SJC edited the manuscript and contributed to particular sections. AS supervised and edited the manuscript, and contributed to multiple critical revisions. All authors read and approved the final manuscript.

Competing interests

The authors declare that they have no competing interests.

Author details

[1]The Kinghorn Cancer Centre, Cancer Research Division, Garvan Institute of Medical Research, Darlinghurst, NSW 2010, Australia. [2]St Vincent's Clinical School, Faculty of Medicine, UNSW, Darlinghurst, NSW 2010, Australia. [3]Epigenetics Research Program, Genomics and Epigenetics Division, Garvan Institute of Medical Research, Darlinghurst, NSW 2010, Australia.

References

1. Visvader JE, Stingl J. Mammary stem cells and the differentiation hierarchy: current status and perspectives. Genes Dev. 2014;28:1143–58.
2. Macias H, Hinck L. Mammary gland development. Wiley Interdiscip Rev Dev Biol. 2012;1:533–57.
3. Stingl J, Eirew P, Ricketson I, Shackleton M, Vaillant F, Choi D, Li HI, Eaves CJ. Purification and unique properties of mammary epithelial stem cells. Nature. 2006;439:993–7.
4. Shackleton M, Vaillant F, Simpson KJ, Stingl J, Smyth GK, Asselin-Labat ML, Wu L, Lindeman GJ, Visvader JE. Generation of a functional mammary gland from a single stem cell. Nature. 2006;439:84–8.
5. Wang D, Cai C, Dong X, Yu QC, Zhang XO, Yang L, Zeng YA. Identification of multipotent mammary stem cells by protein C receptor expression. Nature. 2015;517:81–4.
6. Rios AC, Fu NY, Lindeman GJ, Visvader JE. In situ identification of bipotent stem cells in the mammary gland. Nature. 2014;506:322–7.
7. Van Keymeulen A, Rocha AS, Ousset M, Beck B, Bouvencourt G, Rock J, Sharma N, Dekoninck S, Blanpain C. Distinct stem cells contribute to mammary gland development and maintenance. Nature. 2011;479:189–93.
8. van Amerongen R, Bowman AN, Nusse R. Developmental stage and time dictate the fate of Wnt/beta-catenin-responsive stem cells in the mammary gland. Cell Stem Cell. 2012;11:387–400.
9. Prater MD, Petit V, Alasdair Russell I, Giraddi RR, Shehata M, Menon S, Schulte R, Kalajzic I, Rath N, Olson MF, et al. Mammary stem cells have myoepithelial cell properties. Nat Cell Biol. 2014;16:942–50. 941-947
10. Wuidart A, Ousset M, Rulands S, Simons BD, Van Keymeulen A, Blanpain C. Quantitative lineage tracing strategies to resolve multipotency in tissue-specific stem cells. Genes Dev. 2016;30:1261–77.
11. Galliot B, Ghila L. Cell plasticity in homeostasis and regeneration. Mol Reprod Dev. 2010;77:837–55.
12. Chaffer CL, Marjanovic ND, Lee T, Bell G, Kleer CG, Reinhardt F, D'Alessio AC, Young RA, Weinberg RA. Poised chromatin at the ZEB1 promoter enables breast cancer cell plasticity and enhances tumorigenicity. Cell. 2013;154:61–74.
13. Holliday R, Pugh JE. DNA modification mechanisms and gene activity during development. Science. 1975;187:226–32.
14. Smith ZD, Meissner A. DNA methylation: roles in mammalian development. Nat Rev Genet. 2013;14:204–20.
15. Luger K, Mader AW, Richmond RK, Sargent DF, Richmond TJ. Crystal structure of the nucleosome core particle at 2.8 A resolution. Nature. 1997;389:251–60.
16. Bannister AJ, Kouzarides T. Regulation of chromatin by histone modifications. Cell Res. 2011;21:381–95.
17. Skulte KA, Phan L, Clark SJ, Taberlay PC. Chromatin remodeler mutations in human cancers: epigenetic implications. Epigenomics. 2014;6:397–414.
18. Liang G, Zhang Y. Embryonic stem cell and induced pluripotent stem cell: an epigenetic perspective. Cell Res. 2013;23:49–69.
19. Sharma S, Gurudutta G. Epigenetic regulation of hematopoietic stem cells. Int J Stem Cells. 2016;9:36–43.
20. Sharma S, Kelly TK, Jones PA. Epigenetics in cancer. Carcinogenesis. 2010;31: 27–36.
21. Bestor TH. The DNA methyltransferases of mammals. Hum Mol Genet. 2000; 9:2395–402.

22. Laurent L, Wong E, Li G, Huynh T, Tsirigos A, Ong CT, Low HM, Kin Sung KW, Rigoutsos I, Loring J, et al. Dynamic changes in the human methylome during differentiation. Genome Res. 2010;20:320–31.

23. Huang K, Fan G. DNA methylation in cell differentiation and reprogramming: an emerging systematic view. Regen Med. 2010;5:531–44.

24. Bogdanovic O. Tet proteins: master regulators of vertebrate body plan formation? Epigenomics. 2017;9:93–6.

25. Huh SJ, Clement K, Jee D, Merlini A, Choudhury S, Maruyama R, Yoo R, Chytil A, Boyle P, Ran FA, et al. Age- and pregnancy-associated DNA methylation changes in mammary epithelial cells. Stem Cell Rep. 2015;4:297–311.

26. Dos Santos CO, Dolzhenko E, Hodges E, Smith AD, Hannon GJ. An epigenetic memory of pregnancy in the mouse mammary gland. Cell Rep. 2015;11:1102–9.

27. Bloushtain-Qimron N, Yao J, Snyder EL, Shipitsin M, Campbell LL, Mani SA, Hu M, Chen H, Ustyansky V, Antosiewicz JE, et al. Cell type-specific DNA methylation patterns in the human breast. Proc Natl Acad Sci U S A. 2008; 105:14076–81.

28. Maruyama R, Choudhury S, Kowalczyk A, Bessarabova M, Beresford-Smith B, Conway T, Kaspi A, Wu Z, Nikolskaya T, Merino VF, et al. Epigenetic regulation of cell type-specific expression patterns in the human mammary epithelium. PLoS Genet. 2011;7:e1001369.

29. Gascard P, Bilenky M, Sigaroudinia M, Zhao J, Li L, Carles A, Delaney A, Tam A, Kamoh B, Cho S, et al. Epigenetic and transcriptional determinants of the human breast. Nat Commun. 2015;6:6351.

30. Lee HJ, Hinshelwood RA, Bouras T, Gallego-Ortega D, Valdes-Mora F, Blazek K, Visvader JE, Clark SJ, Ormandy CJ. Lineage specific methylation of the Elf5 promoter in mammary epithelial cells. Stem Cells. 2011;29:1611–9.

31. Berdasco M, Esteller M. DNA methylation in stem cell renewal and multipotency. Stem Cell Res Ther. 2011;2:42.

32. Britt K, Ashworth A, Smalley M. Pregnancy and the risk of breast cancer. Endocr Relat Cancer. 2007;14:907–33.

33. Pathania R, Ramachandran S, Elangovan S, Padia R, Yang P, Cinghu S, Veeranan-Karmegam R, Arjunan P, Gnana-Prakasam JP, Sadanand F, et al. DNMT1 is essential for mammary and cancer stem cell maintenance and tumorigenesis. Nat Commun. 2015;6:6910.

34. Hebbes TR, Thorne AW, Crane-Robinson C. A direct link between core histone acetylation and transcriptionally active chromatin. EMBO J. 1988;7:1395–402.

35. Liang G, Lin JC, Wei V, Yoo C, Cheng JC, Nguyen CT, Weisenberger DJ, Egger G, Takai D, Gonzales FA, et al. Distinct localization of histone H3 acetylation and H3-K4 methylation to the transcription start sites in the human genome. Proc Natl Acad Sci U S A. 2004;101:7357–62.

36. Black JC, Van Rechem C, Whetstine JR. Histone lysine methylation dynamics: establishment, regulation, and biological impact. Mol Cell. 2012;48:491–507.

37. Bernstein BE, Mikkelsen TS, Xie X, Kamal M, Huebert DJ, Cuff J, Fry B, Meissner A, Wernig M, Plath K, et al. A bivalent chromatin structure marks key developmental genes in embryonic stem cells. Cell. 2006;125:315–26.

38. Calo E, Wysocka J. Modification of enhancer chromatin: what, how, and why? Mol Cell. 2013;49:825–37.

39. Pal B, Bouras T, Shi W, Vaillant F, Sheridan JM, Fu N, Breslin K, Jiang K, Ritchie ME, Young M, et al. Global changes in the mammary epigenome are induced by hormonal cues and coordinated by Ezh2. Cell Rep. 2013;3:411–26.

40. Pellacani D, Bilenky M, Kannan N, Heravi-Moussavi A, Knapp DJ, Gakkhar S, Moksa M, Carles A, Moore R, Mungall AJ, et al. Analysis of normal human mammary epigenomes reveals cell-specific active enhancer states and associated transcription factor networks. Cell Rep. 2016;17:2060–74.

41. Locke WJ, Zotenko E, Stirzaker C, Robinson MD, Hinshelwood RA, Stone A, Reddel RR, Huschtscha LI, Clark SJ. Coordinated epigenetic remodelling of transcriptional networks occurs during early breast carcinogenesis. Clin Epigenetics. 2015;7:52.

42. Lim E, Wu D, Pal B, Bouras T, Asselin-Labat ML, Vaillant F, Yagita H, Lindeman GJ, Smyth GK, Visvader JE. Transcriptome analyses of mouse and human mammary cell subpopulations reveal multiple conserved genes and pathways. Breast Cancer Res. 2010;12:R21.

43. Lim E, Vaillant F, Wu D, Forrest NC, Pal B, Hart AH, Asselin-Labat ML, Gyorki DE, Ward T, Partanen A, et al. Aberrant luminal progenitors as the candidate target population for basal tumor development in BRCA1 mutation carriers. Nat Med. 2009;15:907–13.

44. Fu NY, Rios AC, Pal B, Law CW, Jamieson P, Liu R, Vaillant F, Jackling F, Liu KH, Smyth GK, et al. Identification of quiescent and spatially restricted mammary stem cells that are hormone responsive. Nat Cell Biol. 2017;19: 164–76.

45. Sauvageau M, Sauvageau G. Polycomb group proteins: multi-faceted regulators of somatic stem cells and cancer. Cell Stem Cell. 2010;7:299–313.

46. van Kruijsbergen I, Hontelez S, Veenstra GJ. Recruiting polycomb to chromatin. Int J Biochem Cell Biol. 2015;67:177–87.

47. Schwartz YB, Pirrotta V. A new world of Polycombs: unexpected partnerships and emerging functions. Nat Rev Genet. 2013;14:853–64.

48. Zhou W, Zhu P, Wang J, Pascual G, Ohgi KA, Lozach J, Glass CK, Rosenfeld MG. Histone H2A monoubiquitination represses transcription by inhibiting RNA polymerase II transcriptional elongation. Mol Cell. 2008;29:69–80.

49. Li X, Gonzalez ME, Toy K, Filzen T, Merajver SD, Kleer CG. Targeted overexpression of EZH2 in the mammary gland disrupts ductal morphogenesis and causes epithelial hyperplasia. Am J Pathol. 2009;175:1246–54.

50. Michalak EM, Nacerddine K, Pietersen A, Beuger V, Pawlitzky I, Cornelissen-Steijger P, Wientjens E, Tanger E, Seibler J, van Lohuizen M, et al. Polycomb group gene Ezh2 regulates mammary gland morphogenesis and maintains the luminal progenitor pool. Stem Cells. 2013;31:1910–20.

51. Yoo KH, Oh S, Kang K, Hensel T, Robinson GW, Hennighausen L. Loss of EZH2 results in precocious mammary gland development and activation of STAT5-dependent genes. Nucleic Acids Res. 2015;43:8774–89.

52. Pietersen AM, Evers B, Prasad AA, Tanger E, Cornelissen-Steijger P, Jonkers J, van Lohuizen M. Bmi1 regulates stem cells and proliferation and differentiation of committed cells in mammary epithelium. Curr Biol. 2008;18:1094–9.

53. Liu S, Dontu G, Mantle ID, Patel S, Ahn NS, Jackson KW, Suri P, Wicha MS. Hedgehog signaling and Bmi-1 regulate self-renewal of normal and malignant human mammary stem cells. Cancer Res. 2006;66:6063–71.

54. Nottke A, Colaiacovo MP, Shi Y. Developmental roles of the histone lysine demethylases. Development. 2009;136:879–89.

55. Yamane K, Tateishi K, Klose RJ, Fang J, Fabrizio LA, Erdjument-Bromage H, Taylor-Papadimitriou J, Tempst P, Zhang Y. PLU-1 is an H3K4 demethylase involved in transcriptional repression and breast cancer cell proliferation. Mol Cell. 2007;25:801–12.

56. Scibetta AG, Santangelo S, Coleman J, Hall D, Chaplin T, Copier J, Catchpole S, Burchell J, Taylor-Papadimitriou J. Functional analysis of the transcription repressor PLU-1/JARID1B. Mol Cell Biol. 2007;27:7220–35.

57. Catchpole S, Spencer-Dene B, Hall D, Santangelo S, Rosewell I, Guenatri M, Beatson R, Scibetta AG, Burchell JM, Taylor-Papadimitriou J. PLU-1/JARID1B/KDM5B is required for embryonic survival and contributes to cell proliferation in the mammary gland and in ER+ breast cancer cells. Int J Oncol. 2011;38:1267–77.

58. Zou MR, Cao J, Liu Z, Huh SJ, Polyak K, Yan Q. Histone demethylase jumonji AT-rich interactive domain 1B (JARID1B) controls mammary gland development by regulating key developmental and lineage specification genes. J Biol Chem. 2014;289:17620–33.

59. Yamamoto S, Wu Z, Russnes HG, Takagi S, Peluffo G, Vaske C, Zhao X, Moen Vollan HK, Maruyama R, Ekram MB, et al. JARID1B is a luminal lineage-driving oncogene in breast cancer. Cancer Cell. 2014;25:762–77.

60. Klein BJ, Piao L, Xi Y, Rincon-Arano H, Rothbart SB, Peng D, Wen H, Larson C, Zhang X, Zheng X, et al. The histone-H3K4-specific demethylase KDM5B binds to its substrate and product through distinct PHD fingers. Cell Rep. 2014;6:325–35.

61. Kawazu M, Saso K, Tong KI, Mizuno T, Goto K, Son DO, Wakeham A, Miyagishi M, Mak TW, Okada H. Histone demethylase JMJD2B functions as a co-factor of estrogen receptor in breast cancer proliferation and mammary gland development. PLoS One. 2011;6:e17830.

62. Yoo KH, Oh S, Kang K, Wang C, Robinson GW, Ge K, Hennighausen L. Histone demethylase KDM6A controls the mammary luminal lineage through enzyme-independent mechanisms. Mol Cell Biol. 2016;36:2108–20.

63. Belenkaya TY, Han C, Standley HJ, Lin X, Houston DW, Heasman J, Lin X. Pygopus encodes a nuclear protein essential for wingless/Wnt signaling. Development. 2002;129:4089–101.

64. Gu B, Sun P, Yuan Y, Moraes RC, Li A, Teng A, Agrawal A, Rheaume C, Bilanchone V, Veltmaat JM, et al. Pygo2 expands mammary progenitor cells by facilitating histone H3 K4 methylation. J Cell Biol. 2009;185:811–26.

65. Gu B, Watanabe K, Sun P, Fallahi M, Dai X. Chromatin effector Pygo2 mediates Wnt-notch crosstalk to suppress luminal/alveolar potential of mammary stem and basal cells. Cell Stem Cell. 2013;13:48–61.

66. Bouras T, Pal B, Vaillant F, Harburg G, Asselin-Labat ML, Oakes SR, Lindeman GJ, Visvader JE. Notch signaling regulates mammary stem cell function and luminal cell-fate commitment. Cell Stem Cell. 2008;3:429–41.

67. Visvader JE. Cells of origin in cancer. Nature. 2011;469:314–22.

68. Locke WJ, Clark SJ. Epigenome remodelling in breast cancer: insights from an early in vitro model of carcinogenesis. Breast Cancer Res. 2012;14:215.

69. Robertson KD. DNA methylation and human disease. Nat Rev Genet. 2005;6: 597–610.
70. Jones PA, Issa JP, Baylin S. Targeting the cancer epigenome for therapy. Nat Rev Genet. 2016;17:630–41.
71. Pathania R, Ramachandran S, Mariappan G, Thakur P, Shi H, Choi JH, Manicassamy S, Kolhe R, Prasad PD, Sharma S, et al. Combined inhibition of DNMT and HDAC blocks the tumorigenicity of cancer stem-like cells and attenuates mammary tumor growth. Cancer Res. 2016;76:3224–35.
72. Kleer CG, Cao Q, Varambally S, Shen R, Ota I, Tomlins SA, Ghosh D, Sewalt RG, Otte AP, Hayes DF, et al. EZH2 is a marker of aggressive breast cancer and promotes neoplastic transformation of breast epithelial cells. Proc Natl Acad Sci U S A. 2003;100:11606–11.
73. Guo BH, Feng Y, Zhang R, Xu LH, Li MZ, Kung HF, Song LB, Zeng MS. Bmi-1 promotes invasion and metastasis, and its elevated expression is correlated with an advanced stage of breast cancer. Mol Cancer. 2011;10:10.
74. Paranjape AN, Balaji SA, Mandal T, Krushik EV, Nagaraj P, Mukherjee G, Rangarajan A. Bmi1 regulates self-renewal and epithelial to mesenchymal transition in breast cancer cells through Nanog. BMC Cancer. 2014;14:785.
75. Noguchi-Yachide T. BET bromodomain as a target of epigenetic therapy. Chem Pharm Bull. 2016;64:540–7.
76. Nagarajan S, Bedi U, Budida A, Hamdan FH, Mishra VK, Najafova Z, Xie W, Alawi M, Indenbirken D, Knapp S, et al. BRD4 promotes p63 and GRHL3 expression downstream of FOXO in mammary epithelial cells. Nucleic Acids Res. 2016;45: 3130–45
77. Shu S, Lin CY, He HH, Witwicki RM, Tabassum DP, Roberts JM, Janiszewska M, Huh SJ, Liang Y, Ryan J, et al. Response and resistance to BET bromodomain inhibitors in triple-negative breast cancer. Nature. 2016;529:413–7.
78. Soysal SD, Tzankov A, Muenst SE. Role of the tumor microenvironment in breast cancer. Pathobiology. 2015;82:142–52.
79. Dunn J, Rao S. Epigenetics and immunotherapy: the current state of play. Mol Immunol. 2017;87:227–39.
80. Emens LA. Breast cancer immunotherapy: facts and hopes. Clin Cancer Res. 2018;24:511–20.
81. Bach K, Pensa S, Grzelak M, Hadfield J, Adams DJ, Marioni JC, Khaled WT. Differentiation dynamics of mammary epithelial cells revealed by single-cell RNA sequencing. Nat Commun. 2017;8:2128.
82. Clark SJ, Lee HJ, Smallwood SA, Kelsey G, Reik W. Single-cell epigenomics: powerful new methods for understanding gene regulation and cell identity. Genome Biol. 2016;17:72.

3

NDRG1 regulates neutral lipid metabolism in breast cancer cells

Christopher J. Sevinsky[1], Faiza Khan[1], Leila Kokabee[1], Anza Darehshouri[2], Krishna Rao Maddipati[3] and Douglas S. Conklin[1]* ⓘD

Abstract

Background: Altered lipid metabolism is an emerging hallmark of aggressive breast cancers. The N-myc downstream regulated gene (NDRG1) gene plays a critical role in peripheral nervous system myelination, as inactivating mutations cause severe demyelinating neuropathy. In breast cancer, elevated NDRG1 expression has been linked to clinical outcomes, but its functional role in breast cancer physiology has remained unclear.

Methods: A meta-analysis of NDRG1 expression in multiple large publicly available genomic databases was conducted. Genome-wide expression correlation and Cox proportional hazards and Kaplan-Meier modeling of clinical outcomes associated with elevated expression were assessed. To study NDRG1 function, gene silencing and overexpression phenotypic studies were carried out in a panel of cell lines representing all major breast cancer molecular subtypes. Changes in cell proliferation, morphology, and neutral lipid accumulation due to altered NDRG1 expression were assessed by high throughput, quantitative microscopy. Comprehensive lipidomics mass spectrometry was applied to characterize global changes in lipid species due to NDRG1 silencing. Labeled fatty acids were used to monitor cellular fatty acid uptake and subcellular distribution under nutrient replete and starvation culture conditions.

Results: NDRG1 overexpression correlated with glycolytic and hypoxia-associated gene expression, and was associated with elevated rates of metastasis and patient mortality. Silencing NDRG1 reduced cell proliferation rates, causing lipid metabolism dysfunction including increased fatty acid incorporation into neutral lipids and lipid droplets. Conversely, NDRG1 expression minimized lipid droplet formation under nutrient replete and starvation conditions.

Conclusions: Here we report that NDRG1 contributes to breast cancer aggressiveness by regulating the fate of lipids in cells that exhibit an altered lipid metabolic phenotype. In line with its role in promoting myelination and its association with altered metabolism in cancer, our findings show that NDRG1 is a critical regulator of lipid fate in breast cancer cells. The association between NDRG1 and poor prognosis in breast cancer suggests it should play a more prominent role in patient risk assessment. The function of NDRG1 in breast cancer lipid metabolism may represent a promising therapeutic approach in the future.

Keywords: Marker, Lipogenic, Metabolism, Metabolomics, Aggressiveness

Background

Elevated N-myc downstream regulated gene (NDRG1) messenger RNA (RNA) and protein expression is found in a subset of many solid tumors, including breast cancer. Autosomal recessive NDRG1 null mutations result in Charcot-Marie-Tooth disease type 4D (CMT4D), a severe demyelinating peripheral neuropathy disorder [1]. CMT4D pathology is thought to be caused by dysfunctional lipid metabolism in Schwann cells, the glia of the peripheral nervous system [2]. However, little functional evidence has been advanced in support of this hypothesis. The NDRG proteins possess an inactive α/β hydrolase fold flanked by intrinsically disordered N and C termini [3], which are subject to extensive post-translational modification. NDRG1 is distinguished from other family members by its transcriptional upregulation in response to stress, including hypoxia, and by its distinctive structural features including a C-terminal

* Correspondence: dconklin@albany.edu
[1]Cancer Research Center, Department of Biomedical Sciences, State University of New York, University at Albany, CRC 342, One Discovery Drive, Rensselaer, NY 12144-3456, USA
Full list of author information is available at the end of the article

metal-binding decapeptide triple repeat that is heavily phosphorylated, and a putative phosphopantetheine attachment site in the core α/β hydrolase domain [4]. The lack of an active site has complicated interpretation of studies exploring NDRG1 function, and insights from studies of NDRG1 in a variety of model systems implicate NDRG1 in several unrelated cellular processes [5–8].

NDRG1 as a prognostic factor in breast cancer remains controversial, as it continues to be cited as both a biomarker of negative prognosis and as a metastasis suppressor [9–13]. Although its function is poorly defined, NDRG1 is a direct transcriptional target of hypoxia inducible factor 1α (Hif1α), Hif2α, and X-box binding protein 1 (XBP1) [12, 14, 15]. NDRG1 protein expression has been associated with high uptake of 18-fluorodeoxyglucose and estrogen receptor (ER)-negative breast cancers in vivo [16], but rather than a role in glycolysis, physical interactors and physiological consequences of NDRG1 malfunction suggest a poorly defined role related to lipid biology in cancer [2, 6, 7, 17]. Like most cancers, aggressive breast cancer subtypes [18] are dependent on elevated glycolytic metabolism [19, 20]. A consequence of the well-characterized dependence on glycolysis of breast cancer cells, de novo lipogenesis is increasingly recognized as a central feature of this metabolism [21–23]. Here, we show that NDRG1 is expressed in a Warburg-like metabolic gene expression program common to many solid tumors, including breast cancer. Several lines of evidence show that NDRG1 performs an important pro-survival function in regulating the fate of lipids in breast cancer cells.

Methods

Tissue culture

Cells were purchased from American Type Culture Collection (ATCC) (Manassas, VA, USA): SKBR3 (HTB-30), MCF7 (HTB-22), HCC1569 (CRL-2330), BT474 (HTB20), MDA-MB-231 (CRM-HTB-26), MDA-MB-468 (HTB-132), HEK293T (CRL-3216). Cells were cultured in DMEM/high glucose with L-glutamine, and sodium pyruvate (Hyclone SH30243.01), supplemented with 10% fetal bovine serum (Sigma), in a standard humidified incubator (5% CO_2), or under hypoxic conditions (1% O_2). All cells cultured under hypoxia conditions were harvested 24 h after exposure to low oxygen. All cell lines were authenticated in March 2016 by the SUNY-Albany Center for Functional Genomics Molecular Core Facility using a short tandem repeat method (Promega GenePrint 10 system).

Gene expression manipulation

For lentivirus production, HEK293T cells were transfected using X-treme gene HP transfection reagent (Roche) with Gag/pol, Rev., VsVG (Invitrogen Virapower), and NDRG1 shRNA pLKO.1 plasmids (Dharmacon/GE Healthcare

TRC short hairpin RNAs (shRNAs): TRCN0000084043, TRCN0000084044, TRCN0000084045, TRCN0000084046, TRCN0000084047), or negative control plasmids: empty vector (RHS4080) and nontargeting eGFP shRNA (RHS684). Virus infection was performed with 8 µg/ml polybrene (Sigma) and cells selected in medium containing 1 µg/ml puromycin (Sigma). For retrovirus production, ΦNX-Ampho cells [24] were transfected with Flag-tagged versions of NDRG1 cloned in the MarxIV vector [25] and empty MarxIV vector was used as a control. Cells were selected with 200 µg/ml hygromycin B and expression confirmed with anti-Flag antibody (SIGMA mouse M2 antibody produced in mouse). The NDRG1 complementary DNA (cDNA) was obtained in pDSRED N2 [6]. A point mutation (L237P) was found in the NDRG1 coding sequence in this construct and corrected using site-directed mutagenesis before generation of other wild-type and mutant expression plasmids.

Fluorescence microscopy

For immunofluorescence, fixed cells were permeabilized in PBS + 0.1% Triton X-100 for 15 min at room temperature. All antibodies were diluted in standard antibody diluent: PBS, 0.1% Tween-20, 5% bovine serum albumin. All primary antibody incubations were carried out overnight at 4 °C, followed by three 5-min washes in 200 µl PBS. Secondary antibodies were diluted to 5 µg/ml, and applied to cells for 1 h at room temperature. Cells were then washed once in 200 µl PBS containing 1 µg/ml Hoechst dye (10 min), followed by two consecutive 5-min washes in 200 µl PBS to eliminate unbound antibody and dye, and remaining PBS was aspirated from wells and replaced with fresh PBS for imaging.

Antibodies included mouse anti-FLAG M2 antibody (SIGMA, cat# F1804), rabbit anti-NDRG1 (Cell Signaling Inc., cat# 9485), rabbit anti-pNDRG1 T346 (Cell Signaling Inc., cat# 5482). Rabbit anti-pNDRG1 S330 (Abcam, cat# ab124713), rabbit anti-glyceraldehyde-3-phosphate dehydrogenase (anti-GAPDH) (Cell Signaling Inc., cat# 5174), rabbit anti-cleaved caspase-3 (Asp175) (Cell Signaling Inc., cat #9579) and rabbit anti-phospho-histone H3 S10 (Cell Signaling Inc., cat #9701). Secondary antibodies were from Jackson Immunoresearch and included donkey anti-rabbit IgG (H + L) Cy3 (cat# 711-166-152) and donkey anti-rabbit IgG (H + L) Alexa 647 (cat# 711-606-152).

Images were acquired at × 20 magnification on an inverted fluorescence microscope (Olympus IX-81) fitted with a Retiga 6000 CCD Camera using Metamorph software or on the InCell Analyzer 2200 high content microscopy platform (GE Healthcare). All images were acquired using the same exposure time to allow quantitative analysis and comparison of staining intensity. For cells imaged using the IN Cell Analyzer 2200 (GE Healthcare), a minimum of four images per well from a minimum of three wells were collected for each condition, and data were summarized at the well-level for statistical comparisons. Exposure times were set to allow quantitative analysis of intensity using statistical tests comparing the brightness of objects (e.g., lipid droplets). Images were analyzed using GE Healthcare In Cell Analyzer software granule and nuclei counting algorithms. For lipid droplet granules, sensitivity was set to the most stringent threshold to reduce nonspecific granule counting. Particle size was set to the range 0.1–2 μm^2. Nuclei were also counted - minimum size 40 μm^2. For the analysis of pNDRG1 puncta dynamics in response to endoplasmic reticulum stress, 5–250 pixel foci with circularity of 0.25–1.0 were segmented using the triangle algorithm, and divided by the total number of nuclei in each image to express puncta per cell.

For live cell imaging, cells transduced with green fluorescent protein (GFP) and NDRG1 targeting virus were plated in 6-well plates, allowed to attach for 24 h, refed, and monitored by phase contrast microscopy for 48 h. Live cell microscopy was conducted using the Invitrogen EVOS FL Auto Cell Imaging System with a pre-warmed, humidified, and 5% CO_2 equilibrated incubation chamber. Images were acquired at 10-min intervals with autofocus on.

Transmission electron microscopy

Hs578T cells expressing three different shNAs targeting NDRG1 and one targeting enhanced (e)GFP were collected at one week post selection. Cells were grown in 10-cm dishes to 80–90% confluence and fixed in 0.1 M cacodylate pH 7.4, 2.5% glutaraldehyde (Electron Microscopy Sciences). Cells were fixed at 37 °C for 15 min, followed by scraping of cells, collection by centrifugation at × 100 g, and resuspension in 10 ml fresh fixation buffer and storage at 4 °C. After three rinses with 0.1 M sodium cacodylate buffer, cell pellets were embedded in 3% agarose and sliced into small blocks (1mm³), rinsed with the same buffer three times and post-fixed with 1% osmium tetroxide and 0.8% potassium ferricyanide in 0.1 M sodium cacodylate buffer for 1.5 h at room temperature. Cells were rinsed with water and stained en bloc with 4% uranyl acetate in 50% ethanol for 2 h. Cells were dehydrated with increasing concentration of ethanol, transitioned into propylene oxide, infiltrated with Embed-812 resin and polymerized in an oven at 60 °C overnight. Blocks were sectioned with a diamond knife (Diatome) on a Leica Ultracut 6 ultramicrotome (Leica Microsystems) and collected onto copper grids, post-stained with 2% aqueous uranyl acetate and lead citrate. Images were acquired on a Tecnai G2 spirit transmission electron microscope (FEI) equipped with a LaB6 source using a voltage of 120 kV.

Lipidomics mass spectrometry

SKBR3 cells transduced with shRNAs targeting NDRG1 or eGFP were grown to 80%–90% confluence and harvested by trypsinization at 14 days post selection (including 7 days in culture without puromycin). As soon as cells lifted, they were immediately suspended in ice cold medium and kept on ice while a small fraction was counted. Cells were then divided into 1 or 2 million cell aliquots (shotgun versus targeted analysis, respectively), rinsed twice in ice cold PBS by low-speed centrifugation at 4 °C and wash was aspirated, and pellets frozen in a dry ice/ethanol bath and stored at – 80 °C until analysis. Silencing levels and lipid droplet quantities were determined in a sample of cells grown in microtiter plates as described above, by anti-NDRG1 immunofluorescence and boron-dipyrromethene (BODIPY) staining, respectively.

Lipid classes were analyzed by the multiple precursor ion scanning (MPIS) method for triacylglycerides, diacylglycerides, phophatidylcholines, phosphatidylethanolamines, phsophatidylserines, phosphatidylglycerols, phosphatidic acids, and phosphatidylinositols following published protocols [26, 27]. Monoacylglycerols, cholesterol esters, sphingomyelins, and ceramides were analyzed by LC-MS methods using multiple reaction monitoring (MRM) methods [28, 29]. To generate a heatmap for visualization of various lipid levels, data were first standardized by normalizing to row means as a fold difference and species not detected in all samples, and extreme outliers were removed (n = 142 species remaining). The online cluster analysis tool CIMiner was used to generate heatmaps using Euclidian distance and colors were represented using quantiles (https://discover.nci.nih.gov/cimminer/home.do).

Targeted LC MS/MS analysis of cholesterol esters was from five biological replicates for each condition, and represented as ng lipid/million cells. Targeted LC MS/MS analysis of triglycerides was from six biological replicates per condition, and represented as micrograms of lipid/micrograms of protein. Individual species were compared using the two-sided Student's t test. Each lipid class (e.g., cholesterol esters, triacylglycerol) was also analyzed as an aggregate of all individual species detected and also compared using the two-sided Student's t test.

mRNA expression analysis

The breast-cancer-specific mRNA expression characteristics were examined for genes coexpresssed or anti-correlated with NDRG1 expression in order to better understand relationships between NDRG1 and markers reflecting intrinsic molecular subtypes. The cBio portal was accessed in order to analyze global gene expression patterns across 18 human solid tumor types [30]. The online tool KM plotter was used to establish query criteria and generate KM plots, hazard ratios, 95% confidence intervals, and p values [31]. Additional cohorts were analyzed by accessing independent patient cohorts with the online tool SurExpress (http://bioinformatica.mty.itesm.mx:8080/Biomatec/SurvivaX.jsp). NDRG1, NDRG1 + MYC, or the 42-member NDRG1-associated gene signature was queried for relationships with adverse outcomes (metastasis-free survival, or recurrence-free survival). The mRNA expression of *NDRG1* in > 1000 cell lines was downloaded from the Broad Institute CCLE portal: https://portals.broadinstitute.org/ccle/home. Breast cancer cell lines were filtered, ranked according to expression level, and plotted to evaluate the range of expression in characterized cell lines. Cell lines chosen for in vitro studies are indicated.

Microarray analysis of SKBR3 cells expressing NDRG1 shRNA1 or vector control were performed with biotin-labeled cDNA from three independent biological replicates hybridized over 16 h to Affymetrix Gene 2.0 ST arrays and scanned on an Affymetrix Scanner 3000 7G using AGCC software. The resulting CEL files were analyzed for quality using Affymetrix Expression Console software and were imported into GeneSpring GX11.5 (Agilent Technologies) where the data were quantile normalized using PLIER and baseline transformed to the median of the control samples. Data sets are available at GEO, Accession number: GSE112841.

Fatty acid conjugated BODIPY tracer experiments

The sixteen carbon BODIPY FL C16 (Invitrogen, cat# D3821) was used to study fatty acid uptake and intracellular distribution in stable shNDRG1 and shGFP expressing SKBR3 cells (cultured as in lipidomics experiments described above). A 2 mM stock solution was prepared in culture medium supplemented with 0.1% fatty acid free bovine serum albumin (Goldbio cat# A-421-100), and diluted in DMEM/high glucose with L-glutamine, and sodium pyruvate + 10% FBS to achieve the desired concentrations. Cells were seeded at 10,000 viable cells per well, allowed them to adhere for 24 h, and medium was replaced with C16-BODIPY at 100 μM, 50 μM, 25 μM and 12.5 μM in complete DMEM and cells were cultured under normal conditions for 16 h in the presence of the tracer. After 16 h, excess tracer was removed by three consecutive washes in complete DMEM, followed by the fixation protocol described above.

To quantify total tracer uptake, an image analysis routine was established to measure the intensity of cell-sized objects above a background threshold. Cell nuclei were counted, and average C-16 BODIPY signal was expressed as the ratio of overall signal divided by the number of nuclei in each field of view. To quantify lipid-droplet-specific signal, the granule counting and measurement algorithm described above was used. The ratio of lipid-droplet-specific C-16 BODIPY signal to total C-16 BODIPY signal was computed to reflect the flow of tracer fatty acid to lipid droplets.

In MCF7 cells, a protocol to induce lipid droplet formation and live cell tracer incorporation through starvation in Hanks buffered saline solution (HBSS) was developed based on published methods [32]. HBSS consists of 0.137 M NaCl, 5.4 mM KCl, 0.25 mM Na2HPO4, 0.63 mM glucose, 0.44 mM KH2PO4, 1.3 mM CaCl2, 1.0 mM MgSO4, and 4.2 mM NaHCO3. Stable MCF7 cell lines transduced with retroviral full length NDRG1–3X FLAG and retroviral empty vector were plated as described above cultured in ether complete medium or HBSS. For live cell experiments, BODIPY 558/568 C12 (C12-BODIPY) was added to initial culture medium at 100 μM to allow cellular uptake, and followed by extended chase periods. Samples were fixed and stained for lipid droplets as described above. To elaborate the time dependence of the phenomenon and rule out tracer specific effects, lipid droplet formation by cells grown without C12-BODIPY tracer were monitored over the course of 4 days by staining with BODIPY 493/503 using analysis methods described above.

Results

NDRG1 is a biomarker of aggressive breast cancers

Previous studies of NDRG1 expression in cancer have been performed on cohorts of limited sizes, and have led to the conclusion that NDRG1 is a metastasis suppressor [9–11, 33]. However, several lines of evidence contradict NDRG1 as a suppressor of metastasis [12, 13]. So that we might resolve questions on the link between NDRG1 expression and disease outcome, we examined large, recently established, public repositories of clinical breast cancer data. A large meta-analysis was conducted examining the association between NDRG1 expression and recurrence-free survival in 23 publicly available breast cancer mRNA expression data sets representing 3554 subjects with breast cancer assessed as a single aggregated cohort [31]. Because *NDRG1* copy number or mRNA expression is altered in approximately 25% of all breast cancers in the The Cancer Genome Atlas (TCGA) data set (Additional file 1: Figure S1), patients in the upper quartile of NDRG1 mRNA expression were compared with patients in the lower three quartiles. Subjects expressing high *NDRG1* exhibit an almost twofold higher risk of disease recurrence 5 years after diagnosis in this aggregate cohort (Fig. 1a). The 23 individual cohorts were also analyzed individually to assess potential bias: 19/23 cohorts show that high *NDRG1* is associated with decreased time to recurrence, 3 show no separation of Kaplan-Meier curves, and a small cohort (*n* = 77 subjects) exhibits an association between high *NDRG1* and positive outcome (Additional file 1: Figure S2).

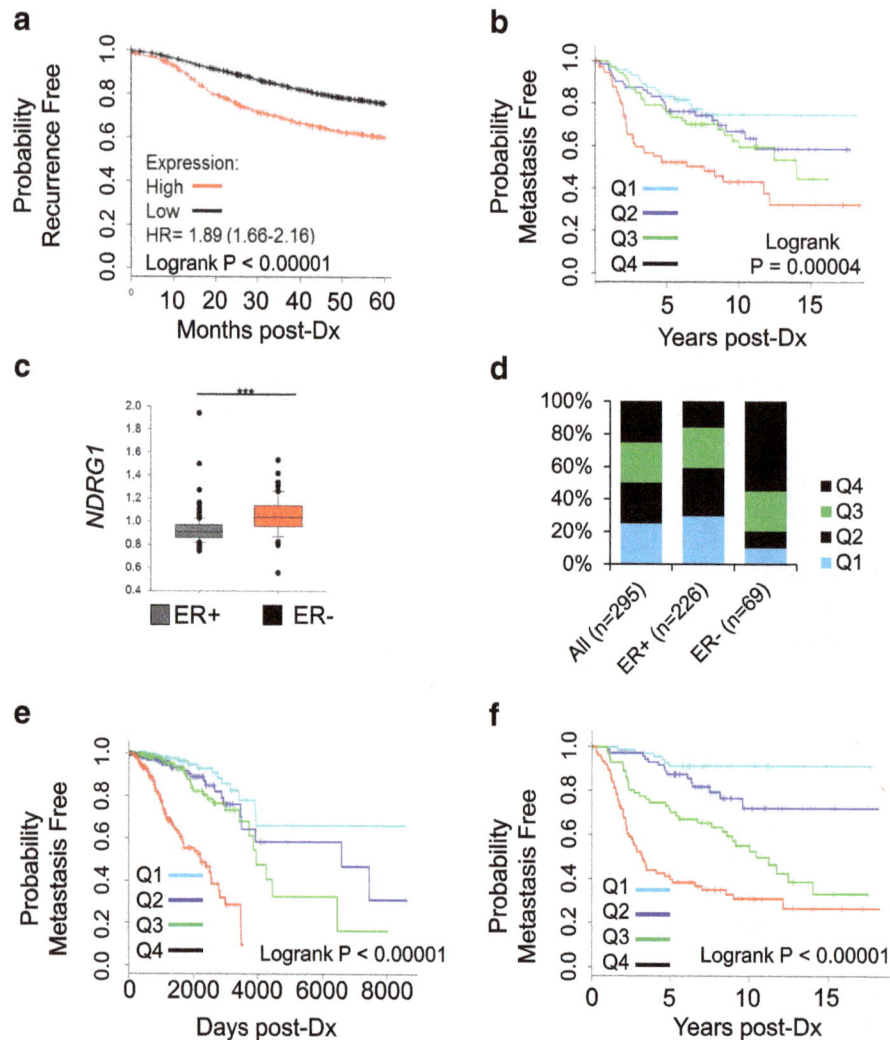

Fig. 1 *NDRG1* expression is associated with adverse outcomes and altered metabolism in breast cancer. **a** Meta-analysis of 23 distinct breast cancer cohorts (*n* = 3554 subjects). Kaplan-Meier curve of recurrence-free survival analysis of *NDRG1* mRNA expression (upper quartile (Q) versus lower three quartiles). Post-DX, Post-diagnosis. **b** Metastasis-free survival of *NDRG1* quartiles in the Van't Veer cohort (*n* = 295). **c** *NDRG1* expression in estrogen receptor (ER)+/− groups of the the Van't Veer cohort. **d** The distribution of total Van't Veer cohort NDRG1 expression quartiles in ER+ and ER- tumors. The unequal distribution further reflects the data in (**c**). **e, f** Metastasis-free survival using the 42-gene signature in The Cancer Genome Atlas breast cancer cohort (*n* = 962), and the Van't Veer breast cancer cohort (n = 295)

An independent cohort of 295 patients in whom metastasis was tracked was examined to evaluate the relationship between metastasis and *NDRG1* expression in more detail [34]. Again, *NDRG1* mRNA expression level stratified patients into poor and favorable prognostic subsets (Fig. 1b). Importantly, elevated NDRG1 expression is a more consistent biomarker of negative prognosis than the genomically co-amplified *MYC* oncogene, ruling out a simple confluence of high *NDRG1* expression with *MYC* amplification as a driver of poor prognosis (Additional file 1: Figure S3A-C). This meta-analysis significantly strengthens the link between elevated *NDRG1* expression and poor prognosis in breast cancer.

NDRG1 is correlated with an aggressive metabolic gene expression profile in breast cancer and other solid tumor types

Genome-wide *NDRG1* coexpression patterns were assessed to investigate links between expression levels and recurrent genetic alterations and previously described intrinsic molecular subtypes were present. Pairwise mRNA expression-level correlation between NDRG1 and all other genes analyzed in the TCGA data set were examined. The estrogen receptor (*ESR1*) is near the top of the list of negatively correlated genes. Other negatively correlated genes include well-established markers of luminal breast cancer: *GATA3*, *FOXA1*, and *PGR* (Additional file 2: Table S1). Positive correlation was common between *NDRG1* and genes associated with angiogenesis, glycolysis, hypoxia, and basal cell lineage, illustrating that high *NDRG1* expression is more common in ER$^-$ breast cancers (Fig. 1c, d, Additional file 2: Table S2). Previous work has shown *NDRG1* expression to be part of an angiogenesis-related gene signature associated with metastasis in breast cancer [12]. These correlations indicate that *NDRG1* expression is strongly associated with breast tumors with high glycolytic and angiogenic gene expression.

The TCGA breast cancer analysis included quantification of the Thr346 phosphorylated form of NDRG1, but not the total protein, by reverse phase protein array [18]. Proteins negatively correlated with phospho-NDRG1 mirrored the results of the mRNA associations (Additional file 2: Table S3), as did an analysis of mRNA levels in *NDRG1* altered and unaltered cases (Additional file 2: Table S4), corroborating a link between NDRG1 and aggressive forms of breast cancer.

Analysis of *NDRG1* mRNA correlation was extended to include 18 solid tumor types analyzed by the TCGA (Data set S1) to reveal common elements of an underlying biological process, illuminating the physiological action of *NDRG1*. In each cancer type, genes with mRNA with a Pearson's product moment correlation coefficient $(R) \geq 0.40$ were identified as NDRG1-associated genes: 41 genes with expression that was correlated with *NDRG1* in at least six individual data sets ($\geq 33\%$) were found to encode nine of ten common glycolysis pathway enzymes, glycolysis regulatory proteins, and downstream regulators of tricarboxylic acid cycle (TCA) cycle entry; regulators of angiogenesis; and several oxidoreductases implicated in oxidative protein folding and signaling under endoplasmic reticulum stress and hypoxic conditions (Additional file 2: Table S5). This pan-cancer correlation with hallmarks of metabolic adaptations underscores the link between NDRG1 and altered cancer metabolism, and the gene list is a potent prognostic signature in breast cancer and several other solid tumors (Fig. 1e, f, and data not shown).

NDRG1 expression is highly variable in breast cancer cell lines and displays distinct subcellular localization

Since the role of NDRG1 in altered cancer metabolism is poorly characterized, in vitro studies of NDRG1 were carried out in a range of breast cancer cell lines to assess its function. Expression of NDRG1 in vivo is dynamic and dependent on microenvironment cues such as hypoxia or iron limitation [12, 14, 15]; nevertheless, in vitro studies represent the most direct approach to examine protein function in cancer cells. *NDRG1* mRNA expression in the 59 breast cell lines characterized by the Cancer Cell Line Encyclopedia (CCLE) was assessed

[35]. Expression levels varied widely, and seven cell lines were selected with a range of *NDRG1* mRNA expression spanning 17-fold (Fig. 2a). The cell lines also represent the full spectrum of major intrinsic molecular subtypes of breast cancer (Additional file 2: Table S6). A wide range of NDRG1 protein expression was also verified. Immunoblots show that HCC1569 expresses the highest level of NDRG1 protein, followed by Hs578T, SKBR3, MDA-MB-231, MDA-MB468, BT474, and MCF7 (Fig. 2b). Similar trends are apparent in immunofluorescence analysis of fixed cells and immunoblots of phosphorylated proteins (Fig. 2c and Additional file 1: Figure S4A). The observed expression profiles are mostly consistent with mRNA levels from the CCLE, and also agree with the preponderance of evidence linking high levels of NDRG1 expression with ER-negative tumors (Fig. 1c, d and Additional file 2: Tables S1–S4).

In addition to total protein levels, we noted differential localization of two phosphorylated forms of NDRG1. The C-terminus of NDRG1 has been shown to be phosphorylated on at least 29 residues [36, 37], but differential phosphorylation states linked with divergent localization or function have not been reported. The total protein, NDRG1 phospho-Thr346 (unique to NDRG1 decapeptide triple repeat), and NDRG1 phospho-Ser330 (conserved in all NDRG proteins) were probed by immunofluorescence microscopy. Immunofluorescence analysis of NDRG1 phospho-Ser330 exhibits an even cellular distribution. NDRG1 phospho-Thr346 in SKBR3 cells showed punctate cytoplasmic patterns consistent with localization to an organelle/endosome/vesicle, suggesting at least partial exclusivity with the Ser330 phosphorylated pool. Remarkably, in addition to upregulation of the total protein, pNDRG1 Ser330 redistributed almost entirely to the nucleus when iron was deprived by chelation with deferoxamine (DFO), which mimics hypoxia, while NDRG1 phospho-Thr346 remained cytoplasmic (Fig. 2d, e and Additional file 1: Figure S4B-D). Because NDRG1 has been implicated in endosomal trafficking, tunicamycin and thapsigargin were used to assess the sensitivity of these structures to inhibition of the endo-lysosomal system [6, 38]. A brief thapsigargin treatment dispersed puncta completely, while tunicamycin had no effect in the acute setting (Fig. 2f). These differences between modified forms of NDRG1 show that distinct pools are sensitive to distinct stimuli, which may explain some of the divergent and apparently unrelated functions attributed to NDRG1 [39].

NDRG1 expression is critical to breast cancer cell proliferation, viability, and morphology

To study NDRG1 function in breast cancer cells, lentiviral shRNAs targeting NDRG1 and corresponding GFP targeting controls were used to study the

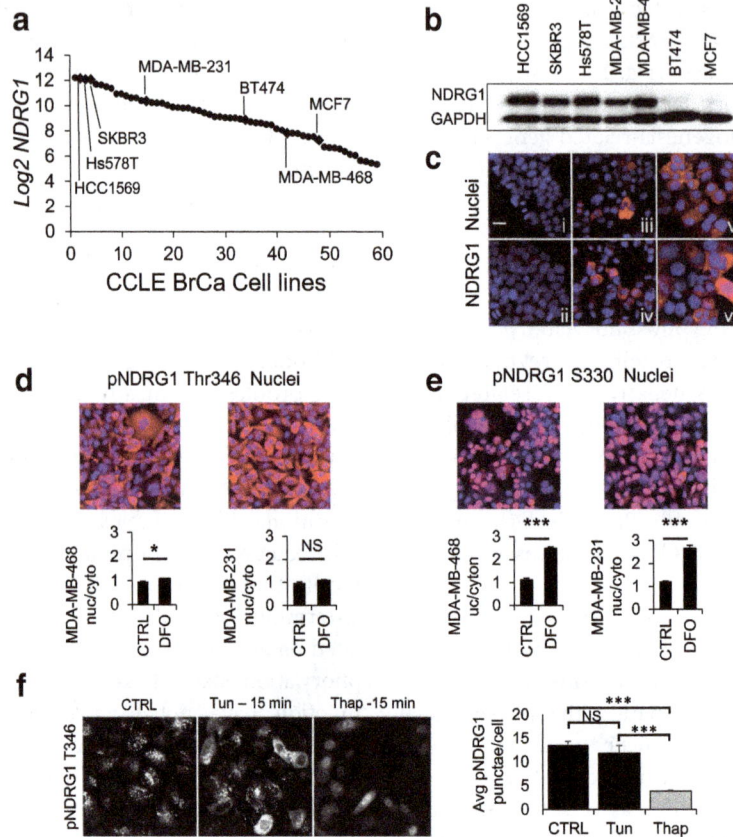

Fig. 2 NDRG1 expression level and localization variability in breast cancer cell lines. **a** Cancer Cell Line Encyclopedia (CCLE)-analyzed breast cancer cell lines ordered by *NDRG1* expression level - cell lines selected for in vitro analysis are indicated. **b** Immunoblots of NDRG1 and GAPDH loading control from crude lysates (10 µg total protein/lane). **c** Immunofluorescence analysis of NDRG1 in breast cancer cell lines, scale = 25 µm: **i** MCF7, **ii** BT474, **iii** MDA-MB-231, **iv** MDA-MB-468, **v** SKBR3, **vi** HCC1569. **d, e** NDRG1 pT346 and pS330 immunofluorescence and localization in MDA-MB-231 and MDA-MB-468 cells treated with 100 µM deferoxamine (DFO): nucleus:cytoplasm ratio is shown: $N = 3$/group. **f** pNDRG1 T346 immunofluorescence localization to puncta in SKBR3 cells: thapsigargin (Thap) (1 µM) but not tunicamycin (Tun) treatment (5 µg/ml) disperses puncta. Data are represented as mean ratio +/− SD. *$p < 0.001$, ***$p < 1 \times 10^{-10}$. CRTL, control; NS, not significant

effect of reducing NDRG1 protein levels by silencing its expression (Fig. 3a and Additional file 1: Figure S4A). Beginning at 5 days post-selection, proliferation rates of NDRG1 silenced and control shRNA cells were monitored by comparing nuclei counts at different time points with initial population sizes. SKBR3, MCF7 and BT474 were monitored at 7 days and HCC1569 at 4 days after plating (Fig. 3b), and a series of SKBR3, MDA-MB-231, and MDA-MB-468 time points were also monitored over 7–9 days (Additional file 1: Figure S4E-G). An NDRG1 silencing-dependent reduction in cell proliferation was observed in each of the six cell lines. The magnitude of reduced proliferation was variable, but roughly followed endogenous expression levels, with the most modest effects observed in MCF7, and the greatest effects seen in SKBR3, HCC1569, and MDA-MB-231.

Markers of apoptosis and mitosis were assayed by immunofluorescence microscopy to determine the mechanism of reduced cell proliferation. Silencing NDRG1 in SKBR3 cells increases the cleaved caspase 3 immunofluorescence positive area fraction by 4.5–7-fold (Fig. 3c). This indicates that NDRG1 contributes to cell survival in SKBR3 cells, but the actual fraction of apoptotic cells is small, and NDRG1-depleted cells continue to proliferate. We also analyzed SKBR3 mitotic cell fractions in fixed cells and monitored cell division rates by live cell microscopy. Live cell microscopy showed that NDRG1 depleted SKBR3 cells exhibit a twofold reduction in cell division rates. In addition, a significant morphology change in NDRG1-depleted SKBR3 cells is observed (Fig. 3d, Additional files 3, 4, 5, 6, 7 and 8: Movies S1–S6). Analysis of the mitotic cell marker Histone H3 phospho-Ser10 showed that NDRG1

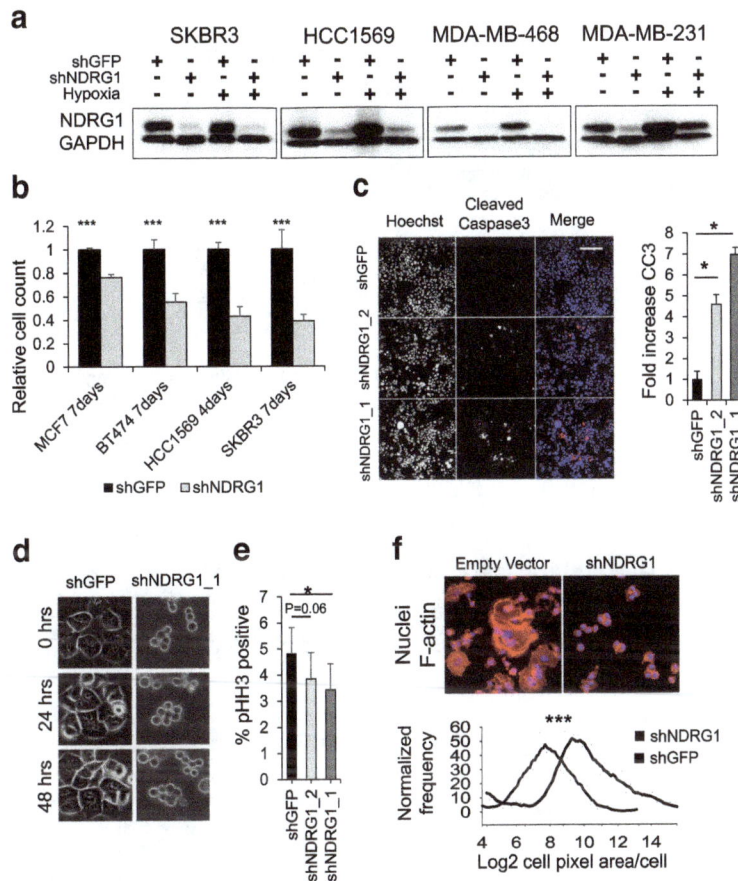

Fig. 3 NDRG1 is required for normal breast cancer cell proliferation, viability and morphology. **a** Immunoblots of NDRG1 and GAPDH loading control after selection of four stable lentiviral transduced shRNA expressing cell lines. A green fluorescent protein (GFP) targeting shRNA serves as negative control, and silencing was verified at 1% O_2. **b** Cell proliferation assays: cell number was compared by comparing NDRG1 silenced cell numbers to control at the times indicated: ***$p < 0.0001$, $N = 3$/group - see Additional file 1: Figure S5. **c** Cleaved caspase 3 (CC3) immunofluorescence analysis of stable shRNA expressing SKBR3 cells at 1 week post selection. CC3 positive area was normalized to total cell area and each population compared: shNDRG1_1 $p = 2.5 \times 10^{-6}$, shNDRG1_2 $p = 1.2 \times 10^{-4}$, scale = 100 μm, $N = 12$/group. **d** Individual frames from a 48 h live cell microscopy analysis of SKBR3 cells expressing the indicated shRNAs: $N = 3$/group, see Additional files 3, 4, 5, 6, 7 and 8: Movies S1–S6. **e** Mitotic cell fractions comparing the percentage of histone H3 phsopho-serine10 positive cells in the indicated shRNA expressing cell lines: shNDRG1_1 $p = 0.02$, shNDRG1_2 $p = 0.06$, $N = 12$/group. **f** Comparison of individual cell two-dimensional area based on phalloidin stain ($p < 0.001$, Mann-Whitney U test, $N = > 650$ cells each group). Log2 two-dimensional area is shown. All bar graphs represent means +/− SD. Comparisons were by two-sided Student's t test unless indicated otherwise

depletion results in a significant reduction in the mitotic cell population size with one shRNA and a trend toward reduction with a second shRNA (Fig. 3e). We also noted that NDRG1-depleted SKBR3 cells appear smaller, and retain a round morphology throughout the cell cycle, while control hairpin-expressing cells undergo repetitive cycles of post-mitosis flattening, followed by rounding upon entry into mitosis (Fig. 3d and Additional files 3, 4, 5, 6, 7 and 8: Movies S1–S6). In fixed F-actin and nuclear counterstained cells, analysis of single cell populations showed that NDRG1 depletion results in approximately twofold reduction in median F-actin area/cell relative to control (Fig. 3f). Thus, NDRG1 expression is essential to the maintenance of cell proliferation rates, viability, and morphology in breast cancer cells, especially in cell lines with high expression levels.

NDRG1 affects lipid metabolism in breast cancer cells

The demyelinating peripheral neuropathy Charcot Marie Tooth disease type 4D (CMT4D) is caused by homozygous null mutations in the NDRG1 gene [1]. Since myelination is a lipid metabolism-intensive and trafficking-intensive process, we investigated the impact of decreased NDRG1 levels on lipid metabolism in SKBR3 cells by shotgun mass spectrometry lipidomics. Quantities of several diverse lipid species including structural, storage, biosynthetic intermediates and signaling molecules are increased due to NDRG1 depletion, whereas very few lipids are reduced due to silencing (Fig. 4a and Additional file 1: Figure S5). Consistent with the lack of a catalytic active site, changes in individual species reveal no obvious links between NDRG1 silencing and the inhibition or acceleration of a single biochemical

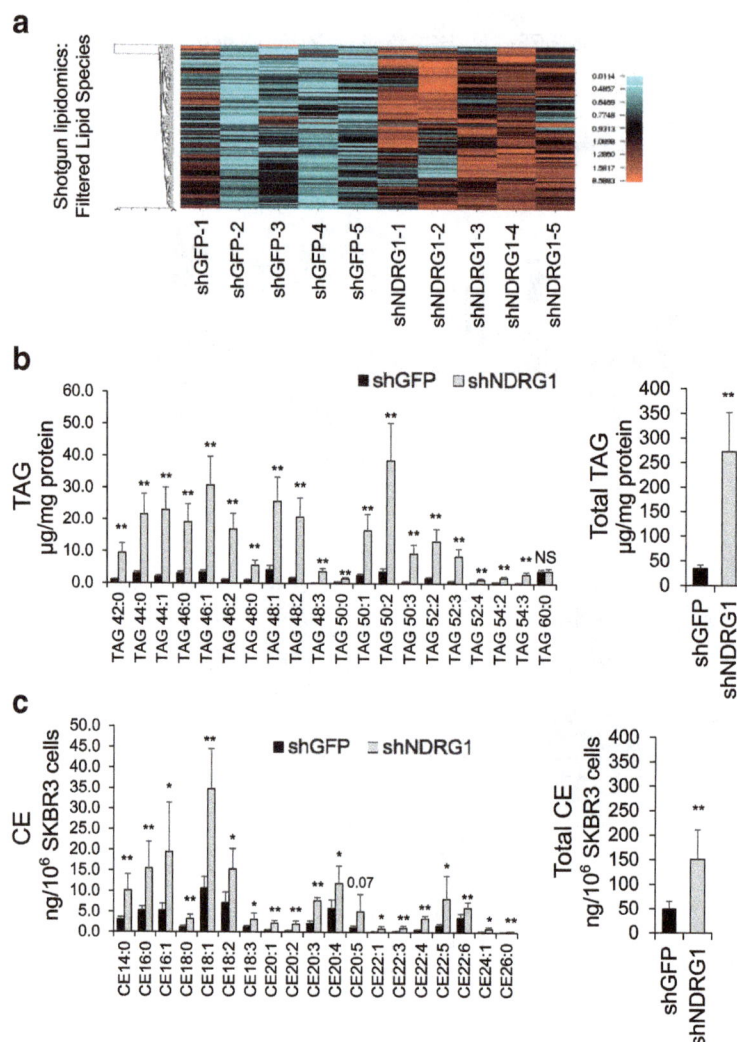

Fig. 4 NDRG1 depletion causes increased levels of major lipid species. **a** Semi-quantitative shotgun LC MS/MS of major lipid species in SKBR3 cells. Heatmap represents fold differences in species detected in all samples standardized relative to row means. Color range 0.01–8-fold relative to row mean, $N = 5$ per group. See Additional file 1: Figure S5 for quantification of an independent analysis (**b**) in micrograms of triacylglycerol/mg protein. Individual species and sums are plotted separately (**c**) in nanograms of cholesterol ester per million cells. Sums of individual species and cholesterol ester (CE) species are plotted separately: $N = 6$ for TAG and $N = 5$ for CE analysis. Data represent mean +/− SD, comparisons were by the two-sided t test: **$p < 0.01$, ***$p < 0.00001$. TAG, triacylglycerols; GFP, green fluorescent protein

reaction. Analysis of changes in aggregate lipid species performed by comparing the sums of each lipid class between cell lines show the largest effects on the two main storage lipids in NDRG1 silenced cells, triacylglycerols (TAG) and cholesterol esters (CE), with smaller but significant increases in other species (Fig. 4a and Additional file 1: Figure S5).

TAGs and CEs were analyzed by quantitative targeted LC MS/MS, extending the depth of species analyzed within each class of lipid. In accordance with the shotgun analysis, overall TAG abundance increased 7.8-fold, and nearly every species showed a significant increase in the NDRG1-depleted cells (Fig. 4b). Aggregate CE levels increased threefold, and each individual species

exhibited increased abundance as well (Fig. 4c). This indicates that NDRG1 regulates neutral lipid storage in SKBR3 cells and that NDRG1-dependent lipid homeostasis in breast cancer cells is important for optimal cell viability.

NDRG1 depletion results in increased lipid droplet formation in breast cancer cells

As neutral lipids are primarily stored in lipid droplets, quantitative high-content microscopy analysis was applied to characterize the relationship between NDRG1 expression and lipid droplet formation in several additional cell lines. Lipid droplets are composed of a neutral lipid core of mainly TAGs and/or CEs surrounded by a protein and phospholipid monolayer [40]. The fluorescent neutral lipid stain BODIPY 493/503 was used together with an automated granule segmentation and quantification image analysis algorithm to characterize neutral lipid foci in NDRG1 silenced cells [41].

Image analysis results from the BODIPY lipid droplet assay consistently showed that NDRG1 depletion causes increases in lipid droplet formation and intensity relative to control shRNA in all cell lines examined. This effect was largest in SKBR3 cells, where NDRG1 depletion caused a 3.3-fold increase in lipid droplet staining intensity (Fig. 5a, b). NDRG1-depleted HCC1569, Hs578T, and BT474 cell lines also exhibited a significant increase in lipid droplet staining intensity, with 1.8, 2.6, and 2.9-fold increases relative to control, respectively (Fig. 5b). Microarray analysis of transcriptional changes in NDRG1-depleted cells did not reveal significant changes in lipid droplet binding or lipid synthetic pathway genes. The top downregulated gene in NDRG1 knockdown cells was Spot14 [42], which plays an incompletely understood regulatory role in stimulating the lipid synthetic process in breast cancer cells [43]. This result is consistent with a feedback inhibitory mechanism in cells that already have a high lipid level.

MCF7 cells normally express low levels of NDRG1 (Fig. 2b), and form few lipid droplets under normal culture conditions. NDRG1 expression is increased in MCF7 cells cultured under hypoxic conditions, which induces lipid droplet formation in other cell lines [44, 45]. While NDRG1 depletion has little effect on lipid droplet quantity in MCF7 cells under normal conditions, lipid droplet formation was stimulated by hypoxia (1% O_2, 24 h) and further enhanced 1.8-fold by NDRG1 depletion, both of which are conditions favoring lipogenesis (Fig. 5b). Two additional shRNAs confirmed that NDRG1 depletion causes lipid droplet formation in Hs578T cells, and electron microscopy affirmed the presence of lipid droplets at the ultrastructural level (Additional file 1: Figure S6C and Fig. 5d). Thus, multiple cell lines respond to NDRG1 depletion by increasing neutral lipid storage, especially under conditions that rely on a lipogenic metabolism.

In addition to silencing NDRG1, we generated stable SKBR3 cell lines overexpressing wild-type and truncation mutants lacking the N or C terminus (ΔN-NDRG1 and ΔC-NDRG1). The N and C termini of NDRG1 are predicted to be intrinsically disordered, and are known to be subject to post-translational modification. Notably, the N-terminus has been shown to be ubiquitinylated and SUMOylated, while the C-terminus is subject to extensive phosphorylation [36]. Guided by the structure of NDRG2 and its sequence alignment with NDRG1 [3], the N and C termini were excised to isolate their contribution to the lipid storage phenotype. Both ΔN-NDRG1 and ΔC-NDRG1 overexpressing SKBR3 cells exhibited increased lipid storage relative to the wild-type overexpressing control, but the increase was higher in ΔN-NDRG1 than in ΔC-NDRG1, showing 2.1-fold and 1.3-fold increases relative to the full-length control (Fig. 5c). These results suggest that the N-terminus of NDRG1 is particularly important in maintaining lipid homeostasis, and are consistent with the involvement of NDRG1 in minimizing lipid storage and promoting lipid homeostasis in breast cancer cells.

Dysregulated lipid metabolism has been linked with increased endoplasmic reticulum stress in breast cancer [46, 47] and increased lipid droplet formation is a conserved consequence of endoplasmic reticulum stress [47, 48]. Since we observed that NDRG1 regulates lipid droplet formation and since NDRG1 overexpression is induced in response to endoplasmic reticulum stress [49], we tested whether loss of NDRG1 impacted response to agents that induce endoplasmic reticulum stress. We found that cell death was enhanced twofold in NDRG1-depleted SKBR3 cells subjected to 48 h exposure with either thapsigargin or tunicamycin at 1 μM and 5 μg/ml, respectively (Additional file 1: Figure S7A). Importantly, treatment with the ATP competitive mTOR inhibitor Ku-0063794 (1 μM) had little effect on cell survival (Additional file 1: Figure S7A). In a series of doses spanning three orders of magnitude, NDRG1-depleted SKBR3 cells are more sensitive at each concentration, with reduced lethal dose 50% (LD50) values for each compound of ~ 100 fold for thapsigargin and ~ 75 fold for tunicamycin (Fig. 5e, f, Additional file 1: Figure S7). These results show that NDRG1 depletion sensitizes SKBR3 cells to agents with distinct mechanisms of endoplasmic reticulum stress induction [46] and suggest that NDRG1 functions in part to counteract endoplasmic reticulum stress.

NDRG1 controls cellular fatty acid distribution

In order to better understand the impact of NDRG1 function on fatty acid trafficking and metabolism, BODIPY-labeled fatty acids were employed to trace their fate in living cells. Several BODIPY fatty acid conjugates are known to enter fatty acid metabolic pathways, including esterification to TAGs and phospholipids such as phosphatidylcholine, making them useful tools to study fatty acid uptake, metabolism, and distribution [32].

SKBR3 cells exhibited dramatic subcellular distributions of the fluorescent 16-carbon palmitate analog C16 BODIPY 493/503 that depended on NDRG1 expression and dosage of the tracer (Fig. 6a). Cells were fed a dilution series of albumin-coupled C16 BODIPY (12.5–100 μM), and total signal was quantified in segmented cells to compare overall cellular tracer uptake levels. Control and NDRG1-silenced SKBR3 cells showed dose-dependent

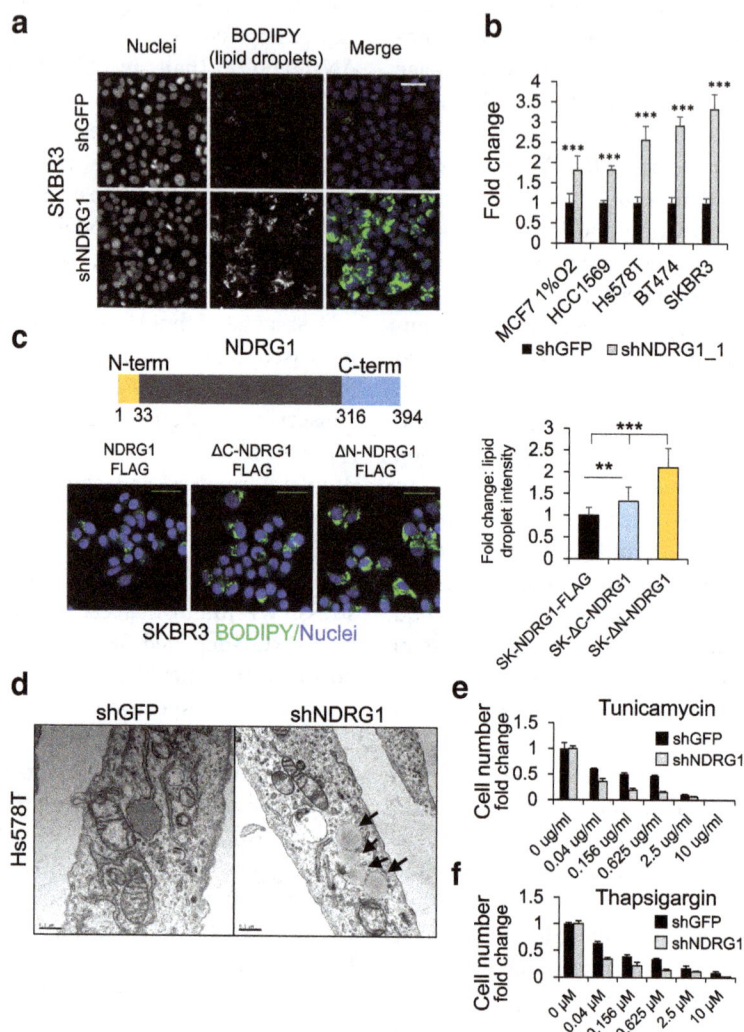

Fig. 5 NDRG1 depletion increases neutral lipid storage in lipid droplets. **a** Boron-dipyrromethene (BODIPY) 493/503 and Hoechst-stained stable SKBR3 cells expressing NDRG1 or green fluorescent protein (GFP) targeting shRNA at 2 weeks post selection. Scale bar = 25 μm. **b** Comparison of BODIPY-positive lipid droplet specific signal/cell in stable SKBR3, MCF7 1% O_2, MDA-MB-231, MDA-MB-468, and HCC1569 expressing the indicated shRNAs: all N = 6 and ***p < 0.00001. See Additional file 1: Figure S6 for related data. **c** Comparison of lipid droplet signal in stable SKBR3 cells expressing FLAG tagged full-length NDRG1 and N and C terminal truncations as indicated. N = 12, **p < 0.01, ***p < 0.00000001, scale bar = 25 μm. **d** Electron microscopy analysis of Hs578T cells +/− NDRG1 depletion. Arrows indicate lipid droplets. Scale bar = 0.5 μm. **e-f** Analysis of thapsigargin and tunicamycin and survival by counting Hoechst-stained nuclei 48 h post stable SKBR3 +/− NDRG1 depletion. Plots represent surviving cell fraction compared to untreated cells, N = 3. All bar graphs represent mean +/− SD and comparisons were by the two-sided t test. Scale bars = 25 μm

increases in C16 BODIPY uptake (Fig. 6b), in line with experiments demonstrating that albumin-coupled oleic acid stimulates comparable increases in lipid droplet formation (Additional file 1: Figure S6A, B). NDRG1-depleted cells take up less of the tracer but overall signal intensity was similar at the highest dose (Fig. 6b), eliminating the possibility that NDRG1-silencing-dependent increases in neutral lipid storage are due to increased fatty acid uptake.

The intracellular distribution of C16 BODIPY showed surprising dose-dependent and NDRG1 status-dependent differences that suggest that NDRG1 helps distribute lipids within cells. C16 BODIPY localized to

lipid droplets was quantified (Fig. 6c) and compared to overall uptake, yielding the fraction of tracer in droplets relative to that in the whole cell. In the NDRG1-depleted cell line, the relative balance of lipid droplet and total signal remained constant across all concentrations, and strong colocalization between lipid droplets and the tracer was maintained (Fig. 6a and d). Unexpectedly, as the dose of C16 BODIPY increased, the relative distribution of tracer signal changed in control cells, and a notable shift in tracer signal away from lipid droplets and into other parts of the cell was observed (Fig. 6a and d). In control cells, the proportion

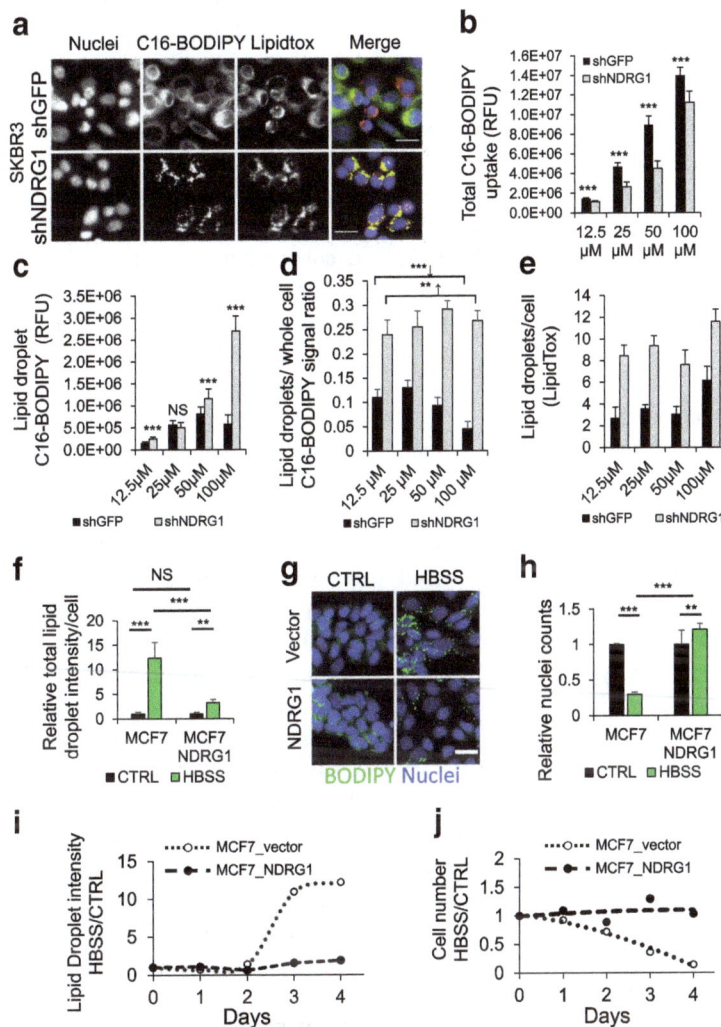

Fig. 6 Fluorescent fatty acid tracers reveal NDRG1 suppresses fatty acid incorporation Into neutral lipids and storage in lipid droplets. **a** Fluorescence micrographs of stable NDRG1 SKBR3 +/− NDRG1 depletion fed the 16-carbon boron-dipyrromethene (BODIPY) palmitate (BODIPY C16–100 μM, 16 h), fixed. Lipid droplets and nuclei counterstained with LipidTox Deep Red and Hoechst, respectively. **b** Quantification of total BODIPY C16 uptake in SKBR3 cells +/− NDRG1 depletion. Graphs represent average total signal per cell at indicated tracer concentrations. **c** Quantification of lipid droplet specific BODIPY C16 by segmentation of small granules. **d** Relative distribution of BODIPY C16 signal representing droplet/whole cell signal. **e** LipidTox stained lipid droplet numbers represented as objects per cell. **f** Comparison of lipid droplet intensities of starved and fed controls at day 3 in stable BODIPY 558/568 C12 loaded MCF7 cells. Complete medium versus Hank's buffered saline (HBSS). **g** BODIPY 493/503 counterstaining of NDRG1-FLAG overexpressing and control cells fed complete medium or HBSS for 3 days. **h** Analysis of cell survival due to starvation in stable BODIPY 558/568 C12-fed MCF7 cells transduced with NDRG1-FLAG or empty vector after 3 days of culture in HBSS. **i, j** Time course of changes in lipid droplet formation and cell count due to HBSS starvation in stable MCF7 cells transduced with the indicated constructs. Values represent HBSS/complete medium. All bar graphs represent mean +/− SD and comparisons were by two-sided t test. $N = 12$/group for all. Scale bars = 25 μm. CTRL, control

of tracer signal in lipid droplets actually decreased at the 50 μM and 100 μM doses, relative to the 25 μM dose, as total lipid droplet-specific signal gain was outpaced by total uptake and distribution to non-lipid droplet destinations (Fig. 6b–d). In contrast, the NDRG1-depleted cells consistently increased tracer signal in lipid droplets in accord with overall uptake (Fig. 6c). That the distribution of tracer was less dynamic in cells with decreased NDRG1 levels was confirmed by counter staining with LipidTOX Deep Red to quantify number and visualize localization of lipid droplets in C16-BODIPY-fed cells after 16 h. Although found in all treatment groups, LipidTOX-positive lipid droplets are largely distinct from C16 BODIPY stained droplets in control cells indicating redistribution of C16 BODIPY tracer after uptake. In NDRG1-depleted cells, a high degree of C16 BODIPY and LipidTOX Deep Red staining overlap was maintained at all C16 BODIPY levels (Fig. 6a). The average number of lipid droplets in each cell remained constant at 12.5, 25, and 50 µM C16 BODIPY doses, but increases in both cell lines at the 100 µM dose (shGFP 2-fold and shNDRG1 1.5-fold (Fig. 6e)). This shows that C16 BODIPY tracer feeding does not reduce lipid droplet numbers in either cell line, eliminating alternative explanations involving an NDRG1-dependent reduction in lipid droplet number at the 100 µM dose as grounds for the observed effect. Taken together, these results indicate that NDRG1 function influences pathways dictating the flow of fatty acids into storage and structural lipid pathways in breast cancer cells.

Ectopic overexpression protects cells with low endogenous NDRG1 levels from starvation-mediated lipid droplet formation and cell death

NDRG1 expression is induced in response to metabolic limitations imposed by oxygen and iron deprivation, suggesting that it may play an important role in the altered metabolism associated with poorly perfused tumor microenvironments [17, 50–52]. Since lipid storage has been shown in a number of cell types to occur as a response to metabolic limitations of hypoxia [44] and glucose starvation [32, 53] and since our results showed that NDRG1 limits neutral lipid storage (Fig. 4), we tested whether NDRG1 expression protects breast cancer cells from conditions found in poorly perfused tumor microenvironments. MCF7 cells, which ordinarily express very low levels of NDRG1 (Fig. 3a) and do not produce high levels of lipids endogenously [21–23], were engineered to overexpress NDRG1 and empty vector control. These cells were pulsed overnight with the 12-carbon BODIPY fatty acid analog C12 BODIPY Red (100 µM), followed by a chase under tracer-free conditions. One population was cultured in HBSS for 3 days to mimic the nutrient starvation found in poorly perfused tumor microenvironments, and controls were cultured in complete medium. Both populations exhibited similar ubiquitous distributions of the tracer under normal culture conditions in complete medium. However, when NDRG1 overexpressing and vector control MCF7 cells were subjected to starvation in HBSS for 3 days, a striking shift in the tracer to lipid droplets was evident. The control cells, but not MCF7-NDRG1 cells, exhibited an acute shift in C12 BODIPY Red localization to lipid droplets. NDRG1 overexpressing cells appeared relatively unchanged over the course of starvation (Fig. 6f and g). In addition to attenuating lipid droplet formation, NDRG1 overexpression protected MCF7 cells from starvation-induced cell death. Starvation in HBSS for 72 h decreased control MCF7 cell numbers to 30% of fed control populations, while MCF7-NDRG1 cells maintained cell populations similar to fed controls under the same conditions (Fig. 6h). Similar results were

observed with other cell types. SKBR3 cells expressing NDRG1 shRNAs displayed increased sensitivity to combined glucose, serum, and glutamine limitation (data not shown).

To understand the temporal nature of this process, and to rule out adverse effects due to the tracer, nutrient starvation was analyzed in unlabeled cells over a 4-day period. Interestingly, the spike in lipid droplet formation occurred between the 48 h and 72 h time points, and consistent with tracer results was coincident with the steepest period of decline in cell number in tracer-free conditions. Comparatively minor increases in lipid droplets were seen in MCF7-NDRG1 cells. Lipid droplet formation analysis showed 10-fold and 12-fold increases in lipid droplet staining intensity per cell in the control after 72 and 96 h of starvation, with comparatively small 1.5-fold and 1.8-fold increases in MCF7-NDRG1 cells at the same time points (Fig. 6i and j). Cell number decreases occurred in concert with lipid droplet formation in the control cells, and NDRG1 overexpressing cells remained at levels consistent with the fully fed control. Thus, NDRG1 overexpression both protects MCF7 cells from nutrient starvation induced cell death and attenuates starvation- induced lipid droplet formation. These results suggest that NDRG1 protects cancer cells from death in ill-perfused, nutrient-poor tumor microenvironments by optimizing lipid utilization. As NDRG1 is typically expressed in hypoxic microenvironments, however, it is likely that unlike most normal cells [32, 53], the lipids in breast cancer cells are ultimately likely to have fates other than beta oxidation.

Discussion

Altered lipid metabolism is a common accessory pathway to the well-characterized increased dependence on glycolysis seen in breast cancer cells. This study defined a new function for the disease-associated protein NDRG1, and solidified its role as a negative prognostic marker in breast cancer. We showed that high *NDRG1* expression is a common feature of poor prognosis in breast cancer and that elevated expression is correlated with an aggressive metabolic gene signature and portends a high likelihood of disease recurrence and metastasis in several independent patient cohorts (Fig. 1a, b and Additional file 1: Figure S2). In vitro studies indicate that NDRG1 promotes optimal lipid composition and distribution in breast cancer cells, as depleting NDRG1 increases both lipid droplet and endosome formation and reduces viability, and overexpression protects cells from lipid droplet formation and starvation-induced cell death. Fluorescent fatty acid pulse-chase experiments show that NDRG1 plays a major role in directing the intracellular fate of fatty acids, favoring ubiquitous intracellular distribution in cells expressing high levels of

NDRG1, or localization to lipid droplets and vesicles in cells with low levels of NDRG1. Although the precise role of NDRG1 may be impacted by other molecules or cells in the tumor microenvironment, these findings would appear to have significant implications for the understanding of lipid metabolism and cell survival under conditions including aerobic glycolysis (Warburg metabolism) and ill-perfused breast cancer microenvironments. The lipid management function described here is also consistent with the NDRG1 mutation-related defects in Schwann cell biology seen in CMT4D and impacts on cell size, which may be regulated directly by lipid availability [54].

Until now, elevated NDRG1 expression has alternately been referred to as both a biomarker of metastasis, and a metastasis suppressor, although in vivo experimental confirmation has been lacking. Our meta-analysis of the relationship between NDRG1 mRNA expression and prognosis in large populations of patients with breast cancer is definitive: overexpression of NDRG1 mRNA is a significant negative prognostic factor in breast cancer. Genomic expression analysis confirmed that elevated NDRG1 levels are associated with a metabolic gene expression profile that is a potent signature of aggressive disease in the most common solid tumor types, including breast cancer (Fig. 1e, f and data not shown). Similarly, the notion that the role of NDRG1 in the altered breast cancer metabolism associated with aggressive cells is in lipid management is supported by previous functional genomic studies [6, 8, 17] and that the lipid synthesis regulator Spot14 [42] is the most significantly downregulated gene in NDRG1 silenced SKBR3 cells. The fact that other genes related to lipid synthesis are not upregulated may be due to the high basal lipid synthesis activity of these cells. Expression of genes related to lipid-induced endoplasmic reticulum stress for example are already maximally induced in many human epidermal growth factor receptor 2 (HER2)-positive cell lines.

In addition to its binding partners, structural features suggest two means by which NDRG1 might participate in lipid trafficking in breast cancer cells. First, the inactive α/β hydrolase fold of NDRG1 could retain fatty acid binding activity in the substrate binding cleft or in a manner similar to the CGI-58 protein [55]. CGI-58 is an inactive α/β hydrolase recently shown to interact with lipid droplets through a lipid droplet anchor sequence composed of three clustered tryptophan residues. We note that among the NDRG family, only NDRG1 possesses a similar sequence of clustered tryptophans in alpha helix 6. Although the precise role of CGI-58 is incompletely understood, it appears to play some role in recruiting adipose triglyceride lipase (ATGL) to the surface of lipid droplets [55]. A similar mechanism for NDRG1 is consistent with our data, although more work

would is needed to confirm this. Intriguingly, in a study examining NDRG1 and lipid binding, recombinant purified NDRG1 was shown to bind phosphatidylinositol 4-phosphate [6]. Second, NDRG1 encodes a consensus phosphopantetheine modification site. Direct evidence of this post-translational modification of NDRG1 has not been reported, but if modified, NDRG1 could support fatty acid trafficking or metabolism by reversibly binding fatty acids. One study examining the effect of NDRG1 on lipid trafficking in the epidermoid carcinoma cell line A431 showed NDRG1 silencing-altered multivesicular body morphology, reduced low density lipoprotein uptake due to mislocalization of the LDL receptor, and decreased cholesterol ester levels, while increasing ceramide levels [7]. Although the results differ, this study also points to altered lipid management in NDRG1-deficient cells. Further study is needed to determine whether NDRG1 directly binds additional fatty acids or complex lipids in a physiological setting.

NDRG1 has been implicated in divergent processes in a number of studies, complicating the interpretation of its function [56]. NDRG1 exhibits varied localization in tissues and cultured cell lines [57]. It is mainly cytoplasmic in breast cancer cells, but hypoxia or iron chelation causes dramatic redistribution of the pNDRG1 Ser330 pool to the nucleus in multiple cell types. Under both conditions, phospho-Thr346 NDRG1 remains cytoplasmic. These distinct modified forms may reconcile seemingly unrelated and even contradictory reports of NDRG1 function. In addition to lipid trafficking and metabolism, NDRG1 has also been implicated in DNA repair in the nucleus [8], and the phospho-Ser330 form may be the key player. In any event, fully deciphering NDRG1 regulation by post-translational modification will be extremely complex, as NDRG1 has been shown to be phosphorylated on at least 29 residues [36].

Conclusions

The central role of NDRG1 in regulating fatty acid metabolic fate, neutral lipid storage, and cell viability in breast cancer cells establishes strong evidence of its function in cancer cell metabolism. In addition, these findings may be relevant to the NDRG1 mutation dependent Schwann cell pathology that leads to the characteristic demyelinating phenotype of CMT4D. Lipid synthesis is linked with glycolysis, and is a required component of transformed cell physiology [58]. Our previous work suggests that de novo fatty acid synthesis supports central carbon metabolism via redox coupling with malic enzyme 1 catalyzed conversion of malate to pyruvate in HER2-positive breast cancer cells [22]. In addition to the critical role of de novo fatty acid synthesis, Ras transformation, hypoxia, and TSC2 deficiency have all been linked to defects in fatty acid desaturation, necessitating alternative means of acquiring these fatty acids for the synthesis of structural lipids [59, 60]. Relatively little is known about factors regulating the fidelity of downstream lipid biosynthesis and trafficking pathways in cancer cells. NDRG1 expression correlates with glycolytic metabolism and poor outcomes in breast cancer. NDRG1 is expressed in all subtypes but is more likely to be constitutively expressed in ER-negative breast cancers, and dynamically expressed in response to microenvironment oxygen gradients in ER-positive breast cancers, suggesting it plays a smaller, but not insignificant, role in this setting. Our data place NDRG1 in the pathway dictating fatty acid utilization by the cell, downstream of both fatty acid synthesis and exogenous uptake, in which NDRG1 negatively regulates fatty acid storage in neutral lipids, and promotes alternative fates in cancer cells.

Abbreviations

BODIPY: Boron-dipyrromethene; cDNA: Complementary DNA; CCLE: Cancer Cell Line Encyclopedia; CE: Cholesterol esters; CMT4D: Charcot-Marie-Tooth disease type 4D; Ctrl: Control; DFO: Deferoxamine; DMEM: Dulbecco's modified Eagle's medium; eGFP: Enhanced green fluorescent protein; ER/ESR1: Estrogen receptor; FBS: Fetal bovine serum; GAPDH: Glyceraldehyde-3-phosphate dehydrogenase; GFP: Green fluorescent protein; HBSS: Hank's buffered saline solution; HER2: Human epidermal growth factor receptor 2; HMECs: Human mammary epithelial cells; LC-MS: Liquid chromatography-mass spectrometry; mRNA: Messenger RNA; NDRG1: N-myc downstream regulated gene; PBS: Phosphate-buffered saline; SDS-PAGE: Sodium dodecylsulfate polyacrylamide gel electrophoresis; shRNA: Short hairpin RNA; TAG: Triacylglycerols; TBS: Tris buffered saline

Acknowledgements

We thank Dr Xianhui Wang and other members of the Conklin laboratory and UAlbany CRC for helpful discussions. We thank Dr Sushant Kachhap from Johns Hopkins Medical School for the NDRG1 template plasmid and Dr Sridar Chittur for help with microarray results.

Funding

This work was supported by NCI award R01CA136658-03 to DSC. The funding body was not involved in the design of the study and collection, analysis, and interpretation of data, or in writing the manuscript.

Authors' contributions

CJS performed the bioinformatics data mining and most experiments, KRM performed lipidomics and assisted in data interpretation, AD performed electron microscopy and assisted in data interpretation, FK and LK performed additional experiments, and DSC and CJS conceived and designed the study, interpreted the data and drafted the manuscript. All authors read and approved the final manuscript.

Competing interests

The authors declare that they have no competing interests.

Author details

[1]Cancer Research Center, Department of Biomedical Sciences, State University of New York, University at Albany, CRC 342, One Discovery Drive, Rensselaer, NY 12144-3456, USA. [2]Electron Microscopy Core Facility, The University of Texas Southwestern Medical Center, 5323 Harry Hines Boulevard, Dallas, TX 75390, USA. [3]Lipidomics Core Facility, Wayne State University, 435 Chemistry Bldg., Detroit, MI 48202, USA.

References

1. Kalaydjieva L, Gresham D, Gooding R, Heather L, Baas F, de Jonge R, Blechschmidt K, Angelicheva D, Chandler D, Worsley P, et al. N-myc downstream-regulated gene 1 is mutated in hereditary motor and sensory neuropathy-Lom. Am J Hum Genet. 2000;67:47–58.
2. Hunter M, Angelicheva D, Tournev I, Ingley E, Chan DC, Watts GF, Kremensky I, Kalaydjieva L. NDRG1 interacts with APO A-I and A-II and is a functional candidate for the HDL-C QTL on 8q24. Biochem Biophys Res Commun. 2005;332:982–92.
3. Hwang J, Kim Y, Kang HB, Jaroszewski L, Deacon AM, Lee H, Choi W-C, Kim K-J, Kim C-H, Kang BS, et al. Crystal structure of the human N-Myc downstream-regulated gene 2 protein provides insight into its role as a tumor suppressor. J Biol Chem. 2011;286:12450–60.
4. Shi X-H, Larkin JC, Chen B, Sadovsky Y. The expression and localization of N-myc downstream-regulated gene 1 in human trophoblasts. PLoS One. 2013;8
5. Croessmann S, Wong HY, Zabransky DJ, Chu D, Mendonca J, Sharma A, Mohseni M, Rosen DM, Scharpf RB, Cidado J, et al. NDRG1 links p53 with proliferation-mediated centrosome homeostasis and genome stability. Proc Natl Acad Sci U S A. 2015;112:11583–8.
6. Kachhap SK, Faith D, Qian DZ, Shabbeer S, Galloway NL, Pili R, Denmeade SR, DeMarzo AM, Carducci MA. The N-myc down regulated gene1 (NDRG1) is a Rab4a effector involved in vesicular recycling of E-cadherin. PLoS One. 2007;2:e844.
7. Pietiäinen V, Vassilev B, Blom T, Wang H, Nelson J, Bittman R, Bäck N, Zelcer N, Ikonen E. NDRG1 functions in LDL receptor trafficking by regulating endosomal recycling and degradation. J Cell Sci. 2013;126:3961–71.
8. Weiler M, Blaes J, Pusch S, Sahm F, Czabanka M, Luger S, Bunse L, Solecki G, Eichwald V, Jugold M, et al. mTOR target NDRG1 confers MGMT-dependent resistance to alkylating chemotherapy. Proc Natl Acad Sci U S A. 2014;111:409–14.
9. Bandyopadhyay S, Pai SK, Gross SC, Hirota S, Hosobe S, Miura K, Saito K, Commes T, Hayashi S, Watabe M, et al. The Drg-1 gene suppresses tumor metastasis in prostate cancer. Cancer Res. 2003;63:1731–6.
10. Bandyopadhyay S, Pai SK, Hirota S, Hosobe S, Takano Y, Saito K, Piquemal D, Commes T, Watabe M, Gross SC, et al. Role of the putative tumor metastasis suppressor gene Drg-1 in breast cancer progression. Oncogene. 2004;23:5675–81.
11. Guan RJ, Ford HL, Fu Y, Li Y, Shaw LM, Pardee AB. Drg-1 as a differentiation-related, putative metastatic suppressor gene in human colon cancer. Cancer Res. 2000;60:749–55.
12. Hu Z, Fan C, Livasy C, He X, Oh DS, Ewend MG, Carey LA, Subramanian S, West R, Ikpatt F, et al. A compact VEGF signature associated with distant metastases and poor outcomes. BMC Med. 2009;7:9.
13. Ring BZ, Seitz RS, Beck R, Shasteen WJ, Tarr SM, Cheang MCU, Yoder BJ, Budd GT, Nielsen TO, Hicks DG, et al. Novel prognostic immunohistochemical biomarker panel for estrogen receptor-positive breast cancer. J Clin Oncol Off J Am Soc Clin Oncol. 2006;24:3039–47.

14. Chen X, Iliopoulos D, Zhang Q, Tang Q, Greenblatt MB, Hatziapostolou M, Lim E, Tam WL, Ni M, Chen Y, et al. XBP1 promotes triple-negative breast cancer by controlling the HIF1α pathway. Nature. 2014;508:103–7.

15. Piperi C, Adamopoulos C, Papavassiliou AG. XBP1: a pivotal transcriptional regulator of glucose and lipid metabolism. Trends Endocrinol Metab. 2016;27:119–22.

16. Sood A, Miller AM, Brogi E, Sui Y, Armenia J, McDonough E, Santamaria-Pang A, Carlin S, Stamper A, Campos C, et al. Multiplexed immunofluorescence delineates proteomic cancer cell states associated with metabolism. JCI Insight. 2016;1

17. Askautrud HA, Gjernes E, Gunnes G, Sletten M, Ross DT, Børresen-Dale AL, Iversen N, Tranulis MA, Frengen E. Global gene expression analysis reveals a link between NDRG1 and vesicle transport. PLoS One. 2014;9:e87268.

18. Cancer Genome Atlas Network. Comprehensive molecular portraits of human breast tumours. Nature. 2012;490(7418):61–70.

19. Ahn SG, Park JT, Lee HM, Lee HW, Jeon TJ, Han K, Lee SA, Dong SM, Ryu YH, Son EJ, et al. Standardized uptake value of 18F-fluorodeoxyglucose positron emission tomography for prediction of tumor recurrence in breast cancer beyond tumor burden. Breast Cancer Res. 2014;16:502.

20. Liberti MV, Locasale JW. The Warburg effect: how does it benefit cancer cells? Trends Biochem Sci. 2016;41:211–8.

21. Baumann J, Sevinsky C, Conklin DS. Lipid biology of breast cancer. Biochim Biophys Acta. 2013;1831(10):1509–17.

22. Kourtidis A, Jain R, Carkner RD, Eifert C, Brosnan MJ, Conklin DS. An RNA interference screen identifies metabolic regulators NR1D1 and PBP as novel survival factors for breast cancer cells with the ERBB2 signature. Cancer Res. 2010;70(5):1783–92.

23. Menendez JA, Lupu R. Fatty acid synthase and the lipogenic phenotype in cancer pathogenesis. Nat Rev Cancer. 2007;7:763–77.

24. Hitoshi Y, Lorens J, Kitada SI, Fisher J, LaBarge M, Ring HZ, Francke U, Reed JC, Kinoshita S, Nolan GP. Toso, a cell surface, specific regulator of Fas-induced apoptosis in T cells. Immunity. 1998;8(4):461–71.

25. Hannon GJ, Sun P, Carnero A, Xie LY, Maestro R, Conklin DS, Beach D. MaRX: an approach to genetics in mammalian cells. Science. 1999;283(5405):1129–30.

26. Ejsing CS, Duchoslav E, Sampaio J, Simons K, Bonner R, Thiele C, Ekroos K, Shevchenko A. Automated identification and quantification of glycerophospholipid molecular species by multiple precursor ion scanning. Anal Chem. 2006;78(17):6202–14.

27. Ekroos K, Chernushevich IV, Simons K, Shevchenko A. Quantitative profiling of phospholipids by multiple precursor ion scanning on a hybrid quadrupole time-of-flight mass spectrometer. Anal Chem. 2002;74(5):941–9.

28. Shaner RL, Allegood JC, Park H, Wang E, Kelly S, Haynes CA, Sullards MC, Merrill AH Jr. Quantitative analysis of sphingolipids for lipidomics using triple quadrupole and quadrupole linear ion trap mass spectrometers. J Lipid Res. 2009;50(8):1692–707.

29. Liebisch G, Binder M, Schifferer R, Langmann T, Schulz B, Schmitz G. High throughput quantification of cholesterol and cholesteryl ester by electrospray ionization tandem mass spectrometry (ESI-MS/MS). Biochim Biophys Acta. 2006;1761(1):121–8.

30. Cerami E, Gao J, Dogrusoz U, Gross BE, Sumer SO, Aksoy BA, Jacobsen A, Byrne CJ, Heuer ML, Larsson E, et al. The cBio Cancer Genomics Portal: an open platform for exploring multidimensional cancer genomics data. Cancer Discov. 2012;2:401–4.

31. Györffy B, Lanczky A, Eklund AC, Denkert C, Budczies J, Li Q, Szallasi Z. An online survival analysis tool to rapidly assess the effect of 22,277 genes on breast cancer prognosis using microarray data of 1,809 patients. Breast Cancer Res Treat. 2010;123:725–31.

32. Rambold AS, Cohen S, Lippincott-Schwartz J. Fatty acid trafficking in starved cells: regulation by lipid droplet lipolysis, autophagy and mitochondrial fusion dynamics. Dev Cell. 2015;32:678–92.

33. Jin R, Liu W, Menezes S, Yue F, Zheng M, Kovacevic Z, Richardson DR. The metastasis suppressor NDRG1 modulates the phosphorylation and nuclear translocation of β-catenin through mechanisms involving FRAT1 and PAK4. J Cell Sci. 2014;127:3116–30.

34. van 't Veer LJ, Dai H, van de Vijver MJ, He YD, Hart AAM, Mao M, Peterse HL, van der Kooy K, Marton MJ, Witteveen AT, et al. Gene expression profiling predicts clinical outcome of breast cancer. Nature. 2002;415:530–6.

35. Barretina J, Caponigro G, Stransky N, Venkatesan K, Margolin AA, Kim S, Wilson CJ, Lehár J, Kryukov GV, Sonkin D, et al. The Cancer Cell Line Encyclopedia enables predictive modelling of anticancer drug sensitivity. Nature. 2012;483:603–7.

36. Hornbeck PV, Zhang B, Murray B, Kornhauser JM, Latham V, Skrzypek E. PhosphoSitePlus, 2014: mutations, PTMs and recalibrations. Nucleic Acids Res. 2015;43:D512–20.

37. Murray JT, Campbell DG, Morrice N, Auld GC, Shpiro N, Marquez R, Peggie M, Bain J, Bloomberg GB, Grahammer F, et al. Exploitation of KESTREL to identify NDRG family members as physiological substrates for SGK1 and GSK3. Biochem J. 2004;384:477–88.

38. Sahni S, Bae D-H, Lane DJR, Kovacevic Z, Kalinowski DS, Jansson PJ, Richardson DR. The metastasis suppressor, N-myc downstream-regulated gene 1 (NDRG1), inhibits stress-induced autophagy in cancer cells. J Biol Chem. 2014;289:9692–709.

39. Fang BA, Kovačević Ž, Park KC, Kalinowski DS, Jansson PJ, Lane DJR, Sahni S, Richardson DR. Molecular functions of the iron-regulated metastasis suppressor, NDRG1, and its potential as a molecular target for cancer therapy. Biochim Biophys Acta. 2014;1845:1–19.

40. Walther TC, Farese RV. Lipid droplets and cellular lipid metabolism. Annu Rev Biochem. 2012;81:687–714.

41. Baumann JM, Kokabee L, Wang X, Sun Y, Wong J, Conklin DS. Metabolic assays for detection of neutral fat stores. Bio Protoc. 2015;5(12)

42. Kinlaw WB, Quinn JL, Wells WA, Roser-Jones C, Moncur JT. Spot 14: a marker of aggressive breast cancer and a potential therapeutic target. Endocrinology. 2006;147(9):4048–55.

43. Park S, Hwang I-W, Makishima Y, Perales-Clemente E, Kato T, Niederländer NJ, Park EY, Terzic A. Spot14/Mig12 heterocomplex sequesters polymerization and restrains catalytic function of human acetyl-CoA carboxylase 2. J Mol Recognit. 2013;26:679–88.

44. Bensaad K, Favaro E, Lewis CA, Peck B, Lord S, Collins JM, Pinnick KE, Wigfield S, Buffa FM, Li J-L, et al. Fatty acid uptake and lipid storage induced by HIF-1α contribute to cell growth and survival after hypoxia-reoxygenation. Cell Rep. 2014;9:349–65.

45. Boström P, Magnusson B, Svensson P-A, Wiklund O, Borén J, Carlsson LMS, Ståhlman M, Olofsson S-O, Hultén LM. Hypoxia converts human macrophages into triglyceride-loaded foam cells. Arterioscler Thromb Vasc Biol. 2006;26:1871–6.

46. Baumann J, Wong J, Sun Y, Conklin DS. Palmitate-induced ER. stress increases trastuzumab sensitivity in HER2/neu-positive breast cancer cells. BMC Cancer. 2016;16:551.

47. Volmer R, Ron D. Lipid-dependent regulation of the unfolded protein response. Curr Opin Cell Biol. 2015;33:67–73.

48. Fei W, Wang H, Fu X, Bielby C, Yang H. Conditions of endoplasmic reticulum stress stimulate lipid droplet formation in Saccharomyces cerevisiae. Biochem J. 2009;424:61–7.

49. Kokame K, Kato H, Miyata T. Homocysteine-respondent genes in vascular endothelial cells identified by differential display analysis GRP78/BiP and novel genes. J Biol Chem. 1996;271:29659–65.

50. Cangul H. Hypoxia upregulates the expression of the NDRG1 gene leading to its overexpression in various human cancers. BMC Genet. 2004;5:27.

51. Lai L-C, Su Y-Y, Chen K-C, Tsai M-H, Sher Y-P, Lu T-P, Lee C-Y, Chuang EY. Down-regulation of NDRG1 promotes migration of cancer cells during reoxygenation. PLoS One. 2011;6:e24375.

52. Lane DJR, Saletta F, Rahmanto YS, Kovacevic Z, Richardson DR. N-myc downstream regulated 1 (NDRG1) is regulated by eukaryotic initiation factor 3a (eIF3a) during cellular stress caused by iron depletion. PLoS One. 2013;8:e57273.

53. Singh R, Kaushik S, Wang Y, Xiang Y, Novak I, Komatsu M, Tanaka K, Cuervo AM, Czaja MJ. Autophagy regulates lipid metabolism. Nature. 2009;458:1131–5.

54. Rao MJ, Srinivasan M, Rajasekharan R. Cell size is regulated by phospholipids and not by storage lipids in Saccharomyces cerevisiae. Curr Genet. 2018;1831(10):1509–17. https://doi.org/10.1007/s00294-018-0821-0

55. Boeszoermenyi A, Nagy HM, Arthanari H, Pillip CJ, Lindermuth H, Luna RE, Wagner G, Zechner R, Zangger K, Oberer M. Structure of a CGI-58 motif provides the molecular basis of lipid droplet anchoring. J Biol Chem. 2015;290(44):26361–72.

56. Ellen TP, Ke Q, Zhang P, Costa M. NDRG1, a growth and cancer related gene: regulation of gene expression and function in normal and disease states. Carcinogenesis. 2008;29:2–8.

57. Lachat P, Shaw P, Gebhard S, van Belzen N, Chaubert P, Bosman FT. Expression of NDRG1, a differentiation-related gene, in human tissues. Histochem Cell Biol. 2002;118:399–408.

58. Pavlova NN, Thompson CB. The emerging hallmarks of cancer metabolism. Cell Metab. 2016;23:27–47.

59. Kamphorst JJ, Cross JR, Fan J, de Stanchina E, Mathew R, White EP, Thompson CB, Rabinowitz JD. Hypoxic and Ras-transformed cells support growth by scavenging unsaturated fatty acids from lysophospholipids. Proc Natl Acad Sci U S A. 2013;110:8882–7.

60. Young RM, Ackerman D, Quinn ZL, Mancuso A, Gruber M, Liu L, Giannoukos DN, Bobrovnikova-Marjon E, Diehl JA, Keith B, et al. Dysregulated mTORC1 renders cells critically dependent on desaturated lipids for survival under tumor-like stress. Genes Dev. 2013;27(10):1115–31.

4

Immune characterization of breast cancer metastases: prognostic implications

Maria Vittoria Dieci[1,2]* ⓘ, Vassilena Tsvetkova[1], Enrico Orvieto[3], Federico Piacentini[4], Guido Ficarra[5], Gaia Griguolo[1,2], Federica Miglietta[1,2], Tommaso Giarratano[2], Claudia Omarini[6], Serena Bonaguro[1], Rocco Cappellesso[7], Camillo Aliberti[8], Grazia Vernaci[1,2], Carlo Alberto Giorgi[2], Giovanni Faggioni[2], Giulia Tasca[1,2], Pierfranco Conte[1,2] and Valentina Guarneri[1,2]

Abstract

Background: Tumor-infiltrating lymphocytes (TILs) evaluated in primary breast cancer (BC) convey prognostic information. Limited data in the metastatic setting are available.

Methods: Secondary lesions from 94 BC patients, 43 triple-negative (TN) and 51 HER2-positive, were evaluated for TILs and expression of CD8, FOXP3, and PD-L1 by immunohistochemistry.

Results: TILs levels on metastasis were generally low (median 5%) and did not differ between TN and HER2+ tumors. Younger patients showed significantly lower TILs ($p = 0.002$). In HER2+ patients, TILs were higher in lung metastases as compared to other sites ($p = 0.038$). TILs composition was different across metastatic sites: skin metastases presented higher FOXP3 ($p = 0.002$) and lower CD8/FOXP3 ratio ($p = 0.032$). Patients treated for metastatic BC prior to biopsy had lower CD8 (overall: $p = 0.005$, HER2+: $p = 0.011$, TN: $p = 0.075$).

In TN patients, median overall survival (OS) was 11.8 and 62.9 months for patients with low and high TILs, respectively (HR 0.29, 95%CI 0.11–0.76, log-rank $p = 0.008$). CD8/FOXP3 ratio was also prognostic in TN patients (median OS 8.0, 13.2, and 54.0 months in 1st, 2nd and 3th tertile, log-rank $p = 0.019$). Both TILs and CD8/FOXP3 ratio were independent factors at multivariate analysis. Counterintuitively, in HER2+ BC, low TILs tumors showed better prognosis (median OS 53.7 vs 39.9 months in TILs low and TILs high, not statistically significant).

Conclusions: Our findings indicate the relevance of TILs as prognostic biomarker for TNBC even in the advanced setting and provide novel hypothesis-generating data on potential sources of immune heterogeneity of metastatic BC.

Keywords: Metastatic breast cancer, Tumor-infiltrating lymphocytes, PD-L1, Triple negative, HER2

Background

Tumor-infiltrating lymphocytes (TILs) are believed to reflect the immunogenicity of breast cancer (BC), with rapidly accumulating evidence suggesting the clinical validity and potential utility of TILs as a biomarker [1]. Most of available data focus on early BC, where TILs have proved to retain a strong prognostic value especially in triple-negative (TN) and human epidermal growth factor receptor-2 (HER2) positive BC, when assessed on hematoxylin and eosin-stained (HES) sections of primary tumor in accordance with International Immuno-Oncology Biomarker Working Group recommendations [2–9]. In addition, an association between TILs and response to preoperative chemotherapy (plus anti-HER2 agents if HER2-positive) has been reported [10–15].

In contrast to the early setting, little is known on the prognostic role of TILs in advanced disease for patients treated with standard therapies currently available. In this context, prospective-retrospective data come from translational analyses of two trials evaluating combinations of chemotherapy and anti-HER2 agents as first-line for HER2-positive metastatic breast cancer patients [16, 17]. In the Cleopatra trial (trastuzumab+docetaxel vs pertuzumab+trastuzumab+docetaxel), longer OS was observed in patients with high TILs levels [16], whereas in the MA.31 trial (trastuzumab+taxane vs

* Correspondence: mariavittoria.dieci@unipd.it
[1]Department of Surgery, Oncology and Gastroenterology, University of Padova, Via Gattamelata 64, 35128 Padova, Italy
[2]Medical Oncology 2, Istituto Oncologico Veneto IRCCS, Via Gattamelata 64, 35128 Padova, Italy
Full list of author information is available at the end of the article

lapatinib+taxane) poorer prognosis was observed in case of low CD8-positive TILs on tumor samples from patients treated in the lapatinib arm relative to those receiving trastuzumab [17]. However, as a main limitation of these studies, TILs were assessed almost exclusively on primary tumor samples. Thus, it remains largely unexplored whether the evaluation of TILs in secondary lesions could provide more accurate information on the actual immunological balance between tumor and host. Indeed, available evidence suggests that immune microenvironment may differ between primary tumor and its paired secondary lesions in terms of both TILs levels and composition [18–21].

In the present study we aim to assess TILs levels, immune infiltrate composition and programmed death-ligand 1 (PD-L1) expression in metastatic lesions and to evaluate their prognostic impact for patients with TN and HER2+ advanced BC.

Methods
Study population
We retrospectively included 94 patients with HER2+ or TN (HR-/HER2-) metastatic BC diagnosed before 2015 at IRCCS Istituto Oncologico Veneto in Padua and Modena University Hospital for whom histologic material obtained with surgical resection or biopsy of regional or distant recurrence was available (lymphoid tissue metastasis were excluded).

Patients were identified from a prospectively maintained institutional database, in which clinicopathological characteristics (including histological type, tumor grade, hormonal receptor, HER2 status and clinical stage at diagnosis), time and site of recurrence and follow-up data were recorded.

Patients with ipsilateral in-breast recurrences were excluded given the difficulty in discriminating between a recurrence and a new primary lesion.

The study protocol was approved by local ethics committee.

Pathology assessments
Formalin-fixed paraffin-embedded tumor samples from metastatic sites and, when available, matched primary tumor samples were retrieved.

Estrogen receptor (ER) and progesterone receptor (PgR) were considered positive if immunohistochemistry (IHC) staining is positive in ≥10% of tumor cells. HER2 was considered negative if it was present in IHC staining of 0/1+ and/or FISH non-amplified.

TILs evaluation
Hematoxylin and eosin-stained (HES) slides were retrieved from Institutional Pathology archives. Stromal TILs were assessed according to consensus guidelines

[3, 22] by two independent investigators (MVD and FM), blinded for clinical data. The average value was used for analyses.

Immunohistochemistry
CD8 and FOXP3 IHC staining was performed by using the fully automated stainer BOND III (Leica, Wetzler, Germany). Paraffin slides were deparaffinized in xylene and rehydrated through graded alcohols. Antigen retrieval was performed with slides heated in EDTA buffer (pH 9.0) for 20 min at 100 °C.

After antigen retrieval, the slides were allowed to cool. The slides were rinsed with Tris-buffered saline (TBS) and the endogenous peroxidase was inactivated with 3% hydrogen peroxide block at room temperature. After protein block, the slides were incubated with primary antibody to human CD8 (Monoclonal Mouse Anti-Human CD8, Clone C8/144B, dilution 1:100, Dako Cytomation, Glostrup, Denmark) and FOXP3 (Monoclonal Mouse Anti-Human FOXP3, Clone 236A/E7, dilution 1:200, Abcam, Cambridge, MA, USA) for 15 min. The sections were rinsed in TBS and incubated for 8 min with the Post-Primary Antibody (Leica Biosystems). Then, the sections were rinsed in TBS and incubated for 8 min with Polymer (Leica Biosystems). Finally, peroxidase reactivity was visualized using a Mixed DAB Refine, then the sections were counterstained with hematoxylin for 15 min and mounted.

PD-L1 IHC staining was performed by using the Ventana automated immunostainer BenchMark ULTRA. (Ventana Medical Systems, Tucson, AZ, USA). The slides were dried at 60 °C for 1 h and deparaffinized using EZ Prep (Ventana Medical Systems) at 72 °C. Cell conditioning was performed using ULTRA CC1 solution (Ventana Medical Systems) at 100 °C for 64 min. Ventana PD-L1 Primary Antibody (rabbit monoclonal, clone SP263 ref. 790–4905, Ventana Medical Systems) was incubated at 36 °C for 16 min. Signals were detected using the OptiView DAB IHC Detection Kit (Ventana Medical Systems). Counterstaining was performed with Hematoxylin II and Bluing reagent (Ventana Medical Systems).

CD8, FOXP3 and PD-L1 scoring
Evaluation of CD8, FOXP3 and PD-L1 expression was performed by a pathologist, blinded for clinical data.

For CD8 and FOXP3, five fields of 2–3 mm of diameter were analyzed at ×40 for each sample. The five field were selected within the area identified for the evaluation of TILs according to available recommendations [3, 22] and were in the area exhibiting tumor invasion. The number of positive immune cells in the five selected fields was counted on a light microscope. For each sample, the average number of stained immune cells across the evaluated fields was calculated.

PD-L1 expression was assessed on the entire section. PD-L1 was evaluated on tumor cells (% of cells positively stained/total tumor cells) and on stromal/immune cells in tumor stroma (% of cells positively stained/total cells in tumor stroma).

PD-L1 expression was found to be predominant in stromal/immune cells rather than tumor cells, mean expression on tumor cells was 7%, mean expression on stromal/immune cells was 15%, t test $p = 0.003$. Expression in the two cells compartments was strongly and positively correlated (Spearman's coefficient 0.554, $p < 0.001$). Therefore, we decided to consider stromal/immune cells expression for further analyses in this study.

Statistical analysis

Statistical analysis was carried out using IBM SPSS (version 24) software (IBM Corp, Armonk, NY, USA).

Descriptive statistics were performed for patient demographics and clinical characteristics. For continuous variables median, range values and quartiles were computed. The Mann-Whitney nonparametric test was used to study the distribution of continuous variables across groups defined by clinicopathologic characteristics.

The Spearman's rank correlation coefficient was used to study the correlation between continuous variables.

Overall survival (OS) was defined as the time from first relapse to death from any cause. Alive patients were censored at the date of last follow-up. Median OS was estimated using the Kaplan–Meier method and reported with 95% confidence intervals (95% CIs). The Kaplan–Meier method was used to estimate survival curves, the log-rank test was used to compare between groups. Univariate and multivariate Cox regression modeling for proportional hazards was used to calculate HR and 95% CI. All reported p values are two-sided, and significance level was set at $p < 0.05$.

The association between TILs levels as continuous variable and OS was tested. The prognostic value of TILs levels categorized using a 10% cutoff [16, 20, 23] was also evaluated. The prognostic value of CD8/FOXP3 ratio was tested using tertiles.

We tested two distinct cutoffs for PD-L1 expression in stromal/immune cells (1% and 5%) and its association with OS.

Results

Clinicopathologic characteristics and association with TILs levels

In the present study, tumor samples of BC recurrences obtained from 94 patients were assessed ($n = 43$ TN and $n = 51$ HER2+) for TILs.

Patients' baseline characteristics are reported in Table 1. Median time from relapse to sample collection was 0 months, the majority of patients ($n = 70$, 74%)

underwent biopsy of recurrent BC before starting any systemic treatment for advanced disease. Most of the patients received prior neoadjuvant systemic treatment (86% of patients received chemotherapy, 59% of HER2+ patients received trastuzumab). The majority of tumor samples were obtained from distant relapses (57%).

Median TIL levels in the overall population was 5% (Q1 2%; Q3 10%), with similar results in TN and HER2+ patients (median 5%, Q1 2.25% to Q3 10% for TN and median 5%, Q1 2% to Q3 11% for HER2+; $p = 0.885$), as shown in Table 2.

Although TILs were not significantly different across biopsy sites, lung samples showed the highest levels among all sites. The comparison of TILs in lung versus other metastatic sites (all together) was of borderline significance in the overall cohort ($p = 0.084$) and reached statistical significance in the HER2+ cohort ($p = 0.038$). In the entire cohort, skin samples showed the lowest median TILs levels among all metastatic sites (3.5%), with similar results in the TN and HER2+ cohorts separately. However, when comparing skin versus other metastatic sites altogether, results were not statistically significant ($p = 0.312$ in the entire cohort, $p = 0.418$ in the TN cohort and $p = 0.548$ in the HER2+ cohort).

Women who were younger at the time of BC diagnosis (≤ 50 years) showed significantly lower TILs on metastasis than older patients (> 50 years) both in the overall population ($p = 0.002$) and when each tumor subtype was considered separately ($p = 0.037$ and $p = 0.010$ and for TN and HER2+ patients, respectively).

In the HER2+ population, TILs were significantly lower in case of HR+ disease ($p = 0.029$).

In the TN cohort, there was a nonsignificant trend for lower TILs for patients who received chemotherapy for metastatic disease prior to metastasis biopsy, as compared to patients undergoing biopsy before starting first-line treatment (median 2%, Q1 2% to Q3 5%; median 5%, Q1 23% to Q3 10%, respectively; $p = 0.104$).

Matched primary tumors were available for only 55 patients. TILs were not significantly different in primary versus matched metastasis (median 5%, Q1 2.5% to Q3 12.5% and median 6.25, Q1 2% to Q3 12.5%, $p = 0.925$). In the TN cohort ($n = 27$), TILs tended to decrease in metastasis, although not significantly (median 7.5%, Q1 2.5% to Q3 20% in primary and median 6.25, Q1 2% to Q3 11% in metastasis, $p = 0.477$). In HER2+ patients TILs were nonsignificantly higher in metastases (median 2.5%, Q1 2% to Q3 7% in primary and median 6%, Q1 2% to Q3 14% in metastasis, $p = 0.452$).

TILs composition

CD8 and FOXP3 were assessed on 64 biopsies ($n = 36$ HER2+, $n = 28$ TN), while PD-L1 expression was

Table 1 Patients' baseline characteristics: overall and according to tumor subtype

	Population evaluated for TILs levels			Population evaluated for CD8, FOXP3, PD-L1		
	Overall n (%)	TN n (%)	HER2+ n (%)	Overall n (%)	TN n (%)	HER2+ n (%)
Tot, n	94	43	51	64	28	36
Age at BC diagnosis, yrs. median (Q1–Q3)	49 (42–57)	51 (44–61)	46 (39–53)	51 (43–59)	54 (45–63)	47 (41–57)
Time to relapse, mos median (Q1–Q3)	27 (15–43)	19 (11–38)	31 (19–60)	27 (16–47)	18 (11–34)	31 (21–55)
Time from relapse to biopsy, mos median (Q1–Q3)	0 (0–5)	0 (0–2)	0 (0–11)	0 (0–6)	0 (0–2)	0 (0–15)
Histotype						
Ductal	81 (86)	36 (84)	43 (84)	56 (88)	22 (79)	34 (94)
Lobular	5 (5)	1 (2)	4 (8)	2 (3)	1 (4)	1 (3)
Other	8 (9)	6 (14)	2 (4)	6 (9)	5 (17)	1 (3)
Grade						
1–2	13 (14)	3 (7)	10 (20)	9 (14)	2 (7)	7 (19)
3	78 (86%)	39 (93)	39 (80)	54 (86)	25 (83)	29 (81)
HR status						
HR+	37 (39)	0 (0)	37 (72)	26 (41)	0 (0)	26 (72)
HR-	57 (61%)	43 (100)	14 (28)	38 (59)	28 (100)	10 (28)
Stage at diagnosis						
I–II	50 (55)	27 (66)	23 (46)	33 (52)	17 (63)	16 (44)
III	38 (42)	13 (32)	25 (50)	27 (43)	9 (33)	18 (50)
IV	3 (3)	1 (2)	2 (4)	3 (5)	1 (4)	2 (6)
Type of recurrent BC sample						
Locoregional relapse	40 (43)	23 (53)	17 (33)	25 (39)	13 (46)	12 (33)
Distant relapse	54 (57)	20 (47)	34 (67)	39 (61)	15 (54)	24 (67)
Organ/site of biopsy						
Liver	24 (25)	5 (12)	19 (37)	15 (23)	4 (14)	11 (31)
Skin	38 (40)	21 (49)	17 (33)	26 (41)	13 (47)	13 (36)
Lung	12 (13)	7 (16)	5 (10)	8 (13)	4 (14)	4 (11)
CNS	9 (10)	4 (9)	5 (10)	9 (14)	4 (14)	5 (14)
Other	11 (12)	6 (14)	5 (10)	6 (9)	3 (11)	3 (8)
Neo/adjuvant chemotherapy						
No	13 (14)	3 (7)	10 (20)	9 (14)	3 (11)	6 (17)
Yes	81 (86)	40 (93)	41 (80)	55 (86)	25 (89)	30 (83)
Neo/adjuvant trastuzumab						
No	–	–	21 (41)	–	–	12 (33)
Yes	–	–	30 (59)	–	–	24 (67)
Pre-biopsy systemic treatment for MBC						
No	70 (74)	36 (88)	34 (67)	46 (72)	25 (89)	21 (58)
Yes	24 (26)	7 (17)	17 (33)	18 (28)	3 (11)	15 (42)

Abbreviations: *TILs* tumor-infiltrating lymphocytes, *TN* triple negative, *HER2* human epidermal growth factor receptor-2, *n* number, *tot* total, *BC* breast cancer, *yrs* years, *mos* months, *Q1* first quartile, *Q3* third quartile, *HR* hormone receptor, *CNS* central nervous system, *MBC* metastatic breast cancer

available for 62 cases (*n* = 35 HER2+, n = 27 TN). Patients' baseline characteristics are reported in Table 1.

Figure 1 shows a heatmap with Spearman's coefficients and *p* values for the correlation between immune markers. In the entire cohort, CD8, FOXP3, PD-L1, and TILs showed a significant positive correlation with each other. The Spearman's coefficients showed generally a moderate correlation between the variables, with the exception of weak correlations between TILs and FOXP3, PD-L1 and CD8, and PD-L1 and FOXP3.

Table 2 TILs distribution according to tumor subtype and clinical characteristics

	TILs %, median (Q1 – Q3): all patients 5 (2–10)					
	Overall	p value	TN	p value	HER2+	p value
Tumor phenotype						
TN	5 (2–10)		–		–	
HER2+	5 (2–11)	0.855	–	–	–	–
Age at BC diagnosis						
≤ 50 years	3 (2–8)	**0.002**	3 (2–10)	**0.037**	4 (2–8)	**0.010**
> 50 years	8 (5–15)		7 (4–11)		9 (5–18)	
HR status						
Negative	–	–	–	–	9 (5–15)	**0.029**
Positive	–		–		4 (2–8)	
Organ/site of biopsy						
Liver	5 (2–8)	0.277	5 (5–11)	0.936	5 (2–8)	0.119
Skin	3(2–10)		3 (2–10)		4 (2–10)	
Lung	9 (5–18)		8 (3–10)		18 (6–19)	
CNS	6 (3–11)		4 (3–38)		11 (5–11)	
Other	5 (2–8)		5 (2–19)		5 (2–8)	
Pre-biopsy systemic treatment for MBC						
No	5 (3–11)	0.563	5 (3–10)	0.104	4 (2–13)	0.652
Yes	5 (2–8)		2 (2–5)		6 (5–9)	

Abbreviations: *TILs* tumor-infiltrating lymphocytes, *Q1* first quartile, *Q3* third quartile, *p* p value, significant values in bold, *TN* triple negative, *HER2* human epidermal growth factor receptor-2, *BC* breast cancer, *HR* hormone receptor, *CNS* central nervous system, *MBC* metastatic breast cancer

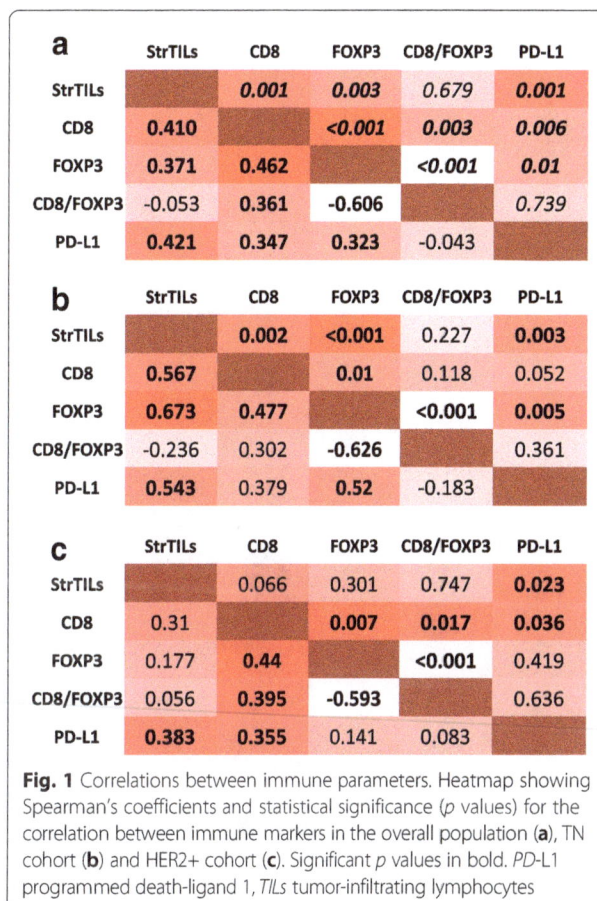

Fig. 1 Correlations between immune parameters. Heatmap showing Spearman's coefficients and statistical significance (*p* values) for the correlation between immune markers in the overall population (**a**), TN cohort (**b**) and HER2+ cohort (**c**). Significant *p* values in bold. *PD*-L1 programmed death-ligand 1, *TILs* tumor-infiltrating lymphocytes

The highest Spearman's correlation coefficients between TILs, CD8, FOXP3, and PD-L1 were observed in the TN cohort. The correlations were mostly moderate, with the exception of a strong correlation between TILs and FOXP3 and a weak correlation between CD8 and PD-L1.

In the HER2 cohort, correlation coefficients between TILs, CD8, FOXP3, and PD-L1 were the lowest. Correlations were very weak to weak, with the exception of the one between CD8 and FOXP3 that showed a Spearman's coefficient of 0.440.

CD8/FOXP3 ratio was obviously positively and negatively correlated with CD8 and FOXP3, respectively, and did not correlate with TILs or PD-L1.

Full data regarding distribution of CD8, FOXP3, CD8/FOXP3 ratio, and PD-L1 according to tumor subtype and other clinical variables is detailed in (Additional file 1: Tables S1; Additional file 2: Table S2; Additional file 3: Table S3; and Additional file 4: Table S4).

Distribution of these parameters did not vary significantly according to tumor subtype.

Levels of FOXP3 were significantly different across site of biopsy (0.046). In particular, FOXP3 was significantly higher in skin metastases as compared to other metastatic sites considered all together (*p* = 0.002).

Accordingly, CD8/FOXP3 ratio was the lowest in skin biopsies as compared to other metastatic sites (*p* = 0.032). This trend was seen both in the HER2+ and TN subgroup, though it only reached statistical significance in the HER2 + subgroup, as shown in Fig. 2.

Patients who underwent biopsy of metastatic lesion prior to start first-line treatment showed significantly higher CD8+ infiltrating lymphocytes as compared to patients who previously received systemic treatment for advanced disease: *p* = 0.005 for overall population and *p* = 0.011 for HER2+ tumors. The analysis in the TN cohort (*p* = 0.075) was limited by the fact that only three patients underwent metastasis biopsy prior to first-line therapy. Most of the HER2+ patients who received systemic therapy for metastatic disease prior to biopsy received both chemotherapy and anti-HER2 (13/17, 76.5%).

CD8/FOXP3 ratio was higher in HR+/HER2+ as compared to HR-/HER2+ patients (*p* = 0.052); however, this might in part be confounded by the fact that more HR-/HER2+ patients had skin metastasis biopsies than HR+/HER2+ patients (43% vs 27%, *p* = 0.277).

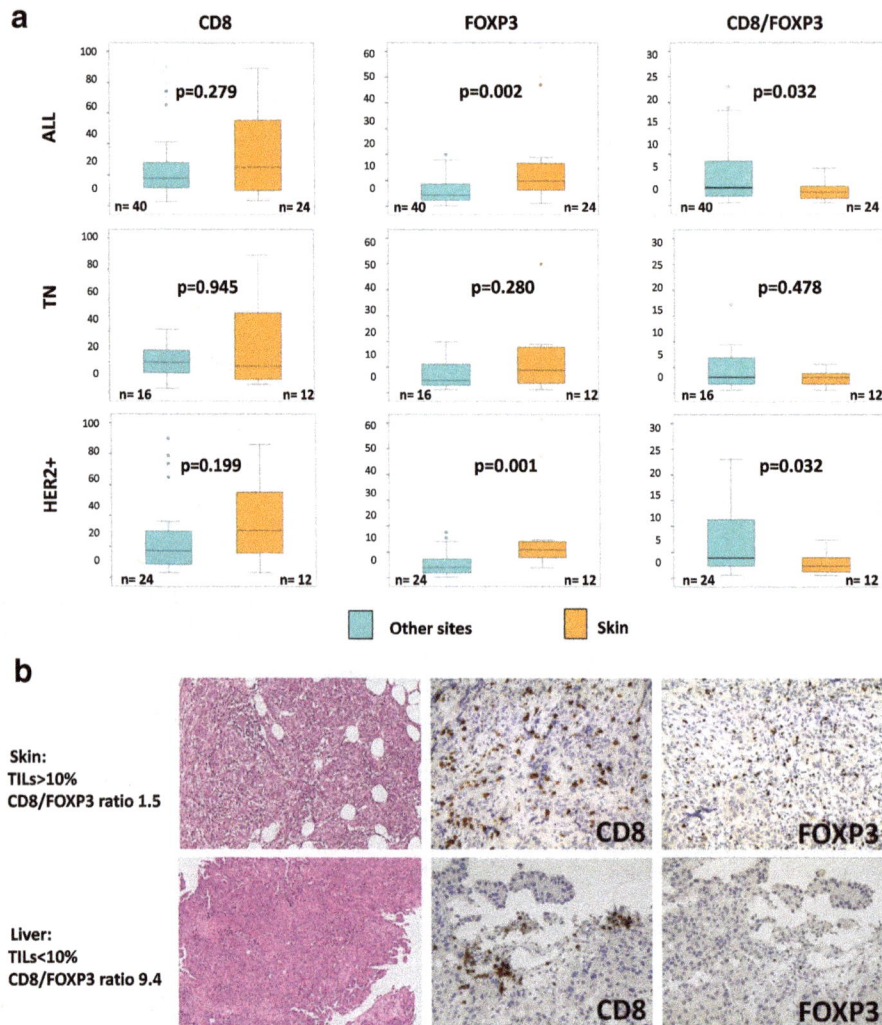

Fig. 2 CD8, FOXP3, and CD8/FOXP3 ratio in skin versus other metastasis sites. Boxplots comparing CD8, FOXP3, and CD8/FOXP3 ratio in skin versus other metastasis sites in all patients and in TN and HER2+ cohorts separately (a). Pictures showing a skin metastasis with high TILs and low CD8/FOXP3 ratio and a liver metastasis with low TILs and high CD8/FOXP3 ratio (b). *HER2* human epidermal growth factor receptor-2, *TILs* tumor-infiltrating lymphocytes, *TN* triple negative.

Impact on survival

Due to profound differences in disease course and therapeutic options, the prognostic value of immune biomarkers was assessed separately in the TN and HER2+ cohorts.

In the TN population, TILs had a significant prognostic impact on OS (median OS 11.8 months vs 62.9 months for TILs low and TILs high, respectively; HR 0.29, 95% CI 0.11–0.76, $p = 0.012$) (Fig. 3a). Each 1% increase in TILs was associated with a 3% reduction in the risk of death (HR 0.97, 95% CI 0.94–1.00, $p = 0.075$). Since we did not show significantly different TILs levels between primary and metastasis in the 27 TN cases with available samples, we explored, in this subgroup, the prognostic value of TILs in primary tumor and in metastasis. TILs in metastasis were significantly associated

with OS (HR 0.29, 95% CI 0.09–0.91, $p = 0.033$), whereas TILs in primary tumor did not (HR 0.50, 95% CI 0.19–1.34, $p = 0.170$). In addition, CD8/FOXP3 ratio on metastasis also showed a prognostic role in TN patients (median OS 8.0, 13.2 and 54.0 months in the first, second and third tertile, respectively; $p = 0.019$) (Fig. 3b). TILs and CD8/FOXP3 ratio were weakly correlated (Fig. 1), indeed, biopsies with high CD8/FOXP3 ratios (third tertile) were almost exclusively characterized by low TILs (eight out of nine cases with high CD8/FOXP3 ratio). In a multivariate Cox regression analysis both TILs and CD8/FOXP3 ratio maintained an independent prognostic value in TN tumors (Table 3) and the combined use of TILs and CD8/FOXP3 ratio allowed refining the prognostic ability of single biomarkers (median OS 8.0 months for tumors with low TILs and low CD8/

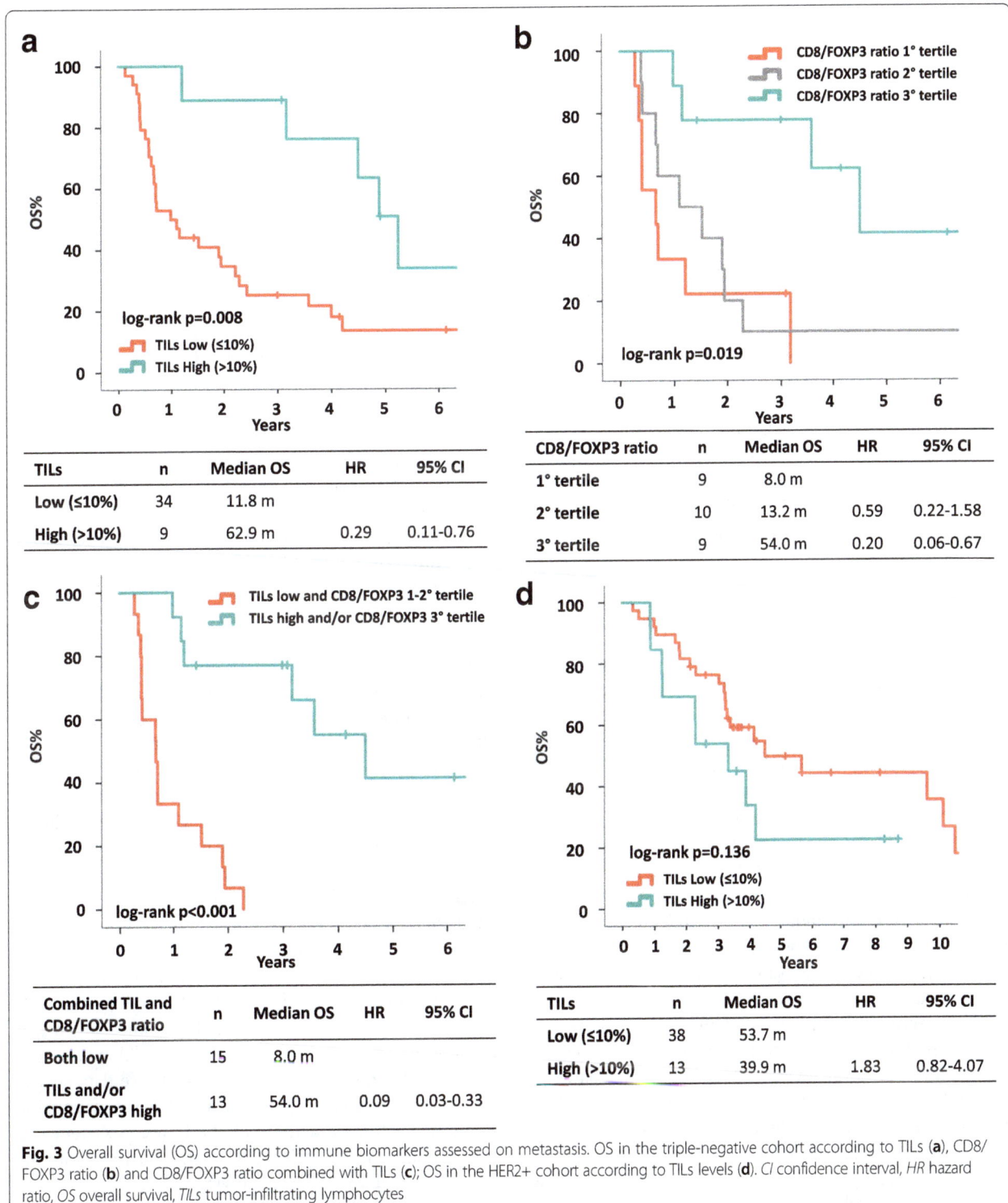

Fig. 3 Overall survival (OS) according to immune biomarkers assessed on metastasis. OS in the triple-negative cohort according to TILs (**a**), CD8/FOXP3 ratio (**b**) and CD8/FOXP3 ratio combined with TILs (**c**); OS in the HER2+ cohort according to TILs levels (**d**). *CI* confidence interval, *HR* hazard ratio, *OS* overall survival, *TILs* tumor-infiltrating lymphocytes

FOXP3 ratio vs 54.0 months for tumors with high TILs and/or high CD8/FOXP3 ratio, $p < 0.001$, Fig. 3c).

In the HER2+ population, an inverse relationship between TILs and prognosis was observed, with patients with lower TILs showing better prognosis (not statistically significant): median OS was 53.7 months vs 39.9 months for TILs low and TILs high, respectively; $p = 0.136$ (Fig. 3d). Results were similar in HR-/HER2+ and HR+/HER2+ patients, although the analysis was limited by reduced sample size. In HR-/HER2+, median OS was 50.3 months vs 15.1 months for patients with low and high TILs, respectively (HR 2.45, 95%CI 0.54–

Table 3 OS univariate and multivariate analysis of immune parameters evaluated on metastasis biopsies of triple-negative breast cancer

		Median OS months (95%CI)	Univariate HR (95%CI)	p	Multivariate HR (95%CI)
TILs	Low ≤10%	11.8 (4.1–19.5)	ref	**0.012**	ref
	High > 10%	62.9 (52.3–73.5)	0.29 (0.11–0.76)		0.06 (0.01–0.29)
CD8/FOXP3 ratio	1st tertile	8.0 (0.0–17.1)	ref	**0.020**	ref
	2nd tertile	13.2 (0.0–28.3)	0.59 (0.22–1.58)		0.17 (0.05–0.59)
	3rd tertile	54.0 (32.4–75.7)	0.20 (0.06–0.67)		0.03 (0.004–0.15)

Abbreviations: OS overall survival, HR hazard ratio, p p value, TILs tumor-infiltrating lymphocytes
Significant p values in bold

11.16). In HR+/HER2+ patients median OS was 68.9 and 47.1 months in case of low and high TILs, respectively (HR 1.54, 95% CI 0.55–4.28). CD8/FOXP3 ratio did not show any prognostic role (Additional file 5: Figure S1).

PD-L1 expression in tumor stroma was not prognostic in TN and in HER2+ tumors when considering a 5% cutoff (Additional file 6: Figure S2). Similar results were obtained with a 1% cutoff (data not shown).

Discussion

This article reports the assessment of immune-related biomarkers for patients with TN and HER2+ metastatic breast cancer. The series of samples analyzed in this work represents the largest published series of metastatic breast cancer samples analyzed for immune biomarkers. In our study, TILs were generally low. It is now recognized that patients with HER2+ and TN early BC with high levels of TILs on primary tumor have a lower recurrence rate [2–9], therefore suggesting that BC recurrences might be enriched in low TILs tumors. Moreover, previous reports showed lower TIL levels in secondary lesions as compared to primary tumors [16, 18, 19]. We only found a nonsignificant decrease in TILs from primary to metastasis in the TN cohort of our study, however, the sample size of patients with matched samples was small.

We observed that host-dependent factors are associated with TILs on metastasis. In particular, younger women showed lower levels of TILs than older patients. This is the first time that such correlation is reported for patients with metastatic disease. The reason for lower TILs levels in younger patients is largely unknown. A potential underexplored hypothesis is that younger patients present higher levels of circulating estrogens, which might have an immunosuppressive action [24, 25]. However, most of the patients had received neoadjuvant chemotherapy, which might have induced iatrogenic menopause and, unfortunately, it was not possible to capture the menopausal status of these patients at the time of metastatic disease onset. Other host-related factors such as race have been also shown

to be associated with differing levels of immune infiltrate in a previous study [16].

We found in our analysis that the characteristics of the tumor immune infiltrate may be different across metastatic sites. We observed the highest TILs levels in lung metastasis and the lowest levels in skin secondary lesions, which is consistent with previous data [16, 20]. Interestingly, we also could appreciate differences in immune infiltrate composition. In particular, skin metastasis presented significantly higher FOXP3 levels and lower CD8/FOXP3 ratio, as compared to other biopsy sites. This may suggest that cutaneous tissue might harbor a more permissive immune microenvironment for tumor growth. A physiological mitigation of the cytotoxic immune activity in skin tissue through different immunosuppressive mechanisms, a process known as "immune privilege", has been described by several authors [26, 27]. The immune heterogeneity across metastatic sites deserves to be further explored, due to potential relevance in explaining heterogeneous response to standard treatments and to immunotherapy.

Another factor that was found to be significantly related to TILs composition is previous treatment. Having received CT or anti-HER2 therapy in the metastatic setting prior to biopsy was associated with lower CD8+ TILs. Recently, Loi et al. reported lower levels of TILs for TN patients treated with multiple lines of chemotherapy as compared to patients who did not receive treatment for metastatic disease [20]. These data suggest that heavily pretreated patients might have an impaired antitumor cytotoxic activity of the immune system thus possibly explaining, at least in part, data from immune checkpoint inhibitor trials showing better response rates in first-line treatment than in subsequent lines [28–30].

TILs showed a strong prognostic value in TN BC, further corroborating the relevance of TILs as a biomarker in this disease subtype across different settings. TILs were significantly correlated with CD8, FOXP3, and PD-L1 in TN disease in our study, suggesting that the levels of TILs in TN reflect a general activation of the immune system. This observation supports TILs as a simple method to appreciate the immune activation status of a TN tumor. Indeed, given the availability of a standardized methodology for TILs assessment in the metastatic setting, the evaluation of this immune marker is technically simple and clinically reliable [22]. In addition, CD8/FOXP3 ratio was capable of identifying an additional subgroup of TN BC patients at good prognosis, which were not captured by the high TILs group. This hypothesis-generating result highlights that a finer evaluation of tumor microenvironment may be worthy of investigation in future studies.

Other well-known immune-related markers, such as PD-L1 expression, did not significantly affect outcome.

The clinical utility of TILs may not be confined to its prognostic value; in fact in recent studies of immune check-point inhibitors for metastatic TN BC patients, TILs rather than PD-L1 are a better predictor of response to immunotherapy [20, 23].

A different scenario was observed in HER2+ BC, where we did not observe any favorable impact of high TILs on OS. This result may appear in conflict with data from Cleopatra study [16], where higher TIL values were associated with improved OS. However, our HER2+ population was mostly represented by patients previously treated with anti-HER2 agents (60%) with samples obtained from metastases, while in the Cleopatra trial only a small proportion of patients was pretreated with anti-HER2 therapy (10.9%) and the majority of samples analyzed came from the primary tumor. As previously discussed, pretreatment with CT or HER2-targeted therapy may modify tumor immune microenvironment leading to impaired antitumor cytotoxic activity of the immune system.

Conclusions

The main results of this study further stress the relevance of TILs as a prognostic biomarker for TN even in the advanced setting and provide novel hypothesis-generating data with regards to immune composition across different metastatic sites and the influence of previous treatments. Finally, the more complex interplay between the immune system and HER2+ BC deserve further exploration in the metastatic setting.

Additional files

Additional file 1: Table S1. CD8 levels distribution according to tumor subtype and clinicopathological features. (DOCX 18 kb)

Additional file 2: Table S2. FOXP3 levels distribution according to tumor subtype and clinicopathological features. (DOCX 18 kb)

Additional file 3: Table S3. CD8/FOXP3 ratio distribution according to tumor subtype and clinicopathological features. (DOCX 18 kb)

Additional file 4: Table S4. PD-L1 levels distribution according to tumor subtype and clinicopathological features (DOCX 17 kb)

Additional file 5: Figure S1. Overall survival for HER2+ patients according to CD8/FOXP3 ratio. (PPTX 80 kb)

Additional file 6: Figure S2. Overall survival according to PD-L1 expression in HER2+ patients (2A) and TN patients (2B). (PPTX 91 kb)

Funding
This study was supported by a grant from University of Padova (DOR1721185/17) and a grant from Istituto Oncologico Veneto IRCCS (L02P28).

Authors' contributions
MVD conceived, designed and supervised the study, and participated in data acquisition, analysis and interpretation. VT, EO, GF (fifth author), SB, and RC provided material for the study, participated in pathology assessments, provided technical support, and participated in data analysis and interpretation. FP and CO provided material for the study and participated in data acquisition. GG, FM, TG, CA, GV, CAG, GF (fifth author), and GT participated in data acquisition. PFC and VG participated in data acquisition, analysis, and interpretation. All authors were involved in manuscript writing and reviewing, gave their final approval and agreed to be accountable for all aspects of the work.

Competing interests
The authors declare that they have no competing interests.

Author details
[1]Department of Surgery, Oncology and Gastroenterology, University of Padova, Via Gattamelata 64, 35128 Padova, Italy. [2]Medical Oncology 2, Istituto Oncologico Veneto IRCCS, Via Gattamelata 64, 35128 Padova, Italy. [3]Department of Pathology, Azienda Ospedaliera di Padova, Padova, Italy. [4]Department of Medical and Surgical Sciences of Mother, Child and Adult, University of Modena and Reggio Emilia, Modena, Italy. [5]Division of Pathology, University Hospital of Modena, Modena, Italy. [6]Department of Medical Oncology, University Hospital of Modena, Modena, Italy. [7]Surgical Pathology and Cytopathology Unit, Department of Medicine, University of Padova, Padova, Italy. [8]Radiology, Istituto Oncologico Veneto IRCCS, Padova, Italy.

References
1. Savas P, Salgado R, Denkert C, Sotiriou C, Darcy PK, Smyth MJ, et al. Clinical relevance of host immunity in breast cancer: from TILs to the clinic. Nat Rev Clin Oncol. 2016;13(4):228–41.
2. Dieci MV, Criscitiello C, Goubar A, Viale G, Conte P, Guarneri V, et al. Prognostic value of tumor-infiltrating lymphocytes on residual disease after primary chemotherapy for triple-negative breast cancer: a retrospective multicenter study. Ann Oncol. 2014;25(3):611–8.
3. Salgado R, Denkert C, Demaria S, Sirtaine N, Klauschen F, Pruneri G, et al. The evaluation of tumor-infiltrating lymphocytes (TILs) in breast cancer: recommendations by an international TILs working group 2014. Ann Oncol. 2015;26(2):259–71.
4. Loi S, Sirtaine N, Piette F, Salgado R, Viale G, Van Eenoo F, et al. Prognostic and predictive value of tumor-infiltrating lymphocytes in a phase III randomized adjuvant breast cancer trial in node-positive breast cancer comparing the addition of docetaxel to doxorubicin with doxorubicin-based chemotherapy: BIG 02-98. J Clin Oncol. 2013;31(7):860–7.
5. Loi S, Michiels S, Salgado R, Sirtaine N, Jose V, Fumagalli D, et al. Tumor infiltrating lymphocytes are prognostic in triple negative breast cancer and

predictive for trastuzumab benefit in early breast cancer: results from the FinHER trial. Ann Oncol. 2014;25(8):1544–50.

6. Perez EA, Ballman KV, Tenner KS, Thompson EA, Badve SS, Bailey H, et al. Association of stromal tumor-infiltrating lymphocytes with recurrence-free survival in the N9831 adjuvant trial in patients with early-stage HER2-positive breast cancer. JAMA Oncol. 2016;2(1):56–64.

7. Adams S, Gray RJ, Demaria S, Goldstein L, Perez EA, Shulman LN, et al. Prognostic value of tumor-infiltrating lymphocytes in triple-negative breast cancers from two phase III randomized adjuvant breast cancer trials: ECOG 2197 and ECOG 1199. J Clin Oncologia. 2014;32(27):2959–66.

8. Dieci MV, Mathieu MC, Guarneri V, Conte P, Delaloge S, Andre F, et al. Prognostic and predictive value of tumor-infiltrating lymphocytes in two phase III randomized adjuvant breast cancer trials. Ann Oncol. 2015;26(8): 1698–704.

9. Dieci MV, Radosevic-Robin N, Fineberg S, van den Eynden G, Ternes N, Penault-Llorca F, et al. Update on tumor-infiltrating lymphocytes (TILs) in breast cancer, including recommendations to assess TILs in residual disease after neoadjuvant therapy and in carcinoma in situ: a report of the international Immuno-oncology biomarker working group on breast cancer. Semin Cancer Biol. 2017.

10. Denkert C, Loibl S, Noske A, Roller M, Muller BM, Komor M, et al. Tumor-associated lymphocytes as an independent predictor of response to neoadjuvant chemotherapy in breast cancer. J Clin Oncol. 2010;28(1): 105–13.

11. Salgado R, Denkert C, Campbell C, Savas P, Nuciforo P, Aura C, et al. Tumor-infiltrating lymphocytes and associations with pathological complete response and event-free survival in HER2-positive early-stage breast cancer treated with lapatinib and trastuzumab: a secondary analysis of the NeoALTTO trial. JAMA Oncol. 2015;1(4):448–54.

12. Issa-Nummer Y, Darb-Esfahani S, Loibl S, Kunz G, Nekljudova V, Schrader I, et al. Prospective validation of immunological infiltrate for prediction of response to neoadjuvant chemotherapy in HER2-negative breast cancer–a substudy of the neoadjuvant GeparQuinto trial. PLoS One. 2013;8(12): e79775.

13. Dieci MV, Prat A, Tagliafico E, Pare L, Ficarra G, Bisagni G, et al. Integrated evaluation of PAM50 subtypes and immune modulation of pCR in HER2-positive breast cancer patients treated with chemotherapy and HER2-targeted agents in the CherLOB trial. Ann Oncol. 2016;27(10):1867–73.

14. West NR, Milne K, Truong PT, Macpherson N, Nelson BH, Watson PH. Tumor-infiltrating lymphocytes predict response to anthracycline-based chemotherapy in estrogen receptor-negative breast cancer. Breast Cancer Res. 2011;13(6):R126.

15. Denkert C, von Minckwitz G, Darb-Esfahani S, Ingold Heppner B, Klauschen F, Furlanetto F, et al. Evaluation of tumor-infiltrating lymphocytes (TILs) as predictive and prognostic biomarker in different subtypes of breast cancer treated with neoadjuvant therapy. Abstract S1-09. Presented at SABCS2016, San Antonio, TX, USA, 2016.

16. Luen SJ, Salgado R, Fox S, Savas P, Eng-Wong J, Clark E, et al. Tumour-infiltrating lymphocytes in advanced HER2-positive breast cancer treated with pertuzumab or placebo in addition to trastuzumab and docetaxel: a retrospective analysis of the CLEOPATRA study. Lancet Oncol. 2017;18(1):52–62.

17. Liu S, Chen B, Burugu S, Leung S, Gao D, Virk S, et al. Role of cytotoxic tumor-infiltrating lymphocytes in predicting outcomes in metastatic HER2-positive breast cancer: a secondary analysis of a randomized clinical trial. JAMA Oncol. 2017;3(11):e172085.

18. Cimino-Mathews A, Ye X, Meeker A, Argani P, Emens LA. Metastatic triple-negative breast cancers at first relapse have fewer tumor-infiltrating lymphocytes than their matched primary breast tumors: a pilot study. Hum Pathol. 2013;44(10):2055–63.

19. Ogiya R, Niikura N, Kumaki N, Bianchini G, Kitano S, Iwamoto T, et al. Comparison of tumor-infiltrating lymphocytes between primary and metastatic tumors in breast cancer patients. Cancer Sci. 2016;107(12):1730–5.

20. Loi S, Adams S, Schmid P, Cortes J, Cescon D, Winer E, et al. Relationship between tumor infiltrating lymphocyte levels and response to pembrolizumab in metastatic triple-negative breast cancer: results from Keynote-086 trial. 2017. Presented at: European Society of Medical Oncology (ESMO) 2017 Congress; Madrid, Spain: September 8–12, 2017. Abstract LBA13

21. Sobottka B, Pestalozzi B, Fink D, Moch H, Varga Z. Similar lymphocytic infiltration pattern in primary breast cancer and their corresponding distant metastases. Oncoimmunology. 2016;5(6):e1153208.

22. Hendry S, Salgado R, Gevaert T, Russell PA, John T, Thapa B, et al. Assessing tumor-infiltrating lymphocytes in solid tumors: a practical review for pathologists and proposal for a standardized method from the international Immuno-oncology biomarkers working group: part 2: TILs in melanoma, gastrointestinal tract carcinomas, non-small cell lung carcinoma and mesothelioma, endometrial and ovarian carcinomas, squamous cell carcinoma of the head and neck, genitourinary carcinomas, and primary brain tumors. Adv Anat Pathol. 2017;24(6):311–35.

23. Schmid P, Cruz C, Braiteh F, Eder J, Tolaney S, Kuter I, et al. Atezolizumab in metastatic TNBC: long-term clinical outcomes and biomarker analyses. Presented at AACR Annual Meeting 2017, April 1–5, 2017; Washington, DC, USA.

24. Svoronos N, Perales-Puchalt A, Allegrezza MJ, Rutkowski MR, Payne KK, Tesone AJ, et al. Tumor cell-independent estrogen signaling drives disease progression through mobilization of myeloid-derived suppressor cells. Cancer Discov. 2017;7(1):72–85.

25. Dieci MV, Griguolo G, Miglietta F, Guarneri V. The immune system and hormone-receptor positive breast cancer: is it really a dead end? Cancer Treat Rev. 2016;46:9–19.

26. Gilhar A, Paus R, Kalish RS. Lymphocytes, neuropeptides, and genes involved in alopecia areata. J Clin Invest. 2007;117(8):2019–27.

27. Wang X, Marr AK, Breitkopf T, Leung G, Hao J, Wang E, et al. Hair follicle mesenchyme-associated PD-L1 regulates T-cell activation induced apoptosis: a potential mechanism of immune privilege. J Invest Dermatol. 2014;134(3):736–45.

28. Adams S, Diamond J, Hamilton E. Phase Ib trial of atezolizumab in combination with nab-paclitaxel in patients with metastatic triple-negative breast cancer (mTNBC). Presented at ASCO Annual Meeting 2016, Chicago, Il, USA, Abstract 1009.

29. Adams S, Schmid P, Rugo H, Winer E, Loirat D, awada A, et al. Phase 2 study of pembrolizumab montherapy for previously treated metastatic triple-negative breast cancer: KEYNOTE-086 cohort A. Presented at ASCO 2017, Chicago, Il, USA, Abstract 1008.

30. Adams S, Loi S, Toppmeyer D, Cescon D, De Laurentis M, Nanda R, et al. Phase 2 study of pembrolizumab as first-line therapy for PD-L1-positive metastatic triple-neative breast cancer: Preliminary data from Keynote-086 cohort B. Presented at ASCO 2017, Chicago, Il, USA, Abstract 108.

5

A phase Ib study of pictilisib (GDC-0941) in combination with paclitaxel, with and without bevacizumab or trastuzumab, and with letrozole in advanced breast cancer

Patrick Schöffski[1,2*], Sara Cresta[3], Ingrid A. Mayer[4], Hans Wildiers[1], Silvia Damian[3], Steven Gendreau[5], Isabelle Rooney[6], Kari M. Morrissey[7], Jill M. Spoerke[5], Vivian W. Ng[8], Stina M. Singel[6] and Eric Winer[9]

Abstract

Background: This phase Ib study (NCT00960960) evaluated pictilisib (GDC-0941; pan-phosphatidylinositol 3-kinase inhibitor) plus paclitaxel, with and without bevacizumab or trastuzumab, or in combination with letrozole, in patients with locally recurrent or metastatic breast cancer.

Methods: This was a three-part multischedule study. Patients in parts 1 and 2, which comprised 3 + 3 dose escalation and cohort expansion stages, received pictilisib (60–330 mg) plus paclitaxel (90 mg/m^2) with and without bevacizumab (10 mg/kg) or trastuzumab (2–4 mg/kg). In part 3, patients received pictilisib (260 mg) plus letrozole (2.5 mg). Primary objectives were evaluation of safety and tolerability, identification of dose-limiting toxicities (DLTs) and the maximum tolerated dose (MTD) of pictilisib, and recommendation of a phase II dosing regimen. Secondary endpoints included pharmacokinetics and preliminary antitumor activity.

Results: Sixty-nine patients were enrolled; all experienced at least one adverse event (AE). Grade ≥ 3 AEs, serious AEs, and AEs leading to death were reported in 50 (72.5%), 21 (30.4%), and 2 (2.9%) patients, respectively. Six (8.7%) patients reported a DLT, and the MTD and recommended phase II pictilisib doses were established where possible. There was no pictilisib–paclitaxel drug–drug interaction. Two (3.4%) patients experienced complete responses, and 17 (29.3%) patients had partial responses.

Conclusions: Combining pictilisib with paclitaxel, with and without bevacizumab or trastuzumab, or letrozole, had a manageable safety profile in patients with locally recurrent or metastatic breast cancer. The combination had antitumor activity, and the additive effect of pictilisib supported further investigation in a randomized study.

Keywords: Pictilisib, GDC-0941, PI3K

Background

Despite improvements in treatment outcomes for patients with metastatic breast cancer, there is a continued unmet need to improve therapies for this patient population. Breast cancer is a heterogeneous disease, and current treatment strategies are based on disease type. Hormone receptor-positive, recurrent, or stage IV breast cancer in postmenopausal women is often managed with endocrine therapies, such as the nonsteroidal aromatase inhibitor letrozole [1], whereas primary treatment options for patients with human epidermal growth factor receptor 2 (HER2)-negative locally recurrent or metastatic breast cancer include single-agent cytotoxic chemotherapeutic agents, such as paclitaxel [1, 2]. Addition of the monoclonal antibody bevacizumab, which blocks angiogenesis by inhibiting vascular endothelial growth factor A,

* Correspondence: patrick.schoffski@uzleuven.be
[1]Department of General Medical Oncology, Leuven Cancer Institute, University Hospitals Leuven, Leuven, Belgium
[2]Department of Oncology, Faculty of Medicine, Laboratory of Experimental Oncology, KU Leuven, Herestraat 49, B-3000 Leuven, Belgium
Full list of author information is available at the end of the article

to paclitaxel has been shown to improve progression-free survival (PFS) and objective response rate (ORR) in patients with first-line metastatic breast cancer [1, 3]. In patients with HER2-positive locally recurrent or metastatic breast cancer, therapies include the antibody–drug conjugate ado-trastuzumab emtansine and the combination of the monoclonal antibodies trastuzumab and pertuzumab, both of which target HER2, with either docetaxel or paclitaxel [1, 2].

The phosphatidylinositol 3-kinase (PI3K) signaling pathway is deregulated in a wide variety of cancers, including breast cancer [4–6], and plays a key role in cell growth, survival, and migration [7]. The PI3K lipid kinases are grouped according to substrate specificity, structure, and mechanism of action into three classes (IA, IB, II, and III) [8]. Activating mutations of the catalytic subunit of PI3K (phosphatidylinositol-4,5-bisphosphate 3-kinase catalytic subunit alpha [PIK3CA]), which belongs to the class IA PI3K family, are frequently observed in breast cancer [9, 10], and approximately 35–45% of cases of hormone receptor-positive breast cancer harbor mutations in this gene [11, 12]. Preclinical data suggest that activation of the PI3K pathway, via mutation of PIK3CA, loss of phosphatase and tensin homolog (PTEN) expression, or HER2 overexpression, may promote resistance to antiestrogen therapy and hormonal independence in estrogen receptor (ER)-positive models of breast cancer [13–15]. In addition, results from three clinical trials suggest that inhibition of both the PI3K/mammalian target of rapamycin (mTOR) and estrogen-signaling pathways may provide improved efficacy compared with single-agent endocrine therapies [16–18]. Thus, inhibition of the PI3K pathway has emerged as a promising strategy for treatment of breast cancer.

Pictilisib (GDC-0941) is a potent and selective oral inhibitor of class I PI3K [19] that prevents the formation of phosphatidylinositol (3,4,5)-trisphosphate, a key component of the PI3K pathway, by binding to the adenosine triphosphate-binding pocket of PI3K [19]. Pictilisib is a pan-PI3K inhibitor that inhibits all four isoforms of class I PI3Ks (p110α, p110β, p110δ, and p110γ subunits) [19] with rapid absorption following oral administration and a dose-proportional pharmacokinetic (PK) profile [20]. Pan-PI3K inhibitors may be better suited to combination therapy than inhibitors of mammalian target of rapamycin complex 1/2, and there is evidence that their activity may not be restricted to tumor types with PIK3CA mutations [21]. In contrast, isoform-specific PI3K inhibitors such as alpelisib (BYL719) and taselisib (GDC-0032), which both selectively target PI3Kα [22, 23], offer the potential specifically to block their target while limiting toxicities associated with a broader inhibition [21].

In preclinical studies, pictilisib had antitumor activity in breast cancer models harboring PIK3CA mutations and/or amplification of HER2, although several models without these mutations were also sensitive to pictilisib treatment [24]. Pictilisib was found to increase the antitumor activity of taxanes, with an associated increase in apoptotic cell death, in multiple breast cancer xenografts [25] and, in combination with trastuzumab, synergistically inhibited cell proliferation and the PI3K signaling pathway in HER2-amplified breast cancer cell lines [26]. Pictilisib was also reported to inhibit the growth of activated human endothelial cells, suggesting the potential for antiangiogenic activity [27].

Single-agent pictilisib was well tolerated and showed evidence of antitumor activity in a phase I study of 60 patients with solid tumors at doses ≥ 100 mg [20]. In addition, the PK profile of single-agent pictilisib was dose-proportional, with a maximum tolerated dose (MTD) of 330 mg administered orally daily [20]. Several studies have investigated the effect of PI3K inhibition in patients with breast cancer and alterations of the PI3K pathway. The phase III BOLERO-2 trial demonstrated that the mTOR inhibitor everolimus, when combined with an aromatase inhibitor, improved PFS in hormone receptor-positive advanced breast cancer previously treated with nonsteroidal aromatase inhibitors [17], although there was no statistically significant improvement in overall survival [28].

This open-label, multischedule phase Ib study aimed to evaluate the safety and PK of pictilisib in combination with paclitaxel, with and without bevacizumab or trastuzumab, or letrozole, in patients with locally recurrent or metastatic breast cancer. In addition, we sought to establish a recommended phase II dose for each treatment combination regimen.

Methods

Patients

Eligible patients were ≥ 18 years with histologically or cytologically confirmed locally recurrent or metastatic adenocarcinoma of the breast. Inclusion criteria specified that patients had HER2-negative tumors, unless in the cohort that received trastuzumab, where all patients were required to have HER2-positive tumors and an Eastern Cooperative Oncology Group Performance Status (ECOG PS) of 0 or 1. Patients who received letrozole were postmenopausal and required to have hormone receptor-positive disease. Adequate hematologic and end-organ function was required, in addition to disease measurable by Response Evaluation Criteria In Solid Tumors (RECIST) v1.0.

Patients who had received more than two prior chemotherapy regimens for locally recurrent or metastatic breast cancer were not eligible for inclusion in the arms that received pictilisib + paclitaxel ± bevacizumab or trastuzumab treatment (parts 1 and 2). Patients were eligible for enrollment in the pictilisib + letrozole arm (part 3) if they were currently receiving letrozole for the treatment of advanced or metastatic breast cancer, but they were excluded if they had received more than one prior chemotherapy regimen or more than two prior endocrine therapy regimens for locally recurrent or metastatic breast cancer. Patients with known hypersensitivity to paclitaxel were excluded.

Patients were not eligible for bevacizumab treatment if they had inadequately controlled hypertension, significant vascular disease within 6 months prior to the first dose of study treatment, history of hemoptysis within 1 month prior to the first dose of study treatment, or evidence of bleeding diathesis or significant coagulopathy. Patients were not eligible for trastuzumab treatment if they had a history of grade ≥ 3 hypersensitivity to the antibody, or grade ≥ 1 with the most recent trastuzumab infusion before study entry, or continued requirement for prolonged trastuzumab infusions (> 30 minutes) to prevent infusion-related reactions. Patients with a history of exposure to anthracyclines (cumulative doses > 500 mg doxorubicin, > 900 mg liposomal doxorubicin, > 900 mg epirubicin, > 120 mg mitoxantrone, and > 90 mg idarubicin; if another anthracycline or more than one anthracycline was used, the cumulative dose could not exceed the equivalent of 500 mg doxorubicin) and cardiopulmonary dysfunction were also excluded.

Study design and treatment

This was an open-label, multicenter, phase Ib dose escalation study (ClinicalTrials.gov registration number NCT00960960) performed in three parts. Parts 1 and 2 comprised two stages (a 3 + 3 dose escalation stage and a cohort expansion stage), with the dose escalation stage designed to evaluate the safety, tolerability, and PK of pictilisib in combination with paclitaxel, or with paclitaxel plus bevacizumab or trastuzumab. Part 3 had a 3 + 3 dose escalation enrollment design and assessed the combination of pictilisib and letrozole. Patients were assigned in the order in which they were enrolled.

In part 1, patients received oral pictilisib (at an initial dose of 60 mg) administered daily on days 1–21 of each 28-day cycle ("21 + 7" schedule) and 90 mg/m^2 intravenous paclitaxel (cohort 1) or 90 mg/m^2 intravenous paclitaxel plus 10 mg/kg intravenous bevacizumab (all subsequent cohorts). On study treatment days, pictilisib was administered prior to paclitaxel or bevacizumab. Paclitaxel was administered on days 1, 8, and 15 of each 28-day cycle, and bevacizumab was administered on days 1 and 15 of each 28-day cycle.

In part 2, patients received oral pictilisib (daily for 5 of 7 consecutive days ["5 + 2" schedule]) in combination with 90 mg/m^2 intravenous paclitaxel. Once the MTD had been established, two additional arms were opened to determine the MTD for pictilisib in combination with

paclitaxel plus 10 mg/kg intravenous bevacizumab or 2–4 mg/kg intravenous trastuzumab. The starting dose for pictilisib in combination with paclitaxel plus bevacizumab was at or below the MTD for pictilisib plus paclitaxel, whereas the starting dose for pictilisib in combination with paclitaxel plus trastuzumab was at least one dose level below the MTD for pictilisib plus paclitaxel alone. Paclitaxel was administered on days 1, 8, and 15 of each 28-day cycle; bevacizumab was administered on days 1 and 15 of each 28-day cycle; and trastuzumab was administered on days 1, 8, 15, and 22 of each 28-day cycle.

In part 3, patients were treated with 260 mg pictilisib plus 2.5 mg letrozole by continuous daily dosing in 28-day cycles.

Either the MTD or a lower dose was selected as the recommended phase II dose. This was dependent on both the MTD-defining dose-limiting toxicities (DLTs) and the adverse events (AEs) reported during the DLT observation period and beyond in all patients treated at a given dose. Study treatment was discontinued in patients who experienced disease progression or unacceptable toxicity or who were not compliant with the study protocol.

Tumor assessments were performed according to RECIST v1.0. In parts 1 and 2, assessments were performed at screening and at the end of cycles 2, 5, 8, and 11 and every three cycles thereafter for patients who were on the study for > 1 year. Objective responses were confirmed ≥ 4 weeks after the initial documentation. In part 3, assessments were performed at screening and on day 1 of cycle 4 (± 7 days) and on day 1 (± 7 days) every three cycles thereafter.

Safety assessment

AEs were graded according to the National Cancer Institute Common Terminology Criteria for Adverse Events, version 3.0 [29]. AEs were recorded until 30 days after the last dose of study treatment or until initiation of another anticancer therapy, whichever occurred first.

DLT was defined as one of the following AEs, if occurring during the DLT assessment window (following the first dose of pictilisib and including evaluations prior to dosing on day 1 of cycle 2) and considered by the investigator to be related to study treatment: grade ≥ 3 nonhematologic, nonhepatic major organ AE; grade ≥ 4 thrombocytopenia lasting > 48 hours or associated with clinically significant bleeding; grade ≥ 3 fasting hyperglycemia; grade ≥ 4 neutropenia lasting ≥ 7 days; grade ≥ 3 febrile neutropenia; grade ≥ 3 total bilirubin, alkaline phosphatase (ALP), or hepatic transaminases (alanine aminotransferase or aspartate aminotransferase); grade ≥ 2 lung diffusing capacity concomitant with a decrease of $\geq 20\%$ from baseline.

AEs that were not considered DLTs included grade 3 nausea, vomiting, or diarrhea that resolved to grade ≤ 1 with optimal medical management within 3 days, grade 3 hypertension for patients receiving bevacizumab, grade 3 fasting hyperglycemia that resolved to grade ≤ 1 within 7 days (with or without antihyperglycemic therapy), and grade 3 fasting hyperglycemia within 3 days of gluco-corticoid use. For patients with grade 1 hepatic transaminase levels at baseline, a hepatic transaminase elevation > 7.5 times the upper limit of normal (ULN) was considered a DLT. For patients with grade 1 ALP levels at baseline, an elevation > 7.5 times the ULN was considered a DLT.

The DLT assessment window followed the first dose of pictilisib and included evaluations prior to dosing on day 1 of cycle 2. The MTD was exceeded if a DLT was observed in at least one-third of patients or if greater than one-third of patients in a cohort missed ≥ 5 days of pictilisib for drug-related AEs.

PK analysis
Blood samples were collected after single and multiple doses of pictilisib, paclitaxel, and letrozole for PK evaluations. Plasma concentrations of pictilisib, paclitaxel, 6α-hydroxy paclitaxel (6α-OH-paclitaxel; cytochrome P450 2C8 [CYP2C8]-formed metabolite of paclitaxel), and letrozole were determined using validated liquid chromatography-tandem mass spectrometry (LC-MS/MS) methods, and PK parameters were estimated using noncompartmental analysis (WinNonlin 6.4; Pharsight, Mountain View, CA USA).

Outcomes
The primary endpoints for the treatment combinations of pictilisib with letrozole alone, paclitaxel alone, and paclitaxel in combination with bevacizumab or trastuzumab, were safety and tolerability, DLTs, MTD, and identification of a recommended phase II dosing regimen. The secondary endpoints were PK of pictilisib and preliminary antitumor activity (ORR, duration of response [DoR], and PFS). Exploratory objectives included exploration of the potential relationship between PI3K pathway alterations and antitumor activity, as well as identification of the potential role of polymorphisms in drug metabolism enzyme and transporter genes in the PK disposition, and/or response to pictilisib, standard-of-care chemotherapy regimens, or antiestrogen agents.

Biomarker assessments
Mutational analysis of *PIK3CA* was performed using RT-PCR assays as previously described [30]. Nucleotide substitutions in the amino acids E542 (K), E545 (A, G, D, or K), Q546 (E, K, L, or R), and H1047 (L, R, or Y) or the wild-type alleles were detected. PTEN expression

was examined with immunohistochemistry as previously described (clone 138G6; Cell Signaling Technology, Danvers, MA, USA), and an H-score was assigned to each sample on the basis of the percentage of cells staining at four different levels of intensity (0, 1+, 2+, or 3+) [31].

Statistical methods
Final analysis was performed on cumulative clinical data collected until the last patient's last visit. The efficacy-evaluable population, which was the basis for ORR analysis, was defined as treated patients with baseline measurable disease and at least one postbaseline tumor assessment, or discontinuation of the study due to disease progression or death within 30 days of treatment initiation. All analyses were based on the safety-evaluable population, which was defined as all enrolled patients who received any dose of pictilisib. This study was designed not with regard to explicit power and type I error considerations, but to obtain preliminary safety and PK information in this patient population. The data cutoff for all analyses was December 1, 2015.

Results
Patient characteristics
Overall, 69 patients were enrolled in the study (August 2009 to December 2015), with 20 patients in part 1 (pictilisib + paclitaxel ± bevacizumab), 18 patients in part 2A (pictilisib + paclitaxel), 15 patients in part 2B (pictilisib + paclitaxel + bevacizumab), 9 patients in part 2C (pictilisib + paclitaxel + trastuzumab), and 7 patients in part 3 (pictilisib + letrozole) (Fig. 1). At final analysis, all patients had discontinued study treatment because of an AE (21.7%), progressive disease (58.0%), physician decision (13.0%), patient decision (5.8%), or sponsor termination of the study (1.4%). Baseline characteristics were well balanced among treatment groups (Table 1). The median age of all patients was 54.0 years (range, 30–76 years), and the majority of patients (71.0%) had hormone receptor-positive disease.

Safety
The safety profile of all dosing regimens examined in this dose-finding trial was assessed. All patients experienced at least one AE (Table 2), and the most common AEs (reported in ≥ 30% of patients) were diarrhea (78.3%), nausea (62.3%), fatigue (59.4%), alopecia (52.2%), rash (50.7%), neutropenia (44.9%), stomatitis (37.7%), vomiting (33.3%), decreased appetite (33.3%), and cough (30.4%). The most common AEs related to any study drug (≥ 15% of patients) were diarrhea (75.4%), nausea (58.0%), fatigue (56.5%), alopecia (52.2%), rash (46.4%), neutropenia (44.9%), and stomatitis (36.2%) (Additional file 1: Table S1). The majority of patients experienced a grade ≥ 3 AE (n = 50; 72.5%)

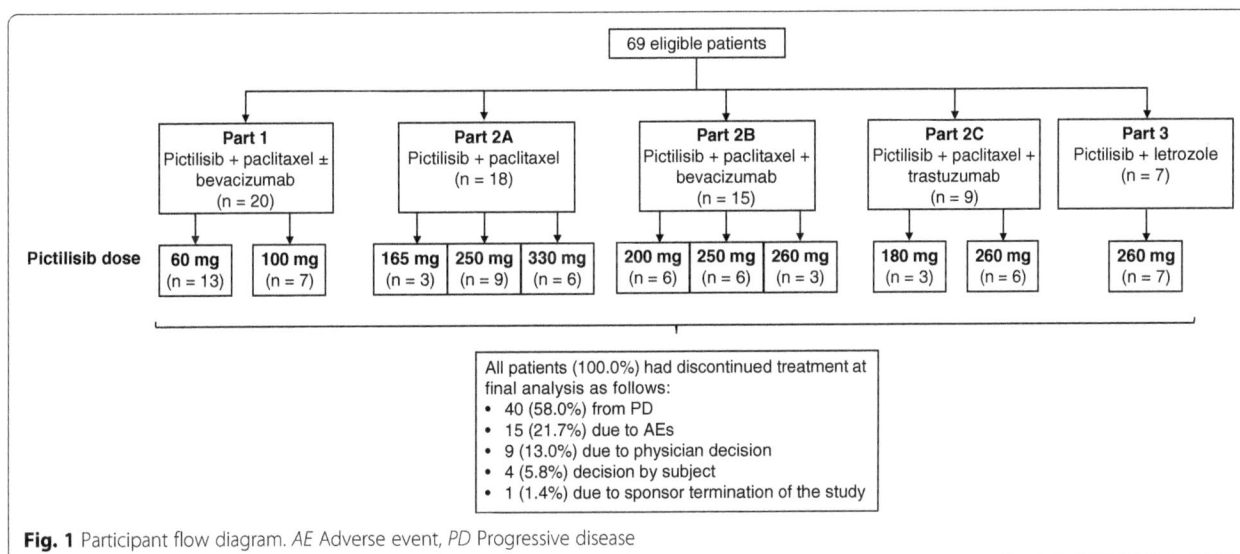

Fig. 1 Participant flow diagram. *AE* Adverse event, *PD* Progressive disease

(Table 2), and the most common (in at least two patients) were neutropenia ($n = 19$), rash ($n = 7$), peripheral neuropathy ($n = 4$), hypophosphatemia ($n = 3$), decreased lung diffusing capacity ($n = 3$), dyspnea ($n = 2$), hypertension ($n = 2$), diarrhea ($n = 2$), nausea ($n = 2$), pneumonia ($n = 2$), increased blood glucose ($n = 2$), decreased appetite ($n = 2$), pulmonary embolism ($n = 2$), nail disorder ($n = 2$), and deep vein thrombosis ($n = 2$). In addition, most patients ($n = 43$; 62.3%) experienced at least one grade ≥ 3 AE related to any study drug (Additional file 1: Table S1). Overall, serious AEs were reported in 30.4% of patients ($n = 21$) (Table 2 and Additional file 1: Table S2) and those reported in at least two patients included pneumonia ($n = 2$), nausea ($n = 2$), decreased lung diffusing capacity ($n = 2$), and pulmonary embolism ($n = 2$).

Fifteen patients (21.7%) had an AE that led to discontinuation of any study drug (Table 2), and the most common were peripheral neuropathy ($n = 5$), decreased lung diffusing capacity ($n = 4$), rash ($n = 3$), neutropenia ($n = 2$), paresthesia ($n = 2$), pulmonary embolism ($n = 2$), deep vein thrombosis ($n = 2$), and hypertension ($n = 2$). In the case of pictilisib, 18 patients (26.1%) experienced AEs leading to withdrawal (Table 2) and those in at least two patients were decreased lung diffusing capacity ($n = 4$), rash ($n = 3$), and deep vein thrombosis ($n = 2$). AEs that led to pictilisib dose reduction included grade 2 neutropenia ($n = 3$) and grades 1 and 3 rash ($n = 1$ and $n = 2$, respectively). Thirty-nine (56.5%) patients had their pictilisib dose interrupted owing to an AE, whereas six patients (8.7%) had their dose reduced (Table 2). Withdrawal of paclitaxel, bevacizumab, and trastuzumab occurred in 21 patients (33.9%), 14 patients (40.0%), and two patients (22.2%), respectively (Table 2).

AEs of special interest included pneumonitis (3 [4.3%] patients), hyperglycemia or increased blood glucose (15 [21.7%] patients), left ventricular dysfunction (1 [1.4%] patient), and decreased carbon monoxide-diffusing capacity (5 [7.2%] patients) (Additional file 1: Table S3). Grade ≥ 3 AEs of special interest in these patients were reported for hyperglycemia or increased blood glucose (4 [5.8%] patients), left ventricular dysfunction (1 [1.4%] patient), and decreased carbon monoxide-diffusing capacity (3 [4.3%] patients) (Additional file 1: Table S3).

Two patients (2.9%) experienced AEs that led to a fatal outcome (Table 2). One patient had grade 5 left ventricular dysfunction, considered by the investigator to be related to pictilisib, bevacizumab, and paclitaxel. The other patient experienced grade 5 worsened ECOG PS, which was considered by the investigator to be related to pictilisib and unrelated to letrozole.

Overall, six patients (8.7%) reported DLTs (Table 2 and Additional file 1: Table S4). In part 1, one DLT was reported with 60 mg pictilisib, whereas none were observed with the 100-mg dose (pictilisib administered on the "21 + 7" dosing schedule and in combination with paclitaxel and bevacizumab). In part 2A, one DLT was observed in a patient treated with 250 mg pictilisib ("5 + 2" dosing schedule and in combination with paclitaxel), whereas there were two DLTs at the next dose level (330 mg pictilisib); thus, the MTD was exceeded. In part 2B, there was one reported DLT in a patient treated with 250 mg pictilisib ("5 + 2" dosing schedule and administered in combination with paclitaxel and bevacizumab), whereas in part 2C a DLT was observed in one patient treated with 260 mg pictilisib ("5 + 2" dosing schedule and administered in combination with paclitaxel plus trastuzumab). There were no DLTs reported in part 3 (260 mg pictilisib administered continuously with letrozole).

The MTD was defined in part 2A as 250 mg pictilisib ("5 + 2" dosing schedule) in combination with paclitaxel

Table 1 Baseline demographics and clinical characteristics

Characteristic	Part 1: pictilisib + paclitaxel ± bevacizumab[a] (n = 20)	Part 2A: pictilisib + paclitaxel (n = 18)	Part 2B: pictilisib + paclitaxel + bevacizumab (n = 15)	Part 2C: pictilisib + paclitaxel + trastuzumab (n = 9)	Part 3: pictilisib + letrozole (n = 7)	All patients (N = 69)
Median age, years (range)	54.0 (41–71)	53.5 (30–76)	49.0 (34–66)	63.0 (42–68)	59.0 (49–69)	54.0 (30–76)
ECOG PS, n (%)						
0	14 (70.0)	6 (33.3)	13 (86.7)	5 (55.6)	4 (57.1)	42 (60.9)
1	5 (25.0)	12 (66.7)	2 (13.3)	4 (44.4)	3 (42.9)	26 (37.7)
Unknown	1 (5.0)	(0.0)	(0.0)	(0.0)	(0.0)	1 (1.4)
ER/PR status, n (%)						
Positive	13 (65.0)	11 (61.1)	10 (66.7)	8 (88.9)	7 (100.0)	49 (71.0)
Negative	7 (35.0)	6 (33.3)	5 (33.3)	1 (11.1)	(0.0)	19 (27.5)
Unknown	(0.0)	1 (5.6)	(0.0)	(0.0)	(0.0)	1 (1.4)
HER2 status, n (%)						
Positive	(0.0)	(0.0)	(0.0)	9 (100.0)	(0.0)	9 (13.0)
Negative	20 (100.00)	18 (100.00)	15 (100.00)	(0.00)	7 (100.00)	60 (87.00)
Prior chemotherapy, n (%)						
Neoadjuvant	6 (30.0)	7 (38.9)	5 (33.3)	3 (33.3)	1 (14.3)	22 (31.9)
Adjuvant setting	12 (60.0)	8 (44.4)	7 (46.7)	4 (44.4)	4 (57.1)	35 (50.7)
Metastatic setting	10 (50.0)	9 (50.0)	8 (53.3)	8 (88.9)	(0.0)	35 (50.7)
Prior treatment, n (%)						
Taxanes	10 (50.0)	10 (55.6)	8 (53.3)	6 (66.7)	3 (42.9)	37 (53.6)
Anti-HER2 therapies	2 (10.0)	1 (5.6)	(0.0)	9 (100.0)	(0.0)	12 (17.4)
Bevacizumab	1 (5.0)	2 (11.1)	1 (6.7)	(0.0)	1 (14.3)	5 (7.2)
Line of therapy (metastatic setting)						
First	3 (15.0)	5 (27.8)	1 (6.7)	(0.0)	2 (28.6)	11 (15.9)
Second or later[b]	17 (85.0)	13 (72.2)	14 (93.3)	9 (100.0)	5 (71.4)	58 (84.1)

Abbreviations: ECOG PS Eastern Cooperative Oncology Group Performance Status, *ER* Estrogen receptor, *HER2* Human epidermal growth factor receptor, *PR* Progesterone receptor
[a]One patient did not receive bevacizumab
[b]Nineteen patients had four to ten prior lines of therapy

and was not established in all other arms. The MTD or maximum administered dose and recommended phase II doses of pictilisib were 100 mg (when administered with paclitaxel and bevacizumab ["21 + 7" dosing schedule]), 250 mg (when administered with paclitaxel or paclitaxel plus bevacizumab ["5 + 2" dosing schedule]), or 260 mg (when administered with paclitaxel and trastuzumab ["5 + 2" dosing schedule] or letrozole [continuous dosing schedule]).

PK analysis

In vitro data suggest that pictilisib has a moderate potential to inhibit the CYP2C8-mediated metabolism of paclitaxel to 6α-OH-paclitaxel. In this study, a consistent 6α-OH-paclitaxel:paclitaxel AUC ratio was observed across all pictilisib dose levels (Fig. 2), suggesting there was no drug–drug interaction between pictilisib and paclitaxel. In addition, no differences in the PK of pictilisib or letrozole were observed in any of the treatment combination regimens compared with historical single-agent data (data not shown).

Clinical activity

Fifty-eight (84.1%) patients were included in the efficacy-evaluable population for ORR analysis. Complete responses were observed in two patients (3.4%) overall, in parts 1 (5.3%; paclitaxel + bevacizumab) and 2A (5.9%; pictilisib + paclitaxel) (Table 3). Partial responses were observed in patients treated with pictilisib + paclitaxel ± bevacizumab (part 1; 21.1%), pictilisib + paclitaxel (part 2A; 17.6%), pictilisib + paclitaxel + bevacizumab (part 2B; 53.8%), pictilisib + paclitaxel + trastuzumab (part 2C; 33.3%), and pictilisib + letrozole (part 3; 33.3%) (Table 3). The majority of patients showed signs of tumor shrinkage (Fig. 3a–d).

The median DoR was 8.9 months (95% CI, 6.47–11.10) among five responders treated with pictilisib + paclitaxel ± bevacizumab (part 1) and 8.8 months (95% CI, 4.40–15.34) among seven responders treated with pictilisib + paclitaxel + bevacizumab (part 2B) (Table 3).

In all treated patients (N = 69), median PFS ranged from 5.0 months (95% CI, 3.71–NE) in patients treated with pictilisib + paclitaxel (part 2A; n = 18) to 14.8 months

A phase Ib study of pictilisib (GDC-0941) in combination with paclitaxel...

61

Table 2 Safety overview (safety population, regardless of causality)

Pictilisib dose n (%)	Part 1: pictilisib + paclitaxel ± bevacizumab[a]		Part 2A: pictilisib + paclitaxel			Part 2B: pictilisib + paclitaxel + bevacizumab			Part 2C: pictilisib + paclitaxel + trastuzumab		Part 3: pictilisib + letrozole	All patients (N = 69)
	60 mg (n = 13)	100 mg (n = 7)	165 mg (n = 3)	250 mg (n = 9)	330 mg (n = 6)	200 mg (n = 6)	250 mg (n = 6)	260 mg (n = 3)	180 mg (n = 3)	260 mg (n = 6)	260 mg (n = 7)	
All-grade AEs	13 (100)	7 (100)	3 (100)	9 (100)	6 (100)	6 (100)	6 (100)	3 (100)	3 (100)	6 (100)	7 (100)	69 (100)
Grades 3–4 AEs	8 (61.5)	7 (100)	3 (100)	7 (77.8)	5 (83.3)	3 (50.0)	5 (83.3)	3 (100)	1 (33.3)	3 (50.0)	3 (42.9)	48 (69.6)
Grade 5 AEs	1 (7.7)[b]	0	0	0	0	0	0	0	0	0	1 (14.3)[c]	2 (2.9)
SAEs	3 (23.1)	1 (14.3)	1 (33.3)	5 (55.6)	5 (83.3)	2 (33.3)	0	0	0	1 (16.7)	3 (42.9)	21 (30.4)
DLTs	1 (7.7)	0	0	1 (11.1)	2 (33.3)	0	1 (16.7)	0	0	1 (16.7)	0	6 (8.7)
Study withdrawal due to AE	3 (23.1)	2 (28.6)	0	1 (11.1)	2 (33.3)	0	1 (16.7)	2 (66.7)	0	2 (33.3)	2 (28.6)	15 (21.7)
Pictilisib withdrawal due to AE	4 (30.8)	2 (28.6)	1 (33.3)	1 (11.1)	2 (33.3)	0	1 (16.7)	3 (100)	0	2 (33.3)	2 (28.6)	18 (26.1) n = 62
Paclitaxel withdrawal due to AE	6 (46.2)	3 (42.9)	2 (66.7)	1 (11.1)	2 (33.3)	0	1 (16.7)	2 (66.7)	1 (33.3)	3 (50.0)	–	21 (33.9) n = 35
Bevacizumab withdrawal due to AE	6 (46.2)	3 (42.9)	–	–	–	2 (33.3)	1 (16.7)	2 (66.7)	–	–	–	14 (40.0) (n = 9)
Trastuzumab withdrawal due to AE	–	–	–	–	–	–	–	–	0	0 2 (33.3)	–	2 (22.2)
Letrozole withdrawal due to AE	–	–	–	–	–	–	–	–	–	–	2 (28.6)	–
Pictilisib dose reduction due to AE	0	0	0	1 (11.1)	1 (16.7)	0	3 (50.0)	1 (33.3)	0	0	0	6 (8.7)
Pictilisib dose interruption due to AE	7 (53.8)	3 (42.9)	2 (66.7)	5 (55.6)	4 (66.7)	4 (66.7)	3 (50.0)	3 (100)	0	4 (66.7)	4 (57.4)	39 (56.5)

Abbreviations: AE Adverse event, *DLT* Dose-limiting toxicity, *ECOG PS* Eastern Cooperative Oncology Group Performance Status, *SAE* Serious adverse event

[a] One patient did not receive bevacizumab
[b] Patient had grade 5 left ventricular dysfunction
[c] Patient had a worsened ECOG PS (grade 5)

(95% CI, 3.52–16.62) in patients treated with pictilisib + paclitaxel + trastuzumab (part 2C; n = 9) (Table 3).

PIK3CA mutation status and PTEN expression were evaluated in 24 formalin-fixed, paraffin-embedded tumor samples from parts 2A, 2B and 2C. Four of the 24 samples were evaluable for PTEN only (n = 2) or *PIK3CA* only (n = 2). PTEN expression was reduced or absent in five of the 22 samples examined, whereas 10 of 22 samples harbored a *PIK3CA* mutation. Among the patients in part 2A and 2B with evaluable tissue and either a *PIK3CA* mutation or PTEN loss, five of 11 (45.5%) had a complete or partial response compared with two of seven (28.6%) patients without these alterations (Fig. 3b).

Discussion

This phase Ib study evaluated the safety and PK of the pan-PI3K inhibitor pictilisib in combination with paclitaxel, with and without bevacizumab or trastuzumab, or letrozole,

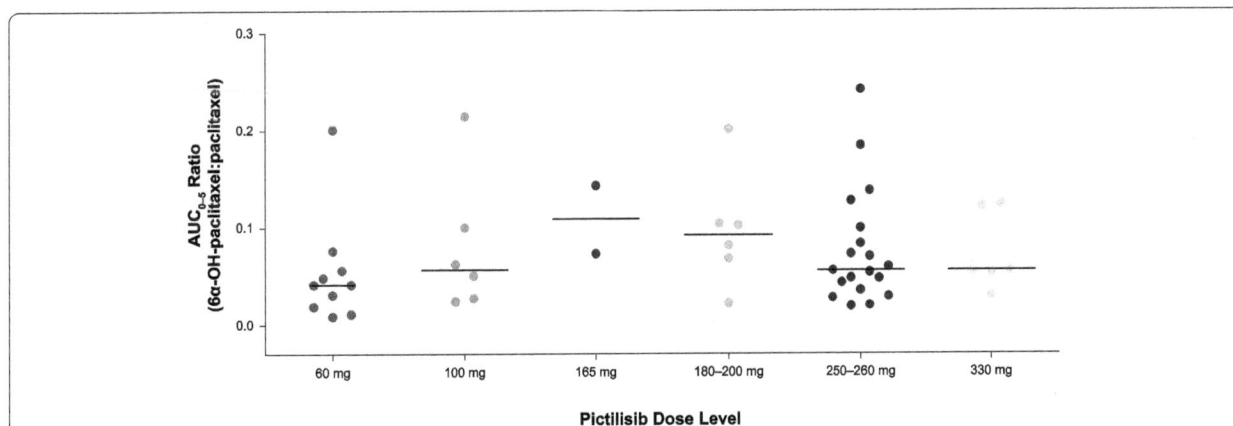

Fig. 2 Plasma 6α-OH-paclitaxel/paclitaxel AUC ratio as a function of pictilisib dose. Patients with evaluable 6α-OH-paclitaxel and paclitaxel PK after multiple doses of paclitaxel and pictilisib were pooled across all paclitaxel treatment arms (parts 1 and 2, n = 49). *Black lines* represent the median ratio for each dose level, and *dots* represent individual subject ratios. *PK* Pharmacokinetics

in patients with locally recurrent or metastatic breast cancer. At a dose of 260 mg, pictilisib had a manageable safety profile, when combined with paclitaxel, with and without bevacizumab or trastuzumab ("21 + 7" or "5 + 2" dosing schedules) or in combination with 2.5 mg letrozole. The MTD of pictilisib was exceeded in patients treated with 330 mg pictilisib plus paclitaxel. Antitumor activity was observed across all treatment arms. The PK analysis suggested no evidence of a clinical drug–drug interaction between agents in each of the evaluated treatment combination regimens. Taking the potential benefit–risk balance into consideration, 260 mg pictilisib was selected as the recommended phase II dose.

Previous clinical trials of pictilisib have reported inconsistent results. The first-in-human phase I trial of single-agent pictilisib in patients with advanced solid tumors demonstrated evidence of antitumor activity in patients with gastrointestinal stromal tumors, cervical cancer, melanoma, colorectal cancer, cholangiocarcinoma, breast cancer, and ovarian cancer, and it showed that pictilisib was well tolerated [20]. Addition of pictilisib to anastrozole in patients with ER-positive, HER2-negative early breast cancer in the OPPORTUNE study significantly decreased tumor cell proliferation [32]. The randomized phase II PEGGY trial (NCT01740336) did not show any benefit from the addition of pictilisib to paclitaxel in patients with hormone receptor-positive, HER2-negative locally recurrent or metastatic breast cancer [33]. Moreover, a randomized phase II trial (FERGI;

NCT01437566) in patients with ER-positive, HER2-negative, endocrine-resistant breast cancer found that the addition of pictilisib to fulvestrant did not significantly improve PFS [34]. Although the phase III BELLE-2 study (NCT01610284) reported modest improvements in median PFS (1.9 months) in patients with hormone receptor-positive metastatic breast cancer treated with the pan-PI3K inhibitor buparlisib (BKM120) in combination with fulvestrant (versus placebo plus fulvestrant) [35], combining a PI3K inhibitor with different therapies is challenging. In both the PEGGY and FERGI studies, efficacy was likely limited by the higher incidence of AEs and dose reductions/discontinuations owing to AEs with pictilisib treatment [33, 34]. As a result, further development of pictilisib by the sponsor is not planned.

Exploratory biomarker analyses in this study showed a numerical difference in ORR between tumors that harbored a *PIK3CA* mutation or had PTEN loss (45.5%) and those without these alterations (28.6%); however, this study was not powered to distinguish antitumor activity between these patient groups, and results were interpreted with caution owing to small patient numbers. Previous studies found little evidence for a link between *PIK3CA* mutations and antitumor activity with pictilisib [32–34].

Although there was evidence of antitumor activity with pictilisib in this patient population, the sample size was limited. Thus, because efficacy was not the primary endpoint and the study was not powered to detect meaningful

Table 3 Clinical activity in patients with measurable disease at baseline (efficacy-evaluable population)

	Part 1: pictilisib + paclitaxel ± bevacizumab[a]	Part 2A: pictilisib + paclitaxel	Part 2B: pictilisib + paclitaxel + bevacizumab	Part 2C: pictilisib + paclitaxel + trastuzumab	Part 3: pictilisib + letrozole	All patients
ORR						
Best confirmed response, n (%)	n = 19	n = 17	n = 13	n = 6	n = 3	n = 58
CR	1 (5.3)	1 (5.9)	(0.0)	(0.0)	(0.0)	2 (3.4)
PR	4 (21.1)	3 (17.6)	7 (53.8)	2 (33.3)	1 (33.3)	17 (29.3)
SD	11 (57.9)	9 (52.9)	6 (46.2)	3 (50.0)	2 (66.7)	31 (53.4)
PD	2 (10.5)	4 (23.5)	(0.0)	(0.0)	(0.0)	6 (10.3)
NE	1 (5.3)	(0.0)	(0.0)	1 (16.7)	(0.0)	2 (3.4)
DoR	n = 5	n = 4	n = 7	n = 2	n = 1	
Patients with an event, n (%)	3 (60.0)	0 (0.0)	5 (71.4)	1 (50.0)	0 (0.0)	–
Median DoR, months	8.9	NE	8.8	NE	NE	–
95% CI	6.47–11.10	NE–NE	4.40–15.34	5.36–NE	NE–NE	–
PFS	n = 20	n = 18	n = 15	n = 9	n = 7	
Patients with an event, n (%)	13 (65.0)	10 (55.6)	10 (66.7)	5 (55.6)	5 (71.4)	–
Median duration of PFS, months	5.8	5.0	7.5	14.8	5.4	–
95% CI	3.52–10.87	3.71–NE	4.60–10.41	3.52–16.62	1.87–NE	–

Abbreviations: CR Complete response, *DoR* Duration of response, *NE* Nonevaluable, *PD* Progressive disease, *PFS* Progression-free survival, *PR* Partial response, *SD* Stable disease
a One patient did not receive bevacizumab

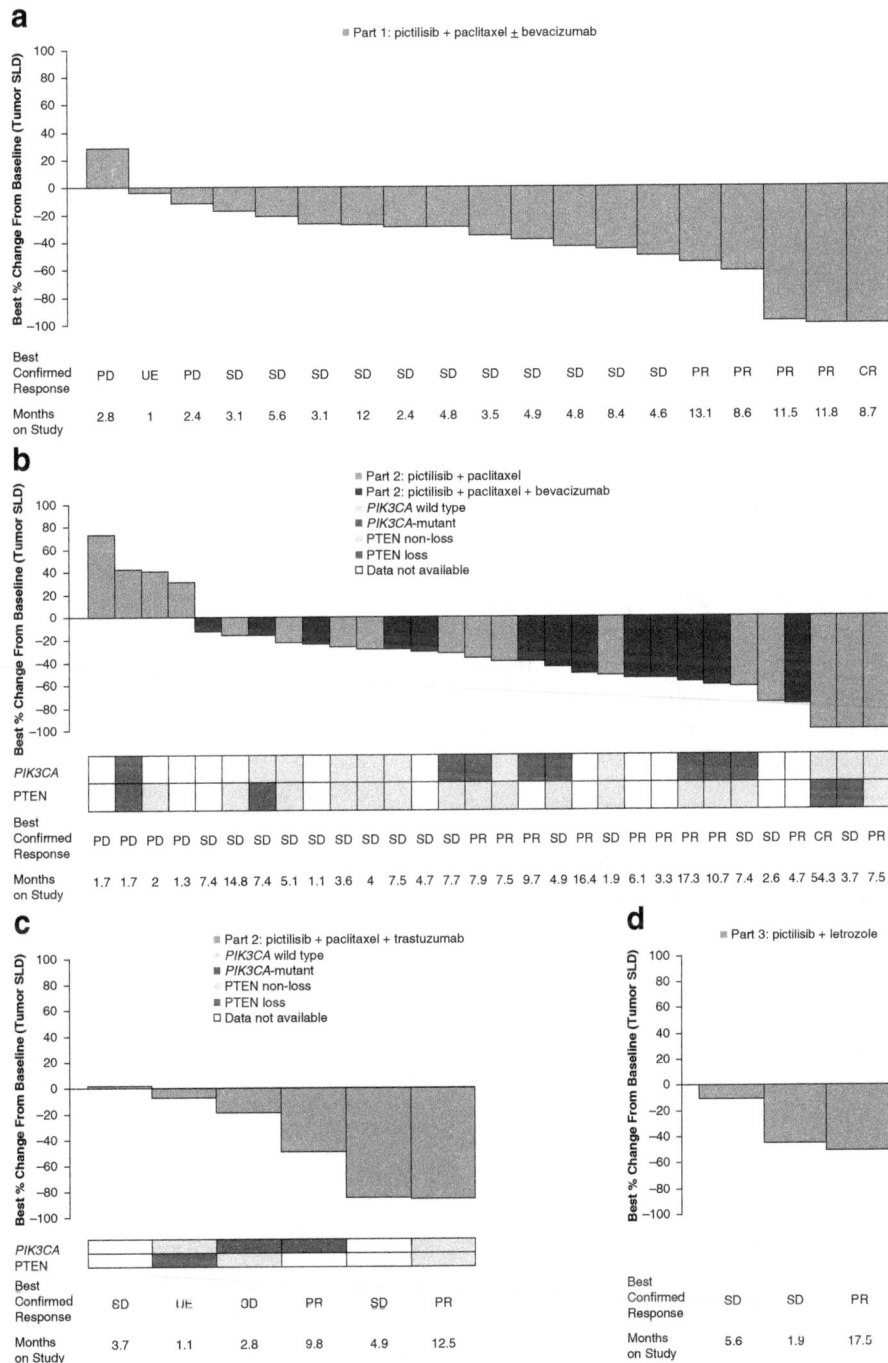

Fig. 3 Waterfall plot of maximum percentage changes from baseline in SLD for target lesions. Maximum percentage changes are shown in (**a**) part 1 (pictilisib + paclitaxel ± bevacizumab), (**b**) parts 2A and B (2A: pictilisib + paclitaxel; 2B: pictilisib + paclitaxel + bevacizumab), (**c**) part 2C (pictilisib + paclitaxel + trastuzumab), and (**d**) part 3 (pictilisib + letrozole). PTEN categories were defined as PTEN loss (PTEN H-score ≥ 0 but ≤ 100) or nonloss (PTEN H-score > 100). *CR* Complete response, *MND* Mutation not detectable, *PD* Progressive disease, *PIK3CA* Phosphatidylinositol-45-bisphosphate 3-kinase catalytic subunit-alpha, *PR* Partial response, *PTEN* Phosphatase and tensin homolog, *SD* Stable disease, *SLD* Sum of the longest diameters, *UE* Unevaluable

differences between study arms, the conclusions of the observed antitumor activity are limited.

Targeting the PI3K pathway with isoform-specific inhibitors may decrease dose modifications caused by toxicity.

Alpelisib showed some single-agent activity, with a favorable safety profile, in patients with *PIK3CA*-mutant advanced breast cancer [36]. In addition, alpelisib in combination with fulvestrant demonstrated clinical activity in

Table 4 Ethical approval: list of independent ethics committees and institutional review boards

Country	Central ethics committee
United States	Dana Farber Cancer Institute Institutional Review Board
Italy	Comitato Etico Indipendente della Fondazione IRCCS Istituto Nazionale dei Tumori di Milano
Belgium	Commissie Medische Ethiek van de Universitaire Ziekenhuizen KU Leuven
United States	Vanderbilt University Institutional Review Board
United States	University of Illinois College of Medicine at Peoria

patients with ER-positive, *PIK3CA*-mutated, locally advanced or metastatic breast cancer [37], whereas alpelisib in combination with letrozole was well tolerated, with evidence of clinical activity in patients with ER-positive metastatic breast cancer that was refractory to endocrine therapy [38]. Taselisib, a potent and selective PI3K inhibitor that has greater selectivity for mutant PI3Kα isoforms than wild-type PI3Kα [23, 39, 40], has single-agent activity in tumors with *PIK3CA* mutations [41]. Thus, taselisib is currently being evaluated in combination with fulvestrant in postmenopausal women with ER-positive, HER2-negative, *PIK3CA*-mutant, locally advanced or metastatic breast cancer (ClinicalTrials.gov identifier NCT02340221) [42].

Conclusions

The combination of pictilisib with paclitaxel, with and without bevacizumab or trastuzumab, or letrozole, in this phase Ib study had an acceptable safety profile with manageable toxicities, with evidence of antitumor activity in patients with locally recurrent or metastatic breast cancer. The effect of pictilisib in combination with paclitaxel supported further investigation in a randomized clinical study.

Abbreviations

6α-OH-paclitaxel: 6α-Hydroxy paclitaxel; AE: Adverse event; ALP: Alkaline phosphatase; CR: Complete response; DLT: Dose-limiting toxicities; DoR: Duration of response; ECOG PS: Eastern Cooperative Oncology Group Performance Status; ER: Estrogen receptor; HER2: Human epidermal growth factor receptor 2; MND: Mutation not detectable; MTD: Maximum tolerated dose; mTOR: Mammalian target of rapamycin; NE: Nonevaluable; ORR: Objective response rate; PD: Progressive disease; PFS: Progression-free survival; PI3K: Phosphatidylinositol 3-kinase; PIK3CA: Phosphatidylinositol-4,5-bisphosphate 3-kinase catalytic subunit alpha; PK: Pharmacokinetics; PR: Partial response; PTEN: Phosphatase and tensin homolog; RECIST: Response Evaluation Criteria In Solid Tumors; SAE: Serious adverse event; SD: Stable disease; SLD: Sum of the longest diameters; UE: Unevaluable; ULN: Upper limit of normal

Acknowledgements

We thank the patients, their families, the nurses, and the investigators who participated in this study. Support for third-party writing assistance, furnished by Islay Steele, PhD, of Health Interactions, was provided by F. Hoffmann-La Roche Ltd.

Funding

This study was funded by Genentech Inc./F. Hoffmann-La Roche Ltd.

Disclosure of prior publication

These analyses were presented previously in part in abstract form [43].

Authors' contributions

PS, SG, and KMM were involved in the conception and design of the study. SG, JMS, and SMS were involved in development of the methodology used. PS, SC, IAM, HW, SD, and EW were involved in acquisition of data (provided animals, acquired and managed patients, provided facilities). PS, HW, SG, KMM, VWN, and SMS were involved in analysis and interpretation of data (e.g., statistical analysis, biostatistics, computational analysis). SG, IR, JMS, VWN, and SMS were involved in administrative, technical, or material support (i.e., reporting or organizing data, constructing databases). SMS and EW were involved in study supervision. All authors were involved in the writing, review, and/or revision of this manuscript. All authors read and approved the final manuscript.

Competing interests

PS has received travel support from Roche for presentation of parts of this work at the 37th San Antonio Breast Cancer Symposium in 2014, institutional research support from Genentech for exploring pictilisib in patient-derived xenograft models of sarcoma, and institutional technical support from Roche (donation of a LightCycler). In addition, and outside the submitted work, PS has received honoraria (institutional support) from Daiichi Sankyo, Eisai, Eli Lilly, Medpace, Novartis, and Swedish Orphan Biovitrium; consulting or advisory role institutional support from Sixth Element Capital, Adaptimmune, Amcure, AstraZeneca, Bayer, Blueprint Medicines, BMS, Boehringer Ingelheim, Cristal Therapeutics, Daiichi Sankyo, Eisai, Eli Lilly, Epizyme, Genzyme, Ipsen, Loxo Oncology, Medpace, Nektar, Novartis, Philogen, PIQUR Therapeutics, and Plexxikon; speaker's bureau institutional support from Bayer, Eisai, Eli Lilly, GSK, Novartis, PharmaMar, and Swedish Orphan Biovitrium; research funding (institutional support) from Bayer, Blueprint Medicines, CoBioRes NV, Exelixis, GSK, Novartis, and Plexxikon; and institutional support for travel, accommodation, and expenses from Sixth Element Capital, Adaptimmune, Amcure, AstraZeneca, Bayer, Blueprint Medicines, BMS, Boehringer Ingelheim, Cristal Therapeutics, Daiichi Sankyo, Eisai, Eli Lilly, Epizyme, Genzyme, GSK, Ipsen, Loxo Oncology, Medpace, Nektar, Novartis, PharmaMar, Philogen, PIQUR Therapeutics, Plexxikon, and Swedish Orphan Biovitrium. IAM has received research support from Novartis and Pfizer and advisory board honoraria from Novartis. HW has received advisory board honoraria, speaker's fees, and travel support from Roche. SG, IR, KMM, JMS, VWN, and SMS are employees of Genentech/Roche. EW has received research support from Genentech, an advisory board honorarium from Genentech, and scientific advisory board support from Leap Pharmaceuticals. SC and SD declare that they have no potential conflicts of interest.

Author details

[1]Department of General Medical Oncology, Leuven Cancer Institute, University Hospitals Leuven, Leuven, Belgium. [2]Department of Oncology, Faculty of Medicine, Laboratory of Experimental Oncology, KU Leuven, Herestraat 49, B-3000 Leuven, Belgium. [3]Department of Medical Oncology, Fondazione IRCCS Istituto Nazionale dei Tumori, Milan, Italy. [4]Department of Medicine, Vanderbilt University Medical Center, Nashville, TN, USA. [5]Oncology Biomarker Development, Genentech Inc, South San Francisco, CA, USA.

A phase Ib study of pictilisib (GDC-0941) in combination with paclitaxel...

65

[6]Product Development Oncology, Genentech Inc, South San Francisco, CA, USA. [7]Clinical Pharmacology, Genentech Inc, South San Francisco, CA, USA. [8]Biostatistics, Genentech Inc, South San Francisco, CA, USA. [9]Department of Medical Oncology, Dana-Farber Cancer Institute, Boston, MA, USA.

References

1. National Comprehensive Cancer Network (NCCN). NCCN Clinical Practice Guidelines in Oncology (NCCN Guidelines®): Breast Cancer. Version 2. 2016. https://www.nccn.org/professionals/physician_gls/pdf/breast.pdf. Accessed 14 Oct 2016.

2. Cardoso F, Costa A, Norton L, Senkus E, Aapro M, André F, et al. ESO-ESMO 2nd International Consensus Guidelines for Advanced Breast Cancer (ABC2). Breast. 2014;23(5):489–502.

3. Miller K, Wang M, Gralow J, Dickler M, Cobleigh M, Perez EA, et al. Paclitaxel plus bevacizumab versus paclitaxel alone for metastatic breast cancer. N Engl J Med. 2007;357(26):2666–76.

4. Yuan TL, Cantley LC. PI3K pathway alterations in cancer: variations on a theme. Oncogene. 2008;27(41):5497–510.

5. Engelman JA. Targeting PI3K signalling in cancer: opportunities, challenges and limitations. Nat Rev Cancer. 2009;9(8):550–62.

6. Ma CX, Ellis MJ. The Cancer Genome Atlas: clinical applications for breast cancer. Oncology (Williston Park). 2013;27(12):1263–9. 1274–1279

7. Cantley LC. The phosphoinositide 3-kinase pathway. Science. 2002; 296(5573):1655–7.

8. Vanhaesebroeck B, Leevers SJ, Panayotou G, Waterfield MD. Phosphoinositide 3-kinases: a conserved family of signal transducers. Trends Biochem Sci. 1997;22(7)):267–72.

9. Bachman KE, Argani P, Samuels Y, Silliman N, Ptak J, Szabo S, et al. The PIK3CA gene is mutated with high frequency in human breast cancers. Cancer Biol Ther. 2004;3(8):772–5.

10. Samuels Y, Wang Z, Bardelli A, Silliman N, Ptak J, Szabo S, et al. High frequency of mutations of the PIK3CA gene in human cancers. Science. 2004;304(5670):554.

11. Stemke-Hale K, Gonzalez-Angulo AM, Lluch A, Neve RM, Kuo WL, Davies M, et al. An integrative genomic and proteomic analysis of PIK3CA, PTEN, and AKT mutations in breast cancer. Cancer Res. 2008;68(15):6084–91.

12. Arthur LM, Turnbull AK, Renshaw L, Keys J, Thomas JS, Wilson TR, et al. Changes in PIK3CA mutation status are not associated with recurrence, metastatic disease or progression in endocrine-treated breast cancer. Breast Cancer Res Treat. 2014;147(1):211–9.

13. Shou J, Massarweh S, Osborne CK, Wakeling AE, Ali S, Weiss H, et al. Mechanisms of tamoxifen resistance: increased estrogen receptor-HER2/neu cross-talk in ER/HER2-positive breast cancer. J Natl Cancer Inst. 2004;96:926–35.

14. Miller TW, Perez-Torres M, Narasanna A, Guix M, Stal O, Perez-Tenorio G, et al. Loss of phosphatase and tensin homologue deleted on chromosome 10 engages ErbB3 and insulin-like growth factor-I receptor signaling to promote antiestrogen resistance in breast cancer. Cancer Res. 2009;69(10):4192–201.

15. Miller TW, Balko JM, Arteaga CL. Phosphatidylinositol 3-kinase and antiestrogen resistance in breast cancer. J Clin Oncol. 2011;29(33):4452–61.

16. Baselga J, Semiglazov V, van Dam P, Manikhas A, Bellet M, Mayordomo J, et al. Phase II randomized study of neoadjuvant everolimus plus letrozole compared with placebo plus letrozole in patients with estrogen receptor-positive breast cancer. J Clin Oncol. 2009;27(16):2630–7.

17. Baselga J, Campone M, Piccart M, Burris HA 3rd, Rugo HS, Sahmoud T, et al. Everolimus in postmenopausal hormone-receptor-positive advanced breast cancer. N Engl J Med. 2012;366(6):520–9.

18. Bachelot T, McCool R, Duffy S, Glanville J, Varley D, Fleetwood K, et al. Comparative efficacy of everolimus plus exemestane versus fulvestrant for hormone-receptor-positive advanced breast cancer following progression/

recurrence after endocrine therapy: a network meta-analysis. Breast Cancer Res Treat. 2014;143(1):125–33.

19. Folkes AJ, Ahmadi K, Alderton WK, Alix S, Baker SJ, Box G, et al. The identification of 2-(1H-indazol-4-yl)-6-(4-methanesulfonyl-piperazin-1-ylmethyl)-4-morpholin-4-yl-thieno[3,2-d]pyrimidine (GDC-0941) as a potent, selective, orally bioavailable inhibitor of class I PI3 kinase for the treatment of cancer. J Med Chem. 2008;51(18):5522–32.

20. Sarker D, Ang JE, Baird R, Kristeleit R, Shah K, Moreno V, et al. First-in-human phase I study of pictilisib (GDC-0941), a potent pan-class I phosphatidylinositol-3-kinase (PI3K) inhibitor, in patients with advanced solid tumors. Clin Cancer Res. 2015;21(1):77–86.

21. Dienstmann R, Rodon J, Serra V, Tabernero J. Picking the point of inhibition: a comparative review of PI3K/AKT/mTOR pathway inhibitors. Mol Cancer Ther. 2014;13(5):1021–31.

22. Fritsch C, Huang A, Chatenay-Rivauday C, Schnell C, Reddy A, Liu M, et al. Characterization of the novel and specific PI3Kalpha inhibitor NVP-BYL719 and development of the patient stratification strategy for clinical trials. Mol Cancer Ther. 2014;13(5):1117–29.

23. Olivero AG, Heffron TP, Baumgardner M, Belvin M, Ross LB, Blaquiere N, et al. Discovery of GDC-0032: a beta-sparing PI3K inhibitor active against PIK3CA mutant tumors [abstract]. Cancer Res. 2013;73(8 Suppl):Abstract DDT02–1.

24. O'Brien C, Wallin JJ, Sampath D, GuhaThakurta D, Savage H, Punnoose EA, et al. Predictive biomarkers of sensitivity to the phosphatidylinositol 3' kinase inhibitor GDC-0941 in breast cancer preclinical models. Clin Cancer Res. 2010;16(14)):3670–83. A published erratum appears in Clin Cancer Res. 2011;17(7):2066–7

25. Wallin JJ, Guan J, Prior WW, Lee LB, Berry L, Belmont LD, et al. GDC-0941, a novel class I selective PI3K inhibitor, enhances the efficacy of docetaxel in human breast cancer models by increasing cell death in vitro and in vivo. Clin Cancer Res. 2012;18(14):3901–11.

26. Junttila TT, Akita RW, Parsons K, Fields C, Phillips GDL, Friedman LS, et al. Ligand-independent HER2/HER3/PI3K complex is disrupted by trastuzumab and is effectively inhibited by the PI3K inhibitor GDC-0941. Cancer Cell. 2009;15(5):429–40.

27. Raynaud FI, Eccles SA, Patel S, Alix S, Box G, Chuckowree I, et al. Biological properties of potent inhibitors of class I phosphatidylinositide 3-kinases: from PI-103 through PI-540, PI-620 to the oral agent GDC-0941. Mol Cancer Ther. 2009;8(7):1725–38.

28. Piccart M, Hortobagyi GN, Campone M, Pritchard KI, Lebrun F, Ito Y, et al. Everolimus plus exemestane for hormone-receptor-positive, human epidermal growth factor receptor-2-negative advanced breast cancer: overall survival results from BOLERO-2. Ann Oncol. 2014;25(12):2357–62.

29. U.S. Department of Health and Human Services, National Institutes of Health (NIH), National Cancer Institute (NCI). Common Terminology Criteria for Adverse Events (CTCAE). Version 3.0. 9 Aug 2006. https://ctep.cancer.gov/protocoldevelopment/electronic_applications/docs/ctcaev3.pdf. Accessed 14 Oct 2016.

30. Patel R, Tsan A, Tam R, Desai R, Spoerke J, Schoenbrunner N, et al. Mutation scanning using MUT-MAP, a high-throughput, microfluidic chip-based, multi-analyte panel. PLoS One. 2012;7:e51153.

31. Spoerke JM, O'Brien C, Huw L, Koeppen H, Fridlyand J, Brachmann RK, et al. Phosphoinositide 3-kinase (PI3K) pathway alterations are associated with histologic subtypes and are predictive of sensitivity to PI3K inhibitors in lung cancer preclinical models. Clin Cancer Res. 2012;18(24):6771–83.

32. Schmid P, Pinder SE, Wheatley D, Macaskill J, Zammit C, Hu J, et al. Preoperative window of opportunity study of the PI3K inhibitor pictilisib (GDC-0941) plus anastrozole vs anastrozole alone in patients with ER+, HER2-negative operable breast cancer (OPPORTUNE study) [abstract]. Cancer Res. 2015;75(9 Suppl):Abstract S2–03.

33. Vuylsteke P, Huizing M, Petrakova K, Roylance R, Laing R, Chan S, et al. Pictilisib PI3Kinase inhibitor (a phosphatidylinositol 3-kinase [PI3K] inhibitor) plus paclitaxel for the treatment of hormone receptor-positive, HER2-negative, locally recurrent, or metastatic breast cancer: interim analysis of the multicentre, placebo-controlled, phase II randomised PEGGY study. Ann Oncol. 2016;27:2059–66.

34. Krop IE, Mayer IA, Ganju V, Dickler M, Johnston S, Morales S, et al. Pictilisib for oestrogen receptor-positive, aromatase inhibitor-resistant, advanced or metastatic breast cancer (FERGI): a randomised, double-blind, placebo-controlled, phase 2 trial. Lancet Oncol. 2016;17:811–21.

35. Baselga J, Im S, Baselga J, Im SA, Iwata H, Cortés J, et al. Buparlisib plus fulvestrant versus placebo plus fulvestrant in postmenopausal, hormone receptor-positive, HER2-negative, advanced breast cancer (BELLE-2): a randomised, double-blind, placebo-controlled, phase 3 trial. Lancet Oncol. 2017;18:904–16.

36. Janku F, Juric D, Cortes J, Rugo H, Burris HA, Schuler M, et al. Phase I study of the PI3Kα inhibitor BYL719 plus fulvestrant in patients with PIK3CA-altered and wild type ER+/HER2-locally advanced or metastatic breast cancer [abstract]. Cancer Res. 2015;75(9 Suppl)):Abstract PD5.

37. Juric D, Gonzalez-Angulo AM, Burris HA, Schuler M, Schellens J, Berlin J, et al. Preliminary safety, pharmacokinetics and anti-tumor activity of BYL719, an alpha-specific PI3K inhibitor in combination with fulvestrant: results from a phase I study. Cancer Res. 2013;73(24 Suppl):Abstract P2–16-14.

38. Mayer IA, Abramson VG, Formisano L, Balko JM, Estrada MV, Sanders ME, et al. A phase Ib study of alpelisib (BYL719), a PI3Kα-specific inhibitor, with letrozole in ER /HER2-negative metastatic breast cancer. Clin Cancer Res. 2017;23(1):26–34.

39. Wallin JJ, Edgar KA, Guan J, Sampath D, Nannini M, Belvin M, et al. The PI3K inhibitor GDC-0032 is selectively potent against PIK3CA mutant breast cancer cell lines and tumors [abstract]. Cancer Res. 2013;73(24 Suppl)):Abstract P2–17-01.

40. Edgar KA, Song K, Schmidt S, Kirkpatrick DS, Phu L, Nannini M, et al. The PI3K inhibitor, taselisib (GDC-0032), has enhanced potency in PIK3CA mutant models through a unique mechanism of action [abstract]. Cancer Res. 2016;76(14 Suppl):Abstract 370.

41. Juric D, Krop I, Ramanathan RK, Xiao J, Sanabria S, Wilson TR, et al. GDC-0032, a beta isoform-sparing PI3K inhibitor: results of a first-in-human phase Ia dose escalation study [abstract]. Cancer Res. 2013;73(8 Suppl):Abstract LB-64.

42. Baselga J, Cortes J, De Laurentiis M, Diéras V, Harbeck N, Hsu JY, et al. SANDPIPER: phase III study of the PI3-kinase (PI3K) inhibitor taselisib (GDC-0032) plus fulvestrant in patients (pts) with oestrogen receptor (ER)-positive, HER2-negative locally advanced or metastatic breast cancer (BC) enriched for pts with PIK3CA mutant tumors [abstract]. Ann Oncol. 2016;27(Suppl 6):Abstract 313TiP.

43. Schöffski P, Cresta S, Mayer IA, Wildiers H, Rooney I, Apt D, Gendreau S, Morrissey K, Lackner M, Spoerke J, Winer E. Tolerability and anti-tumor activity of the oral PI3K inhibitor GDC-0941 in combination with paclitaxel, with and without bevacizumab or trastuzumab in patients with locally recurrent or metastatic breast cancer [abstract]. Cancer Res. 2015;75(9 Suppl):P5-19-10.

6

Atypical ductal hyperplasia: update on diagnosis, management, and molecular landscape

Tanjina Kader[1,2,3], Prue Hill[4], Emad A. Rakha[5], Ian G. Campbell[1,2,6] and Kylie L. Gorringe[2,3,6*]

Abstract

Background: Atypical ductal hyperplasia (ADH) is a common diagnosis in the mammographic era and a significant clinical problem with wide variation in diagnosis and treatment. After a diagnosis of ADH on biopsy a proportion are upgraded to carcinoma upon excision; however, the remainder of patients are overtreated. While ADH is considered a non-obligate precursor of invasive carcinoma, the molecular taxonomy remains unknown.

Main text: Although a few studies have revealed some of the key genomic characteristics of ADH, a clear understanding of the molecular changes associated with breast cancer progression has been limited by inadequately powered studies and low resolution methodology. Complicating factors such as family history, and whether the ADH present in a biopsy is an isolated lesion or part of a greater neoplastic process beyond the limited biopsy material, make accurate interpretation of genomic features and their impact on progression to malignancy a challenging task. This article will review the definitions and variable management of the patients diagnosed with ADH as well as the current knowledge of the molecular landscape of ADH and its clonal relationship with ductal carcinoma in situ and invasive carcinoma.

Conclusions: Molecular data of ADH remain sparse. Large prospective cohorts of pure ADH with clinical follow-up need to be evaluated at DNA, RNA, and protein levels in order to develop biomarkers of progression to carcinoma to guide management decisions.

Keywords: Atypical ductal hyperplasia, Breast neoplasms, Ductal carcinoma in situ, Breast cancer progression, Clonal relationship, Patient care management

Background

The term "benign breast disease" encompasses a heterogeneous group of non-malignant lesions (Fig. 1) [1–5]. With the introduction of population-based mammographic screening programs, there has been an increased detection of these putative precursor lesions. While the detection of invasive ductal carcinoma (IDC) by mammographic screening programs has increased 1.6-fold, the detection of benign lesions has increased two- to four-fold [6], indicating that not all precursor lesions will ever progress to malignancy. Indeed, a recent study with a median of 12 years follow-up showed that only a

minority of women (143 among 698; 20%) with atypical hyperplasia (AH; both atypical ductal hyperplasia (ADH) and atypical lobular hyperplasia (ALH)) eventually progressed to malignancy even without any preventative strategies [7]. Based on their study and other available data the authors concluded that atypical hyperplasia confers an absolute risk of subsequent breast cancer of 30% at 25 years of follow-up [7]. However, the studies shown in Fig. 1 [1–5] show some heterogeneity in the rate of a subsequent breast carcinoma event after a benign biopsy. The variability of associated risk with each type of lesion could be due to multiple factors, including sample size (range 24–336 AH diagnoses), length of follow-up (range 8–17 years), inclusion criteria (e.g., the Nashville study [1] excluded patients who had breast cancer within 6 months of the first biopsy), and in particular the criteria used for atypical hyperplasia diagnosis, which is known to vary as discussed below. Given that

* Correspondence: kylie.gorringe@petermac.org
[2]The Sir Peter MacCallum Department of Oncology, University of Melbourne, Melbourne, VIC, Australia
[3]Cancer Genomics Program, Peter MacCallum Cancer Centre, Melbourne, VIC, Australia
Full list of author information is available at the end of the article

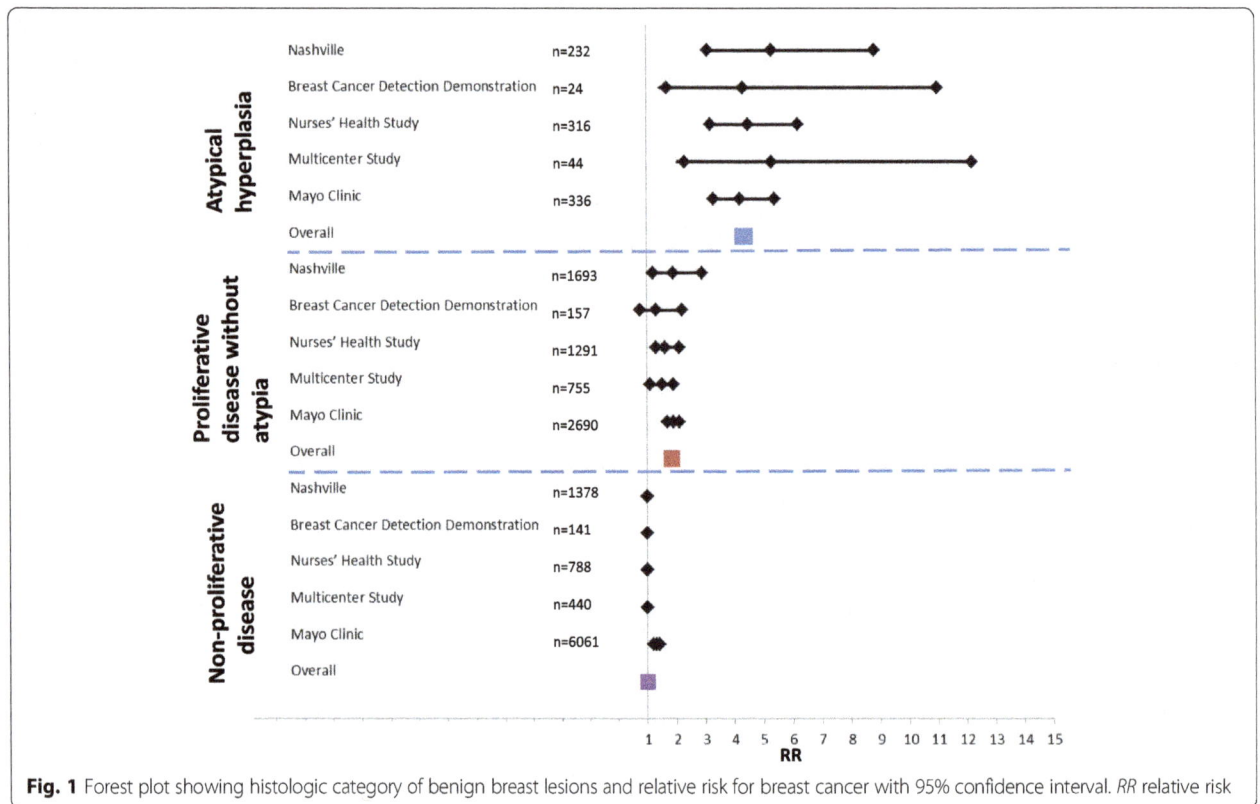

Fig. 1 Forest plot showing histologic category of benign breast lesions and relative risk for breast cancer with 95% confidence interval. *RR* relative risk

each lesion will have variable potential for carcinoma development [5] (Fig. 1), it is important to know which ones are true precursors of breast cancer to facilitate appropriate management. Although both forms of AH, ductal and lobular, carry a similar long-term risk of developing metachronous carcinoma [8, 9], in this review we will particularly focus on ADH, which is histopathologically distinct from ALH [3], presents a more common clinical issue, and has a higher upgrade rate [7].

ADH is not only a risk factor for IDC, it is also considered to be a direct but non-obligate precursor to carcinoma [1]. Diagnosis of ADH carries a four- to fivefold increased risk of developing breast cancer within 5 years that is not limited to the ipsilateral breast [1, 10]. However, Hartmann et al. [7] pointed out that risk estimation has not been calculated as cumulative incidence by the current breast cancer risk prediction tools (such as Gail/Breast Cancer Risk Assessment Tool, International Breast Cancer Intervention Study (IBIS)), and that the lifetime incidence is 25–30% according to multiple large retrospective studies, each with more than 300 AH (both ductal and lobular) diagnoses [7–9, 11].

Strikingly, the risk associated with ADH is doubled with family history, suggesting inherited factors are associated with ADH development. Hoogerbrugge et al. [12] showed that high risk histopathologic lesions, including ADH (39%), were detected in almost 50% of the women

younger than age 40 years with a hereditary predisposition for breast cancer who underwent prophylactic mastectomy, not limited to only *BRCA* mutation carriers.

The occurrence of ADH in the general population varies widely from 3% of benign biopsies [13] (based on 30,953 cases), to 8–10% [14, 15] ($n = 3532$), to 23% [16] ($n = 2833$). These differences could come from the total number of biopsies analyzed and/or when these biopsies have been performed (pre/post-widespread mammographic screening). In the pre-mammographic era, biopsies would likely have been performed only for palpable lesions with concomitant low frequency of ADH (2.1% [17], $n = 10,542$). In the current era of mammographic screening biopsies are additionally performed based on micro-calcifications, for example; therefore, a higher frequency of ADH could be observed [18]. These differences may also reflect geographical or temporal differences in incidence, as ADH is associated with hormone replacement therapy (HRT), use of which varies widely over time [13]. Moreover, the variations in ADH frequency may suggest under- or over-diagnosis of ADH at different centers due to differing definitions or variation arising as a consequence of the number of slides sectioned per specimen. For example, Page et al. reported only 2.1% ADH in their cohort with, on average, one to five slides per specimen (total original biopsies $n = 10,542$) [17] as opposed to 26 slides by de Mascarel et al.

(23% detection rate) ($n = 2833$) [16]. In autopsy studies in the general population, ADH was observed in the breast of 3–13% of women [19], which could well be an underestimate, given limited sampling techniques.

In this review, we focus on the definition, diagnosis, and current management of ADH as well as its molecular alterations. We also mention the strengths and limitations of some previous studies and propose ideas for studies that need to be undertaken in order to better understand breast cancer development associated with ADH.

Definition of ADH

ADH resembles low nuclear grade ductal carcinoma in situ (DCIS) with cytonuclear and architectural atypia but with either partial involvement of the ducts and/or small size for a diagnosis of DCIS. In ADH there are ducts partially filled with abnormally uniform evenly spaced cells with polarization [20] (Fig. 2). ADH and low nuclear grade DCIS (LG DCIS) show not only morphological similarities, including cytological and architectural features, but also immuno-phenotypical overlap (both are estrogen receptor (ER)- and progesterone receptor (PR)-positive and HER2-negative) and especially genomic alterations [21]. ADH has been defined as having "some but not all the requisite features of DCIS" with an involvement of ducts by an architecturally complex proliferation of monotonous cells forming cribriform-like and/or micro-papillary formation with a maximum of two separate spaces [20, 22]. The cells might grow in arcades, rigid bridges, or bars of uniform thickness, micro-papillae, solid or cribriform patterns. The involved spaces might also contain a population of cells with similar characteristics of usual ductal hyperplasia (UDH) or residual normal epithelium [22]. Due to their similar morphological features, ADH and LG DCIS are difficult to reproducibly distinguish; therefore, one other feature was added to differentiate between them—ADH is arbitrarily defined as having a size of ≤ 2 mm [10, 20–22]. Unlike intermediate and high grade DCIS, ADH typically lacks central necrosis and significant nuclear atypia [1].

One of the major impediments to proper management of ADH is the conflicting definitions of ADH and intraobserver variability which make a definitive diagnosis difficult [10, 23]. Ghofrani et al. [23] described instances of the inconsistencies and disagreements of ADH diagnosis among 230 pathologists. For example, one of the scenarios showed that although ADH is defined by having a diameter ≤ 2 mm or only partially involved ducts, when five ducts, each ≤ 2 mm, were involved, 37% of pathologists diagnosed it as DCIS and when > 20 partially involved ducts were involved more than 60% of pathologists diagnosed it as DCIS and recommended excision [23]. Multiple other studies showed a similar lack of concordance in differentiating ADH from LG DCIS among

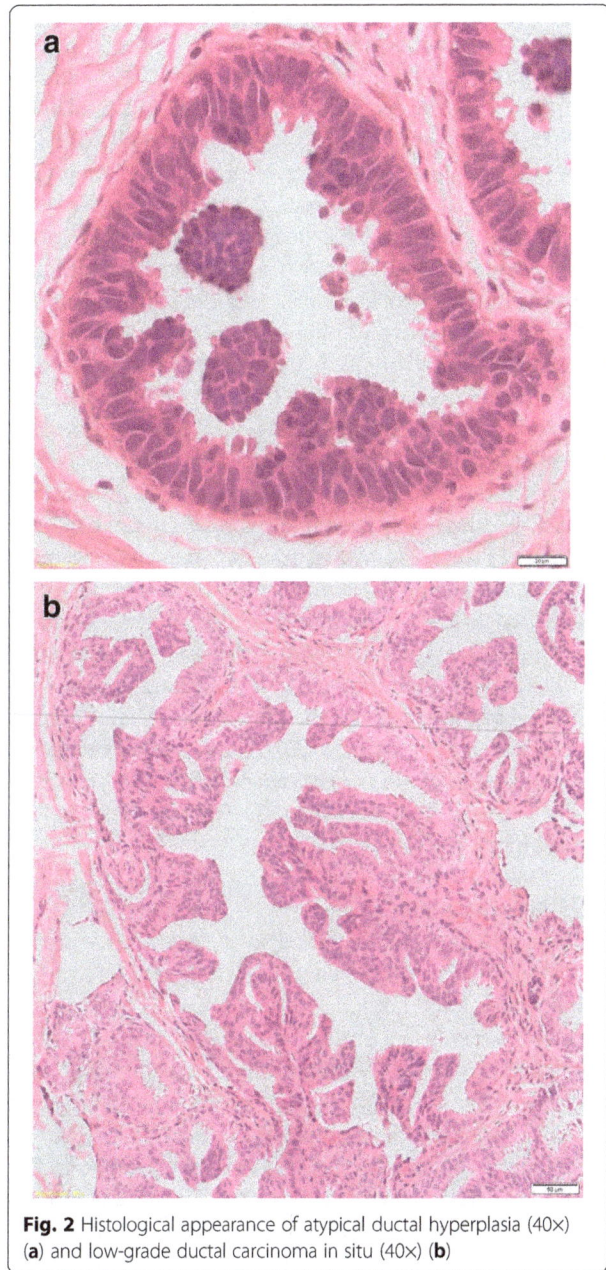

Fig. 2 Histological appearance of atypical ductal hyperplasia (40×) (**a**) and low-grade ductal carcinoma in situ (40×) (**b**)

pathologists, ranging from 58 to 92% (reviewed by Walia et al. [10]). However, when standardized published criteria were followed, particularly with a set of provided teaching slides, the concordance rate was satisfactory (71–92%, six participants) [24]. Moreover, one study with nine participants showed not only lack of concordance between ADH and LG DCIS but also between ADH and UDH; however, this poor concordance can be improved by including data from immuno-histochemical staining with multiple cytokeratins (CK) [25]. Particularly, basal type cytokeratins (CK5/6) were found to be very effective for such differential diagnosis [22, 26]. Low nuclear grade neoplasia in the breast, including ADH, typically shows diffuse strong nuclear ER positivity and lacks high molecular weight cytokeratins, such as CK5/6 expression, in keeping with proliferation of end-differentiated luminal cells, unlike UDH (heterogeneous mosaic pattern). Myoepithelial-specific markers such as p63 and myoid markers such as SMA are helpful to demonstrate preservation of myoepithelial cells at the epithelialstroma interface. Notably, while myoepithelial marker positivity in the proliferative pools is useful in the diagnosis of adenomyoepithelioma and other myoepithelial lesions, this does not aid in the differential diagnosis of epithelial hyperplasia versus epithelial neoplasia/atypia [27]. It is important to note that CK5/6 cannot distinguish ADH from LG DCIS as both show uniformly negative staining for luminal cells [25]. Collectively, these studies suggest that a more objective biomarker for the differential diagnosis of ADH and LG DCIS would be highly desirable since extent alone cannot differentiate an early neoplastic lesion that may not progress to malignancy from those that represent part of a DCIS process that is underrepresented in the examined specimen and are more likely to progress. Molecular studies could play an important role to identify such biomarkers; however, given the above described lack of concordance at assessing ADH [28], any studies related to ADH need to include a strict review procedure by one or more breast pathologists with sufficient experience before inclusion into the study.

ADH diagnosis and management

ADH is usually first identified in a core needle biopsy (CNB), and first designated as a "B3" lesion: i.e., of uncertain malignant potential of the breast. The management of patients diagnosed with ADH on CNB varies not only because of the initial biopsy type/size but also because of the variable reported "upgrade rate". Upgrade of ADH refers to the finding of cancer (DCIS/IDC) in the surgical excision biopsy that was not present in the CNB. One very recent review stated that 22–65% of ADH diagnosed by CNB were upgraded to carcinoma [29]. The surgical excision rate is lower (60%) if the ADH was diagnosed by vacuum assisted biopsy (VAB), since this technique is thought to be more efficient at removing lesion areas than CNB [29]. While most upgrades of ADH are DCIS, upgrades to IDC do happen [30]. In terms of the management of the patients, some clinicians prefer to observe patients diagnosed with ADH. However, this option may put those patients at risk of undertreatment. Given the high upgrade rate, it is not surprising that the majority of clinicians suggest a surgical excision after ADH diagnosis on CNB to rule out concomitant malignancy. For example, if a patient had an area of radiographic abnormality and her CNB showed a focus of atypical cells in keeping with ADH and not sufficient for the diagnosis of LG DCIS, it would

be preferable to perform an excision to examine the whole area of abnormality. Because the abnormal radiological mass might be due to a well-developed DCIS, surgical excision could avoid missing a higher risk lesion requiring more intensive treatment [31]. In this type of upgrade scenario, presumably the most likely explanation for missing a higher risk lesion from a CNB would be sampling limitations. This highlights the important clinical utility of identifying robust biomarkers that can distinguish between pure ADH and ADH that is likely to be associated with a synchronous LG DCIS and thereby avoiding the need for recommending surgical excision for all. Alternatives to surgical excision include treatment with tamoxifen as this has been reported to reduce the risk of developing breast cancer from 21 to 7.5% in 10 years (from 2459 ADH diagnoses) [32]. However, recent studies on breast cancer prevention with endocrine therapy show a very low rate of uptake and even lower rate of persistence due to the side effects, even in women at very high genetic risk [33].

Some parameters may be useful to take into consideration before excision, such as the number of cores, type of needle used, type of lesion, and lesion diameter [7, 10]. It has also been suggested to take into account the number of the foci in the core and how much of the radiographic lesion was removed, with multiple foci requiring a greater area to be removed [34]. Similarly, another recent paper [35] suggested that the radiographic presence of residual lesions after CNB and the maximum lesion size could be predictive of upgrades with 78% sensitivity and 80% specificity. However, this study had only a small and retrospective sample cohort ($n = 151$) and included only those patients already recommended for surgical excision. None of these parameters or suggestions is clinically proven and prospective validation is required to evaluate such prediction tools. Thus, the recommendation and current clinical practice is to perform an open surgical excision on all ADH diagnosed on CNB or VAB unless ADH is a single focus [29, 36]. This practice would certainly overtreat the majority of women diagnosed with ADH and clearly demonstrates the need to identify a robust biomarker to avoid unnecessary surgery and optimal management.

Risk prediction following ADH diagnosis

Unfortunately, risk prediction following ADH diagnosis is controversial [7], and counseling and further screening for these women diagnosed with ADH are therefore probably not adequate. Indeed, Degnim et al. [8, 11] showed that the 25-year risk of developing cancer associated with ADH is at least 25%, and it could be as high as 50–60% if the ADH is both multifocal and calcified ($n = 331$). One possibility is that this combination indicates a lesion already DCIS at a cellular biology level but lacking the extent to be diagnosed as such. Calcification in their study was present in 70% of the ADH cases, and calcification alone didn't have a significant independent association with higher risk [8, 11]. An elevated risk of breast cancer associated with calcification of atypical hyperplasia was, however, reported by Hutchinson et al. ($n = 210$) [37]. In terms of multifocality, a very recent case-control study from Nurses' Health Studies found that multifocality was only a significant risk factor for ALH ($n = 110$) rather than ADH ($n = 173$) [3]; differences in sampling and the level of centralized pathology review between the two studies are potential confounders for these observations. Although the multiple foci of ADH were well defined by the pathologists to distinguish between ADH and LG DCIS in Degnim et al. [8, 11] and the Nurses' Health Studies [3], the location of calcification was not specified (intra-ductal versus stromal) [8, 11] or was unknown [3]. As calcification is one of the common features of ADH [16, 22], it would have been really interesting to see if intra-ductal calcification and/or stromal calcification correlate with different risk. The degree of atypia can also vary in ADH, but this is not a feature that has been evaluated in terms of subsequent risk, perhaps because of the difficulty in standardizing such a measure across different pathologists.

Apart from the histologic variables, younger/pre-menopausal women (< 45 years) are at higher risk of developing metachronous carcinoma as found by several studies [8, 38, 39], particularly higher grade cancer [40]. The complexities of analyzing focality, calcification, and atypia in terms of how these are measured emphasizes the importance of understanding the breast biology, as well as the precursor versus risk indicator status of ADH. Given the fact that only a fraction of ADH (9.8–30%) [7, 41] develop metachronous carcinoma, a molecular marker of risk may have the potential to be more objective than clinical symptoms or histopathological features alone for the management of patients.

Thus far, despite the high risk of developing cancer associated with ADH, attempts to identify clinicopathological or molecular biomarkers to predict individual risk have been unsuccessful. Risk reduction strategies remain varied, from active surveillance at one end of the spectrum to prophylactic mastectomy at the other.

Molecular features of ADH

Breast cancer is well known to be a genetic disease, with very frequent somatic copy number changes, a number of driver mutations such as in *PIK3CA* and *TP53*, and widespread transcriptional deregulation [42]. While molecular studies of benign breast disease are fewer, they suggest both similarities to and differences from breast carcinoma.

Genetic events in pure ADH

Very few studies have described the molecular genetic features of ADH (Table 1) and these are further limited because most were carried out on small numbers of samples using low resolution methodology, such as microsatellite marker-based loss of heterozygosity (LOH) or allelic imbalance (AI) analysis and cytogenetic comparative genomic hybridization (CGH). The latter has a genomic resolution of 5–10 Mb, whereas most LOH studies were carried out using only a few markers, which were chosen based on the location of common regions of AI in IDC. One of the major barriers to studying ADH is the limited amount of DNA available, a problem reported by multiple studies [43, 44]. This limitation can be overcome by using in situ assays, such as fluorescence in situ hybridization (FISH), but at the cost of being highly locus-specific.

An LOH study of 41 ADH samples at 15 genetic loci selected based on the locations of frequently inactivated tumor suppressor genes in IDC, such as *TP53*, *RB1*, and *BRCA1*, reported that 42% of "pure" ADH (without synchronous DCIS/IDC) showed LOH in at least one locus, suggesting that inactivation of these tumor suppressor genes might be an early neoplastic event and related to the subsequent development of IDC [45]. This study identified loss of 16q as an LOH "hot spot" in ADH and also in low-grade DCIS and IDC. Loss of 16q was also confirmed as a common event in breast cancer by other studies (Table 1), signifying that this event might be particularly important in the early development of breast cancer. Indeed, flow cytometry studies have suggested that 15–44% of ADH are aneuploid, indicating that copy number alterations are often present at this premalignant stage [46–50]. A more sensitive FISH study using nine chromosomal probes supported these observations, finding that all ADH had chromosomal aneuploidy, and the number of cells with aneuploidy was higher than in lesions without atypia, although less frequent than in carcinomas [51]. In contrast, two other FISH analyses observed aneuploidy in 1/5 and 0/2 ADH using two and six probes, respectively, whereas carcinomas all carried aneuploidies [52, 53].

Using alternative methods, Gao et al. [54] detected copy number aberrations in 15 pure ADH samples by array CGH and found that although there were similar genetic alterations among ADH, DCIS, and IDC, there were also alterations unique to each lesion. Firstly, they found that gain at 19p and losses at 2p, 6q, 11p, 12q, 22q, and Xq were only present in DCIS and IDC, suggesting that these changes might be a later event in breast cancer progression. Secondly, ADH had a high prevalence of 17q gain [54], although the number of cases studied was small. In addition, this study is the only one in the literature in which ADH showed more copy number changes than DCIS. This unusual feature, along with the pattern of CGH alterations

Table 1 Major genetic features of atypical ductal hyperplasia

Method[a]	Number of samples	Number of loci or genomic resolution	Cases with aberration	Average cases altered per locus	Location of copy number gain[a]	Location of copy number loss/LOH/AI[a]	SNV[a]	Reference
LOH	10[P]	2	50%	38.9%	NA	16q, 17p	NA	[43]
LOH	26[P] 25[S]	15	42%[P] 44%[S]	6.2% 9.5%	NA	11p, 13q, 16q, 17p, 17q	NA	[45]
LOH	23[S]	14	NA	15%	NA	8p,16q,17q	NA	[79]
LOH	16[S]	22	75%	13%	NA	1q, 3p, 11p, 11q, 16q, 17p	NA	[44]
LOH	31[P]	26	65%	6.1%	NA	8q	NA	[67]
LOH total	131 (67[P], 64[S])	2–26	53%[P], 70%[S]	15%	NA	16q (24%), 13q (15%), 17q (12%), 11p (12%), 17p (10%)	NA	
CGH	9[P]	5–10 Mb	55%	NA	1q, 16p, 11q	16q, 17p, 20p	NA	[80]
CGH	2[P]	5–10 Mb	100%	NA	1q, 3p, 6p, 10p, 11q, 12q, 13q, 16p, 17q, 20q, 8q, 14q, 15q	4q, 5q, 1p, 13q, 16q, 17p	NA	[55]
CGH	3[S]	5–10 Mb	100%	NA	3p, 8q, 15q, 16p, 20q, 22q	13q, 16q	NA	[56]
CGH	15[P]	5–10 Mb	93%	NA	1p, 1q, 2q, 8q, 10p, 17q, 20q, 20p, 2q, Xp	8p, 9p, 11q, 13q, 14q, 16q, 21q, Xp	NA	[54]
CGH total	29		80%[P], 100%[S]	NA	8q, 20q, 16p, 17q, 1q	16q, 13q, 17p, 8p	NA	
Targeted sequencing	4	130–296 SNV/case	100%	NA	NA	NA	Lineage heterogeneity	[58]
WGS	2	1 base pair	100%	NA	1q gain early neoplastic event	–	ADH and carcinoma shared SNVs	[57]
FISH[P]	9	8	100%	45.6%	7, 8, 18	–	–	[51]
FISH[S]	13	1	54%	NA	Higher *ERBB2* amplification from ADH to DCIS to IDC	NA	NA	[65]

[a]*LOH* loss of heterozygosity, *AI* allelic imbalance, *CGH* comparative genomic hybridization, *SNV* single nucleotide variant, *WGS* whole-genome sequencing, *FISH* fluorescence in situ hybridization, *NA* not available or not applicable. Gains are considered when chromosomal imbalance is > 1.25 and losses are considered when it is < 0.8 of the normal allelic ratio. AI is considered when the imbalance is > 1.33 or < 0.75 of the normal allelic ratio. Any gains or losses are reported when changes occurred in at least one sample of the cohort. *P* = pure ADH (no synchronous carcinoma), *S* = ADH with synchronous carcinoma

with a high proportion of changes at telomeres, may suggest an imperfect assay, particularly for ADH samples where material would have been limited. Two other CGH studies each showed several copy number gains (Table 1); however, the sample sizes were just two (pure ADH) [55] and three (synchronous) [56].

These genetic studies emphasize the difficulty in analyzing small numbers of cases with varying definitions of ADH, often leading to different conclusions. Nonetheless, despite individual small sample sizes, across all LOH and CGH studies, 16q loss remained the most common cytogenetic event in pure ADH, followed by 1q gain, with other loci being gained and lost at relatively lower and varying frequencies. In addition, collectively these studies show that most pure ADH carry one or more large-scale cytogenetic abnormalities.

ADH as a precursor lesion
As well as evaluating pure ADH, a common strategy has been to study "synchronous" ADH found in the same

breast as carcinoma (DCIS or IDC). The goal of these studies has been to establish whether ADH could be a genetic precursor to carcinoma (and determine which type of carcinoma), and to evaluate whether genetic events are required for progression.

Early studies used LOH to investigate the clonal relationship between ADH and associated cancers; for example, Larson et al. [44] performed a microsatellite analysis of 45 ADH samples with co-existing DCIS or IDC from 16 patients. These studies found that ~ 60% of the cancer cases had a co-existing clonal ADH lesion. More recently, next-generation sequencing approaches have been applied, although only in small numbers of cases so far. For example, Newburger et al. [57] showed that atypical hyperplasia shared a common ancestor with the carcinoma based on somatic mutations, although this was based on only two patient samples [57]. Similarly, Weng et al. [58] assessed the phylogenetic relationship between early neoplasias, including ADH, and DCIS and IDC by studying six breast cancer patients with concurrent neoplasias (four with atypia). This analysis revealed considerable lineage heterogeneity and the authors suggested that the early neoplastic lesions and DCIS were not direct precursors of the co-existing IDC, but rather independent clonal proliferations of cells with a common ancestor. Interestingly, they also found that some neoplasias showed a mixed-lineage origin, referring to the samples whose cells are geographically co-located but have originated from at least two genetically diverse lineages (although often still sharing an ancient common ancestor). The accumulated somatic mutations of those samples could not be explained by a single lineage tree, suggesting existing high intra-individual genetic heterogeneity, which was also observed by Larson et al. [44]. Given that genetic heterogeneity may be a bad prognostic feature in several tumor types [59], its detection in benign lesions could be relevant for patient management. If multiple neoplastic or atypical lesions were detected by high resolution imaging, phylogenetic analysis of carcinoma and concurrent neoplasia/ ADH might change the direction of the patients' management by treating or removing not only cancerous lesions, but also the reservoir of genetically diverse neoplasias to prevent recurrence.

These genetic studies to date support a role for ADH as a precursor of carcinomas identified in the same breast, but they do not explain the risk associated with ADH for the contralateral breast. It has been noted in multiple studies that ipsilateral recurrence is most common (almost twice that of contralateral) in the first 5 years after ADH diagnosis; however, the long-term risk remains high for both breasts [7, 9]. It is important to note that ipsilateral recurrence is not limited to the initial site of diagnosis of ADH and in cases where the carcinoma recurs at a different quadrant, it could be speculated that this would be non-clonal. Indeed, this possibility is supported by Larson et al., who noted that ADH in different tissue blocks to the co-existing carcinoma were less likely to be clonal (75% clonal when in the same block vs 27% when in different blocks) [44]. Interestingly, they also observed the presence of ADH heterogeneity in 46% of cases when there were multiple ADH foci in the same cancer-containing breast, indicating independent origins of the lesions. ADH may therefore also be a marker of elevated risk not associated with clonal recurrence. As suggested by a study of field cancerization effect in epidermoid carcinoma [60], ADH and other benign lesions could be the result of a "field effect" where non-related tumors are co-located within a cancer-prone tissue. Apart from germline predisposition, the cause of such a field effect in the breast is not yet known; however, at least for ER+ tumors, factors suggested by epidemiological studies could play a role— for example, parity, breast feeding, and mammographic breast density [3]. Other environmental risk factors, such as alcohol consumption, smoking, or obesity, could also

contribute to such a "field". These micro-environmental influencers could provide a possible explanation for the initiation of multiple breast lesions over long periods of time, their persistence, and their progression to carcinoma. Particularly, ADH in younger women could be the result of an oncogenic insult and/or extreme susceptibility for the proposed oncogenic estrogen metabolites associated with the premenopausal hormonal environment [8]. Studying the association of atypia with these characteristics could give an insight into identifying patients with a higher risk of recurrence. Interestingly, a very recent study showed no association between mammographic breast density and risk of recurrence in patients diagnosed with atypical hyperplasia [14]. Breast density, therefore, despite being a major indicator of an altered breast microenvironment, appears not to influence subsequent progression to carcinoma after ADH. Similarly, higher BMI, early menarche, and smoking are not associated with a higher risk of developing invasive cancer after a previous breast benign biopsy [61]. Further study is needed to evaluate the different contributions of these factors for disease initiation as distinct from disease progression. The role of the immune system has barely begun to be investigated as a factor controlling disease progression, but could well be crucial.

Early models of breast cancer development, which proposed a direct linear progression from normal epithelium to ductal hyperplasia to ADH to low-grade DCIS and then to low- or high-grade IDC, are now considered to be oversimplified [21]. Instead, distinct low- and high-grade multistep models of breast cancer progression have been hypothesized [21]. The "low-grade like" progression pathway is characterized by recurrent loss of 16q (> 75%), gains of 1q; expression of hormone receptors (ER+, PR+), lack of HER2 overexpression and a low-grade-like gene expression signature [21, 62, 63]. The "high-grade-like" progression pathway is characterized mainly by gains of 8q (75%) and 1q (60%), losses of 1p (60%), 8p (60%), and 17p (60%), and a luminal B, HER2, or basal-like mRNA expression profile [21, 63]. Studies of breast cancer stem cells also suggest that, apart from the claudin-low subtype, the cell of origin for the other intrinsic breast cancer subtypes may originate at different points along the luminal progenitor lineage [64]. It remains unknown if distinct precursors arise from these progenitors since many of the molecular alterations are not necessarily exclusive to each pathway. Where does ADH fit into this new paradigm?

Regarding ADH progression, a prevailing view is that ADH is only a direct precursor of LG and ER-positive carcinoma [21]; however, this is not supported entirely by the literature. On one side, Larson et al. demonstrated that clonality between ADH and synchronous carcinoma was more likely when the carcinoma was low grade and that ADH lacking any AI was most commonly associated with high grade cancer, although these trends were non-significant [44]. However, at least two of the clonal cases studied by Larson et al. must have been of high grade, although this was not explicitly stated. Indeed, few genetic studies have stated the grade of cancer synchronous to ADH. In addition, the later development of breast carcinoma associated with ADH is not limited to LG cancer. Two recent studies [9, 40] showed that about two-thirds of the recurrent breast carcinomas were ER+ intermediate/high grade. It is noteworthy that small subsets of patients diagnosed with ADH developed ER– (9%) and/or HER2+ ductal carcinoma (7%) [40], including ipsilateral recurrences. As the precursor of HG DCIS and/or HG IDC is still unknown, a synchronous ADH genomics study with LG and HG carcinoma and including all intrinsic subtypes of carcinoma, along with detailed histopathological features of the ADH, would be highly desirable to determine the precursor relationship. It would certainly aid in patient management if we could identify the subsets of patients diagnosed with ADH that might develop HG cancer and treat them accordingly. In fact, after the accurate diagnosis of ADH, this question is one of the most challenging unaddressed clinical questions regarding ADH. Degnim et al. [8] showed the importance of both the number of foci of ADH and calcification as features associated with a higher risk of recurrence; however, they did not mention whether any of these features also significantly correlated with grade or ER status of the subsequent breast carcinoma. Correlative studies of tumor type after ADH also do not address the genetic relationship of recurrences to previous ADH: at present, this is entirely unknown, but critical in order to understand the natural history of ADH and to guide therapy choices.

While genetic analysis of ADH with high-grade and/or ER– carcinomas is underrepresented in the literature, HER2 cases have been addressed through the use of FISH. Interestingly, a FISH study of synchronous cases reported that the amplitude of the amplification of ERBB2 increased from ADH to DCIS to IDC [65]. Fifty-four percent of ADH synchronous with HER2+ IDC showed low or moderate ERBB2 amplification, suggesting ERBB2 amplification can be involved early in breast oncogenesis but higher amplification may be required for progression [65]. This result supports ADH as a precursor lesion for HER2+ cancer, consistent with the observation of HER2+ breast cancer arising after an ADH diagnosis [9, 40].

Other studies of ADH synchronous to carcinoma have also attempted to identify genetic events associated with progression, similar to studies comparing pure DCIS to DCIS synchronous with IDC, in which it has been observed that pure DCIS have different molecular profiles to synchronous DCIS, with the latter carrying more copy number changes overall [66]. Similarly, when pure ADH was compared to synchronous ADH, pure ADH showed

less AI compared to cases synchronous with DCIS or IDC, although the power of the studies was limited [45, 67]. However, while DCIS was genetically very similar to synchronous IDC [68, 69], the overlap between synchronous ADH and carcinomas has shown that even when clonally related (~60% of the time) co-existing carcinomas often have additional genetic events [44]. In addition, a sequencing study found that while few driver point mutations were found, patients with atypical hyperplasia shared aneuploidy events with the carcinomas, suggesting that copy number change, particularly the 1q gain commonly observed in IDC [70], might be an early driver of the neoplastic phenotype [57]. Their findings also suggested that early neoplasias can harbor sufficient driver aneuploidy events to progress into carcinoma, possibly with a combination of mutational load and accumulated aneuploidy, as well as epigenetic and stromal changes over time. A similar aneuploidy hypothesis was proposed by Forsberg et al. [71], who observed copy number changes in histologically normal epithelial cells at uninvolved margins of IDC. However, these studies only included cases with synchronous carcinoma, which may not be representative of atypical hyperplasia without co-existing carcinoma. Overall no consistency in specific genetic events can be attributed to progression. This may reflect inter-tumoral genetic heterogeneity and/or that the number and combination of drivers are more important than the order of genetic events. It may not be possible, therefore, to map specific genetic events to the cancer phenotype, although as noted already, the number of cases in the current literature is inadequate to say whether this is indeed the case.

Transcriptional changes in ADH

As well as the genetic events described above, progression to IBC from ADH may be evaluated by gene expression differences, which can also reflect the influence of the local environment. In order to understand the key driver events in breast cancer progression, Brunner et al. [72] carried out expression analysis of matched normal, ADH, and cancer tissue from 16 patients to characterize transcriptional differences. Interestingly, they found a pro-oncogenic gene expression signature in early neoplasia which was distinct from normal tissues and carcinoma (DCIS/IDC) including up-regulation of ERBB2, FOXA1, and GATA3 [72]. The ERBB2 mRNA overexpression was not thought to be due to genomic amplification of the ERBB2 locus since only three cases tested clinically positive for HER2 amplification in the IDC. They suggested that ERBB2 has a role in early stages of breast cancer development independent of gene amplification [72]. However, this conclusion is not supported by two other immunohistochemistry-based studies, which did not identify any overexpression of ERBB2 among 44 and 19 atypical hyperplasias, respectively [73, 74]. The prognostic and predictive factors of *ERBB2* amplification and/or overexpression should be studied extensively in a larger cohort. *GATA3* up-regulation was highly correlated with ER positivity and *FOXA1* expression in this study [72]. As *FOXA1* is one of the early events in the ER pathway activation cascade, it might be possible that the oncogenic nature of ER pathway activation is already established in early neoplasia and continues to IDC as *FOXA1* and *GATA3* are frequently mutated in ER+/luminal breast tumors [42]. Additionally, Brunner et al. [72] reported that several pathways influencing membrane transport, including endocytosis by ABC transporters, fatty acid metabolism, and phenylalanine metabolism, are highly enriched already in early neoplasia compared to normal tissues. Notably, these pathways do not encompass any well-known oncogenes; thus, they should be explored further to elucidate the mechanisms involved.

A second gene expression profiling study of ADH synchronous with cancer (DCIS/IDC) ($n = 31$, eight with ADH) showed that significant alterations are already present in ADH and maintained in DCIS and IDC [75]. All ADH showed a grade 1 gene expression pattern and clustered with low grade DCIS and IDC, confirming the close relationship between ADH and low-grade carcinoma (DCIS/IDC) and that ADH have potential to progress into carcinoma [75]. Interestingly, *GATA3* was differentially expressed in this study, which supports the finding of Brunner et al. [72]; however, *FOXA1* and *ERBB2* were not reported. In addition, other key differentially expressed genes and pathways found in Brunner et al., such as the ABC transporters, were not found in Ma et al. (except *ABCA8* but with a low enrichment) [75]. Only around 60 genes overlapped between these two studies; however, there is a very poor correlation of gene expression profiling reported previously between microarrays and RNA sequencing with formalin-fixed paraffin embedded tissues [76]. In general, however, both studies showed that ADH was clearly different from normal breast epithelium, and additional differences were noted on progression to carcinoma.

While these studies are informative for ADH present in synchrony with carcinoma, the expression profiles of pure ADH have not been adequately assessed in a sufficiently powered study. One study did attempt to profile pure ADH in comparison to ADH associated with carcinoma; however, the tissue used was taken adjacent to the ADH lesion observed histologically, with no certainty that the ADH lesion was in fact present [77]. Nonetheless, some overlap was observed with genes differentially expressed in Ma et al. [75] and the authors proposed MMP-1 as a biomarker for progression to carcinoma. A detailed transcriptional study with a larger cohort consisting of pure ADH with extensive patient outcome data would be very powerful in order to identify new pathways for breast cancer prevention associated with ADH. Such studies are increasingly becoming feasible, as the technology for transcriptional studies from formalin-fixed, paraffin-embedded tissue becomes more robust.

Conclusions

The increasing diagnoses of ADH as a consequence of population-based mammographic screening have created clinical dilemmas for treating physicians. Should ADH always be excised or are other options viable? Understanding the genetics of ADH might lead to effective strategies to prevent development and progression of breast cancer associated with ADH and shed light on the breast cancer progression model, in particular the relationship of ADH with non-low grade as well as ER– carcinoma. In addition to synchronous cases, cases with neoplasia not associated with cancer should be assessed in depth as these could be informative for early diagnosis and preventative therapeutic strategies. The comparison of pure ADH with synchronous ADH and cases where ADH was upgraded to carcinoma on excision may be informative for development of biomarkers to help aid in clinical treatment decisions. Overall, the various limitations of all the previous studies discussed in this review (small sample size, lacking careful selection of ADH with and without carcinoma, low resolution methodology, etc.) need to be overcome in any future study of ADH. With the improvement of next-generation sequencing technologies, a careful selection of a larger cohort of ADH than studied to date (with and without carcinoma of different grades), reviewed by an experienced pathologist, would give an insight into early breast cancer progression. Cases of ADH with at least 25 years follow-up should also be included to differentiate between the cancerized and non-cancerized lineages [78], whereby the former is the subset of ADH that could progress to carcinoma while the latter subset would lack progression capability even when harboring clonal genetic events. The outcome of such a study could reduce the burden of overtreatment associated with ADH.

Abbreviations

ADH: Atypical ductal hyperplasia; AI: Allelic imbalance; CGH: Comparative genomic hybridization; CNB: Core needle biopsy; DCIS: Ductal carcinoma in situ; ER: Estrogen receptor; FISH: Fluorescence in situ hybridisation; IDC: Invasive ductal carcinoma; LG DCIS: Low-grade DCIS; LOH: Loss of heterozygosity; PR: Progesterone receptor; VAB: Vacuum assisted biopsy; WGS: Whole genome sequencing

Funding

The authors would like to acknowledge support by the Australian National Health and Medical Research Council (NHMRC APP1063092). TK was supported by Melbourne International Research Scholarship and Melbourne International Fee Remission Scholarship. KLG was supported by a Victorian Cancer Agency Fellowship.

Authors' contributions

TK performed the literature search, wrote and edited the manuscript, and generated the figures. PH, EAR, and IGC wrote and edited the manuscript. KLG conceptualized the paper, wrote and edited the manuscript, generated the figures, and provided overall supervision and co-ordination of manuscript preparation. All authors were involved in writing the manuscript and approved the submitted version.

Competing interests

The authors declare that they have no competing interests.

Author details

[1]Cancer Genetics Laboratory, Peter MacCallum Cancer Centre, Melbourne, VIC, Australia. [2]The Sir Peter MacCallum Department of Oncology, University of Melbourne, Melbourne, VIC, Australia. [3]Cancer Genomics Program, Peter MacCallum Cancer Centre, Melbourne, VIC, Australia. [4]Department of Anatomical Pathology, St Vincent's Hospital, Fitzroy, VIC, Australia. [5]Department of Histopathology, University of Nottingham and Nottingham University Hospitals NHS Trust, City Hospital, Nottingham, UK. [6]Department of Pathology, University of Melbourne, Parkville, VIC, Australia.

References

1. Dupont WD, Page DL. Risk Factors for Breast Cancer in Women with Proliferative Breast Disease. N Engl J Med. 1985;312(3):146–51.
2. Dupont WD, Parl FF, Hartmann WH, Brinton LA, Winfield AC, Worrell JA, Schuyler PA, Plummer WD. Breast cancer risk associated with proliferative breast disease and atypical hyperplasia. Cancer. 1993;71(4):1258–65.
3. Collins LC, Aroner SA, Connolly JL, Colditz GA, Schnitt SJ, Tamimi RM. Breast cancer risk by extent and type of atypical hyperplasia: an update from the Nurses' Health Studies. Cancer. 2016;122(4):515–20.
4. Kabat GC, Jones JG, Olson N, Negassa A, Duggan C, Ginsberg M, Kandel RA, Glass AG, Rohan TE. A multi-center prospective cohort study of benign breast disease and risk of subsequent breast cancer. Cancer Causes Control. 2010;21(6):821–8.
5. Hartmann LC, Sellers TA, Frost MH, Lingle WL, Degnim AC, Ghosh K, Vierkant RA, Maloney SD, Pankratz VS, Hillman DW, et al. Benign breast disease and the risk of breast cancer. N Engl J Med. 2005;353(3):229–37.
6. Li CI, Anderson BO, Daling JR, Moe RE. Trends in incidence rates of invasive lobular and ductal breast carcinoma. JAMA. 2003;289(11):1421–4.
7. Hartmann LC, Degnim AC, Santen RJ, Dupont WD, Ghosh K. Atypical hyperplasia of the breast—risk assessment and management options. N Engl J Med. 2015;372(1):78–89.
8. Degnim AC, Visscher DW, Berman HK, Frost MH, Sellers TA, Vierkant RA, Maloney SD, Pankratz VS, de Groen PC, Lingle WL, et al. Stratification of breast cancer risk in women with atypia: a Mayo cohort study. J Clin Oncol. 2007;25(19):2671–7.
9. Hartmann LC, Radisky DC, Frost MH, Santen RJ, Vierkant RA, Benetti LL, Tarabishy Y, Ghosh K, Visscher DW, Degnim AC. Understanding the premalignant potential of atypical hyperplasia through its natural history: a longitudinal cohort study. Cancer Prev Res. 2014;7(2):211–7.
10. Walia S, Ma Y, Lu J, Lang JE, Press MF. Pathology and current management of borderline breast epithelial lesions. Am J Hematol/Oncol®. 2017;14(8):24–31.
11. Degnim AC, Dupont WD, Radisky DC, Vierkant RA, Frank RD, Frost MH, Winham SJ, Sanders ME, Smith JR, Page DL, et al. Extent of atypical hyperplasia stratifies breast cancer risk in 2 independent cohorts of women. Cancer. 2016;122(19):2971–8.
12. Hoogerbrugge N, Bult P, LMd W-L, Beex LV, Kiemeney LA, Ligtenberg MJL, Massuger LF, Boetes C, Manders P, Brunner HG. High prevalence of premalignant lesions in prophylactically removed breasts from women at hereditary risk for breast cancer. J Clin Oncol. 2003;21(1):41–5.
13. Menes TS, Kerlikowske K, Jaffer S, Seger D, Miglioretti DL. Rates of atypical ductal hyperplasia have declined with less use of postmenopausal hormone treatment: findings from the Breast Cancer Surveillance Consortium. Cancer Epidemiol Biomarkers Prev. 2009;18(11):2822–8.
14. Vierkant RA, Degnim AC, Radisky DC, Visscher DW, Heinzen EP, Frank RD, Winham SJ, Frost MH, Scott CG, Jensen MR, et al. Mammographic breast density and risk of breast cancer in women with atypical hyperplasia: an observational cohort study from the Mayo Clinic Benign Breast Disease (BBD) cohort. BMC Cancer. 2017;17(1):84.
15. Pearlman MD, Griffin JL. Benign Breast Disease. Obstet Gynecol. 2010;116(3):747–58.
16. de Mascarel I, MacGrogan G, Mathoulin-Pélissier S, Vincent-Salomon A, Soubeyran I, Picot V, Coindre J-M, Mauriac L. Epithelial atypia in biopsies performed for microcalcifications. Practical considerations about 2,833 serially sectioned surgical biopsies with a long follow-up. Virchows Arch. 2007;451(1):1–10.
17. Page DL, Dupont WD, Rogers LW, Rados MS. Atypical hyperplastic lesions of the female breast. A long-term follow-up study. Cancer. 1985;55(11):2698–708.
18. Rubin E, Visscher DW, Alexander RW, Urist MM, Maddox WA. Proliferative disease and atypia in biopsies performed for nonpalpable lesions detected mammographically. Cancer. 1988;61(10):2077–82.
19. Welch H, Black WC. Using autopsy series to estimate the disease "reservoir" for ductal carcinoma in situ of the breast: How much more breast cancer can we find? Ann Intern Med. 1997;127(11):1023–8.
20. Page DL, Dupont WD, Rogers L, Rados M. Atypical hyperplastic lesions of the female breast. A long-term follow-up study. Cancer. 1959;35:2698–2708.
21. Lopez-Garcia MA, Geyer FC, Lacroix-Triki M, Marchio C, Reis-Filho JS. Breast cancer precursors revisited: molecular features and progression pathways. Histopathology. 2010;57(2):171–92.
22. Biopsy Interpretation of the Breast. Wolters Kluwer/Lippincott Williams & Wilkins; Biopsy Interpretation Series. Philadelphia: Epstein JI, series ed. 2009:4.
23. Ghofrani M, Tapia B, Tavassoli FA. Discrepancies in the diagnosis of intraductal proliferative lesions of the breast and its management implications: results of a multinational survey. Virchows Arch. 2006;449(6):609–16.
24. Schnitt SJ, Connolly JL, Tavassoli FA, Fechner RE, Kempson RL, Gelman R, Page DL. Interobserver reproducibility in the diagnosis of ductal proliferative breast lesions using standardized criteria. Am J Surg Pathol. 1992;16(12):1133–43.
25. Jain RK, Mehta R, Dimitrov R, Larsson LG, Musto PM, Hodges KB, Ulbright TM, Hattab EM, Agaram N, Idrees MT. Atypical ductal hyperplasia: interobserver and intraobserver variability. Mod Pathol. 2011;24(7):917.
26. Douglas-Jones A, Shah V, Morgan J, Dallimore N, Rashid M. Observer variability in the histopathological reporting of core biopsies of papillary breast lesions is reduced by the use of immunohistochemistry for CK5/6, calponin and p63. Histopathology. 2005;47(2):202–8.
27. Boecker W, Buerger H. Evidence of progenitor cells of glandular and myoepithelial cell lineages in the human adult female breast epithelium: a new progenitor (adult stem) cell concept. Cell Prolif. 2003;36(Suppl 1):73–84.
28. Rosai J. Borderline epithelial lesions of the breast. Am J Surg Pathol. 1991;15(3):209–21.
29. Rageth CJ, O'Flynn EA, Comstock C, Kurtz C, Kubik R, Madjar H, Lepori D, Kampmann G, Mundinger A, Baege A, et al. First International Consensus Conference on lesions of uncertain malignant potential in the breast (B3 lesions). Breast Cancer Res Treat. 2016;159:203–213.
30. Calhoun BC. Core needle biopsy of the breast: an evaluation of contemporary data. Surg Pathol Clin. 2018;11(1):1–16.
31. Calhoun BC, Collins LC. Recommendations for excision following core needle biopsy of the breast: a contemporary evaluation of the literature. Histopathology. 2016;68(1):138–51.
32. Coopey SB, Mazzola E, Buckley JM, Sharko J, Belli AK, Kim EM, Polubriaginof F, Parmigiani G, Garber JE, Smith BL, et al. The role of chemoprevention in modifying the risk of breast cancer in women with atypical breast lesions. Breast Cancer Res Treat. 2012;136(3):627–33.
33. Skandarajah AR, Thomas S, Shackleton K, Chin-Lenn L, Lindeman GJ, Mann GB. Patient and medical barriers preclude uptake of tamoxifen preventative therapy in women with a strong family history. Breast. 2017;32(Supplement C):93–7.
34. Peña A, Shah SS, Fazzio RT, Hoskin TL, Brahmbhatt RD, Hieken TJ, Jakub JW, Boughey JC, Visscher DW, Degnim AC. Multivariate model to identify women at low risk of cancer upgrade after a core needle biopsy diagnosis of atypical ductal hyperplasia. Breast Cancer Res Treat. 2017;164(2):295–304.
35. Linsk A, Mehta TS, Dialani V, Brook A, Chadashvili T, Houlihan MJ, Sharma R. Surgical upgrade rate of breast atypia to malignancy: An academic center's experience and validation of a predictive model. Breast J. 2018;24:115–119.
36. Morrow M, Schnitt SJ, Norton L. Current management of lesions associated with an increased risk of breast cancer. Nat Rev Clin Oncol. 2015;12(4):227.

37. Hutchinson WB, Thomas DB, Hamlin WB, Roth GJ, Peterson AV, Williams B. Risk of breast cancer in women with benign breast disease. J Natl Cancer Inst. 1980;65(1):13–20.

38. London SJ, Connolly JL, Schnitt SJ, Colditz GA. A prospective study of benign breast disease and the risk of breast cancer. JAMA. 1992;267(7):941–4.

39. Dupont WD, Page DL. Relative risk of breast cancer varies with time since diagnosis of atypical hyperplasia. Hum Pathol. 1989;20(8):723–5.

40. Visscher DW, Frost MH, Hartmann LC, Frank RD, Vierkant RA, McCullough AE, Winham SJ, Vachon CM, Ghosh K, Brandt KR, et al. Clinicopathologic features of breast cancers that develop in women with previous benign breast disease. Cancer. 2016;122(3):378–85.

41. Danforth DN. Molecular profile of atypical hyperplasia of the breast. Breast Cancer Res Treat. 2018;167:9–29.

42. Cancer Genome Atlas N. Comprehensive molecular portraits of human breast tumours. Nature. 2012;490(7418):61–70.

43. Lakhani S, Collins N, Stratton M, Sloane J. Atypical ductal hyperplasia of the breast: clonal proliferation with loss of heterozygosity on chromosomes 16q and 17p. J Clin Pathol. 1995;48(7):611–5.

44. Larson PS, de las Morenas A, Cerda SR, Bennett SR, Cupples LA, Rosenberg CL. Quantitative analysis of allele imbalance supports atypical ductal hyperplasia lesions as direct breast cancer precursors. J Pathol. 2006;209(3):307–16.

45. O'Connell P, Pekkel V, Allred DC, Fuqua SA, Osborne CK, Clark GM. Analysis of loss of heterozygosity in 399 premalignant breast lesions at 15 genetic loci. J Natl Cancer Inst. 1998;90(9):697–703.

46. Stomper P, Stewart C, Penetrante R, Nava M, Tsangaris T. Flow cytometric DNA analysis of excised breast lesions: use of fresh tissue needle aspirates obtained under guidance with mammography of the specimen. Radiology. 1992;185(2):415–22.

47. Niu Y, Wang S, Liu T, Zhang T, Wei X, Wang Y, Jiang L. Expression of centrosomal tubulins associated with DNA ploidy in breast premalignant lesions and carcinoma. Pathol Res Pract. 2013;209(4):221–7.

48. Ruiz A, Almenar S, Callaghan RC, Llombart-Bosch A. Benign, preinvasive and invasive ductal breast lesions. A comparative study with quantitative techniques: morphometry, image-and flow cytometry. Pathol Res Pract. 1999;195(11):741–6.

49. Eriksson E, Schimmelpenning H, Silfverswärd C, Auer G. Immunoreactivity with monoclonal antibody A-80 and nuclear DNA content in benign and malignant human breast disease. Hum Pathol. 1992;23(12):1366–72.

50. Crissman J, Visscher DW, Kubus J. Image cytophotometric DNA analysis of atypical hyperplasias and intraductal carcinomas of the breast. Arch Pathol Lab Med. 1990;114(12):1249–53.

51. Sneige N, Sahin A, Dinh M, El-Naggar A. Interphase cytogenetics in mammographically detected breast lesions. Hum Pathol. 1996;27(4):330–5.

52. Krishnamurthy S, Zhao L, Hayes K, Glassman AB, Cristofanilli M, Singletary SE, Hunt KK, Kuerer HM, Sneige N. Feasibility and utility of using chromosomal aneusomy to further define the cytologic categories in nipple aspirate fluid specimens. Cancer Cytopathol. 2004;102(5):322–7.

53. Visscher DW, Wallis TL, Crissman JD. Evaluation of chromosome aneuploidy in tissue sections of preinvasive breast carcinomas using interphase cytogenetics. Cancer. 1996;77(2):315–20.

54. Gao Y, Niu Y, Wang X, Wei L, Lu S. Genetic changes at specific stages of breast cancer progression detected by comparative genomic hybridization. J Mol Med. 2009;87(2):145–52.

55. Xu S, Wei B, Zhang H, Qing M, Bu H. Evidence of chromosomal alterations in pure usual ductal hyperplasia as a breast carcinoma precursor. Oncol Rep. 2008;19(6):1469–76.

56. Aubele MM, Cummings MC, Mattis AE, Zitzelsberger HF, Walch AK, Kremer M, Höfler H, Werner M. Accumulation of chromosomal imbalances from intraductal proliferative lesions to adjacent in situ and invasive ductal breast cancer. Diagn Mol Pathol. 2000;9(1):14–9.

57. Newburger DE, Kashef-Haghighi D, Weng Z, Salari R, Sweeney RT, Brunner AL, Zhu SX, Guo X, Varma S, Troxell ML. Genome evolution during progression to breast cancer. Genome Res. 2013;23(7):1097–108.

58. Weng Z, Spies N, Zhu SX, Newburger DE, Kashef-Haghighi D, Batzoglou S, Sidow A, West RB. Cell-lineage heterogeneity and driver mutation recurrence in pre-invasive breast neoplasia. Genome Med. 2015;7(1):1.

59. Birkbak NJ, Eklund AC, Li Q, McClelland SE, Endesfelder D, Tan P, Tan IB, Richardson AL, Szallasi Z, Swanton C. Paradoxical relationship between chromosomal instability and survival outcome in cancer. Cancer Res. 2011;71(10):3447–52.

60. Slaughter DP, Southwick HW, Smejkal W. "Field cancerization" in oral stratified squamous epithelium. Clinical implications of multicentric origin. Cancer. 1953;6(5):963–8.

61. Arthur R, Wang Y, Ye K, Glass AG, Ginsberg M, Loudig O, Rohan T. Association between lifestyle, menstrual/reproductive history, and histological factors and risk of breast cancer in women biopsied for benign breast disease. Breast Cancer Res Treat. 2017;165(3):623–31.

62. Bombonati A, Sgroi DC. The molecular pathology of breast cancer progression. J Pathol. 2011;223(2):307–17.

63. Pang JMB, Gorringe KL, Fox SB. Ductal carcinoma in situ–update on risk assessment and management. Histopathology. 2016;68(1):96–109.

64. Visvader JE, Stingl J. Mammary stem cells and the differentiation hierarchy: current status and perspectives. Genes Dev. 2014;28(11):1143–58.

65. Xu R, Perle MA, Inghirami G, Chan W, Delgado Y, Feiner H. Amplification of Her-2/neu gene in Her-2/neu-overexpressing and -nonexpressing breast carcinomas and their synchronous benign, premalignant, and metastatic lesions detected by FISH in archival material. Mod Pathol. 2002;15(2):116–24.

66. Gorringe KL, Hunter SM, Pang JM, Opeskin K, Hill P, Rowley SM, Choong DY, Thompson ER, Dobrovic A, Fox SB, et al. Copy number analysis of ductal carcinoma in situ with and without recurrence. Mod Pathol. 2015;28(9):1174–84.

67. Ellsworth RE, Ellsworth DL, Weyandt JD, Fantacone-Campbell JL, Deyarmin B, Hooke JA, Shriver CD. Chromosomal alterations in pure nonneoplastic breast lesions: implications for breast cancer progression. Ann Surg Oncol. 2010;17(6):1688–94.

68. Iakovlev VV, Arneson NC, Wong V, Wang C, Leung S, Iakovleva G, Warren K, Pintilie M, Done SJ. Genomic differences between pure ductal carcinoma in situ of the breast and that associated with invasive disease: a calibrated aCGH study. Clin Cancer Res. 2008;14(14):4446–54.

69. Johnson CE, Gorringe KL, Thompson ER, Opeskin K, Boyle SE, Wang Y, Hill P, Mann GB, Campbell IG. Identification of copy number alterations associated with the progression of DCIS to invasive ductal carcinoma. Breast Cancer Res Treat. 2012;133(3):889–98.

70. Nik-Zainal S, Van Loo P, Wedge DC, Alexandrov LB, Greenman CD, Lau KW, Raine K, Jones D, Marshall J, Ramakrishna M. The life history of 21 breast cancers. Cell. 2012;149(5):994–1007.

71. Forsberg LA, Rasi C, Pekar G, Davies H, Piotrowski A, Absher D, Razzaghian HR, Ambicka A, Halaszka K, Przewoznik M, et al. Signatures of post-zygotic structural genetic aberrations in the cells of histologically normal breast tissue that can predispose to sporadic breast cancer. Genome Res. 2015;25(10):1521–35.

72. Brunner AL, Li J, Guo X, Sweeney RT, Varma S, Zhu SX, Li R, Tibshirani R, West RB. A shared transcriptional program in early breast neoplasias despite genetic and clinical distinctions. Genome Biol. 2014;15(5):1–16.

73. Coene ED, Schelfhout V, Winkler RA, Schelfhout A-M, Roy NV, Grooteclaes M, Speleman F, Potter CD. Amplification units and translocation at chromosome 17q and c-erb B-2 overexpression in the pathogenesis of breast cancer. Virchows Arch. 1997;430(5):365–72.

74. Eren F, Calay Z, Durak H, Eren B, Çomunoğlu N, Aydin Ö. C-Erb-b2 oncogene expression in intraductal proliferative lesions of the breast. Bosn J Basic Med Sci. 2012;12(1):41.

75. Ma X-J, Salunga R, Tuggle JT, Gaudet J, Enright E, McQuary P, Payette T, Pistone M, Stecker K, Zhang BM. Gene expression profiles of human breast cancer progression. Proc Natl Acad Sci U S A. 2003;100(10):5974–9.

76. Beck AH, Weng Z, Witten DM, Zhu S, Foley JW, Lacroute P, Smith CL, Tibshirani R, Van De Rijn M, Sidow A. 3'-end sequencing for expression quantification (3SEQ) from archival tumor samples. PLoS One. 2010;5(1):e8768.

77. Poola I, DeWitty RL, Marshalleck JJ, Bhatnagar R, Abraham J, Leffall LD. Identification of MMP-1 as a putative breast cancer predictive marker by global gene expression analysis. Nat Med. 2005;11(5):481–3.

78 Curtius K, Wright NA, Graham TA. An evolutionary perspective on field cancerization. Nat Rev Cancer. 2018;18(1):19.

79. Amari M, Suzuki A, Moriya T, Yoshinaga K, Amano G, Sasano H, Ohuchi N, Satomi S, Horii A. LOH analyses of premalignant and malignant lesions of human breast: Frequent LOH in 8p, 16q, and 17q in atypical ductal hyperplasia. Oncol Rep. 1999;6(6):1277–80.

80. Gong G, DeVries S, Chew KL, Cha I, Ljung B-M, Waldman FM. Genetic changes in paired atypical and usual ductal hyperplasia of the breast by comparative genomic hybridization. Clin Cancer Res. 2001;7(8):2410–4.

7

Magnetic resonance imaging and molecular features associated with tumor-infiltrating lymphocytes in breast cancer

Jia Wu[1]* , Xuejie Li[2], Xiaodong Teng[2], Daniel L. Rubin[3,4,5], Sandy Napel[3], Bruce L. Daniel[3] and Ruijiang Li[1]

Abstract

Background: We sought to investigate associations between dynamic contrast-enhanced (DCE) magnetic resonance imaging (MRI) features and tumor-infiltrating lymphocytes (TILs) in breast cancer, as well as to study if MRI features are complementary to molecular markers of TILs.

Methods: In this retrospective study, we extracted 17 computational DCE-MRI features to characterize tumor and parenchyma in The Cancer Genome Atlas cohort ($n = 126$). The percentage of stromal TILs was evaluated on H&E-stained histological whole-tumor sections. We first evaluated associations between individual imaging features and TILs. Multiple-hypothesis testing was corrected by the Benjamini-Hochberg method using false discovery rate (FDR). Second, we implemented LASSO (least absolute shrinkage and selection operator) and linear regression nested with tenfold cross-validation to develop an imaging signature for TILs. Next, we built a composite prediction model for TILs by combining imaging signature with molecular features. Finally, we tested the prognostic significance of the TIL model in an independent cohort (I-SPY 1; $n = 106$).

Results: Four imaging features were significantly associated with TILs ($P < 0.05$ and FDR < 0.2), including tumor volume, cluster shade of signal enhancement ratio (SER), mean SER of tumor-surrounding background parenchymal enhancement (BPE), and proportion of BPE. Among molecular and clinicopathological factors, only cytolytic score was correlated with TILs ($\rho = 0.51$; 95% CI, 0.36–0.63; $P = 1.6\text{E-}9$). An imaging signature that linearly combines five features showed correlation with TILs ($\rho = 0.40$; 95% CI, 0.24–0.54; $P = 4.2\text{E-}6$). A composite model combining the imaging signature and cytolytic score improved correlation with TILs ($\rho = 0.62$; 95% CI, 0.50–0.72; $P = 9.7\text{E-}15$). The composite model successfully distinguished low vs high, intermediate vs high, and low vs intermediate TIL groups, with AUCs of 0.94, 0.76, and 0.79, respectively. During validation (I-SPY 1), the predicted TILs from the imaging signature separated patients into two groups with distinct recurrence-free survival (RFS), with log-rank $P = 0.042$ among triple-negative breast cancer (TNBC). The composite model further improved stratification of patients with distinct RFS (log-rank $P = 0.0008$), where TNBC with no/minimal TILs had a worse prognosis.

Conclusions: Specific MRI features of tumor and parenchyma are associated with TILs in breast cancer, and imaging may play an important role in the evaluation of TILs by providing key complementary information in equivocal cases or situations that are prone to sampling bias.

Keywords: Tumor-infiltrating lymphocytes, Imaging marker, Cytolytic score, Nonsynonymous mutation burden, Breast cancer

---

* Correspondence: jiawu@stanford.edu
[1]Department of Radiation Oncology, Stanford University School of Medicine, 1070 Arastradero Road, Stanford, CA 94305, USA
Full list of author information is available at the end of the article

Background

Immunotherapy for treating patients with cancer has generated much excitement in recent years [1]. Compared with conventional therapies, immune checkpoint blockade (ICB) such as anti-PD1 therapy has achieved durable clinical response and long-term survival benefit in a variety of cancer types [2, 3]. However, only a small proportion of patients respond to current immunotherapy, underscoring the need for predictive biomarkers to identify appropriate patients [4]. One promising biomarker is tumor-infiltrating lymphocytes (TILs), because it is now recognized that a preexisting antitumor immunity is required for the success of ICB-based immunotherapy [5]. In breast cancer, there is strong evidence for the prognostic and predictive value of TILs [6]. Several large clinical trials have demonstrated that TILs are associated with pathological complete response and prognosis after chemotherapy or targeted therapies, particularly in triple-negative breast cancer (TNBC) and human epidermal growth factor receptor 2 (HER2)-positive breast cancer [7–14].

The evaluation of TILs involves visualization and measurement of lymphocytes on H&E-stained histological slides of tumor samples [15]. Current guidelines issued by the International Immuno-Oncology Biomarker Working Group on Breast Cancer recommend that evaluation of TILs be performed in the stromal rather than intraepithelial compartments, and preferably on whole tumor sections over core biopsies [16]. Despite numerous efforts to standardize the evaluation of TILs, this process remains laborious and subjective with inter- and intrarater variability [16]. Moreover, evaluation of TILs in the preoperative neoadjuvant setting is problematic because of heterogeneous tumor shrinkage patterns and sampling bias in a biopsy. A more objective, consistent method to evaluate TILs in breast cancer would be extremely valuable.

Imaging allows noninvasive visualization of the entire tumor and its surrounding tissue. Recent studies have demonstrated associations between specific magnetic resonance imaging (MRI) features and pathological or molecular patterns, such as molecular subtypes [17–22] and gene expression signatures or pathways [23–28]. These data support the underlying pathophysiology of the disease being reflected on imaging at a macroscopic level, and this link may be revealed by a more detailed comprehensive image analysis.

The purpose of this study was to investigate the association between MRI features and TILs in breast cancer. We explored whether computational imaging features could be used to predict TILs. Further, we constructed a composite prediction model by integrating imaging and immune-related molecular features and validated its clinical relevance in an independent cohort.

Methods

Study design

We carried out this institutional review board-approved, Health Insurance Portability and Accountability Act (HIPAA)-compliant retrospective study in three steps (Fig. 1). First, we characterized both tumor and parenchymal enhancement patterns at dynamic contrast-enhanced (DCE) MRI and evaluated their association with TILs. Second, we built a composite model to predict TILs by integrating imaging with molecular and clinicopathological data. Third, we tested the prognostic significance of the TIL model in an independent cohort.

Patient cohorts

We analyzed two breast cancer cohorts from The Cancer Genome Atlas (TCGA) project [29] and the I-SPY 1 (Investigation of Serial Studies to Predict Your Therapeutic Response with Imaging And moLecular Analysis) trial [30]. For this study, the inclusion criteria for TCGA cohort were (1) pathologically proven invasive carcinomas, (2) pretreatment DCE-MRI data available, (3) H&E-stained whole-tumor tissue sections available, and (4) tumor gene expression data from RNA-sequencing (RNA-seq) and mutational data from whole-exome sequencing available. We applied similar inclusion criteria to select patients from the I-SPY 1 cohort, except that outcomes were available, but H&E-stained slides and mutational data were not required. After selection, 126 patients from TCGA and 105 patients from I-SPY 1 were eligible for the proposed study. The detailed selection procedures are shown in Additional file 1: Figure S1. Clinical and imaging data are publicly available for both cohorts from The Cancer Imaging Archive (TCIA) (www.cancerimagingarchive.net).

Evaluation of tumor-infiltrating lymphocytes

TILs were evaluated for TCGA cohort, for which detailed biospecimen collection and processing protocols have been described elsewhere [29]. In brief, the tumor sections were collected from surgical specimens and reviewed by a board-certified pathologist to confirm the presence of invasive carcinoma. The H&E-stained whole-slide tumor sections were digitally scanned and are available from the Cancer Digital Slide Archive (http://cancer.digitalslidearchive.net/).

Two pathologists (XT and XL, with 30 and 5 years of experience, respectively, in reading breast cancer tissue slides) evaluated TILs in consensus based on the recommendations from the International Immuno-Oncology Biomarker Working Group on Breast Cancer [16]. Two pathologists simultaneously reviewed the digital slides of each patient from the Cancer Digital Slide Archive, and the TILs were measured as the percentage of lymphocytes and macrophages in the area of total intratumoral

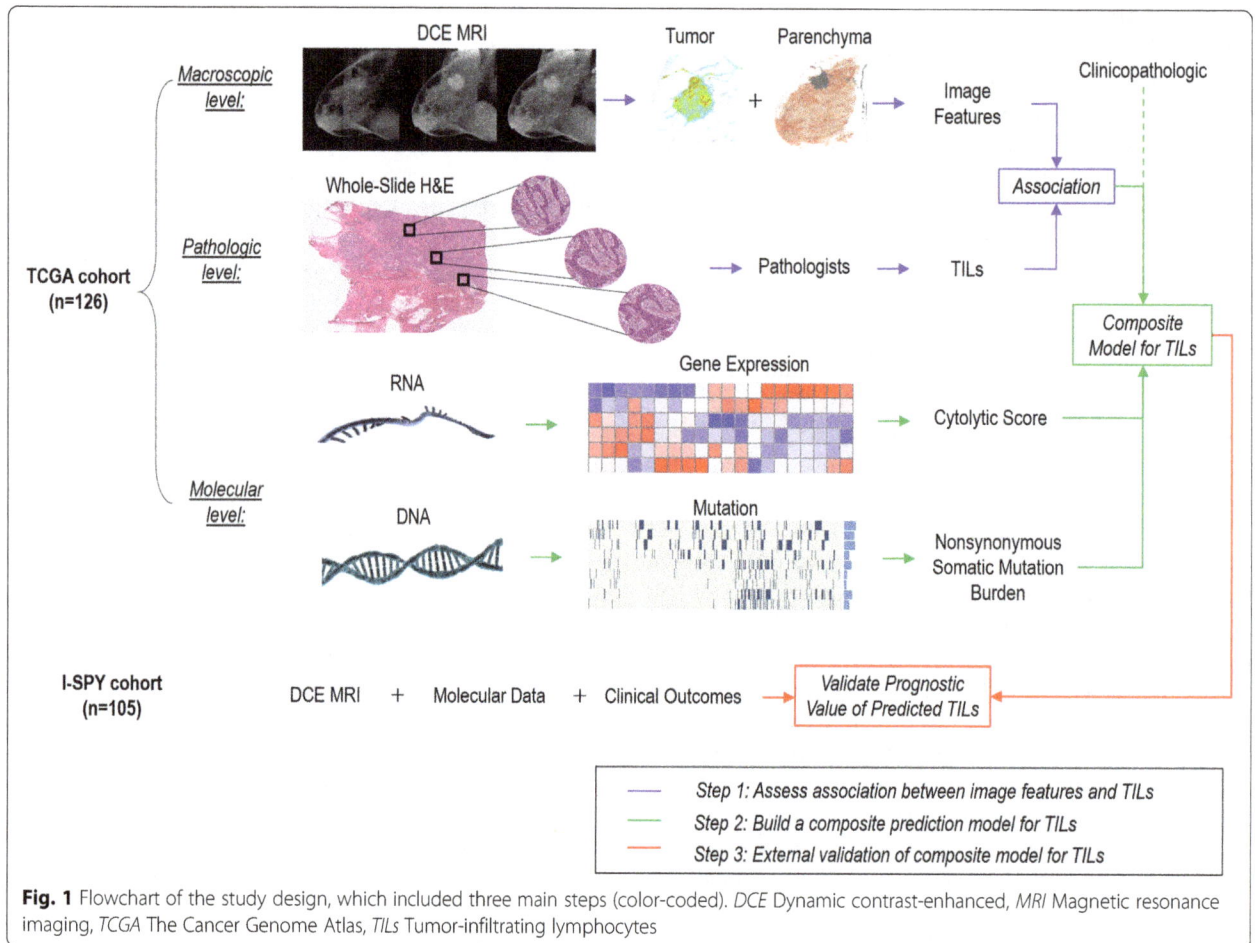

Fig. 1 Flowchart of the study design, which included three main steps (color-coded). *DCE* Dynamic contrast-enhanced, *MRI* Magnetic resonance imaging, *TCGA* The Cancer Genome Atlas, *TILs* Tumor-infiltrating lymphocytes

stromal compartments. In addition, three discrete categories are defined, with ≤ 10%, > 10% to ≤40%, and > 40% to ≤ 90% TILs indicating tumors with no/minimal, intermediate, and high lymphocyte infiltration, respectively [16]. To assess interrater variability, we calculated the intraclass correlation coefficient (ICC) between our TIL percentage and those reported in a previous study focused on TNBC [31] for 15 overlapped cases in TCGA cohort.

Imaging protocols
The detailed imaging protocol for TCGA cohort has been reported elsewhere [27]. In brief, the scans were performed between September 1999 and June 2006 at six participating centers with a 1.5-T or 3-T GE Healthcare (Milwaukee, MI, USA), Siemens (Erlangen, Germany), or Philips (Amsterdam, The Netherlands) whole-body MRI system with a standard double-breast coil. The dynamic protocol of DCE-MRI was in accordance with the American College of Radiology guidelines, which included one precontrast and two to seven postcontrast scans (with a gadolinium-based contrast agent), in either the sagittal or axial view.

The detailed imaging protocol for the I-SPY cohort was reported elsewhere [32, 33]. To match the MRI from TCGA cohort, we focused on the scans acquired before neoadjuvant chemotherapy (i.e., baseline scans). MRI was performed through a 1.5-T GE Healthcare, Siemens, or Philips system, with a dedicated breast radiofrequency coil. The DCE-MRI protocols include one precontrast scan and two postcontrast phases with one ~ 2.5 minutes and another one ~ 7.5 minutes.

Image processing and harmonization
Given the diverse imaging protocols within the multicenter TCGA data and I-SPY 1 cohorts, we developed a pipeline to normalize the imaging data before extracting quantitative feature. First, we applied the N4 bias correction to correct for shading artifacts. Next, we standardized the temporal resolution of DCE-MRI scans in TCGA and I-SPY cohorts. In particular, for each patient, we included DCE-MRI before contrast agent administration and two postcontrast scans, with one having a 2–3-minute delay and the other having an ~7.5-minute delay. Third, to explicitly account for heterogeneous imaging protocols, for each individual, the voxel values of

Magnetic resonance imaging and molecular features associated with tumor-infiltrating...

81

DCE-MRI were normalized by the parenchyma without contrast (i.e., the average value of interquartile voxel from parenchyma before administrating contrast). Finally, the MRI scans were resized to have an isotropic voxel resolution of 1 mm to assure consistent and meaningful computation of 3D textural features.

Tumor and background parenchyma segmentation

The detailed process used for segmentation was reported elsewhere [28, 34]. Briefly, two radiologists with 14 and 11 years of experience, respectively, in breast imaging manually delineated the 3D tumor slice-by-slice and reached consensus regarding 3D tumor contours. The ipsilateral parenchyma was segmented automatically through Fuzzy C-means clustering. The 3D parenchymal segmentation was inspected by two radiologists, and they manually revised it when necessary.

MRI feature exaction

The rationale of feature extraction is to provide a comprehensive characterization of breast cancer at DCE-MRI. We initially extracted 110 computational imaging features as defined in a previous study [28] and removed those with linear ICCs above 0.85. For correlated features, the one that showed highest robustness with respect to tumor contour variations (manual segmentation vs automatic segmentation via Fuzzy C-means clustering) was kept, similar to previous studies [34, 35]. As a result, 17 nonredundant imaging features remained.

The selected features characterize the tumoral and parenchymal phenotypes at DCE-MRI, which include five tumor morphological features, four tumor texture features, two functional tumor volume features, four background parenchymal enhancement (BPE) features, and two tumor-surrounding PE features. The mathematical formulation and the interpretation and clinical relevance [27, 28, 32, 36–38] of these features are elaborated in Table 1. The computation of all imaging features was implemented automatically with MATLAB software (MathWorks, Natick, MA, USA).

Molecular features related to tumor-infiltrating lymphocytes

Tumor mutation burden is an important genetic factor in mediating antitumor immunity. Tumors with a higher mutation load are associated with a higher neoantigen level and thus are more immunogenic and likely to have higher immune infiltration and more TILs [39]. The cytolytic activity reflects local immune effector function and can indicate the presence of TILs. Indeed, cytolytic activity computed from the gene transcript levels of two critical immune cytolytic effectors [40], perforin (*PRF1*) and granzyme A (*GZMA*), has been shown to be closely related to immune infiltration and CD8+ T-cell activation [41, 42]. For TCGA breast cancer cohort, gene expression data from RNA-seq and mutational data from whole-exome sequencing are available in the Genomic Data Commons (https://gdc.cancer.gov/). On the basis

Table 1 Definition and interpretation of 17 computational imaging features extracted from dynamic contrast-enhanced magnetic resonance imaging scans

Type	No.	Definition	Interpretation
Morphology (M)	5	M1: Volume	Tumor shape, size, and boundary smoothness (i.e., descriptors according to BI-RADS classification)
		M2: Sphericity	
		M3: Surface-to-volume ratio	
		M4: Mean of margin sharpness	
		M5: SD of margin sharpness	
Texture of kinetic maps (TEX)	4	TEX1: Correlation of SER	Spatial tumor heterogeneity of the SER map
		TEX2: Cluster shade of SER	
		TEX3: Energy of SER	
		TEX4: Entropy of SER	
Functional tumor volume (FTV)	2	FTV1: Absolute volume of the active tumor with SER > 1.0	Subvolume of tumor with fast contrast uptake and washout
		FTV2: Absolute volume of the active tumor with SER > 1.5	
Ipsilateral background parenchymal enhancement (BPE)	4	BPE1: Absolute volume of BPE with PE > 0.2	Enhanced subvolume of ipsilateral breast parenchyma at the early postcontrast phase, in accordance with the BI-RADS classification
		BPE2: Absolute volume of BPE with PE > 0.6	
		BPE3: Relative volume of BPE with PE > 0.2	
		BPE4: Relative volume of BPE with PE > 0.6	
Tumor surrounding background parenchymal enhancement (TS-BPE)	2	TS-BPE1: Mean value of PE in tumor surrounding parenchyma (2 cm)	Enhancement of parenchyma surrounding the tumor within 2-cm distance
		TS-BPE2: Mean value of SER in tumor surrounding parenchyma (2 cm)	

BI-RADS Breast Imaging Reporting and Data System, *PE* percent enhancement; $PE = \frac{I_{early\ postcontrast} - I_{precontrast}}{I_{precontrast}}$, *SER* signal enhancement ratio; $SER = \frac{I_{early\ postcontrast} - I_{precontrast}}{I_{late\ postcontrast} - I_{precontrast}}$

of these data, we computed the nonsynonymous somatic mutational burden and cytolytic activity score, defined as the geometric mean of the expression of two genes: *GZMA* and *PRF1* [40]. Similarly for the I-SPY 1 cohort, we computed the cytolytic activity score on the basis of microarray gene expression data available from the Gene Expression Omnibus (https://www.ncbi.nlm.nih.gov/geo/ ; [GEO:GSE22226]) [43]. The ComBat algorithm [44] was implemented to harmonize the gene expression data from TCGA and I-SPY.

Association with tumor-infiltrating lymphocytes and predictive modeling

We first evaluated the Pearson linear correlation between individual imaging features and percentage of TILs in TCGA cohort. Next, we built a predictive model for TILs by combining multiple imaging features into an imaging signature. For this purpose, we used linear regression with feature selection via LASSO (least absolute shrinkage and selection operator) [45] to avoid overfitting. In addition, tenfold cross-validation was applied and repeated 100 times to minimize the selection bias. The most frequently selected imaging features (> 90%) were used to fit the final model. Further, we investigated whether combining the imaging signature with immune-related molecular features (cytolytic score and somatic mutation burden) would improve prediction accuracy for TILs by fitting a composite model via multivariate linear regression.

Performance evaluation

To evaluate the prediction models, we calculated the Pearson linear correlation between pathologist-rated and estimated percentage of TILs. In addition, patients were divided into three recognized TIL categories (low, intermediate, and high immune infiltration) [16], and pairwise classification among the three categories was evaluated. We compared the performance of the composite model with molecular features based on cytolytic score and imaging signature. In particular, the ROC analysis and AUC were used to assess the binary prediction accuracy of the models. The threshold used to separate different prediction models was defined on the basis of Youden's J statistics [46], and the corresponding sensitivity, specificity, and accuracy were reported. Finally, we tested prognostic significance of the imaging signature as well as the composite TIL model by assessing their association with recurrence-free survival (RFS) in the entire I-SPY 1 cohort as well as in clinically relevant subgroups according to the receptor status. Because the prognostic value of TILs seems to be strongest in TNBC [11, 13], we expect that the composite model would also be prognostic within the TNBC subgroup in the I-SPY 1 cohort.

Statistical analysis

In univariate analysis, to adjust for multiple statistical testing, the Benjamini-Hochberg method was used to control the false discovery rate (FDR). The Mann-Whitney U statistic was used to assess the statistical significance of binary classification of TIL categories by comparing the prediction models with a random guess with an AUC of 0.5. The DeLong test was used to determine the 95% CIs and compute P values for the comparison of ROC curves. The Cox proportional hazards model was used to build survival models. Kaplan-Meier analysis was used to estimate survival probability. The log-rank test and concordance index were used to assess prognostic performance. All statistical tests were two-sided. P value < 0.05 and FDR < 0.2 were considered to be statistically significant. Statistical analysis was performed in R (R Foundation for Statistical Computing, Vienna, Austria).

Results
Patient characteristics and tumor-infiltrating lymphocyte evaluation

Among 1098 cases in TCGA breast cancer cohort, 126 patients were eligible for our study. A majority ($n = 92$, 73%) of patients had low immune infiltration (0–10% TILs) in their tumor stroma, whereas 20% ($n = 25$) and 7% (n = 9) of patients had intermediate and high immune infiltration, respectively. Clinicopathological characteristics of patients in each of the three TIL categories are shown in Table 2. There was high reproducibility between TILs measured by our pathologists and previously reported values with ICC of 0.80 ($P = 0.002$). For the I-SPY 1 cohort, 105 patients were eligible and included in this study (patient characteristics summarized in Additional file 2: Table S1).

Imaging features associated with tumor-infiltrating lymphocytes

Each of the 17 imaging features independently characterizes the cancer phenotypes, and their pairwise correlation map is shown in Additional file 1: Figure S2. Figure 2 shows the heat map of 17 imaging features for 126 patients in TCGA cohort ranked on the basis of their TILs, monotonically increasing from left to right. In the univariate analysis, 4 of 17 imaging features were significantly associated with the percentage of TILs ($P < 0.05$ and FDR < 0.2), as shown in Fig. 3. Among these four features, the tumor volume was positively correlated with TILs, whereas cluster shade of signal enhancement ratio (SER) map, mean SER of tumor surrounding BPE, and proportion of BPE were negatively correlated with TILs (Additional file 2: Table S2). Next, we built an imaging signature for TILs by fitting a linear model, which consisted of five imaging features: $4.4 \times M1 -$

Table 2 Clinical and pathological Characteristics for Eligible Patients in the TCGA Cohort

Parameter	≤ 10% stromal TILs	> 10 to ≤ 40% stromal TILs	> 40 to ≤ 90% stromal TILs	P value[a]
	Tumor with no/minimal immune cells (n = 92, 73%)	Tumor with intermediate/heterogeneous infiltrate (n = 25, 20%)	Tumor with high immune infiltrate (n = 9, 7%)	
Age, years				
Median (range)	52 (29–82)	56 (38–75)	61 (47–77)	
Mean ± SD	52.8 ± 11.6	55.8 ± 11.1	61.2 ± 8.7	
T				
T1	37 (71)	10 (19)	5 (10)	0.821
T2	47 (65)	15 (23)	3 (5)	0.744
T3	8 (89)	0	1 (11)	0.307
N				
N0	44 (69)	16 (25)	4 (6)	0.726
N1	32 (74)	8 (19)	3 (7)	1
N2	9 (82)	1 (9)	1 (9)	0.748
N3	6 (86)	0	1 (14)	0.290
Nx[b]	1 (100)	0	0	
M				
M0	79 (75)	20 (19)	6 (6)	0.919
Mx[c]	13 (62)	5 (24)	3 (14)	0.361
Stage				
I	22 (73)	6 (20)	2 (7)	1
II	53 (70)	18 (24)	5 (7)	0.826
III	17 (85)	1 (5)	2 (10)	0.204
Histological type				
Invasive ductal carcinoma	80 (75)	19 (18)	7 (7)	0.921
Invasive lobular carcinoma	10 (59)	5 (29)	2 (12)	0.371
Other	2 (67)	1 (33)	0	
Estrogen receptor status				
Positive	79 (75)	19 (18)	7 (7)	0.947
Negative	13 (62)	6 (29)	2 (10)	0.560
Progesterone receptor status				
Positive	71 (76)	16 (17)	6 (6)	0.888
Negative	21 (64)	9 (27)	3 (9)	0.515
Human epidermal growth factor receptor 2 status				
Positive	14 (61)	6 (26)	3 (13)	0.384
Negative	76 (76)	19 (19)	5 (5)	0.790
Equivocal	2 (67)	0	1 (33)	
IHC subtype				
HR+/HER2−	68 (78)	14 (16)	5 (6)	0.824
HER2+	14 (61)	6 (26)	3 (13)	0.571
ER−/PR−/HER2−	10 (63)	5 (31)	1 (6)	0.592
PAM50 intrinsic subtype				
Luminal A	53 (75)	13 (18)	5 (7)	0.966
Luminal B	22 (79)	4 (14)	2 (7)	0.875

Table 2 Clinical and pathological Characteristics for Eligible Patients in the TCGA Cohort *(Continued)*

Parameter	≤ 10% stromal TILs	> 10 to ≤ 40% stromal TILs	> 40 to ≤ 90% stromal TILs	P value[a]
	Tumor with no/minimal immune cells (*n* = 92, 73%)	Tumor with intermediate/heterogeneous infiltrate (*n* = 25, 20%)	Tumor with high immune infiltrate (*n* = 9, 7%)	
HER2	4 (50)	3 (38)	1 (12)	0.219
Basal	10 (63)	5 (31)	1 (6)	0.536
Normal	3 (100)	0	0	

Abbreviations: ER Estrogen receptor, *HER2* Human epidermal growth factor receptor 2, *HR* Hormone receptor, *PR* Progesterone receptor, *TIL* Tumor-infiltrating lymphocyte
[a]Fisher's exact test was used to compare TIL distribution within selected category with TIL distribution of whole population
[b]Lymph node stage is not available
[c]Metastasis cannot be measured

$3.14 \times TEX2 - 2.0 \times TS - BPE2 - 2.62 \times BPE1 - 0.72 \times BPE3 + 13.02$, where $M1$ = tumor volume, $TEX2$ = cluster shade of SER map, $TS\text{-}BPE2$ = mean SER of tumor surrounding BPE (2 cm), $BPE1$ = BPE volume (percentage enhancement or PE > 20%), and $BPE3$ = BPE proportion (PE, > 20%). The mean and SD values of the five selected imaging features are shown in Additional file 2: Table S3. This imaging signature had a moderate linear correlation with TILs (ρ = 0.40; 95% CI, 0.24–0.54; P = 4.2E-6). Moreover, the imaging signature is able to separate three TILs categories in pairwise fashion (Fig. 4a), with

prediction accuracy of 0.73, 0.71, and 0.71, respectively (Table 3). Figure 5 showed the details of three representative patients where there is good agreement between the predicted TILs from proposed imaging signatures and TIL readings by two pathologists.

Relationships between imaging, molecular signatures, and tumor-infiltrating lymphocytes

We evaluated the associations between imaging and immune-related molecular features, as well as the percentage of TILs, in TCGA cohort. In addition to the

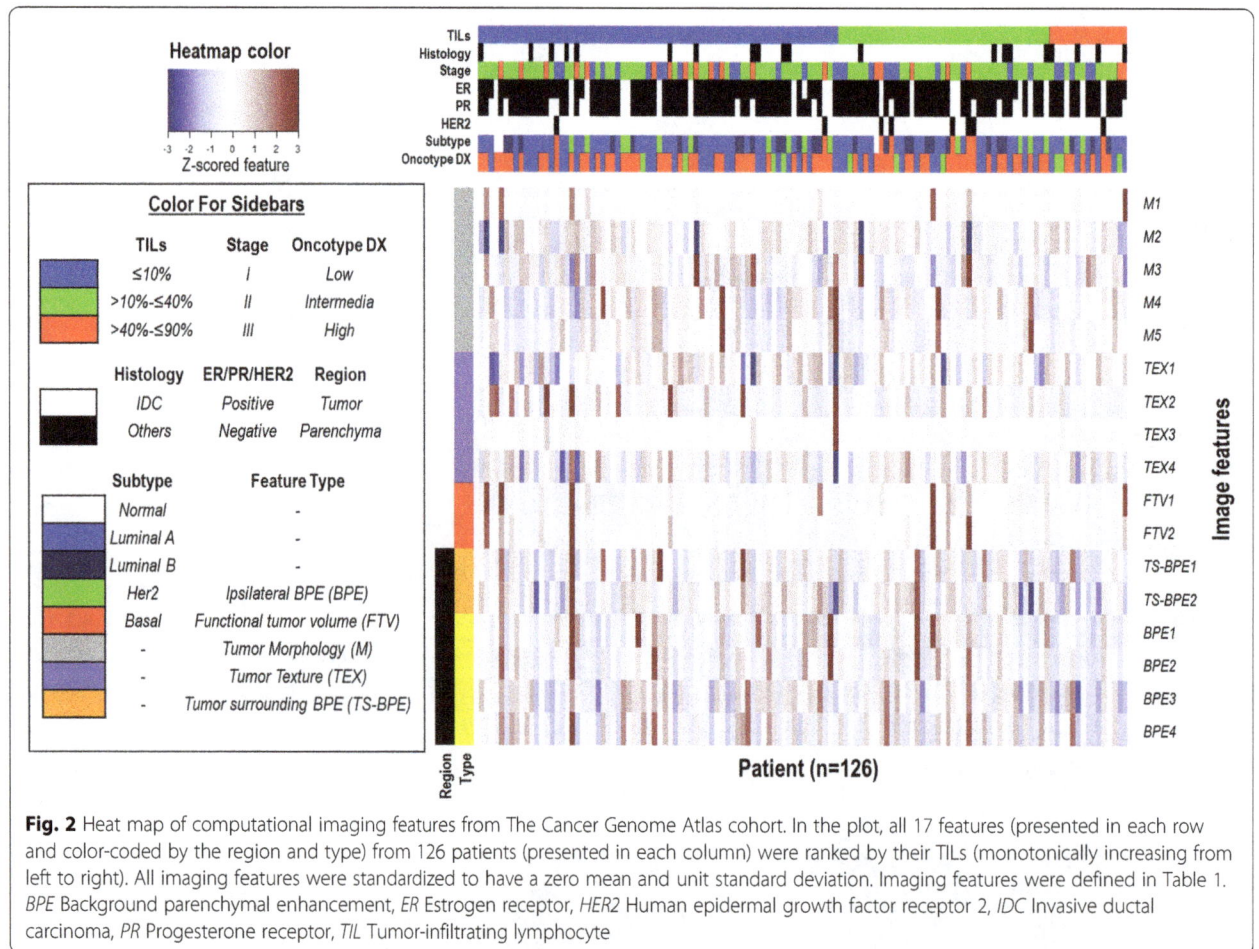

Fig. 2 Heat map of computational imaging features from The Cancer Genome Atlas cohort. In the plot, all 17 features (presented in each row and color-coded by the region and type) from 126 patients (presented in each column) were ranked by their TILs (monotonically increasing from left to right). All imaging features were standardized to have a zero mean and unit standard deviation. Imaging features were defined in Table 1. *BPE* Background parenchymal enhancement, *ER* Estrogen receptor, *HER2* Human epidermal growth factor receptor 2, *IDC* Invasive ductal carcinoma, *PR* Progesterone receptor, *TIL* Tumor-infiltrating lymphocyte

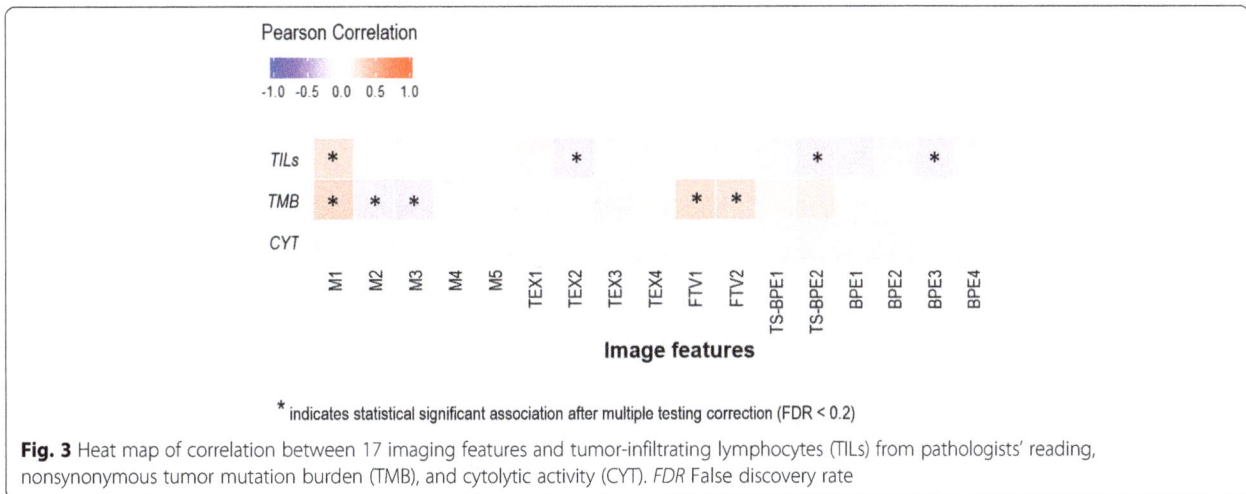

Fig. 3 Heat map of correlation between 17 imaging features and tumor-infiltrating lymphocytes (TILs) from pathologists' reading, nonsynonymous tumor mutation burden (TMB), and cytolytic activity (CYT). *FDR* False discovery rate

imaging signature, cytolytic score was significantly associated with TILs (ρ = 0.51; 95% CI, 0.36–0.63; P = 1.6E-9) (Fig. 4b), whereas none of the clinicopathological factors or the somatic mutation burden were correlated with TILs (Table 4). We found that five imaging features were significantly associated with mutation burden, but none was associated with cytolytic score (Fig. 3, Additional file 2: Table S4). This suggests that imaging and cytolytic score are independent and could be complementary to each other for predicting TILs. For three cases in Fig. 5, the imaging signature can provide more accurate prediction of TILs than the model of cytolytic score.

Composite model for tumor-infiltrating lymphocytes

On multivariate analysis, the imaging signature and cytolytic score remained as independent predictors of TILs (P = 0.004 and P < 0.0001, respectively) after adjusting for stage, estrogen receptor/progesterone receptor/HER2 status, and mutation burden (Table 4). We retained both significant variables and refitted a

composite model for predicting TILs: $5.86 \times Imaging$ $Signature + 7.78 \times Cytolytic\ Score + 13.0$. The linear correlation between the composite model and TILs was improved (ρ = 0.62; 95% CI, 0.50–0.72; P = 9.7E-15). Detailed box plots of inferred TILs from the composite model vs the original pathologists' readings are presented in Fig. 4c.

We tested the composite model for predicting three predefined TILs categories. As shown in Fig. 6a, cytolytic score alone could not differentiate between intermediate and high TILs (AUC, 0.63; P = 0.14). By integrating imaging signature and cytolytic score, the composite model successfully separated these two TILs groups (AUC, 0.76; P = 0.01), and the improvement was statistically significant (DeLong test P = 0.039). Similar results were observed for differentiating low vs high TILs groups (AUC, 0.88 vs 0.94) (Fig. 6b). For distinguishing low and intermediate groups, there was no significant improvement using the composite model over cytolytic score (AUC, 0.77 vs 0.79) (Additional file 1: Figure S3). In addition, we performed a detailed evaluation of the

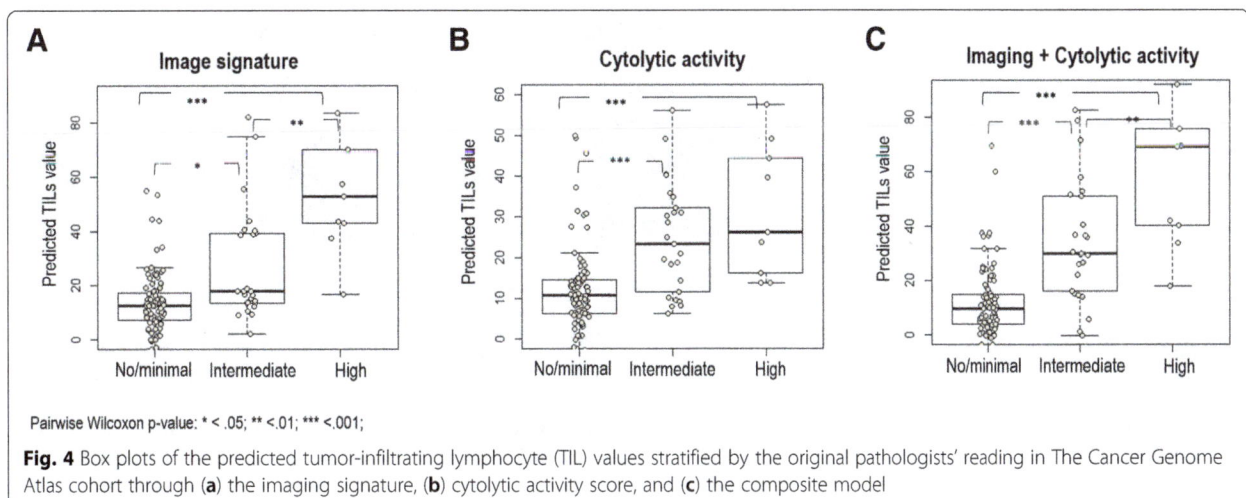

Fig. 4 Box plots of the predicted tumor-infiltrating lymphocyte (TIL) values stratified by the original pathologists' reading in The Cancer Genome Atlas cohort through (a) the imaging signature, (b) cytolytic activity score, and (c) the composite model

Table 3 Model evaluation of three classification models for predicting tumor-infiltrating lymphocyte groups in The Cancer Genome Atlas

	Specificity	Sensitivity	Accuracy
Low vs intermediate TIL groups			
Imaging signature	0.93	0.36	0.73
Cytolytic activity	0.86	0.68	0.83
Imaging + cytolytic activity	0.82	0.68	0.85
Low vs high TIL groups			
Imaging signature	0.70	0.89	0.71
Cytolytic activity	0.68	1	0.71
Imaging + cytolytic activity	0.91	0.88	0.91
Intermediate vs high TIL groups			
Imaging signature	0.64	0.89	0.71
Cytolytic activity	0.84	0.44	0.74
Imaging + cytolytic activity	0.68	0.78	0.75

TIL Tumor-infiltrating lymphocyte

proposed composite model, as in Table 3, where the composite model's accuracy is 0.85, 0.91, and 0.75, respectively.

Clinical validation of the composite model

The previously developed composite model was used to infer TILs based on imaging and molecular data in an independent cohort from the I-SPY 1 trial. We found that hormone receptor-negative (HR−)/HER2− or TNBC had significantly higher predicted TILs than HR+/HER2− breast cancer ($P = 0.049$) (Additional file 1: Figure S4). With the threshold values obtained from the training cohort, we divided the patients into three groups based on the predicted TIL values. Then, we investigated the relationship between predicted TIL groups and outcomes. In TNBC, patients without recurrence had significantly higher predicted TILs than those who developed recurrence ($P = 0.024$) (Fig. 7a). Within the TNBC group, distinct RFS exists between the predicted no/minimal TIL group and the predicted high/intermediate TILs group (log-rank $P = 0.0008$) (Fig. 8a), where the group with lower TILs had significantly worse prognosis. However, predicted TIL groups were not associated with RFS in HR+/HER2− or HER2+ breast cancer (Fig. 7b and c and Fig. 8b and c, respectively).

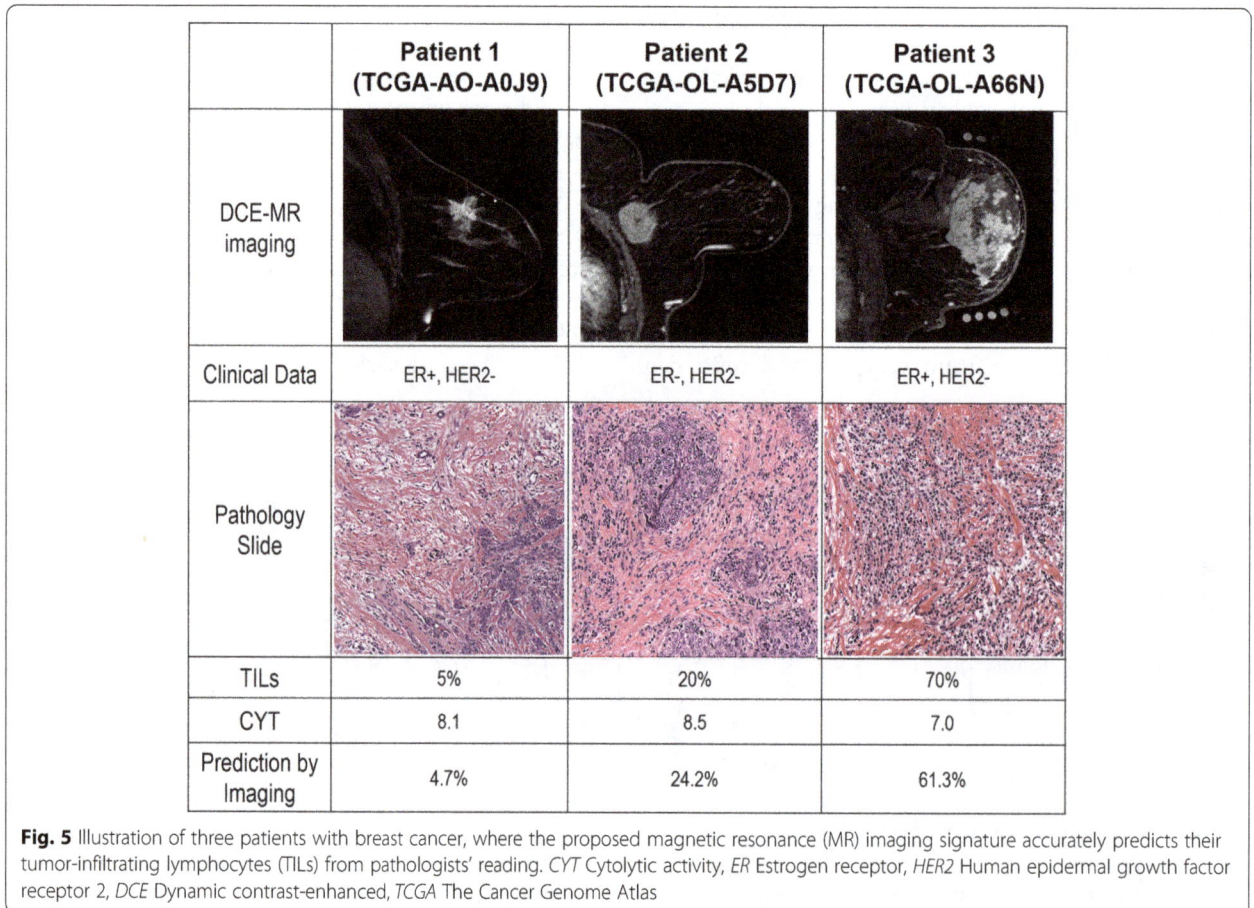

	Patient 1 (TCGA-AO-A0J9)	Patient 2 (TCGA-OL-A5D7)	Patient 3 (TCGA-OL-A66N)
DCE-MR imaging			
Clinical Data	ER+, HER2-	ER-, HER2-	ER+, HER2-
Pathology Slide			
TILs	5%	20%	70%
CYT	8.1	8.5	7.0
Prediction by Imaging	4.7%	24.2%	61.3%

Fig. 5 Illustration of three patients with breast cancer, where the proposed magnetic resonance (MR) imaging signature accurately predicts their tumor-infiltrating lymphocytes (TILs) from pathologists' reading. *CYT* Cytolytic activity, *ER* Estrogen receptor, *HER2* Human epidermal growth factor receptor 2, *DCE* Dynamic contrast-enhanced, *TCGA* The Cancer Genome Atlas

Table 4 Univariate and multivariate analyses of tumor-infiltrating lymphocytes using the imaging signature, clinicopathological factors, and molecular features in The Cancer Genome Atlas Cohort

Predictors	Univariate			Multivariate		
	ρ	95% CI	P value	Coefficient	SE	P value
Imaging signature	0.40	0.24–0.54	< 0.0001[a]	4.78	1.60	0.003[a]
T[b]	–	–	0.269	–	–	–
N[b]	–	–	0.799	–	–	–
M[b]	–	–	0.214	–	–	–
Stage[b]	–	–	0.650	−2.85	1.97	0.151
ER[c]	–	–	0.479	−3.42	6.85	0.618
PR[c]	–	–	0.561	2.71	4.05	0.504
HER2[b]	–	–	0.152	3.51	3.42	0.308
Triple-negative[c]	–	–	0.782	−0.51	7.43	0.945
PAM50 subtype[b]	–	–	0.309	–	–	–
Mutation burden	0.13	−0.05–0.30	0.167	−0.20	1.24	0.870
Cytolytic activity	0.51	0.36–0.63	< 0.0001*	7.69	1.27	< 0.000[a]

Abbreviations: *ER* Estrogen receptor, *HER2* Human epidermal growth factor receptor 2, *PR* Progesterone receptor
[a]$P < 0.05$
[b]For multinomial variables, the Kruskal-Wallis test was used
[c]For binary variables, the t test was used

Additionally, to validate the imaging signature for TILs, we applied it to 44 patients with TNBC who had images publicly available in the I-SPY 1 cohort. Similarly, with the threshold value obtained from the training cohort, we classified the patients into three TIL categories. A trend similar to that for the composite mode was observed, where no/minimal TILs had a significantly worse prognosis than high/intermediate TILs regarding their RFS (log-rank $P = 0.042$) (Fig. 8d).

Discussion

In this study, we aimed to dissect the complex tumor-immune interactions in breast cancer [5, 6] by integrating imaging, genomic, and histological data. In particular, our pilot study showed that the percentage of stromal TILs evaluated on histological tissue sections were significantly associated with specific enhancement patterns of tumor and surrounding parenchyma at DCE-MRI. Our findings are consistent with a recent study that demonstrated a link between heterogeneous enhancement of tumor-adjacent parenchyma on DCE-MRI and dysregulated tumor necrosis factor signaling pathway in breast cancer [47]. Both studies support the role of inflammatory or immune response in breast cancer progression and its relationship to specific parenchymal enhancement patterns at DCE-MRI. Consistent with previous work, we found that TILs were also associated with cytolytic activity but not with tumor

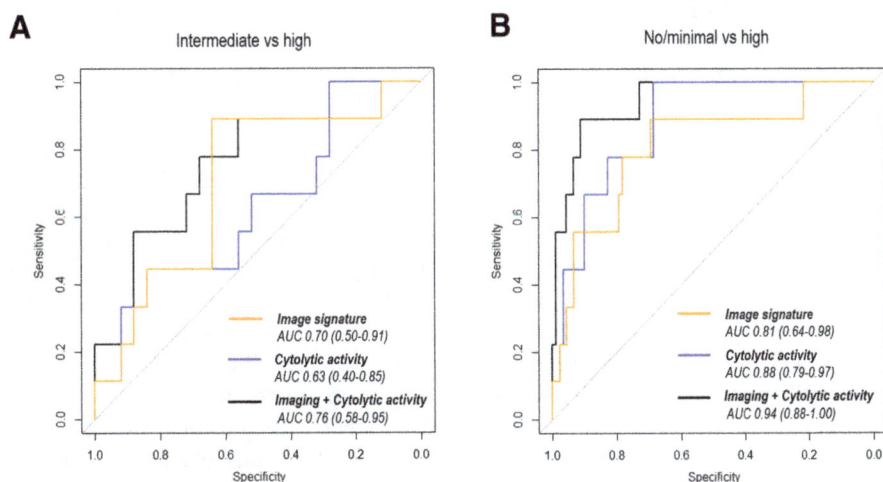

Fig. 6 ROC curves constructed by using imaging signature, cytolytic activity, and the composite model for classification of (**a**) intermediate vs high tumor-infiltrating lymphocyte (TIL) groups and (**b**) no/minimal vs high TIL groups

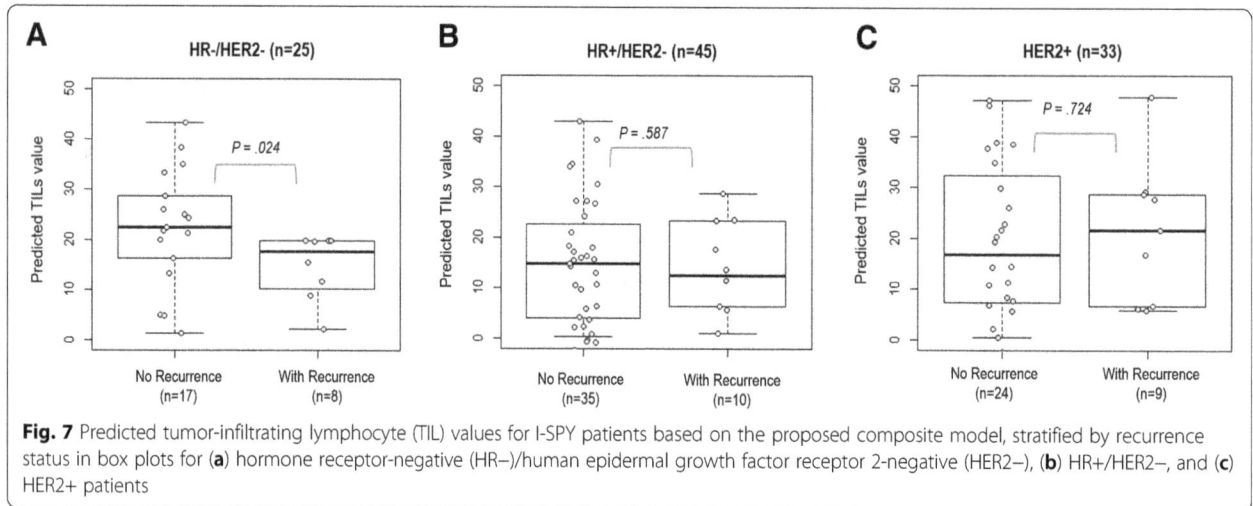

Fig. 7 Predicted tumor-infiltrating lymphocyte (TIL) values for I-SPY patients based on the proposed composite model, stratified by recurrence status in box plots for (**a**) hormone receptor-negative (HR–)/human epidermal growth factor receptor 2-negative (HER2–), (**b**) HR+/HER2–, and (**c**) HER2+ patients

mutational burdens in TCGA breast cancer cohort [48]. In addition to identifying associations, we further developed and evaluated prediction models for TILs that integrated imaging and genomic data. Our results show that a composite model combining an imaging signature and cytolytic score achieved augmented linear correlation with TILs compared with using either alone. The composite model showed good or excellent discriminative ability among low, intermediate, and high TIL groups, with AUCs ranging from 0.76 to 0.94.

The reliable evaluation of TILs has significance and clinical implications in breast cancer. Abundant evidence has demonstrated that TILs have strong prognostic and predictive value in specific breast cancer subtypes [6]. For localized breast cancer, TILs have been shown to be associated with pathological complete response and prognosis after chemotherapy or targeted therapies for localized breast cancer. This suggests that our imaging and molecular signature for TILs could help select patients who will be most likely respond to and benefit from neoadjuvant chemotherapy or targeted therapies in locally advanced breast cancer. On the other hand, they may also be used in combination with established clinical and pathological criteria to identify low-risk patients with a favorable prognosis who might be spared adjuvant chemotherapy in early-stage breast cancer. However, this will require further validation in prospective clinical studies. Although there are yet no U.S. Food and Drug Administration-approved immunotherapies for breast cancer, numerous trials are ongoing with the goal of assessing the clinical activity and potential benefit of ICB [49]. Because the success of ICB hinges on a preexisting antitumor immunity, which is manifested as TILs, TILs could serve as useful predictive biomarkers to select patients who are likely to benefit from immunotherapy.

The current gold standard for evaluating TILs is based on pathologists' visual assessment of H&E-stained whole-tumor tissue sections. This approach is limited mainly by intra- and interrater variability [16]. Gene expression profiles can also reflect antitumor immune response. Recently, a two-gene cytolytic score was proposed to characterize local immune infiltration and cytolytic activity in a large study across 18 tumor types in TCGA [40]. Nonetheless, pathological or molecular evaluation of TILs may be confounded by the spatial intratumoral heterogeneity, especially in the neoadjuvant setting with core biopsies [50]. On the other hand, imaging provides a global, unbiased picture of the entire tumor and its surrounding tissue, potentially allowing more reproducible evaluation for TILs. Our results demonstrate that, compared with cytolytic score, the imaging signature may be particularly useful in distinguishing tumors with high vs intermediate TILs. Although imaging analysis alone cannot replace pathological evaluation for TILs, our study supports imaging playing an important role in this process by providing key complementary information in equivocal cases or situations that are prone to sampling bias (e.g., in core biopsy). In our study, given the tumor contours manually delineated by radiologists, the subsequent imaging analysis was fully automatic. With the rapid advancement of machine learning in radiology [51], we anticipate that much of the process will be automated and that radiological interpretation bias can be minimized. One unique advantage of MRI is that it provides a global view of the whole tumor as well as its surrounding parenchyma, which overcomes the issue of sampling bias in core biopsy.

We validated the clinical relevance of our composite prediction model for TILs in an independent cohort. Consistent with previous findings [52], we showed that TNBC had significantly higher predicted TILs than HR+/HER2– breast cancer. So far, the strongest evidence for the prognostic value of TILs has been in TNBC, whereas its significance is more mixed in HER2+ and

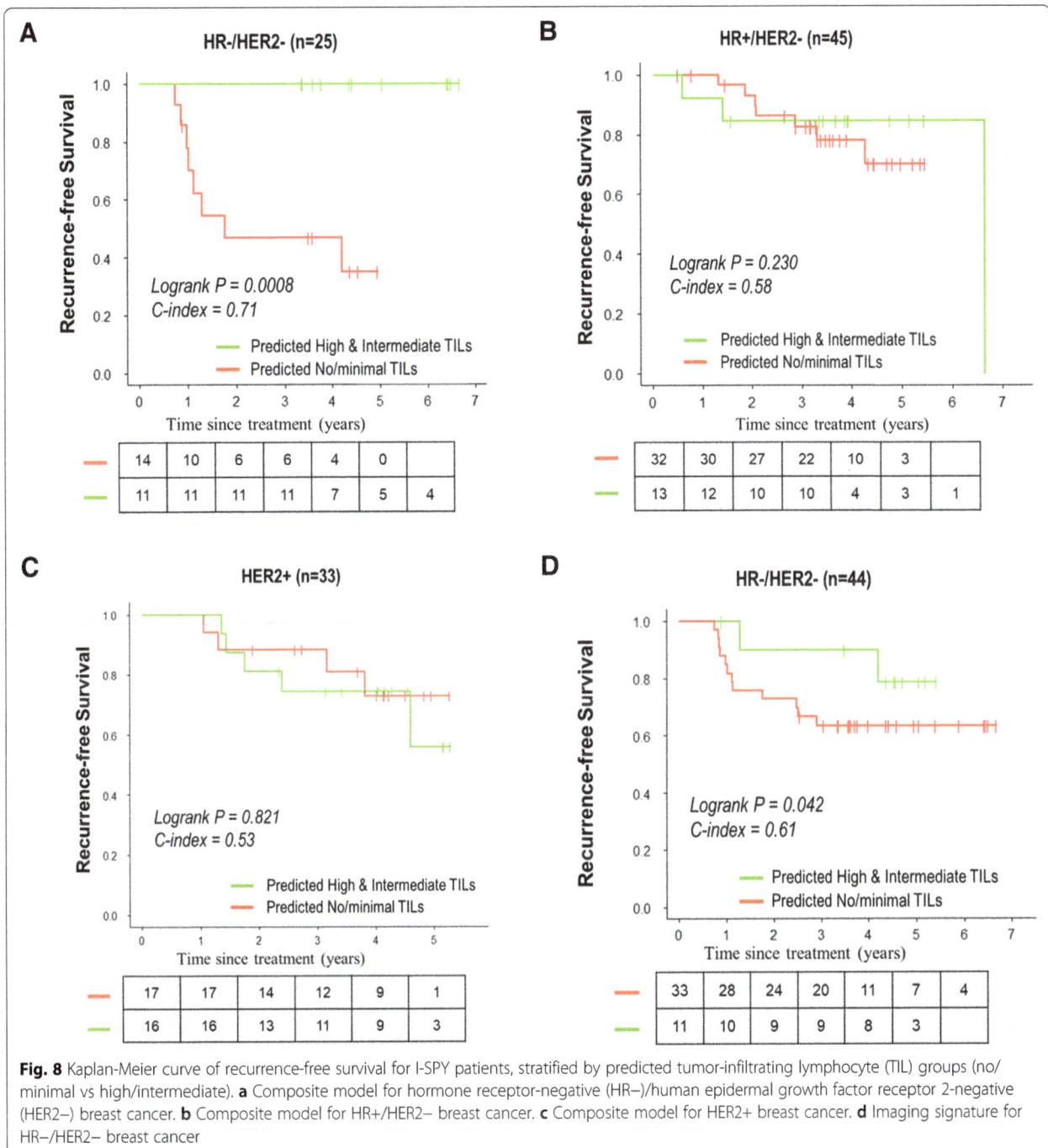

Fig. 8 Kaplan-Meier curve of recurrence-free survival for I-SPY patients, stratified by predicted tumor-infiltrating lymphocyte (TIL) groups (no/minimal vs high/intermediate). **a** Composite model for hormone receptor-negative (HR–)/human epidermal growth factor receptor 2-negative (HER2–) breast cancer. **b** Composite model for HR+/HER2– breast cancer. **c** Composite model for HER2+ breast cancer. **d** Imaging signature for HR–/HER2– breast cancer

seems uncertain in HR+/HER2– subtypes [6]. We confirmed that higher TILs predicted by the composite model were indeed associated with better prognosis and RFS in TNBC, but not among other subtypes. Given the relatively small number of TNBC cases in the I-SPY 1 cohort, it would be important to further validate the model in future studies with more patients.

Our study adds to the growing body of literature where a more detailed comprehensive analysis of imaging phenotypes could reveal the underlying tumor

pathophysiology at the molecular or pathological level [17–28, 53–55]. Different from previous radiogenomic studies that focused on analyses of imaging and genomic properties of the tumor, our study focused on immune infiltration in the stroma and included imaging features of the tumor as well as its surrounding parenchymal tissue. Another distinction is that previous work aimed to find correlation (i.e., similarity) between imaging and molecular data, whereas our study demonstrates that imaging can provide independent value and complement molecular profiles for predicting TILs.

There are several limitations of this study. The images and samples in TCGA cohort were retrospectively collected, which may not be a representative patient population for breast cancer. The association findings in this study should be interpreted as hypothesis-generating, and the composite prediction model for TILs requires validation in large, ideally prospective cohorts. Owing to the limited sample size, our analysis may have been insufficiently powered to detect differences in TILs by receptor status. Future work is needed to confirm the findings in a subtype-specific manner. In addition, there are diverse imaging acquisition protocols in the multi-institutional TCGA cohort, which may have confounded our analysis. Despite our efforts to harmonize imaging data, uncertainty could remain. Finally, we focused on DCE-MRI for association with TILs. Additional imaging modalities such as T2-weighted and diffusion-weighted MRI may be incorporated in future studies.

Conclusions

We showed that specific tumoral and parenchymal imaging features are associated with TILs and that integration of imaging and molecular features allows for better prediction of TILs in breast cancer. These preliminary findings should be validated in additional larger studies.

Acknowledgments
The authors thank The Cancer Imaging Archive (TCIA), the Cancer Digital Slide Archive, the Genomic Data Commons, and Gene Expression Omnibus for providing the breast cancer cases enrolled in The Cancer Genome Atlas (TCGA) study and the I-SPY 1 study.

Funding
This research was partially supported by the National Institutes of Health grants R01 CA222512, R01 CA193730, and K99 CA218667.

Authors' contributions
JW and RL conceived of and designed this research. JW, DLR, and BLD acquired MRI studies and performed preprocessing and feature extraction. XL and XT collected pathological slides and provided evaluation. JW, DLR, SN, and RL integrated and analyzed the data. XL, XT, DLR, and BLD provided expert knowledge. JW and RL wrote the manuscript. All authors edited and approved the final manuscript.

Competing interests
The authors declare that they have no competing interests.

Author details
[1]Department of Radiation Oncology, Stanford University School of Medicine, 1070 Arastradero Road, Stanford, CA 94305, USA. [2]Department of Pathology, First Affiliated Hospital of Zhejiang University, Hangzhou 310058, Zhejiang, China. [3]Department of Radiology, Stanford University School of Medicine, Stanford, CA 94305, USA. [4]Department of Biomedical Data Science, Stanford University School of Medicine, Stanford, CA 94305, USA. [5]Center for Biomedical Informatics Research, Department of Medicine, Stanford University School of Medicine, Stanford, CA 94305, USA.

References
1. Sharma P, Allison JP. The future of immune checkpoint therapy. Science. 2015;348(6230):56–61.
2. Borghaei H, Paz-Ares L, Horn L, Spigel DR, Steins M, Ready NE, Chow LQ, Vokes EE, Felip E, Holgado E. Nivolumab versus docetaxel in advanced nonsquamous non–small-cell lung cancer. N Engl J Med. 2015;373(17):1627–39.
3. Robert C, Long GV, Brady B, Dutriaux C, Maio M, Mortier L, Hassel JC, Rutkowski P, McNeil C, Kalinka-Warzocha E. Nivolumab in previously untreated melanoma without BRAF mutation. N Engl J Med. 2015;372(4):320–30.
4. Topalian SL, Taube JM, Anders RA, Pardoll DM. Mechanism-driven biomarkers to guide immune checkpoint blockade in cancer therapy. Nat Rev Cancer. 2016;16(5):275–87.
5. Fridman WH, Zitvogel L, Sautès-Fridman C, Kroemer G. The immune contexture in cancer prognosis and treatment. Nat Rev Clin Oncol. 2017; 14(12):717–34.
6. Savas P, Salgado R, Denkert C, Sotiriou C, Darcy PK, Smyth MJ, Loi S. Clinical relevance of host immunity in breast cancer: from TILs to the clinic. Nat Rev Clin Oncol. 2016;13(4):228–41.
7. Denkert C, Von Minckwitz G, Brase JC, Sinn BV, Gade S, Kronenwett R, Pfitzner BM, Salat C, Loi S, Schmitt WD. Tumor-infiltrating lymphocytes and response to neoadjuvant chemotherapy with or without carboplatin in human epidermal growth factor receptor 2–positive and triple-negative primary breast cancers. J Clin Oncol. 2014;33(9):983–91.
8. Loi S, Sirtaine N, Piette F, Salgado R, Viale G, Van Eenoo F, Rouas G, Francis P, Crown JP, Hitre E. Prognostic and predictive value of tumor-infiltrating lymphocytes in a phase III randomized adjuvant breast cancer trial in node-positive breast cancer comparing the addition of docetaxel to doxorubicin with doxorubicin-based chemotherapy: BIG 02-98. J Clin Oncol. 2013;31(7):860–7.
9. Salgado R, Denkert C, Campbell C, Savas P, Nuciforo P, Aura C, de Azambuja E, Eidtmann H, Ellis CE, Baselga J. Tumor-infiltrating lymphocytes and associations with pathological complete response and event-free survival in HER2-positive early-stage breast cancer treated with lapatinib and trastuzumab: a secondary analysis of the NeoALTTO trial. JAMA Oncol. 2015; 1(4):448–55.
10. Perez EA, Ballman KV, Tenner KS, Thompson EA, Badve SS, Bailey H, Baehner FL. Association of stromal tumor-infiltrating lymphocytes with recurrence-free survival in the N9831 adjuvant trial in patients with early-stage HER2-positive breast cancer. JAMA Oncol. 2016;2(1):56–64.
11. Loi S, Michiels S, Salgado R, Sirtaine N, Jose V, Fumagalli D, Kellokumpu-Lehtinen P-L, Bono P, Kataja V, Desmedt C. Tumor infiltrating lymphocytes are prognostic in triple negative breast cancer and predictive for trastuzumab benefit in early breast cancer: results from the FinHER trial. Ann Oncol. 2014;25(8):1544–50.
12. Dieci M, Mathieu M, Guarneri V, Conte P, Delaloge S, Andre F, Goubar A. Prognostic and predictive value of tumor-infiltrating lymphocytes in two phase III randomized adjuvant breast cancer trials. Ann Oncol. 2015;26(8):1698–704.
13. Adams S, Gray RJ, Demaria S, Goldstein L, Perez EA, Shulman LN, Martino S, Wang M, Jones VE, Saphner TJ. Prognostic value of tumor-infiltrating lymphocytes in triple-negative breast cancers from two phase III randomized adjuvant breast cancer trials: ECOG 2197 and ECOG 1199. J Clin Oncol. 2014;32(27):2959–66.
14. Wang K, Xu J, Zhang T, Xue D. Tumor-infiltrating lymphocytes in breast cancer predict the response to chemotherapy and survival outcome: a meta-analysis. Oncotarget. 2016;7(28):44288.
15. Luen SJ, Savas P, Fox SB, Salgado R, Loi S. Tumour-infiltrating lymphocytes and the emerging role of immunotherapy in breast cancer. Pathology. 2017; 49(2):141–55.

16. Salgado R, Denkert C, Demaria S, Sirtaine N, Klauschen F, Pruneri G, Wienert S, Van den Eynden G, Baehner FL, Penault-Llorca F. The evaluation of tumor-infiltrating lymphocytes (TILs) in breast cancer: recommendations by an international TILs working group 2014. Ann Oncol. 2014;26(2):259–71.

17. Agner SC, Rosen MA, Englander S, Tomaszewski JE, Feldman MD, Zhang P, Mies C, Schnall MD, Madabhushi A. Computerized image analysis for identifying triple-negative breast cancers and differentiating them from other molecular subtypes of breast cancer on dynamic contrast-enhanced MR images: a feasibility study. Radiology. 2014;272(1):91–9.

18. Sutton EJ, Dashevsky BZ, Oh JH, Veeraraghavan H, Apte AP, Thakur SB, Morris EA, Deasy JO. Breast cancer molecular subtype classifier that incorporates MRI features. J Magn Reson Imaging. 2016;44(1):122–9.

19. Martincich L, Deantoni V, Bertotto I, Redana S, Kubatzki F, Sarotto I, Rossi V, Liotti M, Ponzone R, Aglietta M. Correlations between diffusion-weighted imaging and breast cancer biomarkers. Eur Radiol. 2012;22(7):1519–28.

20. Waugh S, Purdie C, Jordan L, Vinnicombe S, Lerski R, Martin P, Thompson A. Magnetic resonance imaging texture analysis classification of primary breast cancer. Eur Radiol. 2016;26(2):322–30.

21. Blaschke E, Abe H. MRI phenotype of breast cancer: kinetic assessment for molecular subtypes. J Magn Reson Imaging. 2015;42(4):920–4.

22. Wu J, Sun X, Wang J, Cui Y, Kato F, Shirato H, Ikeda DM, Li R. Identifying relations between imaging phenotypes and molecular subtypes of breast cancer: model discovery and external validation. J Magn Reson Imaging. 2017;46(4):1017–27.

23. Yamamoto S, Maki DD, Korn RL, Kuo MD. Radiogenomic analysis of breast cancer using MRI: a preliminary study to define the landscape. Am J Roentgenol. 2012;199(3):654–63.

24. Ashraf AB, Daye D, Gavenonis S, Mies C, Feldman M, Rosen M, Kontos D. Identification of intrinsic imaging phenotypes for breast cancer tumors: preliminary associations with gene expression profiles. Radiology. 2014;272(2):374–84.

25. Yamamoto S, Han W, Kim Y, Du LT, Jamshidi N, Huang DS, Kim JH, Kuo MD. Breast cancer: radiogenomic biomarker reveals associations among dynamic contrast-enhanced MR imaging, long noncoding RNA, and metastasis. Radiology. 2015;275(2):384–92.

26. Sutton EJ, Oh JH, Dashevsky BZ, Veeraraghavan H, Apte AP, Thakur SB, Deasy JO, Morris EA. Breast cancer subtype intertumor heterogeneity: MRI-based features predict results of a genomic assay. J Magn Reson Imaging. 2015;42(5):1398–406.

27. Li H, Zhu Y, Burnside ES, Drukker K, Hoadley KA, Fan C, Conzen SD, Whitman GJ, Sutton EJ, Net JM. MR imaging radiomics signatures for predicting the risk of breast Cancer recurrence as given by research versions of MammaPrint, Oncotype DX, and PAM50 gene assays. Radiology. 2016;281(2):382–91.

28. Wu J, Cui Y, Sun X, Cao G, Li B, Ikeda DM, Kurian AW, Li R. Unsupervised clustering of quantitative image phenotypes reveals breast cancer subtypes with distinct prognoses and molecular pathways. Clin Cancer Res. 2017;23(13):3334–42.

29. Cancer Genome Atlas Network. Comprehensive molecular portraits of human breast tumours. Nature. 2012;490(7418):61–70.

30. Esserman LJ, Berry DA, DeMichele A, Carey L, Davis SE, Buxton M, Hudis C, Gray JW, Perou C, Yau C. Pathologic complete response predicts recurrence-free survival more effectively by cancer subset: results from the I-SPY 1 TRIAL—CALGB 150007/150012, ACRIN 6657. J Clin Oncol. 2012;30(26):3242–9.

31. Lehmann BD, Jovanović B, Chen X, Estrada MV, Johnson KN, Shyr Y, Moses HL, Sanders ME, Pietenpol JA. Refinement of triple-negative breast cancer molecular subtypes: implications for neoadjuvant chemotherapy selection. PLoS One. 2016;11(6):e0157368.

32. Hylton NM, Gatsonis CA, Rosen MA, Lehman CD, Newitt DC, Partridge SC, Bernreuter WK, Pisano ED, Morris EA, Weatherall PT. Neoadjuvant chemotherapy for breast Cancer: functional tumor volume by MR imaging predicts recurrence-free survival—results from the ACRIN 6657/CALGB 150007 I-SPY 1 TRIAL. Radiology. 2016;279(1):44–55.

33. Hylton NM, Blume JD, Bernreuter WK, Pisano ED, Rosen MA, Morris EA, Weatherall PT, Lehman CD, Newstead GM, Polin S. Locally advanced breast cancer: MR imaging for prediction of response to neoadjuvant chemotherapy—results from ACRIN 6657/I-SPY TRIAL. Radiology. 2012;263(3):663–72.

34. Wu J, Cao G, Sun X, Lee J, Rubin DL, Napel S, Kurian AW, Daniel BL, Li R. Intratumoral spatial heterogeneity at perfusion MR imaging predicts

35. Wu J, Aguilera T, Shultz D, Gudur M, Rubin DL, Loo BW Jr, Diehn M, Li R. Early-stage non–small cell lung cancer: quantitative imaging characteristics of 18F fluorodeoxyglucose PET/CT allow prediction of distant metastasis. Radiology. 2016;281(1):270–8.

36. Edwards SD, Lipson JA, Ikeda DM, Lee JM. Updates and revisions to the BI-RADS magnetic resonance imaging lexicon. Magn Reson Imaging Clin N Am. 2013;21(3):483–93.

37. Haralick RM, Shanmugam K, Dinstein IH. Textural features for image classification. IEEE Trans Syst Man Cybern. 1973;SMC-3(6):610–21.

38. Hattangadi J, Park C, Rembert J, Klifa C, Hwang J, Gibbs J, Hylton N. Breast stromal enhancement on MRI is associated with response to neoadjuvant chemotherapy. Am J Roentgenol. 2008;190(6):1630–6.

39. Chen DS, Mellman I. Oncology meets immunology: the cancer-immunity cycle. Immunity. 2013;39(1):1–10.

40. Rooney MS, Shukla SA, Wu CJ, Getz G, Hacohen N. Molecular and genetic properties of tumors associated with local immune cytolytic activity. Cell. 2015;160(1):48–61.

41. Johnson BJ, Costelloe EO, Fitzpatrick DR, Haanen JB, Schumacher TN, Brown LE, Kelso A. Single-cell perforin and granzyme expression reveals the anatomical localization of effector CD8+ T cells in influenza virus-infected mice. Proc Natl Acad Sci U S A. 2003;100(5):2657–62.

42. Herbst RS, Soria JC, Kowanetz M, Fine GD, Hamid O, Gordon MS, Sosman JA, McDermott DF, Powderly JD, Gettinger SN. Predictive correlates of response to the anti-PD-L1 antibody MPDL3280A in cancer patients. Nature. 2014;515(7528):563.

43. Esserman LJ, Berry DA, Cheang MC, Yau C, Perou CM, Carey L, DeMichele A, Gray JW, Conway-Dorsey K, Lenburg ME. Chemotherapy response and recurrence-free survival in neoadjuvant breast cancer depends on biomarker profiles: results from the I-SPY 1 TRIAL (CALGB 150007/150012; ACRIN 6657). Breast Cancer Res Treat. 2012;132(3):1049–62.

44. Leek JT, Johnson WE, Parker HS, Jaffe AE, Storey JD. The sva package for removing batch effects and other unwanted variation in high-throughput experiments. Bioinformatics. 2012;28(6):882–3.

45. Tibshirani R. Regression shrinkage and selection via the lasso. J R Stat Soc Ser B Stat Methodol. 1996;58(1):267–88.

46. Youden WJ. Index for rating diagnostic tests. Cancer. 1950;3(1):32–5.

47. Wu J, Li B, Sun X, Cao G, Rubin DL, Napel S, Ikeda DM, Kurian AW, Li R. Heterogeneous enhancement patterns of tumor-adjacent parenchyma at MR imaging are associated with dysregulated signaling pathways and poor survival in breast cancer. Radiology. 2017;285(2):401–13.

48. Luen S, Virassamy B, Savas P, Salgado R, Loi S. The genomic landscape of breast cancer and its interaction with host immunity. Breast. 2016;29:241–50.

49. Emens LA. Breast cancer immunotherapy: facts and hopes. Clin Cancer Res. 2018;24(3):511–20.

50. Khan AM, Yuan Y. Biopsy variability of lymphocytic infiltration in breast cancer subtypes and the ImmunoSkew score. Sci Rep. 2016;6:36231.

51. Choy G, Khalilzadeh O, Michalski M, Do S, Samir AE, Pianykh OS, Geis JR, Pandharipande PV, Brink JA, Dreyer KJ. Current applications and future impact of machine learning in radiology. Radiology. 2018;288(2):318–28.

52. Stanton SE, Adams S, Disis ML. Variation in the incidence and magnitude of tumor-infiltrating lymphocytes in breast cancer subtypes: a systematic review. JAMA Oncol. 2016;2(10):1354–60.

53. Braman NM, Etesami M, Prasanna P, Dubchuk C, Gilmore H, Tiwari P, Plecha D, Madabhushi A. Intratumoral and peritumoral radiomics for the pretreatment prediction of pathological complete response to neoadjuvant chemotherapy based on breast DCE-MRI. Breast Cancer Res. 2017;19(1):57.

54. Bahl M, Barzilay R, Yedidia AB, Locascio NJ, Yu L, Lehman CD. High-risk breast lesions: a machine learning model to predict pathologic upgrade and reduce unnecessary surgical excision. Radiology. 2018;286(3):810–8.

55. Pinker K, Chin J, Melsaether AN, Morris EA, Moy L. Precision medicine and radiogenomics in breast cancer: new approaches toward diagnosis and treatment. Radiology. 2018;287(3):732–47.

8

Serially transplantable mammary epithelial cells express the Thy-1 antigen

Neethan Amit Lobo[1,2†], Maider Zabala[1†], Dalong Qian[1] and Michael F. Clarke[1*] (ID)

Abstract

Background: Recent studies in murine mammary tissue have identified functionally distinct cell populations that may be isolated by surface phenotype or lineage tracing. Previous groups have shown that $CD24^{med}CD49f^{high}$ cells enriched for long-lived mammary epithelial cells can be serially transplanted.

Methods: Flow cytometry-based enrichment of distinct phenotypic populations was assessed for their gene expression profiles and functional proliferative attributes in vitro and in vivo.

Results: Here, we show Thy-1 is differentially expressed in the $CD24^{med}CD49f^{high}$ population, which allowed us to discern two functionally different populations. The $Thy-1^+CD24^{med}CD49f^{high}$ phenotype contained the majority of the serially transplantable epithelial cells. The $Thy-1^-CD24^{med}CD49f^{high}$ phenotype contains a rare progenitor population that is able to form primary mammary outgrowths with significantly decreased serial in vivo transplantation potential.

Conclusions: Therefore, Thy-1 expression in the immature cell compartment is a useful tool to study the functional heterogeneity that drives mammary gland development and has implications for disease etiology.

Keywords: Tissue-specific stem cells, In vivo serial transplantation, Progenitor cells, Self-renewal

Background

Mammary development is a highly ordered process that is regulated by spatiotemporal cues and directed by local and systemic signals [1]. Seminal studies in murine mammary cell biology revealed that the $CD24^{med}CD49f^{high}CD29^{high}$ cell surface phenotype enriches for mammary repopulating units (MRUs) that have the greatest in vivo proliferative capacity, as measured by serial in vivo transplantation and differentiation into specialized cell types [2, 3]. However, the functional heterogeneity of phenotypically enriched pooled-cell populations complicates descriptions of such populations [4]. Therefore, there remains a need for better phenotypic markers to prospectively enrich for different functional cell populations that can be used to characterize these populations transcriptionally or precisely mark certain populations using lineage-tracing strategies. Thy-1, or CD90, is a GPI-anchored cell surface protein that was originally described as a mouse brain and thymus marker.

Subsequent studies have shown that the Thy-1 antigen is expressed on many cell types, including hematopoietic stem cells (partially reviewed in [5, 6]). Thy-1 is expressed by basal cells in normal human mammary epithelium [7], where stem cells are thought to reside. Using the $Thy-1^+CD24^+$ phenotype, our group prospectively enriched for tumorigenic cells from a subset of MMTV-*Wnt1* murine mammary tumors that share properties with normal murine MRUs (mammary repopulating units, also known as stem cells) [8, 9]. Therefore, we sought to improve upon the current murine MRU cell surface phenotype by functionally assessing the prospective enrichment of serially transplantable mammary cells using Thy-1 expression. Our data revealed that Thy-1 expression on immature cells enriches for serially transplantable MRUs. Interestingly, the immature cells that lack Thy-1 expression enriched for a previously unknown rare population, which we term short-term mammary repopulating units (ST-MRUs), with limited serial proliferative potential in vivo.

* Correspondence: mfclarke@stanford.edu
†Neethan Amit Lobo and Maider Zabala contributed equally to this work.
[1]Institute for Stem Cell Biology and Regenerative Medicine, School of Medicine, Stanford University, 265 Campus Drive, Stanford, CA 94305, USA
Full list of author information is available at the end of the article

Methods

Mouse strains

C57BL/6 and FVB mice were purchased from The Jackson Laboratory, Bar Harbor, ME, USA. pCx-GFP founder mice were kindly provided by Dr. Irving Weissman. All animals were maintained at the Stanford Animal Facility in accordance with the guidelines of both Institutional Animal Care Use Committees.

Mammary gland dissociation and FACS

Six- to 10-week-old mice were euthanized and all fat pads surgically resected. Tissue was digested in Media 199 + 10 mM HEPES + PSA or L-15 for 2 h, and single-cell suspension was obtained as described previously [2] and then processed as described by the manufacturer's instructions for Epicult (Stemcell Technologies, Vancouver, BC, Canada). For all experiments, cells were > 99% viable as assessed by Trypan Blue dye exclusion. Cells were then resuspended at a concentration of 1×10^7 per ml and subjected to staining for flow cytometry. The antibodies CD24-PE, Thy-1.1-APC, Thy-1.1-PE-CY7, Thy-1.2-APC, and Thy-1.2-PE-CY7 were obtained from eBioscience (San Diego, CA, USA), CD45-BIO, Ter119-BIO, CD31-BIO, and CD140α-BIO were obtained from BD Pharmingen (San Jose, CA, USA), and Streptavidin-Pacific Blue was obtained from Invitrogen (Carlsbad, CA, USA). FACS for all experiments was performed on BD FACSAria II equipped with a UV laser. All gating to distinguish positive and negative expression was based upon IgG-isotype color-specific control staining.

In vitro colony-forming assay

Ultra-low attachment 96-well plates (BD, Franklin Lakes, NJ, USA) were prepared with a feeder layer of irradiated L1-WNT3a mixed with 60 µl of growth factor-reduced Matrigel (BD) per well. Sorted cells were then plated into liquid media as previously described [10, 11] 10% FBS, 250 ng/ml Rspo I (R&D Systems, Minneapolis, MN, USA) and 2.5% growth factor-reduced Matrigel were added as supplements. 5 ng/ml purified mouse TGFβ1 ligand (R&D Systems) was added to wells as indicated. Colonies were counted after 7 days in culture in a 5% CO_2 incubator.

In vivo transplants

Sorted cell populations were collected in HBSS + 2% HICS and resuspended at the correct concentration before being injected into the cleared fat pads of 21–28-day-old recipient C57Bl/6 mice as previously described [2]. For all injections of 600 cells and below, cell counts were verified using either a nuclear staining count (1% Trypan Blue/0.1% Triton-X 100 in PBS) or GFP+ cell count. Cells were injected in either 10 or 5 ul volumes of PBS using a 25 ul Hamilton syringe. All

transplants were allowed to grow for at least 5 weeks, but not more than 10 weeks before analysis. In the case of secondary and tertiary transplants, whole glands were dissected under fluorescence to obtain 1–2 mm pieces of tissue that contained GFP+ ductal structures that were transplanted into recipient mice.

Whole mount and immunocytochemistry

Whole mounts stained with carmine alum were processed according to a standard protocol [12]. For immunocytochemistry, mammary glands were fixed in formalin and embedded in paraffin. Three-micrometer sections were dewaxed, hydrated and microwaved for 20 min in Tris-EDTA (0.01 M; pH 9) for antigen retrieval. Tissue sections were incubated overnight at 4 °C with primary antibodies in TBS + 1% BSA. Antibodies were CK6 (Covance, Princeton, NJ, USA), CK5 (Covance), Troma-I (DSHB, Iowa City, IA, USA) and Troma-III (DSHB). Sections were then incubated with anti-rat–Alexa A488 antibody and anti-rabbit–A594 antibody (both from Invitrogen) for 30 min at room temperature. Secondary antibodies were applied at 1:200 dilution. Samples were stained with DAPI and mounted in ProLong before pictures were taken. All images were produced with a Leica (Wetzlar, Germany) microscope and Image Pro Software (Media Cybernetics, Rockville MD, USA).

RNA isolation and RT-PCR

Sorted cell populations were collected in staining media directly and then centrifuged at 5000 rpm for 5 min at 4 °C. Supernatant was then carefully removed from the cell pellet, which was immediately frozen in liquid N_2 and stored at −80 °C until RNA extraction. RNA was extracted from frozen cell pellets by the Trizol method or MirVana kit (Life Technologies, Carlsbad, CA, USA). For RT-PCR, RNA was then converted to cDNA using the Superscript III Reverse Transcriptase system (Invitrogen). qPCR was then performed on fresh cDNA with 2 × SYBR Green Master Mix (Applied Biosystems, Foster City, CA, USA) according to the manufacturer's instructions with primers to amplify specific genes (available upon request).

Microarrays and expression analysis

RNA was then processed for microarray hybridization by the Stanford Protein and Nucleic Acids core facility. RNA was applied to Affymetrix (Santa Clara, CA, USA) GeneChip Mouse Genome 430 2.0 oligonucleotide arrays. The resulting CEL images were then processed using the TIGR TM4 [13, 14] suite of bioinformatic software. Arrays were pre-processed by MIDAS using robust multichip average (RMA) normalization across all samples. Using Cluster 3.0 [15], probes that expressed less than 6.229 (in Log_2 space) in any two of the arrays and whose value was not at least fourfold different in any two arrays were excluded from the analyses. Probes intensities were then mean centered across all arrays as a set. Using MeV (TIGR), Rank products algorithm was then used to compare different populations using two-class unpaired comparisons with a critical p value of 0.01 for differentially expressed probes. Heatmaps are scaled from −3.0 (low) to 3.0 (high) in $\log_2$ space. Microarray data may be found at GenBank under accession GSE89720.

Results

Thy-1 enriches for a molecularly distinct subset of CD24^{med}CD49f^{high} cells

Previous studies have shown CD49f and CD24 are cell surface markers that are able to distinguish self-renewing MRUs (CD24^{med}CD49f^{high}) from basal myoepithelial cells (CD24^{low}CD49f^{med}), CD24^{high}CD49f^{med} colony-forming cells, and CD24^{med}CD49f$^{-/low}$ luminal cells [2, 3]. We found that Thy-1 was expressed on ~30% of luminal cell populations and ~50% of CD24^{med}CD49f^{high} and myoepithelial cells (Fig. 1a, b, c, d). We also found that Thy-1 was expressed by CD24$^{med/high}$CD133$^+$Sca-1$^+$ hormone-sensing luminal progenitor cells [16] as well as CD61$^+$ luminal progenitor cells [17] (Additional file 1: Figure S1A). Real-time PCR confirmed the basal or luminal identity of sorted populations based on the expression of Smaa and Krt14 (basal marker) and Krt18 and Krt19 (luminal marker) genes, respectively (Fig. 1e and f). To test if our enrichment procedures dramatically altered the physiology of the sorted populations, we exposed sorted populations to TGFβ1, a well-studied ligand that is associated with epithelial-to-mesenchymal transition [18]. Sorted populations that expressed basal or luminal gene markers shared similar responses to TGFβ1 exposure (Additional file 1: Figure S1B). Therefore, the sorting paradigm and related procedures effectively enriched for physiologically distinct phenotypic populations.

Numerous studies have linked the transcriptional expression of key genes to the function of cells enriched for by cell surface demarcation or lineage-tracing strategies [16, 19]. For example, Tbx3 is a gene that regulates the development of mammary hormone-sensing cells [20]. Interestingly, we found that all populations except for the Thy-1 expressing CD24^{med}CD49f^{high} cells also expressed Tbx3 (Fig. 1g). This population also had a low transcriptional level of Cdkn1a (Fig. 1h), whose expression is associated with halted cell cycle progression, comparable to luminal CD24^{high}CD49f^{med} cells that have been previously characterized to be highly proliferative. Furthermore, single-cell RNA-Seq data from the Marioni and Khaled laboratories showed that Thy-1 is most highly expressed in cells that are enriched for Procr, a Wnt target gene that has been linked to multipotent mammary stem cells [21] (Fig. 1i). Taken together, these results suggested that Thy-1 does indeed segregate a

functionally distinct subpopulation of CD24^{med}CD49f^{high} cells.

To further investigate the transcriptional differences that define each population, we performed gene expression microarrays on sorted cell populations. We found that Thy-1$^+$CD24^{med}CD49f^{high}, Thy-1$^-$CD24^{med}CD49f^{high}, and CD24^{low}CD49f^{med} cells had unique global gene expression profiles in both C57BL6 and FVB mice (Fig. 2a, b, Additional file 2: Figure S2A and B). There were both strain-specific and distinct genes expressed by sorted populations (Additional file 3). Notably, the Thy-1$^+$CD24^{med}CD49f^{high} cells expressed the highest level of genes that have previously been linked to mammary gland stem cells such as Rarres2 and Aldh1a1 [22, 23] (Fig. 2a). The enriched expression of Rarres1 and Aldh1a1 in both mouse strains' microarray data in the Thy-1$^+$CD24^{med}CD49f^{high} cells was confirmed by real-time PCR and in Procr-enriched cells by single-cell RNA-seq from the Marioni and Khaled laboratories [24] (Additional file 1: Figure S1C, D, E, F). The Thy-1$^+$CD24^{med}CD49f^{high} population was also enriched for the expression of Procr by real-time PCR (Additional file 1: Figure S1E), with the Procr-enriched population expressing high levels of both Procr and Thy-1 by single-cell RNA-seq (Fig. 1i and Additional file 1: Figure S1H). We also observed that CD24^{high}CD49f^{med} luminal cells expressed genes that distinguished this population from CD24^{med}CD49f$^{-/low}$ luminal cells in both the C57BL6 and FVB mouse strains (data not shown, Additional file 2: Figure S2C and Additional file 3). In the BL6 strain, the CD24^{med}CD49f$^{-/low}$ population was enriched for the expression of Elf5, a transcription factor that suppresses mammary stem cell activity [25] (Additional file 3).

Thy-1 enriches for an extensively proliferating subset of CD24^{med}CD49f^{high} cells

Murine mammary stroma depleted of endogenous epithelium provides an excellent in vivo model system to assess the repopulating potential and frequency of implanted cell populations. We leveraged this system and transplanted sorted cell populations from pCx-GFP transgenic mouse cells that ubiquitously express GFP to distinguish donor outgrowths from any residual endogenous epithelium. We found that 100 Thy-1$^+$CD24^{med}CD49f^{high} and 100 Thy-1$^-$CD24^{med}CD49f^{high} cells were able to produce GFP$^+$ ductal outgrowths that looked morphologically similar to those produced by 100 bulk mammary epithelial cells (MECs) (Fig. 3a). However, neither luminal CD24^{high}CD49f^{med} progenitor cells, CD24^{med}CD49f$^{-/low}$ luminal cells, nor CD49f^{med}CD24^{low} differentiated myoepithelial cells were able to produce extensive outgrowths up to 10,000 cells transplanted (Fig. 3a and data not shown). Limiting dilution transplantation studies revealed that the frequency of engrafting cells in the total

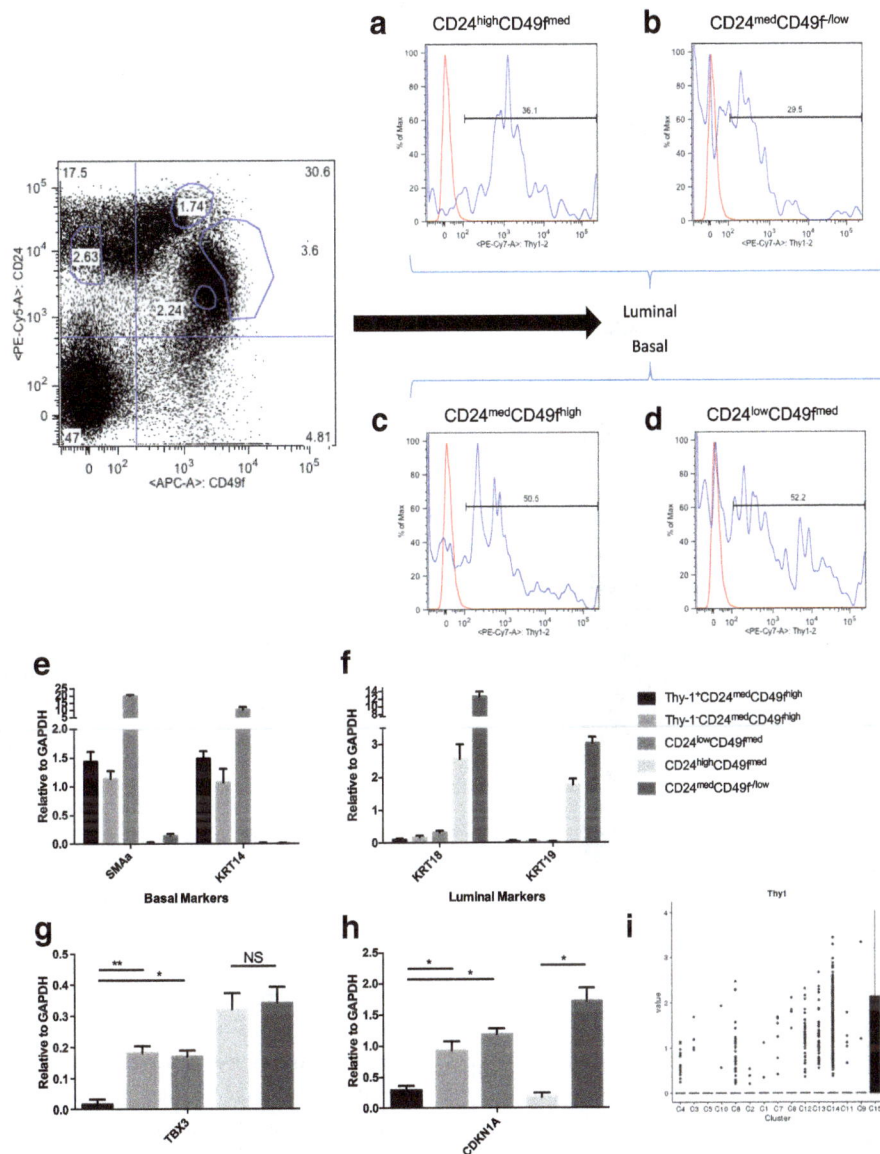

Fig. 1 Thy-1 is differentially expressed in murine mammary epithelium. Freshly dissociated mammary epithelium analyzed for the expression of CD24 and CD49f. Thy-1 expression in (a) CD24^{high}CD49f^{med} MaCFC luminal progenitor (b) CD24^{med}CD49f$^{-/low}$ luminal (c) CD24^{med}CD49f^{high} and (d) CD24^{low}CD49f^{med} myoepithelial cells. e Real-time PCR of sorted populations for basal marker genes' expression. $N = 3$, ± STD. f Real-time PCR of sorted populations for luminal marker genes' expression. $N = 3$, ± STD. g Real-time PCR of sorted populations for Tbx3 expression. $N = 3$, ± STD. **$p < 0.01$, *$p < 0.05$ for an unpaired two-tailed t test. h Real-time PCR of sorted populations for Cdkn1a (p21) expression. $N = 3$, ± STD. *$p < 0.05$ for an unpaired two-tailed t test. i Thy-1 expression in mouse mammary epithelial from single-cell RNA-seq data using the web tool (http://marionilab.cruk.cam.ac.uk/mammaryGland/) from Bach et al. [24]. C15 cells are annotated as Procr-enriched cells

CD24^{med}CD49f^{high} population was 1 in 254 cells, consistent with previous reports (Fig. 3b, c, Additional file 4: Figure S3A). Strikingly, we observed that the majority of the outgrowth-forming ability was confined to CD24^{med}CD49f^{high} cells that also expressed Thy-1 (Fig. 3b, c, Additional file 4: Figure S3A). Single-cell transplantation revealed that one in eight cells from the Thy-1$^+$CD24^{med}CD49f^{high} population were able to produce clonal outgrowths (Fig. 3d).

Previous reports using limiting dilution transplantation studies revealed that the MRU frequency within the CD24^{med}CD49f^{high} phenotype might be influenced by the strain of mice employed [2, 3]. Therefore, we performed another set of limiting dilution transplantation experiments in wild-type (WT) FVB mice (Additional file 4: Figure S3B). Again, we found that CD24^{med}CD49f^{high} cells that also expressed Thy-1 contained most of the outgrowth-forming cells (Additional file 4: Figure S3C). In FVB mice, the Thy-1$^-$CD24^{med}CD49f^{high} cells gave rise to smaller ductal outgrowths that were largely devoid of side branching structures (Additional file 4:

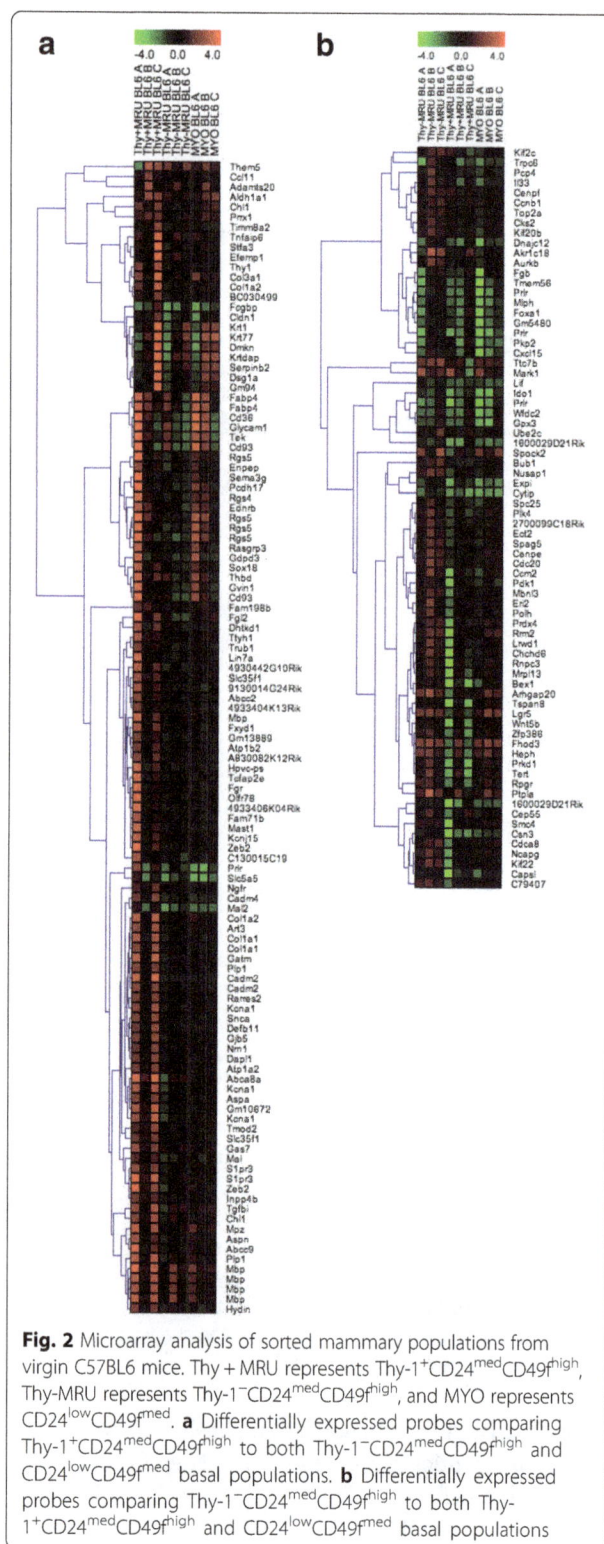

Fig. 2 Microarray analysis of sorted mammary populations from virgin C57BL6 mice. Thy + MRU represents Thy-1$^+$CD24^{med}CD49f^{high}, Thy-MRU represents Thy-1$^-$CD24^{med}CD49f^{high}, and MYO represents CD24^{low}CD49f^{med}. **a** Differentially expressed probes comparing Thy-1$^+$CD24^{med}CD49f^{high} to both Thy-1$^-$CD24^{med}CD49f^{high} and CD24^{low}CD49f^{med} basal populations. **b** Differentially expressed probes comparing Thy-1$^-$CD24^{med}CD49f^{high} to both Thy-1$^+$CD24^{med}CD49f^{high} and CD24^{low}CD49f^{med} basal populations

Figure S3D). The frequency of outgrowth-forming cells in the Thy-1$^+$CD24^{med}CD49f^{high} population was 1 in 156 cells in FVB mice, similar to the frequency in C57BL6 mice (Additional file 4: Figure S3E).

Thy-1$^+$CD24^{med}CD49f^{high} enriches for transplanted outgrowths with serial transplantation potential

MRUs are defined as cells that have both the ability to self-renew and to differentiate into mature luminal and basal cells that give rise to functional milk-secreting epithelium. The presence of MRUs can be detected by serially passaging transplanted cells or tissue fragments in vivo since only cells with extensive proliferative capacity will be able to continually produce outgrowths [3, 26]. Our initial transplantation data showed that the Thy-1$^+$CD24^{med}CD49f^{high} phenotype contained most of the outgrowth-forming cells. We serially transplanted 2 mm^3 fragments of GFP$^+$ donor epithelium from the initial primary outgrowths that were produced by C57BL6 Thy-1$^+$CD24^{med}CD49f^{high}, or Thy-1$^-$CD24^{med}CD49f^{high} GFP$^+$ cells and found these outgrowths grew secondary GFP$^+$ structures (Fig. 4a). A total of 23 out of 33 Thy-1$^+$CD24^{med}CD49f^{high} primary GFP$^+$ epithelial fragments engrafted upon secondary transplantation, giving an engraftment efficiency of about 67% (Additional file 5: Figure S4A). We found that Thy-1$^+$CD24^{med}CD49f^{high} cells were able to give rise to secondary ductal outgrowths that resembled the outgrowths formed from bulk MECs and the phenotypic CD24, CD49f and Thy-1 diversity of WT glands (Figs. 1 and 4c). Thy-1$^+$CD24^{med}CD49f^{high} primary outgrowths were also able to give rise to tertiary outgrowths similar to bulk MECs (Additional file 5: Figure S4B). Strikingly, we found that only 11% of the GFP$^+$ fragments produced by Thy-1$^-$CD24^{med}CD49f^{high} transplanted cells were able to form secondary outgrowths (Additional file 5: Figure S4A). In addition, the secondary outgrowths were much smaller than those produced by initially engrafted GFP$^+$ Thy-1$^+$CD24^{med}CD49f^{hi} cells (Fig. 4a). Unlike the Thy-1$^+$CD24^{med}CD49f^{high} epithelium that produced tertiary outgrowths like bulk MECs, the few GFP$^+$ secondary outgrowths formed by the initially engrafted GFP$^+$Thy-1$^-$CD24^{med}CD49f^{hi} cells were unable to re-engraft a third time (Fig. 4a). These data demonstrated that Thy-1$^+$CD24^{med}CD49f^{high} phenotype enriched for MRUs and that the Thy-1$^-$CD24^{med}CD49f^{hi} phenotype cells were enriched for basal short-term MRUs (ST-MRUs) with less proliferative capacity.

Functionally competent mammary epithelium will be able to give rise to alveolar milk-secreting cells upon pregnancy. We took mice that were engrafted with secondary GFP$^+$ outgrowths produced by bulk MECs and Thy-1$^+$CD24^{med}CD49f^{high} cells at 10 weeks posttransplantation and mated them to determine the milk-producing capability outgrowths. Hematoxylin and eosin staining showed extensive expansion of the ductal epithelium (Additional file 5: Figure S4C). Cytokeratin staining showed CK14, CK8, CK19, and CK6 localization was indistinguishable between WT (non-transplanted), primary, and secondary GFP$^+$ transplanted epithelium

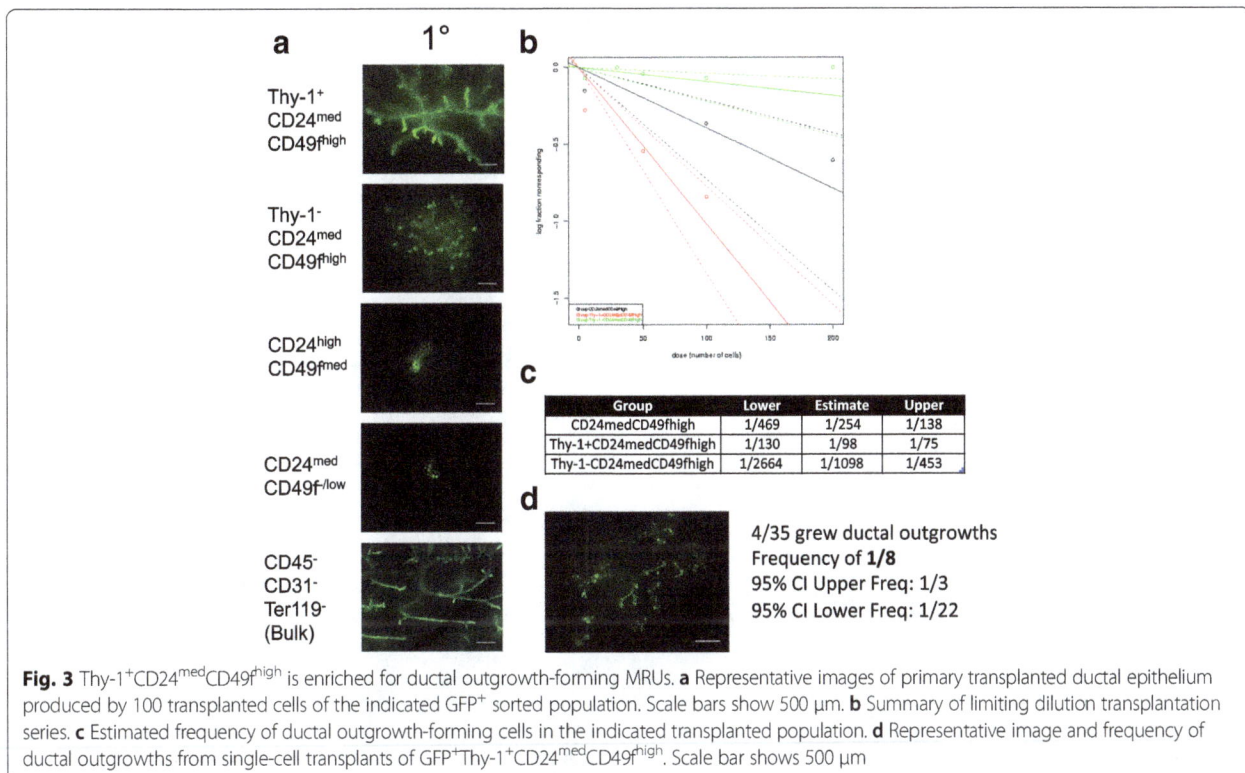

Fig. 3 Thy-1$^+$CD24^{med}CD49f^{high} is enriched for ductal outgrowth-forming MRUs. **a** Representative images of primary transplanted ductal epithelium produced by 100 transplanted cells of the indicated GFP$^+$ sorted population. Scale bars show 500 μm. **b** Summary of limiting dilution transplantation series. **c** Estimated frequency of ductal outgrowth-forming cells in the indicated transplanted population. **d** Representative image and frequency of ductal outgrowths from single-cell transplants of GFP$^+$Thy-1$^+$CD24^{med}CD49f^{high}. Scale bar shows 500 μm

produced by Thy-1$^+$CD24^{med}CD49f^{high} cells (Additional file 5: Figure S4C). In addition, Thy-1$^+$CD24^{med}CD49f^{high} secondary outgrowths underwent pregnancy morphogenesis in a similar fashion to WT epithelium as evaluated by cytokeratin expression, with visual confirmation of milk inside of the lumen of ducts in hematoxylin and eosin staining (Fig. 4c).

Discussion

Prospective isolation studies have shown that mammary tissue contains a distinct cell population of MRUs that is enriched for the ability to establish a functionally competent mammary gland in serial transplantation assays [2, 3]. We found that the Thy-1$^+$CD24^{med}CD49f^{high} phenotype enriches for mammary cells with the highest proliferative capacity as measured by this assay. Surprisingly, we found single-cell transplantation revealed a highly enriched MRU frequency in the Thy-1$^+$CD24^{med}CD49f^{high} cells compared to pooled-cell transplants, which may be due to multiple progenitor cells competing for sparse niche components. We also noted that the Thy-1$^+$CD24^{med}CD49f^{high} cells expressed genes associated with these cells with extensive proliferation capacity [22]. Since the Thy-1$^-$CD24^{med}CD49f^{high} population contains cells with diminished capacity to serially form extensive ductal outgrowths in vivo, these cells may be comparable to multipotent progenitor cells in the hematopoietic system, which also have a lesser proliferative capacity compared to stem cells. To our knowledge, this is the

first report of the existence of a mammary epithelial cell population with short-term MRU capacity. In addition to MRUs, unipotent progenitor cells have been identified and bipotent progenitor cells that lack in vivo transplantation capacity have been previously described [2, 27].

We found that the ortholog of TBX3, a gene mutated in ulnar mammary syndrome (UMS), was expressed in all populations except for Thy-1$^+$CD24^{med}CD49f^{high}. Recent studies have shown that Tbx3 is required for the mammary development and generation of hormone-sensing cells in murine mammary epithelium [28, 29]. Our data suggests that the UMS breast phenotype may be a defect of aberrant specification of cells with the capacity to undergo terminal differentiation. Recent studies have also demonstrated that Elf5 expression is necessary for the differentiation of luminal progenitor cells [25]. Our data showing that the CD24^{med}CD49f$^{-/low}$ compartment expresses Elf5 suggests that this compartment participates in a feedback pathway that instructs mammary epithelial cells to proliferate and differentiate.

Conclusions

Taken together, our data shows that the inclusion of Thy-1 expression to the growing list of phenotypic markers will allow further dissection of the mammary cellular hierarchy and allow for more accurate interpretation of pooled or single-cell analyses.

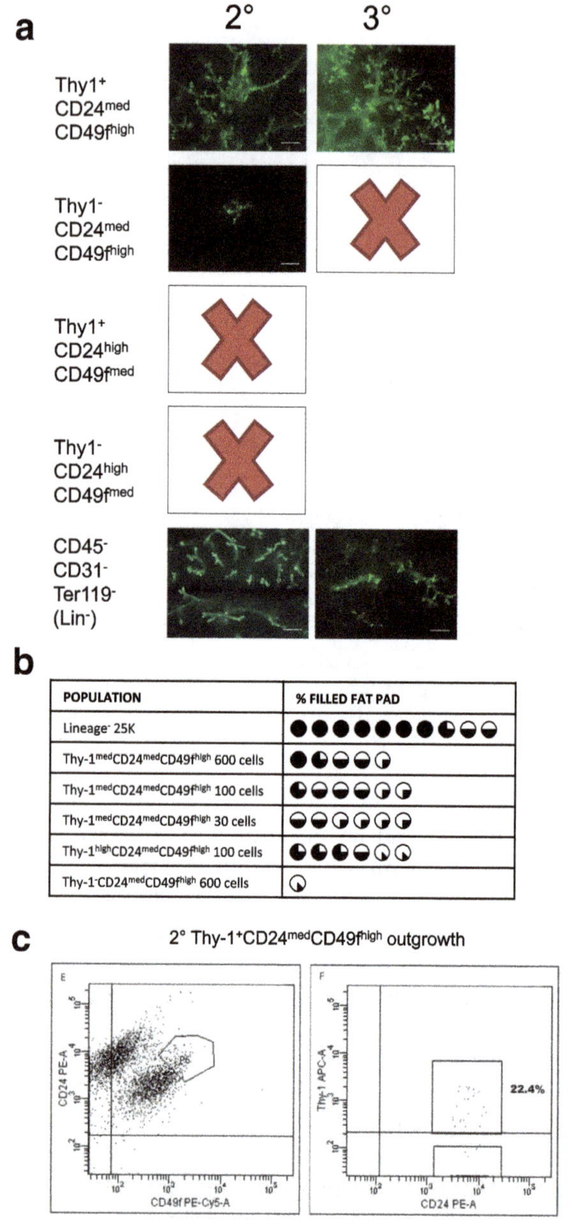

Fig. 4 Thy-1$^+$CD24^{med}CD49f^{high} enriches for self-renewing MRUs. **a** Representative images of secondary and tertiary GFP$^+$ ductal outgrowths produced from the indicated originally sorted populations. Scale bars show 500 μm. **b** Pie-chart representation of the secondary outgrowth formation of the indicated population as a percentage of the total surface area of the engrafted stromal mammary fat pad. **c** Flow cytometric analysis for CD24, CD49f, and Thy-1 expression of representative secondary GFP$^+$ ductal outgrowth produced from a fragment of primary ductal outgrowth originated from GFP$^+$Thy-1$^+$CD24^{med}CD49f^{high} engrafted cells

Additional files

Additional file 1: Figure S1. Phenotypic and physiological analysis of sorted populations. (A) Flow cytometric analysis on luminal cells for Thy-1, CD133, Sca-1, and CD61 expression. (B) Exposure of cultured FACS-enriched mammary populations to TGFB1 ligand. The indicated sorted mammary populations were cultured in three-dimensional self-renewing conditions with and without the addition of 5 ng/ml human TGFB1 ligand. $N = 3$, ± STD. (C) Real-time PCR of sorted populations for Procr expression. N = 3, ± STD. *-$p < 0.05$ for an unpaired two-tailed t test. (D) Procr expression in mouse mammary epithelial from single-cell RNA-seq data using the web tool (http://marionilab.cruk.cam.ac.uk/mammaryGland/) from Bach et al. [24]. C15 cells are annotated as Procr-enriched cells. (E) Real-time PCR of sorted populations for Rarres2 expression. N = 3, ± STD. *$p < 0.05$ for an unpaired two-tailed t test. (F) Rarres2 expression in mouse mammary epithelial from single-cell RNA-seq data using the web tool (http://marionilab.cruk.cam.ac.uk/mammaryGland/) from Bach et al. [24]. C15 cells are annotated as Procr-enriched cells. (G) Real-time PCR of sorted populations for Aldh1a1 expression. N = 3, ± STD. *$p < 0.05$ for an unpaired two-tailed t test. (H) Aldh1a1 expression in mouse mammary epithelial from single-cell RNA-seq data using the web tool (http://marionilab.cruk.cam.ac.uk/mammaryGland/) from Bach et al. [24]. C15 cells are annotated as Procr-enriched cells. (PDF 293 kb)

Additional file 2: Figure S2. Microarray analysis of phenotypically enriched populations isolated from virgin FVB female mice. (A) Differentially expressed probes comparing Thy-1$^+$CD24^{med}CD49f^{high} to both Thy-1$^-$CD24^{med}CD49f^{high} and CD24^{low}CD49f^{med} basal populations. (B) Differentially expressed probes comparing Thy-1$^-$CD24^{med}CD49f^{high} to both Thy-1$^+$CD24^{med}CD49f^{high} and CD24^{low}CD49f^{med} basal populations. (C) Differentially expressed probes comparing CD24^{high}CD49f^{med} to CD24^{med}CD49f$^{-/low}$ luminal cells. (PDF 186 kb)

Additional file 3: Strain and sorted population-specific and overlapping gene sets. Using the microarray data from C57BL6 and FVB mouse strains, each population's significantly enriched genes' expression was compared to determine the overlapping genes as well as the strain-specific genes. File contains tabular sheets of data that correspond to Thy-1$^+$CD24^{med}CD49f^{high}, Thy-1$^-$CD24^{med}CD49f^{high}, CD24^{low}CD49f^{med}, CD24^{high}CD49f^{med}, and CD24^{med}CD49f$^{-/low}$ populations. (XLSX 65 kb)

Additional file 4: Figure S3. Limiting dilution transplantation series in C57BL/6 and FVB mice. (A) Numbers of cells engrafted and ductal outgrowth data from limiting dilution transplantation series in C57BL6 mice from the indicated sorted populations. (B) Numbers of cells engrafted and ductal outgrowth data from limiting dilution transplantation series in FVB mice from the indicated sorted populations. (C) Summary of limiting dilution transplantation series from FVB mice. (D) Representative images of FVB-derived ductal outgrowths from the indicated populations. (E) Estimated frequency of ductal outgrowth forming cells in the indicated transplanted population from FVB mice. (PDF 487 kb)

Additional file 5: Figure S4. Thy-1$^+$CD24^{med}CD49f^{high} MRUs produce functional mammary epithelium. (A) Secondary transplant data from the indicated originally transplanted sorted population. (B) Tertiary transplant data from the indicated originally transplanted sorted population. (C) Hematoxylin and eosin and immunofluorescence staining of the indicated cytokeratin proteins in wild-type (WT) and serially transplanted Thy-1$^+$CD24^{med}CD49f^{high} epithelium. "Preg" denotes recipient mice that hosted donor ductal outgrowths that were mated and tissue analyzed at 11 days into pregnancy. (PDF 1889 kb)

Abbreviations
MEC: Mammary epithelial cell; MRU: Mammary repopulating unit; ST-MRU: Short-term mammary repopulating unit; UMS: Ulnar mammary syndrome; WT: Wild-type

Acknowledgements
We thank Jesse Engreitz and Maximillian Diehn for their bioinformatic advice.

Funding
NIH/NCI grant 5P01 CA139490–05, NIH/NCI grant 5U01CA154209–04, NIH/NCI 5R01 CA100225–09, Department of Defense grant W81XWH-11-1-0287,

Department of Defense/Breast Cancer Research Program (BCRP) Innovator Award W81XWH-13-1-0281, the Breast Cancer Research Foundation, the Ludwig Foundation, and the Breast Cancer Research Program Predoctoral Award DAMD17–03–1-0340.

Authors' contributions
NAL contributed to conception and design, collection and/or assembly of data, data analysis and interpretation, manuscript writing, and final approval of manuscript. MZ contributed to conception and design, collection and/or assembly of data, and data analysis and interpretation. DQ contributed to collection and/or assembly of data. MFC contributed to conception and design, financial support, administrative support, provision of study material or patients, data analysis and interpretation, and final approval of manuscript. All authors read and approved the final manuscript.

Competing interests
The authors declare that they have no competing interests.

Author details
[1]Institute for Stem Cell Biology and Regenerative Medicine, School of Medicine, Stanford University, 265 Campus Drive, Stanford, CA 94305, USA. [2]Cell and Molecular Biology Program, University of Michigan, Ann Arbor, MI, USA.

References
1. Richert MM, Schwertfeger KL, Ryder JW, Anderson SM. An atlas of mouse mammary gland development. J Mammary Gland Biol Neoplasia. 2000;5(2):227–41.
2. Stingl J, Eirew P, Ricketson I, Shackleton M, Vaillant F, Choi D, Li HI, Eaves CJ. Purification and unique properties of mammary epithelial stem cells. Nature. 2006;439(7079):993–7.
3. Shackleton M, Vaillant F, Simpson KJ, Stingl J, Smyth GK, Asselin-Labat ML, Wu L, Lindeman GJ, Visvader JE. Generation of a functional mammary gland from a single stem cell. Nature. 2006;439(7072):84–8.
4. Lobo NA, Shimono Y, Qian D, Clarke MF. The biology of cancer stem cells. Annu Rev Cell Dev Biol. 2007;23:675–99.
5. Haeryfar SM, Hoskin DW. Thy-1: more than a mouse pan-T cell marker. J Immunol. 2004;173(6):3581–8.
6. Herrera-Molina R, Valdivia A, Kong M, Alvarez A, Cardenas A, Quest AF, Leyton L. Thy-1-interacting molecules and cellular signaling in cis and trans. Int Rev Cell Mol Biol. 2013;305:163–216.
7. Eirew P, Stingl J, Raouf A, Turashvili G, Aparicio S, Emerman JT, Eaves CJ. A method for quantifying normal human mammary epithelial stem cells with in vivo regenerative ability. Nat Med. 2008;14(12):1384–9.
8. Cho RW, Wang X, Diehn M, Shedden K, Chen GY, Sherlock G, Gurney A, Lewicki J, Clarke MF. Isolation and molecular characterization of cancer stem cells in MMTV-Wnt-1 murine breast tumors. Stem Cells. 2008;26(2):364–71.
9. Diehn M, Cho RW, Lobo NA, Kalisky T, Dorie MJ, Kulp AN, Qian D, Lam JS, Ailles LE, Wong M, et al. Association of reactive oxygen species levels and radioresistance in cancer stem cells. Nature. 2009;458(7239):780–3.
10. Sato T, Vries RG, Snippert HJ, van de Wetering M, Barker N, Stange DE, van Es JH, Abo A, Kujala P, Peters PJ, et al. Single Lgr5 stem cells build crypt-villus structures in vitro without a mesenchymal niche. Nature. 2009;459(7244):262–5.
11. Zeng YA, Nusse R. Wnt proteins are self-renewal factors for mammary stem cells and promote their long-term expansion in culture. Cell Stem Cell. 2010;6(6):568–77.
12. Plante I, Stewart MK, Laird DW. Evaluation of Mammary Gland Development and Function in Mouse Models. J Vis Exp. 2011;53:e2828. https://doi.org/10.3791/2828.
13. Saeed AI, Bhagabati NK, Braisted JC, Liang W, Sharov V, Howe EA, Li J, Thiagarajan M, White JA, Quackenbush J. TM4 microarray software suite. Methods Enzymol. 2006;411:134–93.
14. Saeed AI, Sharov V, White J, Li J, Liang W, Bhagabati N, Braisted J, Klapa M, Currier T, Thiagarajan M, et al. TM4: a free, open-source system for microarray data management and analysis. Biotechniques. 2003;34(2):374–8.
15. Eisen MB, Spellman PT, Brown PO, Botstein D. Cluster analysis and display of genome-wide expression patterns. Proc Natl Acad Sci U S A. 1998;95(25):14863–8.
16. Sleeman KE, Kendrick H, Robertson D, Isacke CM, Ashworth A, Smalley MJ. Dissociation of estrogen receptor expression and in vivo stem cell activity in the mammary gland. J Cell Biol. 2007;176(1):19–26.
17. Asselin-Labat ML, Sutherland KD, Vaillant F, Gyorki DE, Wu D, Holroyd S, Breslin K, Ward T, Shi W, Bath ML, et al. Gata-3 negatively regulates the tumor-initiating capacity of mammary luminal progenitor cells and targets the putative tumor suppressor caspase-14. Mol Cell Biol. 2011;31(22):4609–22.
18. Xu J, Lamouille S, Derynck R. TGF-beta-induced epithelial to mesenchymal transition. Cell Res. 2009;19(2):156–72.
19. Rios AC, Fu NY, Lindeman GJ, Visvader JE. In situ identification of bipotent stem cells in the mammary gland. Nature. 2014;506(7488):322–7.
20. Kunasegaran K, Ho V, Chang TH, De Silva D, Bakker ML, Christoffels VM, Pietersen AM. Transcriptional repressor Tbx3 is required for the hormone-sensing cell lineage in mammary epithelium. PLoS One. 2014;9(10):e110191.
21. Wang D, Cai C, Dong X, Yu QC, Zhang XO, Yang L, Zeng YA. Identification of multipotent mammary stem cells by protein C receptor expression. Nature. 2015;517(7532):81–4.
22. Soady KJ, Kendrick H, Gao Q, Tutt A, Zvelebil M, Ordonez LD, Quist J, Tan DW, Isacke CM, Grigoriadis A, et al. Mouse mammary stem cells express prognostic markers for triple-negative breast cancer. Breast Cancer Res. 2015;17:31.
23. Eirew P, Kannan N, Knapp DJ, Vaillant F, Emerman JT, Lindeman GJ, Visvader JE, Eaves CJ. Aldehyde dehydrogenase activity is a biomarker of primitive normal human mammary luminal cells. Stem Cells. 2012;30(2):344–8.
24. Bach K, Pensa S, Grzelak M, Hadfield J, Adams DJ, Marioni JC, Khaled WT. Differentiation dynamics of mammary epithelial cells revealed by single-cell RNA sequencing. Nat Commun. 2017;8(1):2128.
25. Chakrabarti R, Wei Y, Romano RA, DeCoste C, Kang Y, Sinha S. Elf5 regulates mammary gland stem/progenitor cell fate by influencing notch signaling. Stem Cells. 2012;30(7):1496–508.
26. Deome KB, Faulkin LJ Jr, Bern HA, Blair PB. Development of mammary tumors from hyperplastic alveolar nodules transplanted into gland-free mammary fat pads of female C3H mice. Cancer Res. 1959;19(5):515–20.
27. Wang C, Christin JR, Oktay MH, Guo W. Lineage-biased stem cells maintain estrogen-receptor-positive and -negative mouse mammary luminal lineages. Cell Rep. 2017;18(12):2825–35.
28. Arendt LM, St Laurent J, Wronski A, Caballero S, Lyle SR, Naber SP, Kuperwasser C. Human breast progenitor cell numbers are regulated by WNT and TBX3. PLoS One. 2014;9(10):e111442.
29. Tarulli GA, Laven-Law G, Shakya R, Tilley WD, Hickey TE. Hormone-sensing mammary epithelial progenitors: emerging identity and hormonal regulation. J Mammary Gland Biol Neoplasia. 2015;20(1–2):75–91.

9

Consistent and reproducible cultures of large-scale 3D mammary epithelial structures using an accessible bioprinting platform

John A. Reid[1], Peter A. Mollica[2], Robert D. Bruno[2]*[†] and Patrick C. Sachs[2]*[†] (iD)

Abstract

Background: Standard three-dimensional (3D) *in vitro* culture techniques, such as those used for mammary epithelial cells, rely on random distribution of cells within hydrogels. Although these systems offer advantages over traditional 2D models, limitations persist owing to the lack of control over cellular placement within the hydrogel. This results in experimental inconsistencies and random organoid morphology. Robust, high-throughput experimentation requires greater standardization of 3D epithelial culture techniques.

Methods: Here, we detail the use of a 3D bioprinting platform as an investigative tool to control the 3D formation of organoids through the "self-assembly" of human mammary epithelial cells. Experimental bioprinting procedures were optimized to enable the formation of controlled arrays of individual mammary organoids. We define the distance and cell number parameters necessary to print individual organoids that do not interact between print locations as well as those required to generate large contiguous organoids connected through multiple print locations.

Results: We demonstrate that as few as 10 cells can be used to form 3D mammary structures in a single print and that prints up to 500 μm apart can fuse to form single large structures. Using these fusion parameters, we demonstrate that both linear and non-linear (contiguous circles) can be generated with sizes of 3 mm in length/diameter. We confirm that cells from individual prints interact to form structures with a contiguous lumen. Finally, we demonstrate that organoids can be printed into human collagen hydrogels, allowing for all-human 3D culture systems.

Conclusions: Our platform is adaptable to different culturing protocols and is superior to traditional random 3D culture techniques in efficiency, reproducibility, and scalability. Importantly, owing to the low-cost accessibility and computer numerical control–driven platform of our 3D bioprinter, we have the ability to disseminate our experiments with absolute precision to interested laboratories.

Keywords: Bioprinting, 3D culture, Organoids, Mammary epithelium, Tissue engineering, Regenerative medicine, Biofabrication

* Correspondence: rbruno@odu.edu; psachs@odu.edu
[†]Robert D. Bruno and Patrick C. Sachs contributed equally to this work.
[2]School of Medical Diagnostic & Translational Sciences, College of Health Sciences, Old Dominion University, 5115 Hampton Blvd, Norfolk, VA 23529, USA
Full list of author information is available at the end of the article

Background

Three-dimensional (3D) culture systems for generating organoid cultures of mammary epithelial cells inside collagen matrices were introduced over four decades ago [1]. In 3D culture, multiple parameters operate together to affect both experimental outcomes and interpretation of experimental results. These parameters include cell type, cell–cell interactions, extracellular matrix (ECM) composition, culture media, and mechanical properties such as matrix stiffness and cell confinement [2–12]. Standard 3D culture procedures involve either mixing dispersed mammary epithelial cells within ECM substrates prior to gelling or culturing cells on top of a pre-formed ECM gel. Once polymerized, the ECM gel can also be left attached to the culture dish or floated. The encapsulated cells will randomly organize into organoids which remodel and reorganize the substrate matrix to generate structures composed of morphologically polarized cells facing an open lumen [13–17]. However, the size and morphology of resulting organoids vary greatly, even within the same ECM gel substrate. While some variability inevitably results from disparities in local environmental conditions, such as collagen fiber anisotropy within specific regions of a gel, a major source of potentially controllable variability results from the random distribution of cells within the gel [18–23]. This variability leads to difficulty in interpreting and reproducing results, especially from laboratory to laboratory. As inter-laboratory reproducibility is a major concern in modern biomedical research, platforms that will allow better control and reproducibility are highly desired [24].

Recent advances in material science have promoted the development of novel synthetic hydrogels with tunable physiochemical properties for cell encapsulation and 3D bioprinting of mammary epithelial cells [25]. However, layer-by-layer methods for 3D cell printing frequently require extrusion nozzles near 300 µm and layer thicknesses of 500 µm, which severely limit the ability to control aspects of the microenvironment at the single-cell scale. We recently described the adaptation of an off-the-shelf 3D printer for the purposes of bioprinting cells within precast 3D substrates [26]. This system uses pulled glass microneedles, which can be designed with tip diameters ranging from 10 to 100 µm, allowing more accurate cell placement down to the single-cell level. We have previously established that multiple needle insertions into a polymerized collagen gel did not disrupt neighboring cell deposits [26]. The glass microneedles used in our system are non-coring and thin enough to allow the gel to seal behind them when removed. Furthermore, because our extrusion apparatus is designed to reliably handle volumes of less than 1 nL, it is unlikely that this volume would significantly alter the local microenvironment associated with a fibrous scaffold,

such as collagen. Our overall goal was to design an accessible, open-access bioprinter that would not be cost-prohibitive to research laboratories. Because of the precision afforded by the computer numerical control (CNC) system and the ability to share the G-Code underlying the printing process, the use of bioprinting in basic research laboratories offers promise for new standards designed to increase internal and intra-laboratory experimental reproducibility. Specifically, the use of CNC systems to control the spatial deposition of cells in 3D structures appears well suited to recreate the tissue-specific contextual cues needed to overcome the limitations of manual pipette patterning [26, 27]. Here, we describe the adaptation and validation of our accessible bioprinter to produce high-fidelity, spatially controlled arrays of human mammary organoids inside 3D collagen matrices. We demonstrate the superiority of our printing process over manual matrix embedding techniques in efficiency and consistency in organoid morphology. We further describe parameters necessary to generate large luminal organoids with shapes dictated by print locations (for example, linear or circular). These data lay the groundwork for adaptation to investigate additional cell types and 3D matrices, thereby providing an ideal method to derive empirical standards aimed to improve the *in vitro* culture of biological processes such as development and tumorigenesis.

Methods

Cell culture

Immortalized non-tumorigenic human breast epithelial cell lines MCF12A and MCF10A were purchased from the American Type Culture Collection (Manassas, VA, USA). MCF12A and MCF10A cells were initially cultured in 2D on tissue culture plastic in a 75-cm^2 flask supplemented with a 1:1 mixture of Dulbecco's modified Eagle's medium and Ham's F12 medium (DMEM/F12), 5% Horse Serum, 20 ng/mL human epidermal growth factor (hEGF), 0.01 mg/mL bovine insulin, 500 ng/mL hydrocortisone, and 1% ABAM (all purchased from Thermo Fisher Scientific, Waltham, MA, USA). Cells were cultured at 37.0 °C and 5.0% carbon dioxide (CO_2). After confluence, the cells were dissociated using TryplcE (Thermo Fisher Scientific) and collected by centrifugation.

Preparation of ECMs and manual cell-matrix embedding

For manual cell-matrix embedding studies, single-cell suspensions of MCF12A or MCF10A cells were mixed with neutralized rat tail collagen I (Corning, Corning, NY, USA) as specified by the manufacturer, unless noted otherwise, to a final concentration of 1.5 mg/mL. Immediately after mixing, 500 µL of neutralized collagen I gel material, containing about 5000 cells, was dispensed into a 24-well plate and allowed to solidify and adhere to the surfaces of the well for 1 h in a laboratory incubator at 37.0 °C and 5.0% CO_2. After gelation (solidification), 500 µL of cell media was added to the wells. Subsequent media changes were performed every 3 days. VitroCol, human collagen I solution (Advanced BioMatrix, San Diego, CA, USA), was prepared in accordance with the recommendations of the manufacturer to a final concentration of 1.0 mg/mL. Hydrogels of growth factor–reduced, LDEV-free Matrigel (Geltrex; Thermo Fisher Scientific) were prepared at 37 °C using the stock solution without dilution in accordance with the protocol of the manufacturer. For all printing experiments, a minimum of 500 µL of collagen gel was dispensed into individual wells of a 24-well plate and allowed to solidify for 1 h in a laboratory incubator at 37.0 °C and 5.0% CO_2. For all experiments, cells were monitored by using a combination of bright-field imaging/fluorescent imaging using a Zeiss axio-observer Z1 fluorescent microscope (Carl Zeiss AG, Oberkochen, Germany) or time-lapse imaging using a Lumascope 620 microscope (Etaluma, Carlsbad, CA, USA).

Bioprinting system

A previously developed bioprinting system was used to robotically insert a microneedle into specified 3D locations of a polymerized collagen gel [26]. Immediately before printing, 2D cultures of MCF12A cells were dissociated into single cells using TrypleE (Thermo Fisher Scientific), centrifuged at 300g, and re-suspended in media to obtain a final "ink" concentration of 60×10^4 cells per milliliter. Shortly thereafter, 50 µL of cell-containing "ink" was loaded into a sterile needle. Printing operations were initiated after the "ink"-containing needle was attached to the print head. The number of cells deposited in a target location was manipulated by varying the volume of cell-containing "bio-ink" extruded from the needle tip, or to equalize volumes, by increasing or decreasing initial cell concentration. Printing operations were optimized to extrude specified numbers of cells with a volume per print of less than 1 nL inside the collagen I gel via a CNC insertion routine which deposited cell-containing media at a specified "target" location inside the polymerized collagen I gel. Users specified intended wells of commercially available tissue culture plates, printing locations, distances among printing locations, and the number of cells per target location. The experiment information was automatically converted into G-Code, loaded into Repetier Host (www.repetier.com), and sent to the three-axis microcontroller of the bioprinter. The bioprinting system was located inside a benchtop biosafety cabinet during all printing operations. The heated print bed was set to 37 °C for all printing operations. Needles used by the bioprinting device were fabricated by using a Sutter P97 programmable pipette puller to have tip diameters of 50 µm. All printing

equipment was sterilized by using a steam autoclave prior to printing procedures. After printing routines were complete, plates were covered with 500 µL of media and placed inside a laboratory incubator at 37 °C, 5% CO_2. After printing, cells were monitored by using a combination of bright-field imaging/fluorescent imaging using a Zeiss axio-observer Z1 fluorescent microscope or time-lapse imaging using a Lumascope 620 microscope (Etaluma). Cell-specific media exchange was performed every 3 days. All experimental conditions were performed in triplicate.

Characterization of organoid growth and morphology

Immediately after printing, the initial quantity of printed cells was verified by using manual counting and image analysis using ImageJ and Matlab. After printing, cells were monitored up to 21 days by using a Zeiss axio-observer Z1 fluorescent microscope. The size of organoids was determined by analyzing bright-field images taken daily for each experimental condition using ImageJ. Within this investigation, organoids were operationally defined as a cluster of cells with no clear cell–cell boundaries or the inability to discern individual cells from neighboring cells. All experiments were performed a minimum of three separate times. All quantitations presented in the results represent total observations across at least three independent experiments.

Immunofluorescence staining

Gels were fixed in 10% neutral buffered formalin, paraffin-embedded, and sectioned. Sections were prepared for staining by deparaffinizing in a xylene substitute, rehydration, and heat-mediated antigen retrieval using pH 9 tris-EDTA with 0.05% tween 20. Sections were blocked in 10% goat serum and incubated with primary antibodies in a humidified chamber at 4 °C overnight. Secondary antibodies were added for 1 h at room temperature. Sections were counterstained with 4′,6-diamidino-2-phenylindole (DAPI). Antibodies were used at the following concentrations: anti-green fluorescent protein (anti-GFP) rabbit IgG Alexa Fluor 488 conjugated (1:75; Invitrogen A21311, Invitrogen, Carlsbad, CA, USA), rabbit polyclonal antibody to GJB1 [Cx32] (1:25; HPA010663, Sigma-Aldrich, St. Louis, MO, USA), biotinylated rabbit polyclonal antibody to red fluorescent protein (RFP) (1:500; Abcam, Cambridge, UK, ab34771), rabbit anti-laminin 1 + 2 (1:100; Abcam, ab7463), and mouse anti-laminin 5 antibody (1:100; Abcam, ab78286), Alexa Fluor 488 and 568 conjugated goat secondary antibodies (1:1000; Thermo Fisher Scientific) or avidin Alexa Fluor 488 (Thermo Fisher Scientific A21370). All sections were counterstained with DAPI and imaged by using a Zeiss axio-observer Z1 fluorescent microscope.

Results

Generation of consistent individual mammary epithelial organoids

As the main aim of this work was to validate experimental bioprinting methods for investigating mammary epithelial biology in 3D culture, we first established baseline behaviors of MCF12A cells using manual cell-matrix embedding techniques. Similar to previous findings [21, 28], we found an extremely high level of inter- and intra-experimental variability, which appears to be mostly independent of culturing conditions. Day 1 after the manual embedding of cells within collagen gels, the cells were similar in morphology, and cells either remained dispersed individually or formed small clusters (data not shown). This activity seemed to correspond with the random nature in which the cells were embedded in the gel—that is, whether cells ended up in close proximity to other cells or not. Noticeable structures emerge by day 5, and by day 8 prominent structural variations appear that by day 14 establish into distinguishable organoids (Fig. 1a). Three common organoid morphologies were observed—sphere-like (Fig. 1b), duct-like (Fig. 1c), and star-like (Fig. 1d)—which ranged in size from 190 to 1235 μm. In manually embedded gels, the initial mixture of 5000 cells per well resulted in an average of 334 ± 66 organoids per well at 7 days and

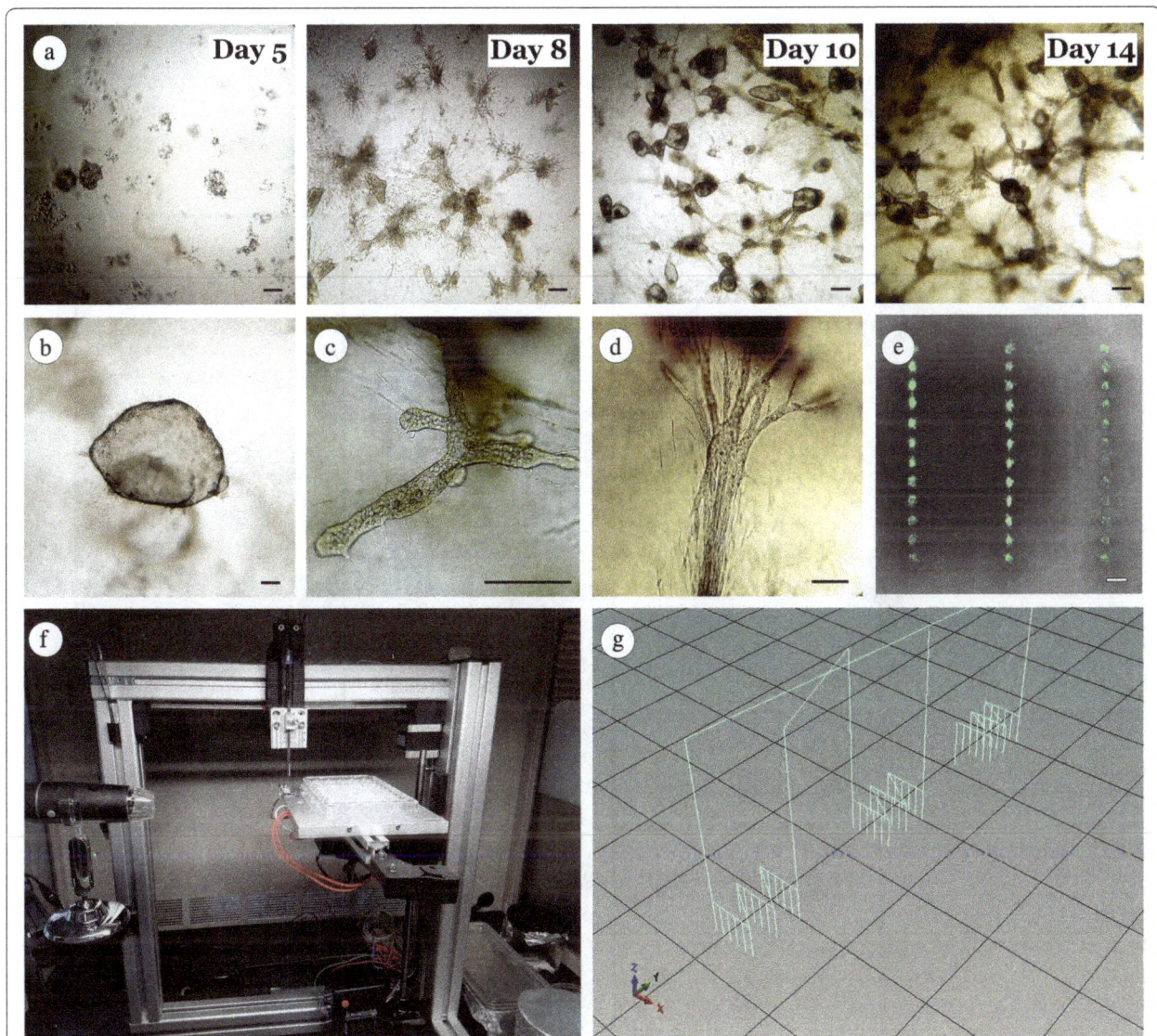

Fig. 1 Manual matrix embedding versus bioprinting of MCF12A cells. (**a**) Example of random organoid dispersion and morphology of MCF12A cells following manual matrix embedding in collagen gels at 5, 8, 10, and 14 days. (**b–d**) Examples of resulting organoid morphologies from manual matrix embedded MCF12a cells: (**b**) "sphere-like", (**c**) "duct-like", (**d**) "star-like". (**e**) Example of controlled and organized growth of MCF12A organoids following three-dimensional (3D) bioprinting. (**f**) Image of our accessible bioprinting platform. (**g**) Visual representation of machine path during insertion routine. Scale bars: **a** = 200 μM, **b–d** = 100 μM, **e** = 500 μM

292 ± 74 organoids per well after 14 days. As noted, the high level of variability resulted in a large discrepancy among the standard deviation values, which further illustrates the difficulty in interpreting experimental findings using traditional embedding techniques.

Using this baseline as our comparator, we next sought to identify the core parameters to reliably generate and guide the formation of organoids using our low-cost bioprinting system (Fig. 1e, f, g) [26]. Our bioprinting method uses CNC processes (Fig. 1g) to guide custom glass capillary microneedles to directly insert cells into 3D locations of polymerized collagen I gels generating a gridded array (Fig. 1e). We have previously shown that these custom glass microneedles impart negligible shear stress on cells and accurately place cells with ranges of 1 to 70 cells with an error rate of less than 10% within less than 1 nL of media [26]. Owing to the non-coring nature of our glass-pulled pipettes, this bioprinting technique confines cell aggregates in specified locations within

pre-cast 3D hydrogels following needle extraction and subsequent gel closure, thus eliminating the random cell distribution commonly observed in layer-by-layer processes and manual cell-matrix embedding procedures (Fig. 1e).

We initially assessed whether the formation frequency of individual human mammary epithelial organoids could be increased by controlling the initial number of singly dissociated cells in a specified location. Using our bioprinting device, we dispensed cell-laden media at equivalent volumes in equally spaced (100 μm) linear arrays inside collagen I gels and tracked them daily for 14 days (Fig. 2).

We found that initial cell injections of not more than 5 (±2) cells formed individual organoids at frequencies of 1 out of 50 and 28 out of 50 at 7 and 14 days, respectively. However, when the initial printed cell number equaled 10 (±3) cells, our system achieved 37 out of 50 and 49 out of 50 organoid efficiency at 7 and 14

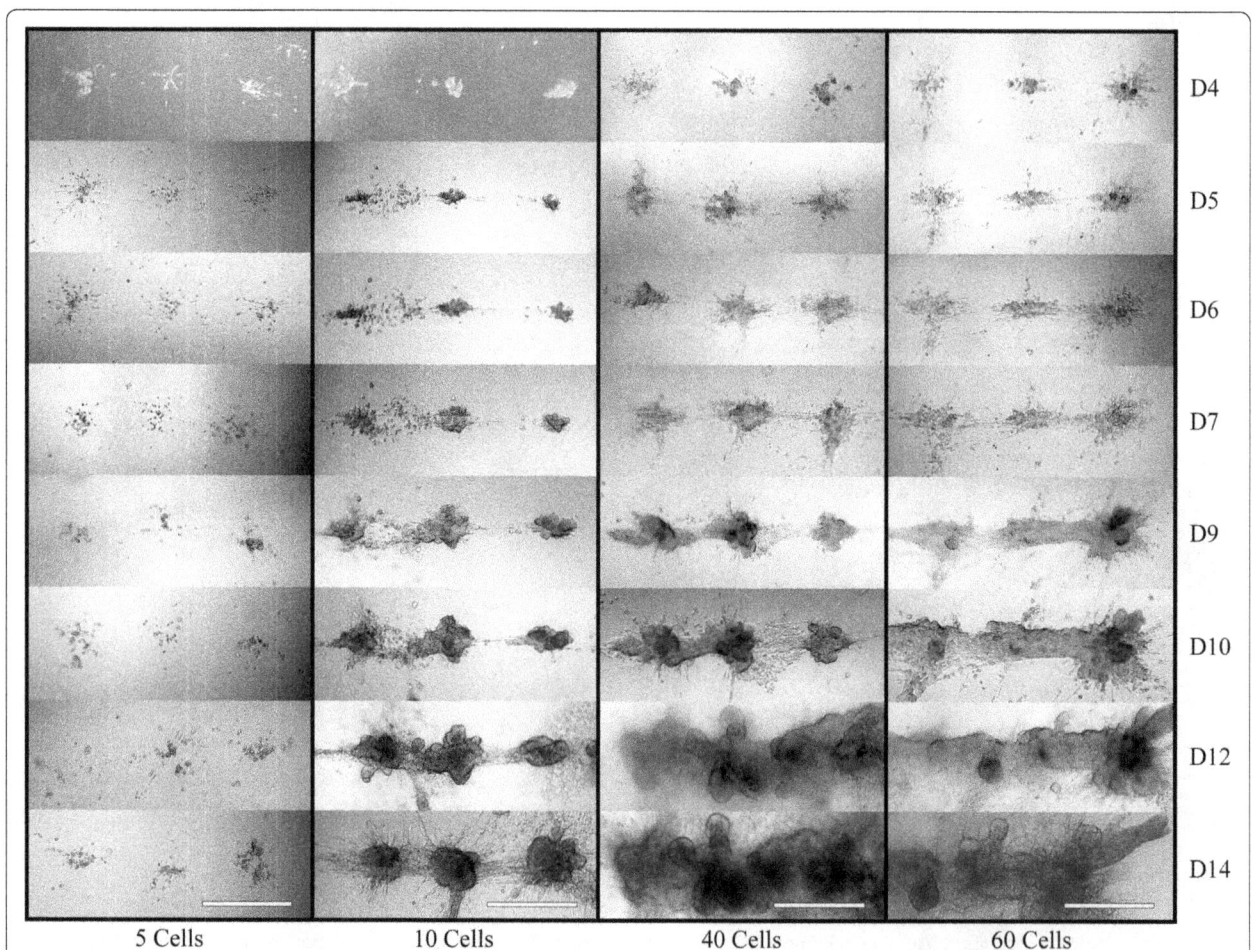

Fig. 2 Bioprinting of as few as 10 cells per print location results in consistent organoid formation. MCF12A cells were printed using initial cell concentration of 5, 10, 40, or 60 cells (columns left to right, respectively) at a distance of 500 μm between print locations. Images were taken at days 4, 5, 6, 7, 9, 10, 12, and 14 (rows top to bottom, respectively). Initial injections of 10 or more cells resulted in consistent organoid formation. Consistent fusion of multiple print locations was seen by day 14 when at least 10 cells were printed per injection site. Scale bar: 500 μm

days, respectively. Using 40 (±4) and 60 (±5) cells resulted in consistent (50 out of 50) organoid formation for both 7 and 14 days. These results indicate that reliable generation of individual organoids can be achieved by increasing the initial number of cells (≥10) in specified locations with a spacing of 500 μm. We also found that printed cell clusters containing cell numbers of at least 10 consistently develop branched processes exclusively pointed toward neighboring organoids by day 10, forming a contiguous structure. Furthermore, the temporal nature of this branching process increased correlative to the addition of more cells within the initial printing event.

Directing the generation of large contiguous mammary epithelial organoids

As the consistent nature of individual organoid formation changed with the variation of cell number, we next sought to determine whether varying distances could evoke a similar impact on the bridged-contiguous organoid formation that we observed in our linear arrays. Specifically, we wished to determine whether organoid spacing could further promote the formation of large-scale contiguous organoids. To this end, we monitored the effect of organoid spacing on growth behavior by printing MCF12A cells along linear arrays of cell deposits containing 40 (± 3) cells in collagen gels (Fig. 3).

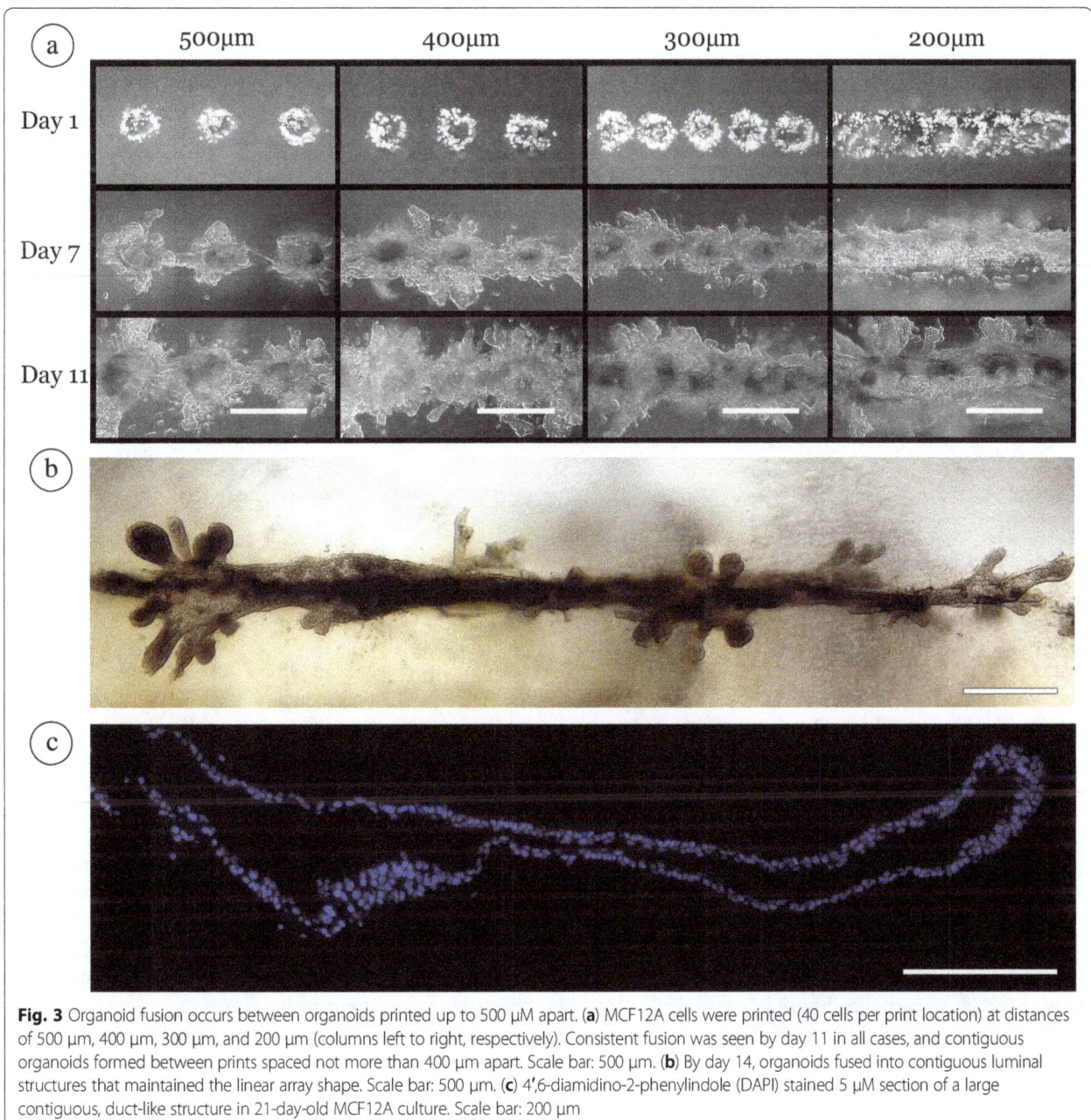

Fig. 3 Organoid fusion occurs between organoids printed up to 500 μM apart. (**a**) MCF12A cells were printed (40 cells per print location) at distances of 500 μm, 400 μm, 300 μm, and 200 μm (columns left to right, respectively). Consistent fusion was seen by day 11 in all cases, and contiguous organoids formed between prints spaced not more than 400 μm apart. Scale bar: 500 μm. (**b**) By day 14, organoids fused into contiguous luminal structures that maintained the linear array shape. Scale bar: 500 μm. (**c**) 4′,6-diamidino-2-phenylindole (DAPI) stained 5 μM section of a large contiguous, duct-like structure in 21-day-old MCF12A culture. Scale bar: 200 μm

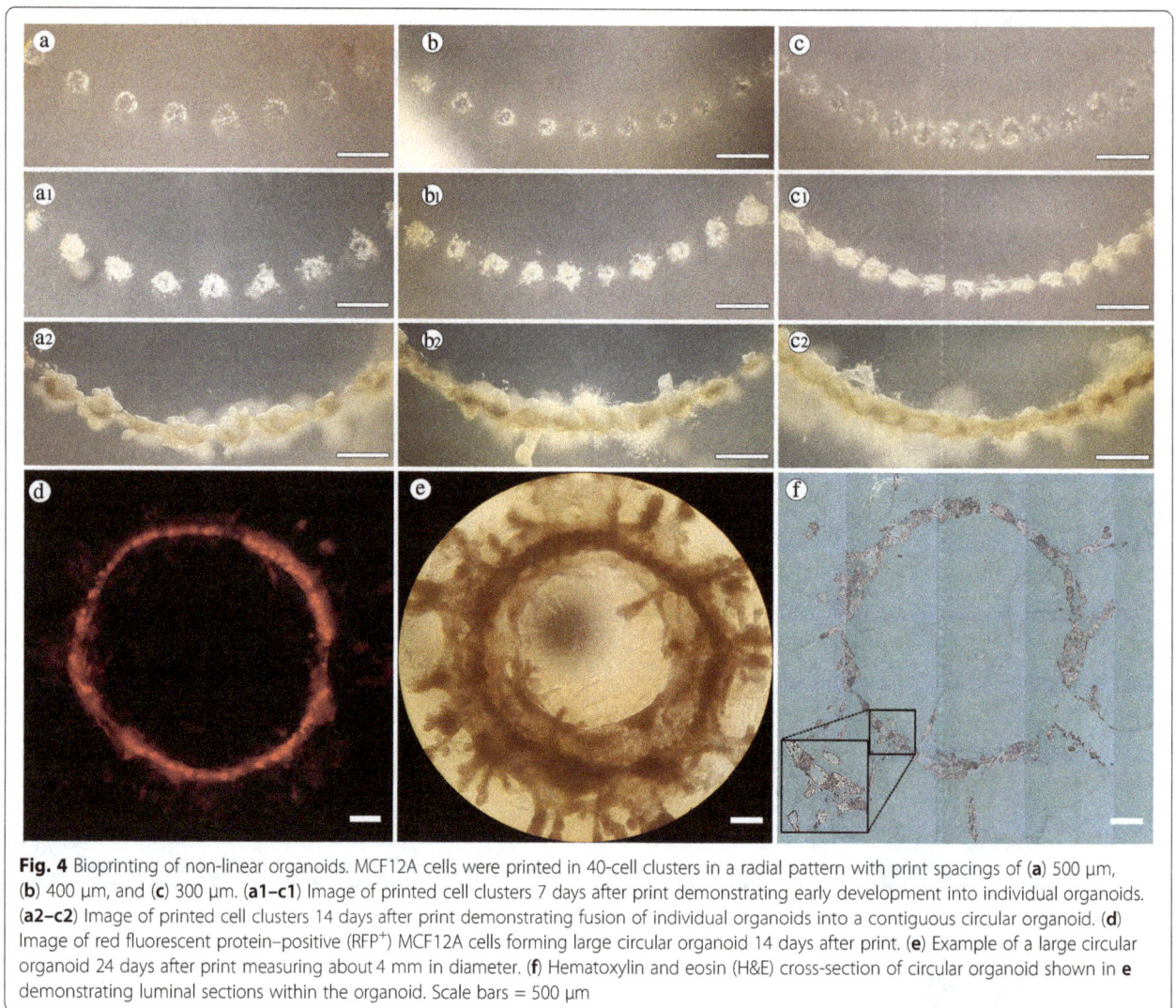

Fig. 4 Bioprinting of non-linear organoids. MCF12A cells were printed in 40-cell clusters in a radial pattern with print spacings of (**a**) 500 μm, (**b**) 400 μm, and (**c**) 300 μm. (**a1–c1**) Image of printed cell clusters 7 days after print demonstrating early development into individual organoids. (**a2–c2**) Image of printed cell clusters 14 days after print demonstrating fusion of individual organoids into a contiguous circular organoid. (**d**) Image of red fluorescent protein–positive (RFP[+]) MCF12A cells forming large circular organoid 14 days after print. (**e**) Example of a large circular organoid 24 days after print measuring about 4 mm in diameter. (**f**) Hematoxylin and eosin (H&E) cross-section of circular organoid shown in **e** demonstrating luminal sections within the organoid. Scale bars = 500 μm

Data indicated that inter-organoid spacing (≤300 μm) directed collective cell growth of all (36 out of 36) organoids into duct-like patterns along the entire length of the linear array (~4 mm) within 7 days after printing (Fig. 3a). At 400 μm, 34 out of 36 organoids fused within 7 days after printing (Fig. 3a). Twenty-three out of 36 organoids spaced 500 μm apart achieved organoid fusion within 7 days; however, 35 out of 36 of these organoids achieved fusion by day 11 (Fig. 3a). When cells were spaced at at least 700 μm, no fusions (0 out of 36) were seen between printed clusters by day 7. Closer examination of the 500-μm print conditions indicated that cell numbers increased during the first 3 days after printing. We observed formation of coordinated branched extensions directed toward neighboring organoids between days 5 and 7 (Additional file 1: Movie S1). It was noted that decreasing organoid spacing appears to promote the initial formation of a central structure corresponding to the axis of the linear array. This also indicated that

individual organoids had a propensity to maintain the linear nature of the initial printed pattern throughout this fusion process (Fig. 3b). Thus, by manipulating the spacing, we can predictably increase the formation of a contiguous structure. This was particularly highlighted where neighboring linear arrays printed at least 700 μm apart were unable to reliably attain directed print geometries within a 14-day observation window. Furthermore, this central structure appears to support the growth of secondary branches, which exclusively radiate from the initial structure (Fig. 3b). DAPI staining of cross-sections of 21-day cultures of MCF12A cells confirmed the presence of contiguous ductal structures resulting from the initial bioprinted cell deposits (Fig. 3c). Of note, some structures were found to have large contiguous lumens. For example, the structure shown in Fig. 3c is over 1 mm in length within a single 5-μm sectional plane. In addition, immunostaining of cross-sections of the resulting structures with antibodies to laminin 1 + 2 and

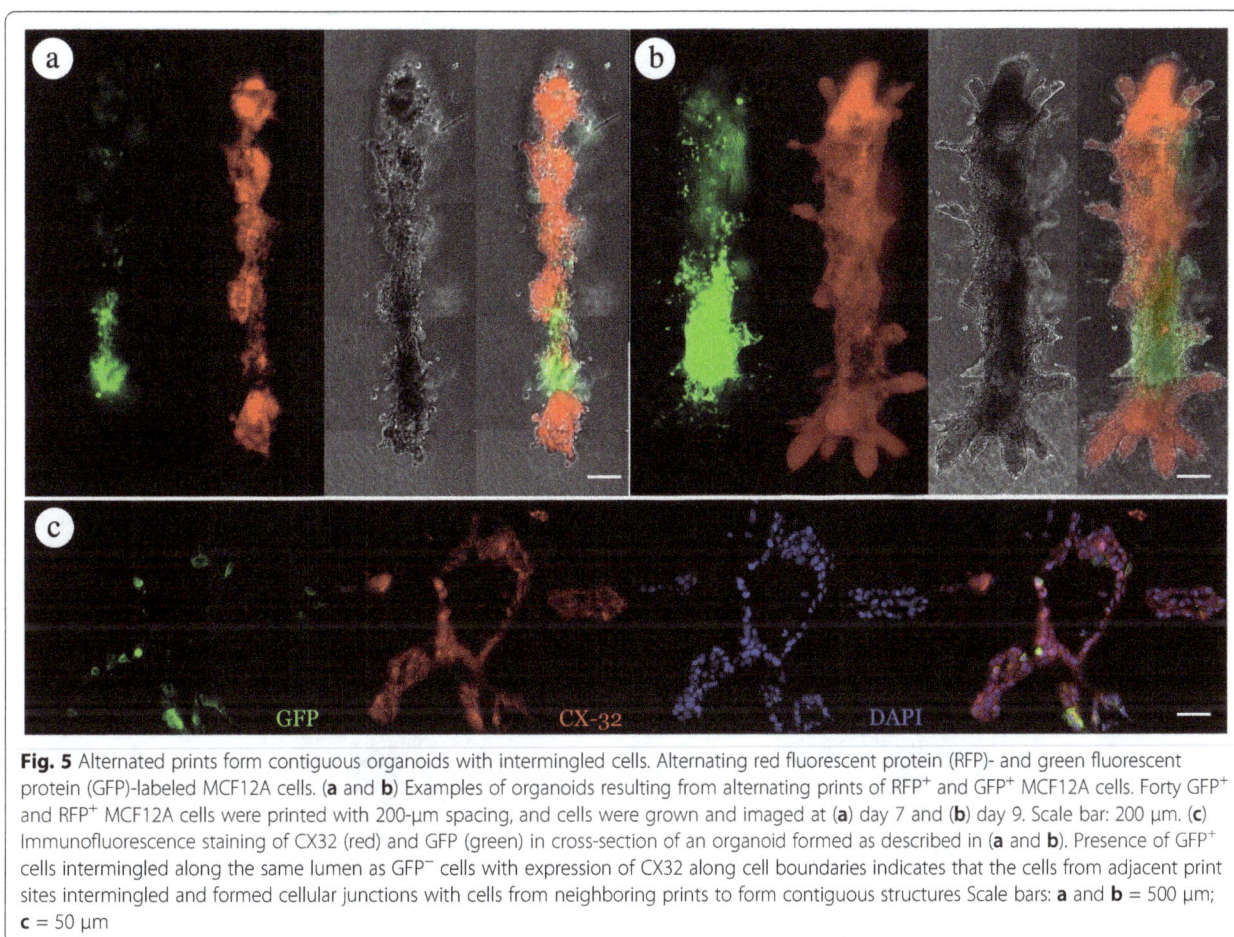

Fig. 5 Alternated prints form contiguous organoids with intermingled cells. Alternating red fluorescent protein (RFP)- and green fluorescent protein (GFP)-labeled MCF12A cells. (**a** and **b**) Examples of organoids resulting from alternating prints of RFP⁺ and GFP⁺ MCF12A cells. Forty GFP⁺ and RFP⁺ MCF12A cells were printed with 200-μm spacing, and cells were grown and imaged at (**a**) day 7 and (**b**) day 9. Scale bar: 200 μm. (**c**) Immunofluorescence staining of CX32 (red) and GFP (green) in cross-section of an organoid formed as described in (**a** and **b**). Presence of GFP⁺ cells intermingled along the same lumen as GFP⁻ cells with expression of CX32 along cell boundaries indicates that the cells from adjacent print sites intermingled and formed cellular junctions with cells from neighboring prints to form contiguous structures Scale bars: **a** and **b** = 500 μm; **c** = 50 μm

laminin 5 demonstrated basal localization of the laminin proteins, consistent with organoid polarization (Additional file 2: Figure S1a,b). These results indicate that methods described here can direct and promote the formation of hollow ductal structures reminiscent of the morphology of a duct formed *in vivo*.

To further explore this, we examined the possibility of directing contiguous luminal structures to conform to alternative shapes. We initially printed 40 cell clusters in a radial pattern within rat tail collagen gels with spacing patterns similar to our linear arrays at 500 μm, 400 μm, and 300 μm (Fig. 4a, b, c). After 7 days, all of the print locations had formed individual organoids (Fig. 4a₁, b₁, c₁), and obvious processes and connections were actively forming among the 300-μm spaced injections. By day 14, again similar to our linear arrays, all groups formed contiguous structures which reflected the intended circular geometry (Fig. 4a₂, b₂, c₂, d). Furthermore, our ability to direct mammary epithelial cell (MEC) structures was maintained throughout 24 days of culture, wherein the cells reacted similarly to the linear arrays and maintained the initial print pattern and formed a contiguous luminal circle about 4 mm in diameter (Fig. 4e, f). These

findings indicate that mammary epithelial migration patterns are not random but rather that the MCF12A cells actively seek neighboring organoid structures to participate in the formation of large structures (Additional file 1: Movie S1 and Additional file 3: Movie S2). Furthermore, these data clearly highlight the tunable nature of our system, where initial cell number can consistently influence the formation of individual organoids. These data also demonstrate that we can print specific cell numbers with the design of consistently generating large contiguous luminal organoids.

Cells from 3D printed individual organoids intermingle and form gap junctions with neighboring organoids

Having established the cell number and individual organoid spacing necessary to form contiguous organoids within 7 days, we next sought to determine to what extent the individual organoids were integrating with their neighbors. To this end, we printed equally spaced 200-μm linear arrays of alternating RFP- and GFP-labeled MCF12A cells in collagen gels. The RFP and GFP printed cells formed contiguous organoids with a central structure and branched extensions with mixed GFP and RFP cells by

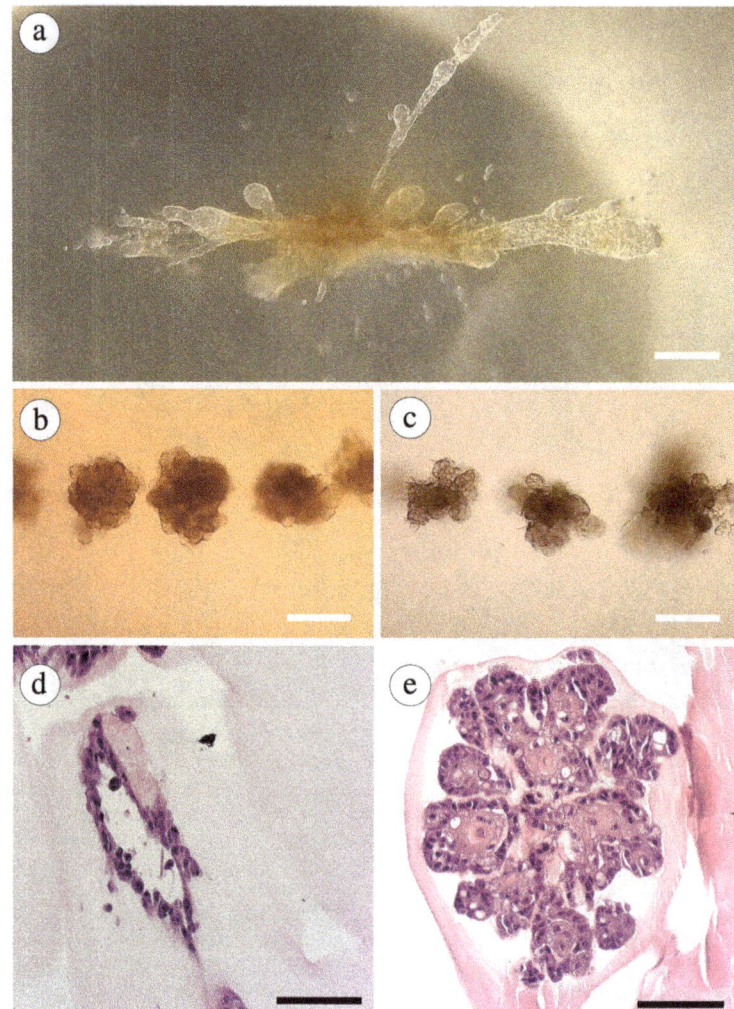

Fig. 6 Adaptation of bioprinting protocol for MCF10A cells and Geltrex hydrogels. (**a**) MCF10A cells growing in rat tail collagen 7 days after printing. Scale bar: 250 μm. (**b** and **c**) MCF10A (**b**) and MCF12A (**c**) cell deposits 7 days after print in Geltrex at 500-μm spacing. Scale bar: 250 μm. (**d**) and (**e**) Hematoxylin and eosin (H&E)-stained cross-sections of MCF10A cells 7 days after printing in rat tail collagen (**d**) and Geltrex (**e**). Scale bar: 100 μm

day 7 (Fig. 5a). Separating the fluorescent channels of these structures revealed the presence of RFP- and GFP-labeled cells intermingling with one another within regions of the larger structure and branched processes at day 14 (Fig. 5b). Indication of coordinated cellular behavior was further supported by positive staining of gap junction protein connexin-32 (CX32) between RFP and GFP MCF12A cells along the same lumen (Fig. 5c).

Printing with MCF10A cells and additional sources of ECM

To provide further comparative data to our MCF12A results, we incorporated MCF10A cells, a commonly used cell type in studies of mammary epithelial biology, into our bioprinting methods. When printed into collagen hydrogels via the same protocol described above, the MCF10A cells formed large structures morphologically similar to those seen with MCF12A cells (Fig. 6a;

Additional file 4: Movie S3). Next, we evaluated our printing system with the commonly used 3D culture substrate growth-factor reduced Matrigel (Geltrex). Unlike organoid growth in collagen gels, both MCF10A and MCF12A cell types displayed a reduced affinity to undergo organoid fusion to form contiguous structures in Geltrex (Fig. 6b–e; Additional file 5: Movie S4). This is consistent with grown patterns previously reported for Matrigel [29]. However, we also observed in a rare incidence the formation of a large contiguous structure with MCF12As similar to that seen in collagen (not shown). These results demonstrate the versatility of our bioprinting system for *in vitro* culture of mammary epithelial cells in various substrates.

Although rodent-derived collagen models recapitulate many features of human mammary gland biology, interspecies variations in ECM composition, organization, density, and function exist [30]. Furthermore, the use of

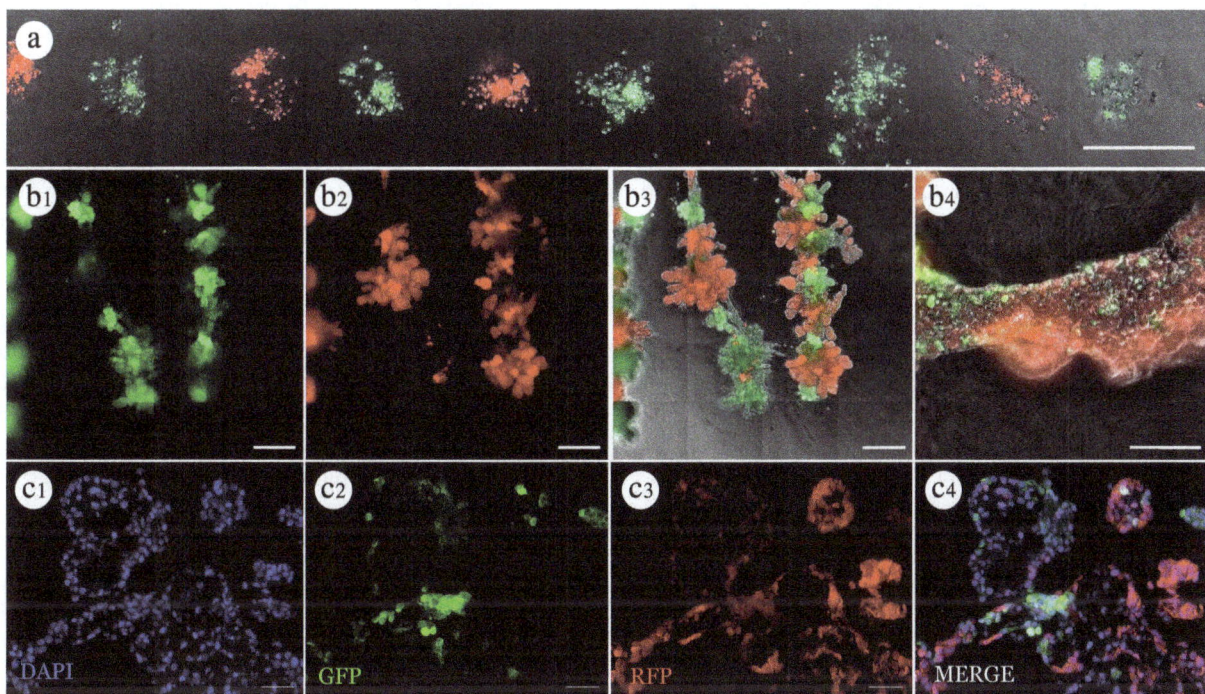

Fig. 7 Breast epithelial morphology in human collagen. (**a**) Bioprinted red fluorescent protein (RFP) and green fluorescent protein (GFP) MCF12A cell deposits in human collagen gel 2 days after printing. (**b**) GFP (**b1**), RFP (**b2**), and merged (**b3** and **b4**) images of organoid formed from alternating prints of GFP and RFP MCF12A cells in human collagen 7 days after printing; higher magnification image (**b4**) demonstrates mix of GFP⁺ and RFP⁺ cells in the same structure. **c**) Immunofluorescent staining of a cross-section of the organoid in (**b**) with 4',6-diamidino-2-phenylindole (DAPI) (**c1**; blue), GFP (**c2**; green), and RFP (**c3**; red). Merged image (**c4**) demonstrates presence of both cell types in the same organoid structure. Scale bars: **a** = 200 μm, **b** = 500 μm, **c** = 100 μM

substrata derived from Engelbreth-Holm-Swarm tumors, commercial preparations, or other non-biomimetic synthetic scaffolds can suffer from batch-to-batch variability. Given our ability to standardize the quantity and spatial distribution of MECs in 3D, we set out to investigate the ability to direct MEC organoid formation in additional sources of ECM by using human-derived collagen gels.

To this end, we again printed RFP- and GFP-labeled MCF12A cells spaced 200 μm apart in linear arrays in human-derived collagen gels (Fig. 7a). After 7 days in culture, both RFP and GFP cells were observed to contribute to the formation of large branched structures (Fig. 7b1–b3). Again, upon closer examination *in situ*, RFP and GFP cells were observed intermingling to form a contiguous organoid structure (Fig. 7b4). Furthermore, data from nine wells, each containing 60 target locations, indicated a total of 528 out of 540 neighboring organoid fusion events within 7 days after printing. Histological staining indicated the presence of GFP- and RFP-labeled cells within the same lumen (Fig. 7c1–c4). These data demonstrate that our bioprinting technique can investigate additional ECM preparations without compromising the number and spatial distribution of printed MECs.

Discussion

The quest for understanding development and disease in higher organisms has been hindered by a lack of investigative tools to accurately and repeatedly control the many variables that impact 3D *in vitro* model systems. A profound example of this is evidenced from the disparate results from laboratory to laboratory in 3D epithelial organoid systems despite the use of biochemically identical ECM matrices and cell types [18, 21, 22, 31]. In the experiments reported herein, we describe a technique to systematically investigate the extent to which cell–cell and cell–ECM interactions act as regulators of normal epithelial cell differentiation into well-organized structures. By standardizing the number and position of cells inside pre-formed gels, we have developed a method to help standardize the analysis of 3D cultures.

It has been noted that organoids resulting from single, primary epithelial cells vary in morphology and formation efficiency compared with organoids derived from primary epithelial cell clusters [32]. Indeed, we expect that the increase in efficiency in our system was due in large part to our ability to define the quantity of cells being placed initially in close proximity to one another. This observation is a likely cause of much of the high variability seen using manual cell-matrix techniques, where we witnessed individual cells preferentially traveling, not clustering, within the gel. In contrast to this, printed cell clusters were prone to quickly begin internal organization into groups and could collectively seek neighboring organoids (Additional file 1: Movie S1, Additional file 3: Movie S2, Additional file 4: Movie S3 and Additional file 5: Movie S4). Our quantitative data bolstered this idea as the formation frequency of organoids increased significantly when we crossed a critical cell number threshold. Furthermore, our data suggest that reliable control over both initial cell number and organoid spacing permits experimenter-directed fabrication of large-scale branched tubular structures of epithelial origin. These data frame the idea that inter-cellular communications that are received when cells are initially introduced into a foreign 3D environment clearly initiate specific sets of response cascades.

It has been shown that following stable adhesion to ECM components, the mechanical interaction between individual cells and ECM results in the transmission of strain patterns which can extend through hundreds of microns of gel [23, 33, 34]. This applied mechanical strain leads collagen fibers to orient along the direction of the strain [18], which results in increased contact guidance. Furthermore, early studies found a preference for MEC organoids to develop along tension lines between adjacent organoids within collagen gels [35]. In a manner similar to which MECs actively seek neighboring organoids in 3D gels, we find that morphological patterns appear to be associated with the relative position of an individual organoid within the printed array. This may explain our observations that organoids seemed to "sense" their neighboring organoids. We observed that cells actively traveling between organoids and extending processes preferentially toward each other ultimately lead to organoid fusion. This process allows us to direct organoid growth by manipulating the distances among initial cell deposits.

Throughout the past decade, testing and controlling microenvironmental aspects of 3D culture systems have enabled researchers to bridge the gap between traditional 2D cell culture systems and animal models for studying development and tumorigenesis. We used our bioprinting device to derive a set of guidelines to enable reliable formation of large-scale, human mammary epithelial organoids in 3D hydrogels. These results demonstrate that epithelial organoid morphology can be directed by initial cell-deposit number, spacing, and overall print geometry. However, the development of actual tissues cannot be reduced to cellular events alone. ECM synthesis and assembly in the mammary gland constitute a dynamic and reciprocal relationship between multiple epithelial cell types, myoepithelial cells, adipocytes, endothelial cells, immune cells, and fibroblasts. Where the

ECM serves to support and instruct cell behavior, cells also continuously modify and synthesize ECM [30]. The methods described here also demonstrate the capability to accurately deposit multiple cell types as neighboring aggregates, which can communicate and synchronize their structure-forming activities. Our approach allows direct control over the generation of *in vitro* constructs large enough for *in vivo* implantation. More importantly, using this system to investigate co-cultures of two or more cell types in a defined microenvironment would greatly increase the ability to develop reliable 3D surrogate models for breast development and carcinogenesis. This is of particular interest to our group, as we have great interest in understanding how the microenvironment controls differentiation of stem and cancer cells [36–45]. We plan to adapt these protocols for the development of chimeric structures containing cancer and normal epithelial cells as *in vitro* models that mimic our previous *in vivo* findings. Furthermore, we expect the processes outlined here to be easily adaptable to other epithelial cell types, including endothelial cells, to study vascularization and development in other tissue types.

Conclusions

In summary, these data demonstrate that our CNC-driven 3D bioprinter is capable of repeatedly and reliably printing mammary epithelial structures. Furthermore, through coordinated cluster placement, our system is capable of generating consistent, large contiguous luminal structures. This 3D bioprinter was developed as an open-source project, where we have disseminated the required data/documents for any biological laboratory to manufacture and use. Thus, through digital transfer of G-Code files, these data could easily be replicated in other laboratories.

Additional files

Additional file 1: Movie S1. MCF12A printed at 500 μm was followed over 1 day from day 7. Cells were seen to collectively branch toward neighboring organoids. Magnification: 20x. (M4V 4232 kb)

Additional file 2: Figure S1. Polarization of bioprinted structures. Laminin 1 + 2 staining (A; green) and laminin 5 (B; red) of bioprinted MCF12A cells show localization of secreted laminins to the basal layer. Nuclei were counterstained with 4',6-diamidino-2-phenylindole (DAPI). Scale bars = 50 μM. (JPG 1048 kb)

Additional file 3: Movie S2. MCF12A printed at 500 μm was followed over 3 days beginning at day 4 after print. Some individual cells can be seen grouping and traveling between organoids. Magnification: 10x. (M4V 2860 kb)

Additional file 4: Movie S3. MCF10A printed at 500 μm in rat tail collagen hydrogels was followed over 8 days beginning at day 4 after print. Magnification: 10x. (MP4 15854 kb)

Additional file 5: Movie S4. MCF10A printed at 500 μm in Geltrex hydrogels was followed over 7 days beginning at day 2 after print. Magnification: 10x. (MP4 11218 kb)

Abbreviations

2D: Two-dimensional; 3D: Three-dimensional; CNC: Computer numerical control; CO_2: Carbon dioxide; CX32: Connexin 32; DAPI: 4′,6-diamidino-2-phenylindole; ECM: Extracellular matrix; GFP: Green fluorescent protein; MEC: Mammary epithelial cell; RFP: Red fluorescent protein

Acknowledgments

We would like to acknowledge Mary Ann Clements and Michael K. Gubler from the Eastern Virginia Medical School Histology Services Lab.

Funding

Funding for this project was provided in part by grants from the Commonwealth Health Research Board, the Jeffress Memorial Trust, and start funds from the Old Dominion University College of Health Sciences to PCS and RDB.

Authors' contributions

JAR designed and performed the experiments, analyzed data, and wrote the manuscript. PMM contributed to the design and execution of the experiments and data interpretation. PCS and RDB equally contributed to the conception of the study, the design of the experiments, interpretation of the data, and writing of the manuscript. All authors read and approved the final manuscript.

Competing interests

The authors declare that they have no competing interests.

Author details

[1]Biomedical Engineering Institute, College of Engineering, Old Dominion University, 5115 Hampton Blvd, Norfolk, VA 23529, USA. [2]School of Medical Diagnostic & Translational Sciences, College of Health Sciences, Old Dominion University, 5115 Hampton Blvd, Norfolk, VA 23529, USA.

References

1. Emerman JT, Pitelka DR. Maintenance and induction of morphological differentiation in dissociated mammary epithelium on floating collagen membranes. In Vitro. 1977;13:316–28.
2. Wozniak MA, Keely PJ. Use of three-dimensional collagen gels to study mechanotransduction in T47D breast epithelial cells. Biol Proced Online. 2005;7:144–61.
3. Overeem AW, Bryant DM, van IJzendoorn SC. Mechanisms of apical-basal axis orientation and epithelial lumen positioning. Trends Cell Biol. 2015;25:476–85.
4. Cassereau L, Miroshnikova YA, Ou G, Lakins J, Weaver VM. A 3D tension bioreactor platform to study the interplay between ECM stiffness and tumor phenotype. J Biotechnol. 2015;193:66–9.
5. Carey SP, Martin KE, Reinhart-King CA. Three-dimensional collagen matrix induces a mechanosensitive invasive epithelial phenotype. Sci Rep. 2017;7:42088.
6. Rodriguez-Fraticelli AE, Martin-Belmonte F. Picking up the threads: extracellular matrix signals in epithelial morphogenesis. Curr Opin Cell Biol. 2014;30:83–90.
7. Glukhova MA, Streuli CH. How integrins control breast biology. Curr Opin Cell Biol. 2013;25:633–41.
8. Manninen A. Epithelial polarity--generating and integrating signals from the ECM with integrins. Exp Cell Res. 2015;334:337–49.
9. Yonemura S. Differential sensitivity of epithelial cells to extracellular matrix in polarity establishment. PLoS One. 2014;9:e112922.
10. Begnaud S, Chen T, Delacour D, Mege RM, Ladoux B. Mechanics of epithelial tissues during gap closure. Curr Opin Cell Biol. 2016;42:52–62.
11. Ravasio A, Cheddadi I, Chen T, Pereira T, Ong HT, Bertocchi C, et al. Gap geometry dictates epithelial closure efficiency. Nat Commun. 2015;6:7683.
12. Inman JL, Bissell MJ. Apical polarity in three-dimensional culture systems: where to now? J Biol. 2010;9:2.
13. Vichas A, Zallen JA. Translating cell polarity into tissue elongation. Semin Cell Dev Biol. 2011;22:858–64.
14. Davis GE, Cleaver OB. Outside in: inversion of cell polarity controls epithelial lumen formation. Dev Cell. 2014;31:140–2.
15. Barcellos-Hoff MH, Aggeler J, Ram TG, Bissell MJ. Functional differentiation and alveolar morphogenesis of primary mammary cultures on reconstituted basement membrane. Development. 1989;105:223–35.
16. Plachot C, Chaboub LS, Adissu HA, Wang L, Urazaev A, Sturgis J, et al. Factors necessary to produce basoapical polarity in human glandular epithelium formed in conventional and high-throughput three-dimensional culture: example of the breast epithelium. BMC Biol. 2009;7:77.
17. O'Brien LE, Zegers MM, Mostov KE. Opinion: building epithelial architecture: insights from three-dimensional culture models. Nat Rev Mol Cell Biol. 2002;3:531–7.
18. Dhimolea E, Maffini MV, Soto AM, Sonnenschein C. The role of collagen reorganization on mammary epithelial morphogenesis in a 3D culture model. Biomaterials. 2010;31:3622–30.
19. Roeder BA, Kokini K, Voytik-Harbin SL. Fibril microstructure affects strain transmission within collagen extracellular matrices. J Biomech Eng. 2009;131:031004.
20. Doyle AD, Carvajal N, Jin A, Matsumoto K, Yamada KM. Local 3D matrix microenvironment regulates cell migration through spatiotemporal dynamics of contractility-dependent adhesions. Nat Commun. 2015;6:8720.
21. Krause S, Maffini MV, Soto AM, Sonnenschein C. A novel 3D in vitro culture model to study stromal-epithelial interactions in the mammary gland. Tissue Eng Part C Methods. 2008;14:261–71.
22. Wozniak MA, Desai R, Solski PA, Der CJ, Keely PJ. ROCK-generated contractility regulates breast epithelial cell differentiation in response to the physical properties of a three-dimensional collagen matrix. J Cell Biol. 2003;163:583–95.
23. Stopak D, Harris AK. Connective tissue morphogenesis by fibroblast traction. I. Tissue culture observations. Dev Biol. 1982;90:383–98.
24. Baker M. 1,500 scientists lift the lid on reproducibility. Nature. 2016;533:452–4.
25. Raphael B, Khalil T, Workman VL, Smith A, Brown CP, Streuli C, et al. 3D cell bioprinting of self-assembling peptide-based hydrogels. Mater Lett. 2017;190:103–6.
26. Reid JA, Mollica PA, Johnson GD, Ogle RC, Bruno RD, Sachs PC. Accessible bioprinting: adaptation of a low-cost 3D-printer for precise cell placement and stem cell differentiation. Biofabrication. 2016;8:025017.
27. Ranga A, Gobaa S, Okawa Y, Mosiewicz K, Negro A, Lutolf MP. 3D niche microarrays for systems-level analyses of cell fate. Nat Commun. 2014;5:4324.
28. Linnemann JR, Miura H, Meixner LK, Irmler M, Kloos UJ, Hirschi B, et al. Quantification of regenerative potential in primary human mammary epithelial cells. Development. 2015;142:3239–51.
29. Lee GY, Kenny PA, Lee EH, Bissell MJ. Three-dimensional culture models of normal and malignant breast epithelial cells. Nat Methods. 2007;4:359–65.
30. Maller O, Martinson H, Schedin P. Extracellular matrix composition reveals complex and dynamic stromal-epithelial interactions in the mammary gland. J Mammary Gland Biol Neoplasia. 2010;15:301–18.
31. Dhimolea E, Soto AM, Sonnenschein C. Breast epithelial tissue morphology is affected in 3D cultures by species-specific collagen-based extracellular matrix. J Biomed Mater Res A. 2012;100:2905–12.
32. Sokol ES, Miller DH, Breggia A, Spencer KC, Arendt LM, Gupta PB. Growth of human breast tissues from patient cells in 3D hydrogel scaffolds. Breast Cancer Res. 2016;18:19.
33. Vanni S, Lagerholm BC, Otey C, Taylor DL, Lanni F. Internet-based image analysis quantifies contractile behavior of individual fibroblasts inside model tissue. Biophys J. 2003;84:2715–27.

34. Rudnicki MS, Cirka HA, Aghvami M, Sander EA, Wen Q, Billiar KL. Nonlinear strain stiffening is not sufficient to explain how far cells can feel on fibrous protein gels. Biophys J. 2013;105:11–20.

35. Foster CS, Smith CA, Dinsdale EA, Monaghan P, Neville AM. Human mammary gland morphogenesis in vitro: the growth and differentiation of normal breast epithelium in collagen gel cultures defined by electron microscopy, monoclonal antibodies, and autoradiography. Dev Biol. 1983;96: 197–216.

36. Bruno RD, Fleming JM, George AL, Boulanger CA, Schedin P, Smith GH. Mammary extracellular matrix directs differentiation of testicular and embryonic stem cells to form functional mammary glands in vivo. Sci Rep. 2017;7:40196.

37. Bruno RD, Boulanger CA, Rosenfield SM, Anderson LH, Lydon JP, Smith GH. Paracrine-rescued lobulogenesis in chimeric outgrowths comprising progesterone-receptor-null mammary epithelium and redirected wild-type testicular cells. J Cell Sci. 2014;127(Pt 1):27–32.

38. Bruno RD, Smith GH. Reprogramming non-mammary and cancer cells in the developing mouse mammary gland. Semin Cell Dev Biol. 2012;23:591–8.

39. Bruno RD, Boulanger CA, Smith GH. Notch-induced mammary tumorigenesis does not involve the lobule-limited epithelial progenitor. Oncogene. 2012;31:60–7.

40. Boulanger CA, Bruno RD, Rosu-Myles M, Smith GH. The mouse mammary microenvironment redirects mesoderm-derived bone marrow cells to a mammary epithelial progenitor cell fate. Stem Cells Dev. 2012;21:948–54.

41. Boulanger CA, Bruno RD, Mack DL, Gonzales M, Castro NP, Salomon DS, et al. Embryonic stem cells are redirected to non-tumorigenic epithelial cell fate by interaction with the mammary microenvironment. PLoS One. 2013;8: e62019.

42. Francis MP, Sachs PC, Elmore LW, Holt SE. Isolating adipose-derived mesenchymal stem cells from lipoaspirate blood and saline fraction. Organogenesis. 2010;6:11–4.

43. Sachs PC, Francis MP, Zhao M, Brumelle J, Rao RR, Elmore LW, et al. Defining essential stem cell characteristics in adipose-derived stromal cells extracted from distinct anatomical sites. Cell Tissue Res. 2012;349:505–15.

44. Zhao M, Sachs PC, Wang X, Dumur CI, Idowu MO, Robila V, et al. Mesenchymal stem cells in mammary adipose tissue stimulate progression of breast cancer resembling the basal-type. Cancer Biol Ther. 2012;13:782–92.

45. Sachs PC, Mollica PA, Bruno RD. Tissue specific microenvironments: a key tool for tissue engineering and regenerative medicine. J Biol Eng. 2017;11:34.

10

Expression of ID4 protein in breast cancer cells induces reprogramming of tumour-associated macrophages

Sara Donzelli[1†], Elisa Milano[1†], Magdalena Pruszko[2], Andrea Sacconi[1], Silvia Masciarelli[3,4], Ilaria Iosue[3,4], Elisa Melucci[5], Enzo Gallo[5], Irene Terrenato[6], Marcella Mottolese[5], Maciej Zylicz[2], Alicja Zylicz[2], Francesco Fazi[3,4*], Giovanni Blandino[1*] and Giulia Fontemaggi[1*] [iD]

Abstract

Background: As crucial regulators of the immune response against pathogens, macrophages have been extensively shown also to be important players in several diseases, including cancer. Specifically, breast cancer macrophages tightly control the angiogenic switch and progression to malignancy. ID4, a member of the ID (inhibitors of differentiation) family of proteins, is associated with a stem-like phenotype and poor prognosis in basal-like breast cancer. Moreover, ID4 favours angiogenesis by enhancing the expression of pro-angiogenic cytokines interleukin-8, CXCL1 and vascular endothelial growth factor. In the present study, we investigated whether ID4 protein exerts its pro-angiogenic function while also modulating the activity of tumour-associated macrophages in breast cancer.

Methods: We performed IHC analysis of ID4 protein and macrophage marker CD68 in a triple-negative breast cancer series. Next, we used cell migration assays to evaluate the effect of ID4 expression modulation in breast cancer cells on the motility of co-cultured macrophages. The analysis of breast cancer gene expression data repositories allowed us to evaluate the ability of ID4 to predict survival in subsets of tumours showing high or low macrophage infiltration. By culturing macrophages in conditioned media obtained from breast cancer cells in which ID4 expression was modulated by overexpression or depletion, we identified changes in the expression of ID4-dependent angiogenesis-related transcripts and microRNAs (miRNAs, miRs) in macrophages by RT-qPCR.

Results: We determined that ID4 and macrophage marker CD68 protein expression were significantly associated in a series of triple-negative breast tumours. Interestingly, ID4 messenger RNA (mRNA) levels robustly predicted survival, specifically in the subset of tumours showing high macrophage infiltration. In vitro and in vivo migration assays demonstrated that expression of ID4 in breast cancer cells stimulates macrophage motility. At the molecular level, ID4 protein expression in breast cancer cells controls, through paracrine signalling, the activation of an angiogenic programme in macrophages. This programme includes both the increase of angiogenesis-related mRNAs and the decrease of members of the anti-angiogenic miR-15b/107 group. Intriguingly, these miRNAs control the expression of the cytokine granulin, whose enhanced expression in macrophages confers increased angiogenic potential.

(Continued on next page)

* Correspondence: francesco.fazi@uniroma1.it; giovanni.blandino@ifo.gov.it;
giulia.fontemaggi@ifo.gov.it
†Sara Donzelli and Elisa Milano contributed equally to this work.
[3]Department of Anatomical, Histological, Forensic & Orthopaedic Sciences,
Section of Histology & Medical Embryology, Sapienza University of Rome, Via
A. Scarpa, 16, 00161 Rome, Italy
[1]Oncogenomics and Epigenetics Unit, IRCCS Regina Elena National Cancer
Institute, Via Elio Chianesi 53, 00144 Rome, Italy
Full list of author information is available at the end of the article

(Continued from previous page)

Conclusions: These results uncover a key role for ID4 in dictating the behaviour of tumour-associated macrophages in breast cancer.

Keywords: ID4, Breast cancer, TAMs, miR-107, HIF-1A, GRN

Background

Breast cancer (BC) is the most common cancer in women worldwide and remains a leading cause of cancer death [1]. It is a heterogeneous disease with multiple subtypes that display different patterns of gene expression, prognosis and response to treatment [2]. Metastasis, which is responsible for over 90% of BC deaths, is regulated to a great extent by reciprocal interactions between cancer cells and immune cells in the tumour microenvironment [3, 4].

Tumour-associated macrophages (TAMs), which are part of the adaptive immune response, constitute a major portion of the leucocyte infiltrate found in breast tumours and tightly control angiogenic switch and progression to malignancy in BC [5]. Tumour cells actively recruit macrophages and educate them to be pro-tumourigenic [6, 7]. TAMs exhibit potent proliferative capacity upon their differentiation from inflammatory monocytes, and the presence of intra-tumoural proliferating macrophages was significantly correlated with high-grade, hormone receptor-negative tumours and a basal-like subtype of BC [7, 8]. The number of proliferating macrophages was also a significant predictor of recurrence and survival [9].

Several reports suggest that TAMs adopt a trophic immunosuppressive phenotype that is functionally reminiscent of the alternatively activated type II (M2) macrophages [10]. However, TAMs present great phenotypic diversity depending on the combinations of stimuli received in the tumour stroma, and it has been proposed that multiple subpopulations of TAMs exist within tumours, which probably change temporally during tumour development and geographically on the basis of their location within the tumour microenvironment [11, 12]. Functionally, TAMs have been shown to facilitate tumour angiogenesis, invasion, intravasation and metastasis in animal models [13, 14] and are now recognised as important therapeutic targets in the treatment of cancer [15].

ID4 is a member of the ID family of proteins (inhibitors of differentiation, ID-1 to ID-4) that act as dominant-negative regulators of basic helix-loop-helix transcription factors [16]. Studies have indicated that ID proteins are associated with loss of differentiation, stemness, unrestricted proliferation, and neoangiogenesis in diverse human cancers. In the context of BC, ID4 is highly expressed in triple-negative breast cancer (TNBC), 70% of which belong to the basal-like breast

cancer (BLBC) molecular subtype [17, 18]. Accordingly, ID4 was repeatedly identified as a component of BLBC-associated molecular signatures [19]. Recent evidence suggests an emerging role for ID4 as a lineage-dependent proto-oncogene that is overexpressed and amplified in BLBCs and is associated with stem-like phenotype and poor prognosis in this subtype and in TNBC [17, 20–23].

At the molecular level, ID4 has been shown to be responsible for the downregulation of BRCA1 promoter activity [24], and consequently, ID4 expression is inversely correlated with that of BRCA1 [20, 23, 25, 26]. In addition, clinical data have indicated preferential ID4 amplification in BRCA1 mutant cases [23, 27]. We previously reported that ID4 protein results in induction of chemokine (C-X-C motif) ligand 1 (CXCL1) and interleukin (IL)-8 pro-angiogenic cytokines and in enhanced angiogenic potential of BC [28, 29]. Moreover, mutant p53 proteins transcriptionally induce ID4, and a complex containing ID4 and mutant p53 proteins is responsible for the synthesis of pro-angiogenic vascular endothelial growth factor (VEGF) isoforms in BC [30].

To fully explore the mechanisms through which ID4 controls BC angiogenesis, we investigated whether it was able to modulate TAM activity. We report that ID4 expression in BC cells is indeed able to reprogramme the expression of angiogenesis-related genes in macrophages through a paracrine VEGF-dependent effect. In particular, we observed the ID4-dependent induction of hypoxia-inducible factor (HIF)-1A, whose expression in macrophages suppresses T-cell function and promotes progression in BC [31], and of granulin (GRN), which was previously reported to control macrophage activity in autoimmune diseases [32]. Of note, microRNAs (miRNAs, miRs) of the miR-15b/107 group, which target these angiogenesis-related factors, were concomitantly downregulated. Our data also showed that high ID4 mRNA expression level is associated with reduced distant metastasis-free survival (DMFS) and overall survival (OS), specifically in patients carrying tumours highly infiltrated by macrophages.

Methods

Cell cultures and transfections

The SKBR3, MDA-MB-468, HL60 and U937 cell lines were grown at 37 °C with 5% CO_2 and maintained in RPMI medium containing 10% heat-inactivated FBS and penicillin/streptomycin. HL60 and U937 cells were differentiated by treatment with 1,25-dihydroxyvitamin D_3 (VitD3) (Sigma-Aldrich, St. Louis, MO, USA) at a concentration of 250 ng/ml. Monocytic differentiation was assessed by fluorescence-activated cell sorting (FACS) as previously reported [33] using allophycocyanin (APC) anti-human CD11b (BD Biosciences, San Jose, CA, USA), PerCP-Cy5.5 (peridinin chlorophyll protein complex-cyanine 5.5) anti-human CD14 (BD Biosciences) and phycoerythrin-immunoglobulin G1 (PE-IgG1) isotype control (eBioscience Inc., San Diego, CA, USA) antibodies for the evaluation of CD11b-CD14 co-expression as a marker of monocytic differentiation. A minimum of 10,000 events were collected for each sample with a flow cytometer (CyAN ADP; Beckman Coulter Life Sciences, Brea, CA, USA) using Summit 4.3 software (Beckman Coulter Life Sciences) for data acquisition and analysis.

An expression vector containing a hemagglutinin (HA)-tagged ID4 coding sequence [28] or control empty vector was transfected in cancer cells using Lipofectamine 2000 reagent (Thermo Fisher Scientific, Waltham, MA, USA) in ID4 overexpression experiments. RNAiMAX reagent (Thermo Fisher Scientific, Waltham, MA, USA) was used to transfect small interfering RNAs (siRNAs) in BC cells. Sequences of siRNAs directed to ID4 were previously reported [30]. Monocytic cell lines were transfected with plasmids, mimic and locked nucleic acid (LNA) oligonucleotides (Dharmacon, Lafayette, CO, USA) using the TransIT-X2® Dynamic Delivery System (Mirus Bio LLC, Madison, WI, USA) following the manufacturer's instructions. Full-length cDNA (including 5′-UTR and 3′-UTR) of human GRN (NM_002087.2), cloned in the pCMV6-XL5 plasmid vector, was generously provided by Dr. Peter Nelson.

Mouse bone marrow-derived macrophage precursors were obtained from rodents by flushing the femurs and tibias with 2% FBS in PBS. Differentiation was induced by culturing precursors in colony-stimulating factor 1 (CSF1)-rich conditioned media (CM) derived from L929 fibroblast cell culture. Differentiation was evaluated by FACS analysis using the following antibodies: anti-mouse F4/80 antigen APC (17-4801; eBioscience), Ly-6G (Gr-1) APC (17-5931; eBioscience, San Diego, CA, USA), CD14 PE (12-0141; eBioscience, San Diego, CA, USA) and CD107b (Mac-3) PE (12-5989; eBioscience, San Diego, CA, USA).

Human peripheral blood-derived monocytes were isolated from blood donors using Lymphoprep solution (Axis-Shield, Dundee, UK) followed by isolation of CD14$^+$ cells with the Monocyte Isolation Kit II (Miltenyi Biotec, Bergisch Gladbach, Germany). Differentiation was achieved through 1-week culturing in RPMI medium containing recombinant CSF1 (human

macrophage colony-stimulating factor, catalogue number 8929SC; Cell Signaling Technology, Danvers, MA, USA).

CM from BC cells were prepared by culturing cells for 24 hours in serum-free RPMI medium. CM were centrifuged to eliminate cell residues before preparation of aliquots and storage at − 80 °C. When si-ID4 BC cells were used to prepare CM, we always collected CM before 48 hours from transfection because of proliferation of cells being delayed after this time point in the si-ID4 condition (Additional file 1: Figure S3).

In vitro and in vivo macrophage migration assays

Migration of mouse bone marrow-derived macrophages in response to SKBR3 cells was evaluated using 3-μm-pore Boyden chambers (Corning Inc., Corning, NY, USA). Infiltration of F4/80$^+$ macrophages in Matrigel plugs containing CM from BC MDA-MB-468 cells was evaluated by subcutaneous inoculation of a solution composed of 500 μl of Matrigel (BD Biosciences) and 50 μl of a 10 × concentration of CM. In the negative control, the CM was replaced with serum-free medium. Plugs were recovered at day 7, fixed for 18–24 hours in 4% (vol/vol) buffered formaldehyde, and then processed with paraffin wax. IHC was performed using F4/80 antibody (MA5-16363; Pierce Biotechnology, Rockford, IL, USA). All procedures involving animals and their care were conducted in conformity with institutional guidelines, which are in compliance with national and international standards.

IHC

Tumours from 62 patients included in this study were previously described in a study by Novelli et al. [34], which was reviewed and approved by the ethics committee of the Regina Elena National Cancer Institute and contained data for which written informed consent was obtained from all patients. Characteristics of these patients are included in Additional file 2: Table S1. BC specimens for IHC analysis were fixed for 18–24 hours in 4% (vol/vol) buffered formaldehyde and then processed with paraffin wax. Anti-ID4 (MAB4393; EMD Millipore, Billerica, MA, USA), anti-oestrogen receptor (clone 6F11; Novocastra, Florence, Italy), anti-progesterone receptor (anti PgR, clone 1A6; Novocastra), and anti-HER2 (A0485; Dako, Milan, Italy) were evaluated by IHC in 5-μm-thick paraffin-embedded tissues. Monoclonal antibodies (mAb) directed against ID4 were incubated at a dilution of 1:200 overnight at 4 °C, and anti-ER and anti-PgR mAb and the polyclonal antibody anti-HER2 were incubated for 60 - minutes at room temperature. Immunoreactions were revealed by a streptavidin-biotin enhanced immunoperoxidase technique (Super Sensitive MultiLink; BioGenex, Fremont, CA, USA) in an autostainer (Bond III; Leica Biosystems, Wetzlar, Germany). Diaminobenzidine (DAB) was used as a chromogenic substrate. Evaluation of the IHC data was performed independently and in a blinded manner by two investigators (EG and EM).

Immunocytochemistry and immunofluorescence

For immunocytochemistry assay, cells were seeded onto glass coverslips (Paul Marienfeld, Lauda-Königshofen, Germany) in 6-well dishes (Corning Inc.) at 4×10^4 cells/well, cultured with RPMI or CM, and fixed with 4% formaldehyde in PBS for 15 minutes at room temperature. Cells were permeabilized with 0.25% Triton X-100 in PBS for 10 minutes. After washing with PBS, the coverslips were incubated with anti-ID4 antibody diluted in 5% bovine serum albumin (BSA)/PBS for 2 hours at room temperature. Cells were incubated with peroxidase inhibitor before primary antibody incubation. Protein staining was revealed through DAB enzymatic reaction, and nuclei were counterstained with haematoxylin.

For immunofluorescence, cells grown in the presence of RPMI or CM (48 hours), as well as cells transfected with mimic oligonucleotides (48 hours), were concentrated onto microscope slides using cytospin and fixed and permeabilized as already described. Slides were blocked for 30 minutes in 5% BSA/PBS at room temperature and then incubated with an anti-HIF-1A antibody (A300-286A; Bethyl Laboratories, Montgomery, TX, USA) diluted in 5% BSA/PBS for 2 hours at room temperature. Cells were incubated with secondary antibody Alexa Fluor 594 (1:500; Thermo Fisher Scientific) for 45 minutes. Nuclei were stained with DAPI (Thermo Fisher Scientific).

Western blotting and antibodies

For the Western blot analysis, cells were lysed in radioimmunoprecipitation assay buffer or 8 M urea. The protein concentration was measured using a Bio-Rad protein assay kit (Bio-Rad Laboratories, Hercules, CA, USA). The lysate was mixed with $4 \times$ Laemmli buffer. Total protein extracts were resolved on polyacrylamide gel and then transferred onto nitrocellulose membrane. The following primary antibodies were used: Gapdh (sc-32,233), ID4 (H70) sc-13047, ID4 (B5) sc-365656, HA (12CA5) sc-57592 (Santa Cruz Biotechnology, Dallas, TX, USA); HIF-1A (A300-286A; Bethyl Laboratories); GRN (PA5-29909), EphB2 (PA5-14607), and Mdk (PA5-30601; Thermo Fisher Scientific). Secondary antibody fused with horseradish peroxidase was used for chemiluminescence detection on a UVITEC instrument (Uvitec, Cambridge, UK). VEGFA blocking antibody (AF-293-NA; R&D Systems, Minneapolis, MN, USA) was added to CM and incubated for 30 minutes at room temperature before being used to culture macrophages, following the manufacturer's instructions.

RNA isolation, RT-qPCR and TaqMan Low Density Arrays

RNA was isolated with TRIzol reagent (Sigma-Aldrich), and its concentration was measured using a NanoDrop 2000 instrument (NanoDrop Technologies, Wilmington, DE, USA). Reverse transcription was performed with Moloney murine leukemia virus reverse transcriptase (Thermo Fisher Scientific). qPCR was carried out on an ABI PRISM 7500 Fast Sequence Detection System (Applied Biosystems, Foster City, CA, USA). Primers used for PCR analyses are available upon request. The expression values of mRNAs were calculated by the standard curve method and normalised with housekeeping control genes (GAPDH, β-actin, H3). qPCR using TaqMan Low Density Arrays (TLDA) Human Angiogenesis (4378725; Thermo Fisher Scientific) was carried out following the manufacturer's instructions on an ABI PRISM 7900HT Sequence Detection System.

Angiogenic assay in zebrafish embryo

Four microlitres of CM was mixed with 4 µl of Growth Factor Reduced Matrigel (BD Biosciences) and 0.5 µl of phenol red. The mixture of CM and Matrigel was injected into the perivitelline space of Tg(fli:EGFP) casper zebrafish embryos at 48 hours post-fertilisation. The injection was performed using glass micropipettes with capillaries of 0.75-mm internal diameter. The following parameters were used for the micropipette puller (P-1000; Sutter Instruments, Novato, CA, USA): heat 510, pull 100, velocity 200, time 40, and pressure 500. The parameters of the PicoPump injector (World Precision Instruments, Sarasota, FL, USA) were set to inject 1 nl of CM. Within 24 hours after injection, the neovascular response originating from the developing subintestinal vessels was observed on a fluorescence stereoscope.

Tube-formation assay

Differentiated U937 cells were transfected with siRNAs directed to GRN mRNA or control siRNAs for 8 hours and subsequently cultured with CM from MDA-MB-468 cells. After 72 hours of culture, CM was collected and used to perform tube-formation assays as described by Pruszko et al. [30].

Cell viability assay

Viability of U937 cells was assessed using the ATPlite assay (PerkinElmer, Waltham, MA, USA) at the indicated time point and according to the manufacturer's instructions. Differentiated U937 cells (1×10^5 cells), previously transfected with GRN expression vector, were seeded into 96-well plates and cultured for 48 hours in CM from MDA-MB-468 cells. Luminescence was read by using the EnSpire® Multimode Plate Reader (PerkinElmer).

Results

ID4 expression correlates with macrophage recruitment in triple-negative breast cancer

We previously demonstrated that ID4 protein expression is associated with high microvessel density in BC. Mechanistically, ID4 promotes the production of pro-angiogenic cytokines in BC cells, leading to enhanced endothelial cell proliferation and migration [28, 30]. Because the onset of angiogenic switch, identified as the formation of a high-density vessel network, is closely associated with the transition to malignancy and is regulated by infiltrating macrophages in primary mammary tumours [5], we investigated whether ID4 promotes angiogenesis by influencing the behaviour of macrophages. We first evaluated whether any association existed between ID4 protein expression and infiltrating TAMs in human BC by staining a series of 62 TNBCs for ID4 protein and for the widely used macrophage marker CD68 [15, 35]. The choice of TNBC was based on evidence that increased ID4 expression is specific to this subtype, characterised by the absence of oestrogen receptor, PgR and HER2 receptors, and mostly attributable to the BLBC molecular subtype, as reviewed by Baker et al. [23]. Expression levels of ID4 in representative TNBC and BLBC cohorts are shown in Additional file 3: Figure S1. Pathological characteristics of the 62 analysed TNBC cases are included in Additional file 2: Table S1.

In agreement with the literature [18, 28], we observed that ID4 protein was detectable in 75% of the analysed specimens. On the basis of protein expression, we divided the analysed tumours into low expressers (comprising negative tumours and tumours scored as 1+) and high expressers (comprising tumours scored as 2+ and 3+). We observed that high CD68 protein expression was significantly associated with the ID4 high expresser group ($P = 0.028$) (Fig. 1a). Representative images of TNBC showing high or low protein levels of ID4 and CD68 are shown in Fig. 1b. ID4 and CD68 proteins were not associated with other pathological characteristics in this group of patients.

ID4 expression predicts survival in tumours highly infiltrated by macrophages

High levels of ID4 expression have been correlated to decreased survival in TNBC and BLBC [17, 20, 21]. Macrophage infiltration has been correlated to angiogenesis in BC, but the study of its prognostic significance has led to contradictory results, probably because of the existence of various intratumoural macrophage populations with different properties [12].

To evaluate ID4 prognostic power in relation to macrophage infiltration, we interrogated the Kaplan-Meier Plotter database (www.kmplot.com) [36], which contains a compendium of studies with gene expression and relative survival data for BLBCs. Interestingly, we observed that high ID4 expression was strongly associated with low probability of DMFS ($n = 232$) and OS ($n = 241$), specifically in the group of tumours characterised by high expression of CD68 (and therefore highly infiltrated by macrophages) (Fig. 1c and Additional file 4: Table S2), whereas no association of ID4 with survival was present in the low-CD68 group (Fig. 1d and Additional file 4: Table S2). A similar result was obtained when a macrophage signature comprising a subset of eight widely used markers (CD14, CD105, CD11b, CD68, CD93, CD33, IL-4R and CD163) for the mononuclear phagocyte system [37] was used to identify tumours highly infiltrated by macrophages (Fig. 1e and f and Additional file 5: Table S3). Analysis of gene expression data from The Cancer Genome Atlas (TCGA) cohort of BLBC confirmed that high ID4 expression is associated to low probability of overall survival specifically in the CD68-high and macrophage signature (MacSig)-high groups (Additional file 6: Figure S2a–d). The TCGA cohort allowed us also to assess that ID4 and CD68 do not associate with the clinical variables T, N and G (as observed in the TNBC cohort analysed by IHC and described in the previous paragraph), whereas ID4 significantly associates with mutated *TP53* status (Additional file 6: Figure S2e). Moreover, because none of the considered patients from the TCGA cohort received neoadjuvant treatment, we can assert that the observed associations are independent of particular treatment regimens. These results indicated that the combination of ID4 and macrophage markers represents a powerful predictive indicator in BLBC.

ID4 expression in breast cancer cells enhances macrophage motility

On the basis of the observed association between ID4 protein expression and TAMs, we wondered whether ID4 expression in BC cells influences macrophage recruitment. To address this, CD34$^+$ progenitors from mouse bone marrow were isolated, differentiated in vitro to macrophages (Fig. 2a), and evaluated for their migratory capacity in response to BC cells with ID4 expression depleted or not (Fig. 2b–c). As shown in Fig. 2c, a lower number of macrophages migrated towards ID4-depleted (si-ID4) BC cells than that for control (si-SCR) cells.

To evaluate if ID4 expression in BC cells influences the recruitment of macrophages in vivo, we performed Matrigel assays. Briefly, Matrigel plugs containing CM from MDA-MB-468 BC cells, transfected with an expression

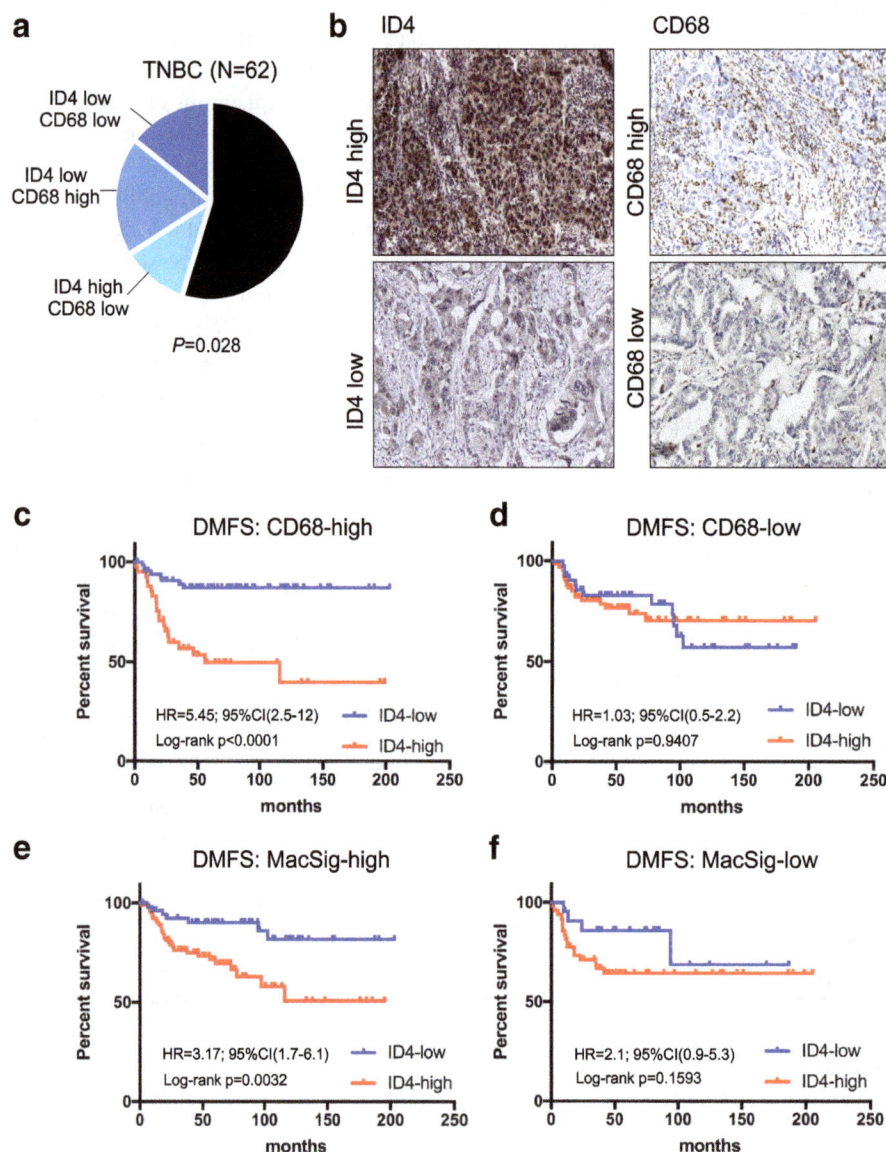

Fig. 1 Inhibitor of differentiation 4 (ID4) protein and macrophage marker CD68 are significantly associated in triple-negative breast cancer (TNBC). **a** and **b** A series of 62 TNBC samples was stained for ID4 protein and for the macrophage marker CD68. ID4 protein expression was considered positive when we observed an immunoreaction in the cytoplasm and/or nucleus. Staining intensity was evaluated as follows: 0 negative, 1+ mild, 2+ moderate, 3+ strong. ID4 was considered overexpressed when more than 10% of neoplastic cells presented a strong immunoreaction. CD68 staining was scored as the infiltration density and was evaluated as follows: 0 absent, 1+ mild, 2+ moderate, 3+ dense. **a** Fisher's exact test demonstrated that high ID4 and CD68 expression are significantly associated ($P = 0.028$). **b** Representative images of TNBC showing high or low protein levels of ID4 or CD68. **c–f** Predictive power of *ID4* messenger RNA expression for distant metastasis-free survival (DMFS) ($N = 232$) was evaluated by Kaplan–Meier analysis in basal-like breast cancer (BLBC) showing high or low CD68 (**c** and **d**) or macrophage signature (MacSig) (**e** and **f**) levels. Macrophage signature is composed of eight widely used markers for the mononuclear phagocyte system (CD14, CD105, CD11b, CD68, CD93, CD33, IL4R, and CD163 [37])

vector for HA-tagged ID4 or an empty vector (Fig. 2d and e), were inoculated subcutaneously in mouse flanks and recovered after 7 days. According to previous reports [38, 39], IHC staining of Matrigel plugs with mouse monocyte/macrophage marker F4/80 showed the presence of F4/80⁺ cells within regions of massive cellular infiltration inside the Matrigel. A higher number of F4/80⁺ cells was observed in

plugs containing CM from ID4-overexpressing cells than that in control plugs (Fig. 2f–g).

ID4 expression in breast cancer cells modulates the activation of a pro-angiogenic programme in macrophages

Because one of the major activities exerted by TAMs is the promotion of angiogenesis, we next analysed

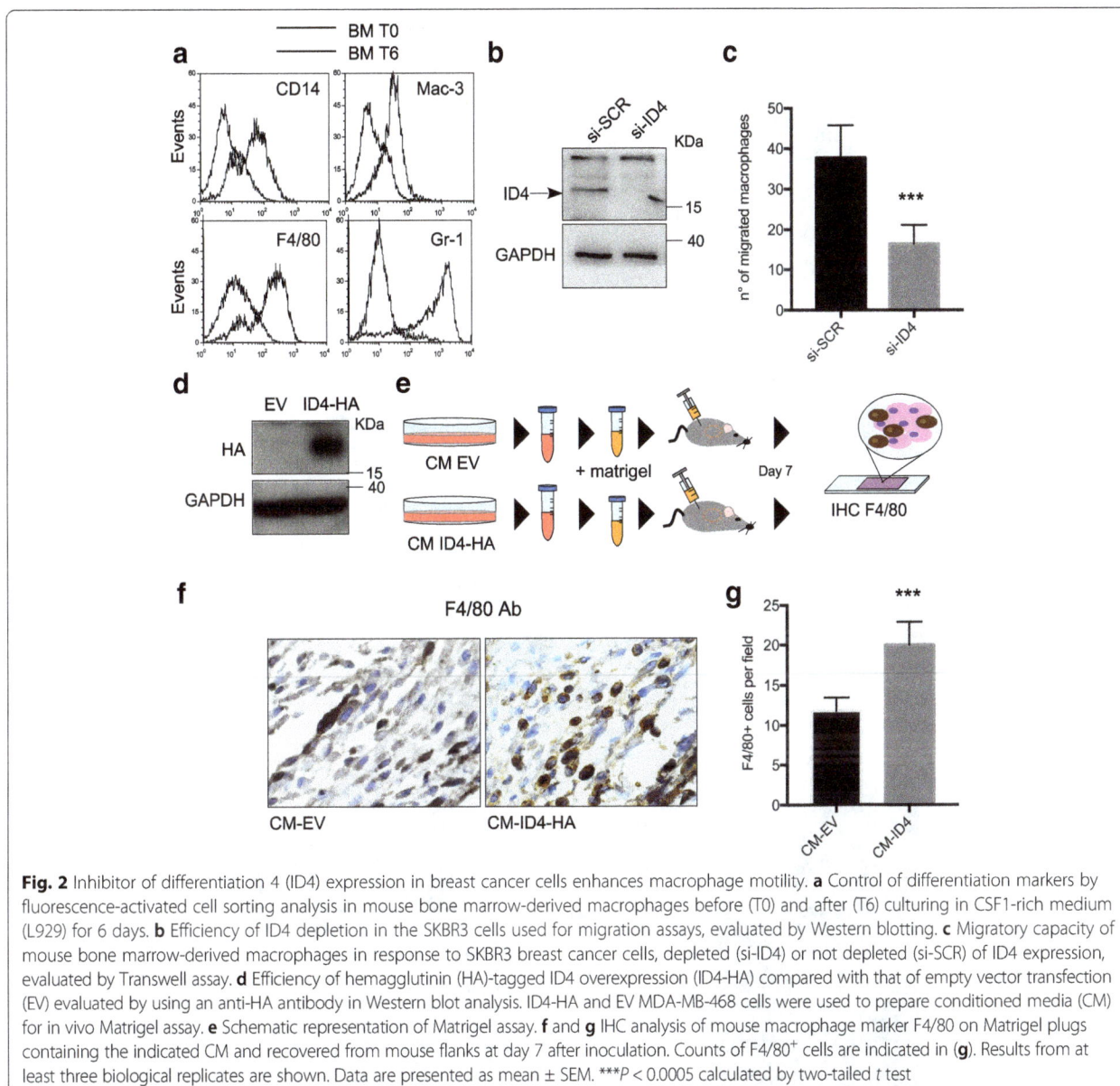

Fig. 2 Inhibitor of differentiation 4 (ID4) expression in breast cancer cells enhances macrophage motility. **a** Control of differentiation markers by fluorescence-activated cell sorting analysis in mouse bone marrow-derived macrophages before (T0) and after (T6) culturing in CSF1-rich medium (L929) for 6 days. **b** Efficiency of ID4 depletion in the SKBR3 cells used for migration assays, evaluated by Western blotting. **c** Migratory capacity of mouse bone marrow-derived macrophages in response to SKBR3 breast cancer cells, depleted (si-ID4) or not depleted (si-SCR) of ID4 expression, evaluated by Transwell assay. **d** Efficiency of hemagglutinin (HA)-tagged ID4 overexpression (ID4-HA) compared with that of empty vector transfection (EV) evaluated by using an anti-HA antibody in Western blot analysis. ID4-HA and EV MDA-MB-468 cells were used to prepare conditioned media (CM) for in vivo Matrigel assay. **e** Schematic representation of Matrigel assay. **f** and **g** IHC analysis of mouse macrophage marker F4/80 on Matrigel plugs containing the indicated CM and recovered from mouse flanks at day 7 after inoculation. Counts of F4/80$^+$ cells are indicated in (**g**). Results from at least three biological replicates are shown. Data are presented as mean ± SEM. ***$P < 0.0005$ calculated by two-tailed t test

whether ID4 expression in BC cells affects the expression of angiogenic genes in macrophages. To this end, we took advantage of a TLDA containing probes for a panel of 94 angiogenesis-related genes. Macrophages obtained from differentiation of HL60 cells [40, 41], cultured with CM from MDA-MB-468 cells transfected with an ID4 expression vector (ID4) or an empty vector (EV), were evaluated along with control macrophages cultured in RPMI medium (Fig. 3a and b). In this experimental setting, we detected 36 expressed genes, 11 of which were modulated in an ID4-dependent manner (1 downregulated and 10 upregulated genes) (Additional file 4: Table S3). The ID4-dependent paracrine induction in macrophages of a subset of these genes, comprising ephrin B2 (*EPHB2*), midkine

(*MDK*), *EDIL3* and *GRN*, was validated by RT-qPCR (Additional file 7: Figure S4a) and Western blotting (Additional file 7: Figure S4b). We verified that ID4 overexpression did not affect the expression of these genes in MDA-MB-468 cells (Additional file 7: Figure S4a, right panel).

Moreover, using an additional macrophage cell line (U937), we observed that the expression of selected ID4-dependent angiogenesis-related genes (*EPHB2*, *GRN* and *NRP2*) was induced in macrophages cultivated in CM compared with RPMI medium (Fig. 3c); as expected, this induction was impaired when CM was derived from si-ID4 BC cells (Fig. 3c–f). Interestingly, analysis of HIF-1A, a master regulator of angiogenesis, revealed that the expression of this transcription factor in

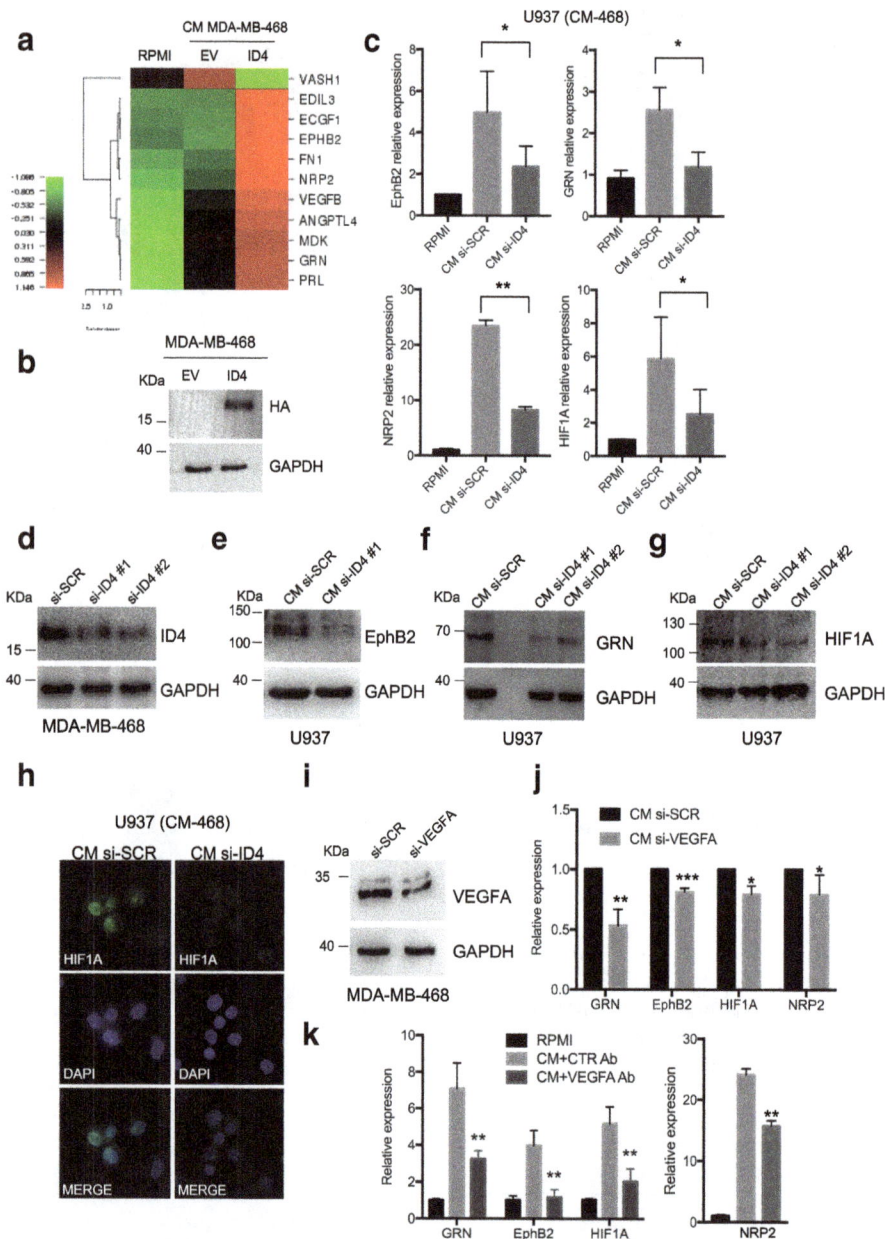

Fig. 3 Inhibitor of differentiation 4 (ID4) expression in breast cancer cells leads to the activation of an angiogenic programme in macrophages. **a** Expression matrix representing a panel of angiogenic factors evaluated using TaqMan Low-Density Arrays (TLDA) in macrophages obtained by 1,25-dihydroxyvitamin D_3 (VitD3)-mediated differentiation of HL60 cells and subsequently cultured in RPMI medium or in conditioned media (CM) from control (EV) or ID4-overexpressing (ID4) MDA-MB-468 breast cancer cells. **b** Western blot showing ID4-HA overexpression in MDA-MB-468 cells. **c** Selected genes modulated in the arrays were evaluated by RT-qPCR in macrophages obtained from VitD3-mediated differentiation of U937 cells and subsequently cultivated in RPMI medium (CTR) or in CM from control (CM si-SCR) or ID4-depleted (CM si-ID4) MDA-MB-468 cells. **d** Western blot analysis showing the level of ID4 protein after transfection of the indicated small interfering RNAs (siRNAs) in MDA-MB-468 cells. **e–g** Western blot analysis of ephrin B2 (EphB2), granulin (GRN) and hypoxia-inducible factor (HIF)-1A proteins in differentiated U937 cells cultured in CM si-SCR or CM si-ID4 from MDA-MB-468 cells. **h** Immunofluorescence analysis of HIF-1A protein performed in differentiated U937 cells cultured in the presence of CM si-SCR or CM si-ID4 from MDA-MB-468 cells. **i** Western blotting showing the efficiency of vascular endothelial growth factor A (VEGFA) depletion by siRNA transfection in MDA-MB-468 cells used to prepare CM used in experiments shown in (**j**). **j** RT-qPCR analysis of the indicated messenger RNAs in U937 macrophages cultivated in the presence of CM from control (si-SCR) or VEGFA-depleted (si-VEGFA) MDA-MB-468 cells. **k** RT-qPCR analysis of the indicated genes in differentiated U937 cells cultivated in RPMI medium or in CM from MDA-MB-468 cells in the presence of VEGFA blocking antibody (Ab) or a control Ab. Specifically, VEGFA blocking Ab or control Ab were incubated with CM for 30 minutes at room temperature and CM plus Ab was subsequently used to culture U937 cells for 48 hours. Results from at least three biological replicates are shown. Data are presented as mean ± SEM. *$P < 0.05$, **$P < 0.005$, ***$P < 0.0005$ calculated by two-tailed t test

macrophages depends on the level of ID4 expression in BC cells (Fig. 3c, g and h and Additional file 7: Figure S4c). Altogether, these results showed that high ID4 expression in BC cells is associated with the activation of a pro-angiogenic programme in macrophages.

Because the expression of the angiogenesis-related genes in macrophages depends on the expression of ID4 in BC cells, we reasoned that a soluble factor, secreted in an ID4-dependent manner from BC cells, is probably responsible for the observed gene expression reprogramming of macrophages. In this regard, we recently reported that ID4 protein promotes the synthesis of pro-angiogenic isoforms of VEGFA at the expense of the anti-angiogenic ones in BC cells [30]. We then explored whether VEGFA was responsible for the observed effects. We first cultured differentiated U937 cells in CM from VEGFA-depleted (si-VEGFA) or control (si-SCR) BC cells. Analysis of a panel of angiogenesis-related factors evidenced a partial decrease of their expression after VEGFA depletion (Fig. 3l and j). Next, we observed that the addition of VEGFA blocking antibody to the CM from BC cells subsequently used to culture U937 cells partially impaired the induction of this panel of angiogenesis-related factors (Fig. 3k). These results indicate that ID4-dependent gene expression modulation in macrophages is at least in part under the control of VEGFA signalling.

ID4 expression in breast cancer cells downregulates anti-angiogenic microRNAs in macrophages

It has been extensively reported that the angiogenic programme is tightly controlled also at the post-transcriptional level by miRNAs in cancer. To explore whether the ID4-dependent reprogramming of macrophages also involved miRNAs, we evaluated the expression of members of the miR-15/107 group, which were previously correlated to angiogenesis in vertebrates and reported to target GRN and HIF-1B [42–47].

We observed that miR-107, miR-15b and miR-195 are downregulated in macrophages cultured with CM from ID4-overexpressing BC cells (CM ID4) compared with macrophages cultured with CM from BC cells with control empty vector (CM EV) (Additional file 5: Figure S5a). On the contrary, expression of these miRNAs was recovered in the presence of CM from si-ID4 BC cells in two macrophage cell lines (Fig. 4a and b and Additional file 8: Figure S5b–e). We evaluated the expression of miR-96, which exhibits oncogenic activity in BC [48], as a control, and we observed that it shows a trend opposite to that of miR-107 (Fig. 4c). Recovery of miR-107, miR-15b and miR-195 expression was also observed in U937 cells cultured in the presence of CM from VEGFA-depleted BC cells (Additional file 8: Figure S5f), indicating that

VEGFA signalling also controls, at least in part, miRNA expression in TAMs.

Time-course analysis of macrophages cultured with CM from BC cells revealed downregulation of these miRNAs (Fig. 4d and e and Additional file 8: Figure S5f). Analysis of pre-miR-107 expression in the same conditions highlighted that decrease of mature miR-107 was accompanied by an accumulation of its precursor (Fig. 4f), suggesting an inhibition of the processing of this miRNA in the presence of CM from BC cells. Altogether, these results indicated that expression of ID4 in BC cells leads to a paracrine downregulation of miR-107, miR-15b and miR-195 in macrophages.

Next, we focused on miR-107, which shows the strongest ID4-dependent paracrine downregulation in macrophages, and evaluated whether it affects the expression of GRN and HIF-1B, two well-established targets [44, 49]. To this end, we inhibited miR-107 in U937 cells by transfecting an LNA oligonucleotide (Fig. 4g). As shown in Fig. 4h, miR-107 inhibition recovered GRN and HIF-1B protein expression, mimicking the effect of si-ID4 BC-derived CM. We also observed induced protein expression of EphB2 and HIF-1A (Fig. 4h), which, as the majority of the angiogenesis-related factors that are activated in an ID4-dependent paracrine manner in macrophages, are predicted to be targeted by the miR-15/107 group members (Additional file 5: Table S3).

To further investigate the relevance of miR-107 downregulation associated with CM, we overexpressed miR-107 using mimic oligonucleotides in macrophages cultured with CM from MDA-MB-468 BC cells (Fig. 4i). As shown in Fig. 4j and k, the forced expression of miR-107 led to decreased GRN mRNA and protein levels. Similar results were observed for HIF-1A (Additional file 8: Figure S5g and h). Our results indicated that the expression of angiogenesis-related genes is strictly controlled by the activity of the ID4-dependent miR-107 in macrophages.

Granulin expression markedly increases the angiogenic potential of macrophages

Among the ID4-dependent angiogenesis-related genes upregulated in macrophages, GRN particularly attracted our attention, because this growth factor is specifically expressed in TNBC and BLBC [50] and has recently been correlated to tumour angiogenesis in mesothelioma [51]. In macrophages, GRN has been reported to control cytokine production [32], but its effect on the angiogenic potential of these cells has not been explored yet.

To evaluate the ability of GRN to confer angiogenic potential to macrophages, we performed in vivo angiogenic assays. To this end, a full-length GRN expression vector, containing 5′- and 3′-UTRs, or control EV was transfected in U937-derived macrophages, which were

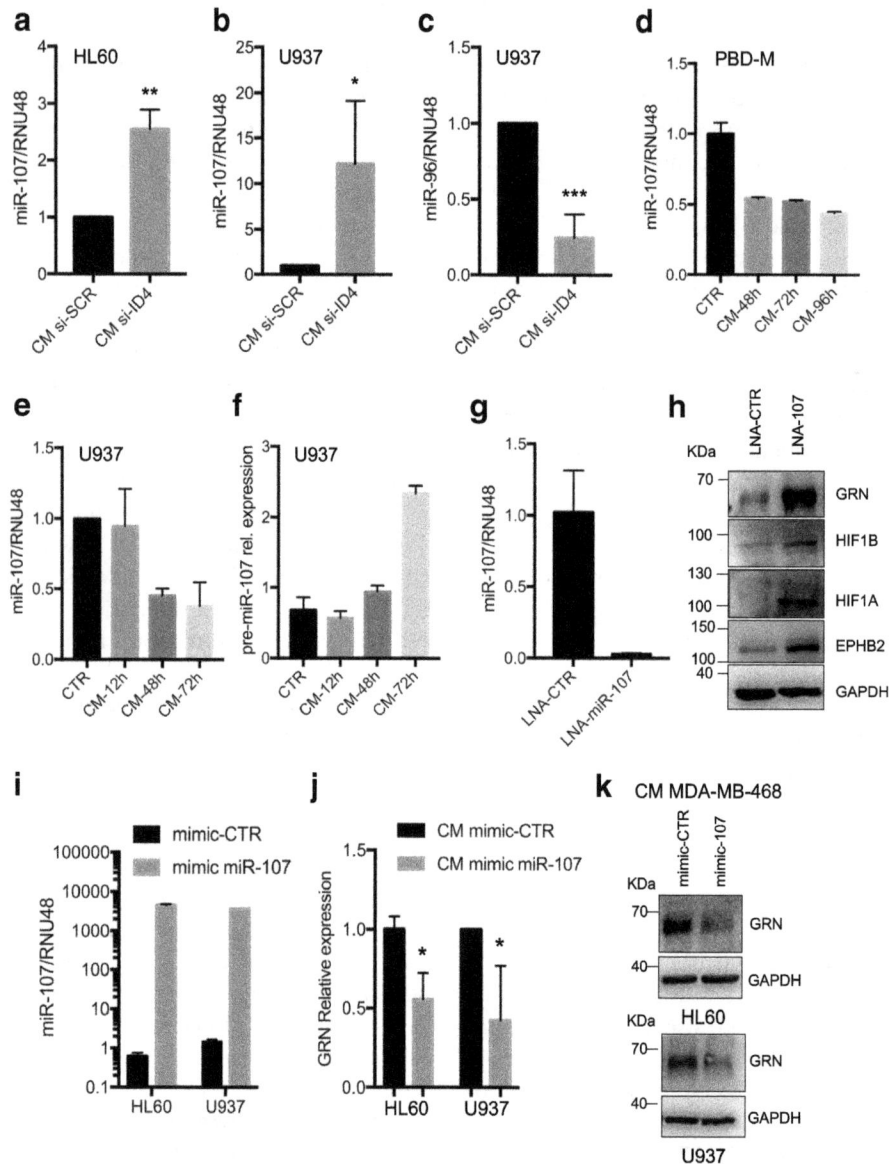

Fig. 4 Inhibitor of differentiation 4 (ID4) expression in breast cancer cells leads to the paracrine downregulation of miR-107 in macrophages. **a** and **b** RT-qPCR analysis to evaluate the expression of miR-107 in macrophages obtained from 1,25-dihydroxyvitamin D₃ (VitD3)-mediated differentiation of HL60 (**a**) and U937 (**b**) cells and subsequently cultivated in conditioned media (CM) from control (si-SCR) or ID4-depleted (si-ID4) MDA-MB-468 cells. **c** RT-qPCR for miR-96 in U937-derived macrophages as in (**b**). **d** and **e** RT-qPCR analysis of miR-107 in peripheral blood-derived macrophages (PBD-M) (**d**) and U937-derived (**e**) macrophages cultivated in RPMI medium (CTR) or in CM from, respectively, SKBR3 and MDA-MB-468 cells for the indicated time points. **f** RT-qPCR for pre-miR-107 in U937 cells as in (**e**). **g** RT-qPCR analysis of miR-107 levels in differentiated U937 cells transfected with locked nucleic acid (LNA) antisense oligonucleotide directed to miR-107. **h** Western blot analysis of the indicated proteins in differentiated U937 cells transfected with LNA antisense oligonucleotide directed to miR-107. **i** and **j** miR-107 (**i**) and granulin (GRN) (**j**) expression levels evaluated by RT-qPCR in HL60 and U937 cells transfected with control mimic or miR-107 mimic oligonucleotides. **k** Western blot analysis of GRN in HL60 and U937 cells transfected with control mimic or miR-107 mimic oligonucleotides. Results from at least three biological replicates are shown. Data are presented as mean ± SEM. *P < 0.05, **P < 0.005, ***P < 0.0005 calculated by two-tailed t test.

then cultured with RPMI or CM from MDA-MB-468 cells. As shown in Fig. 5a and b, although *GRN* mRNA expression levels were comparable between RPMI and CM conditions, GRN protein overexpression was observed only in macrophages cultured with CM. This result further underlined that GRN expression in

macrophages is strictly controlled at the translational level and that its protein expression is obtained only in the presence of CM, possibly as a consequence of miR-107 downregulation (as shown in Fig. 4d and e).

We then evaluated the angiogenic potential of macrophages transfected with GRN or EV and cultured in

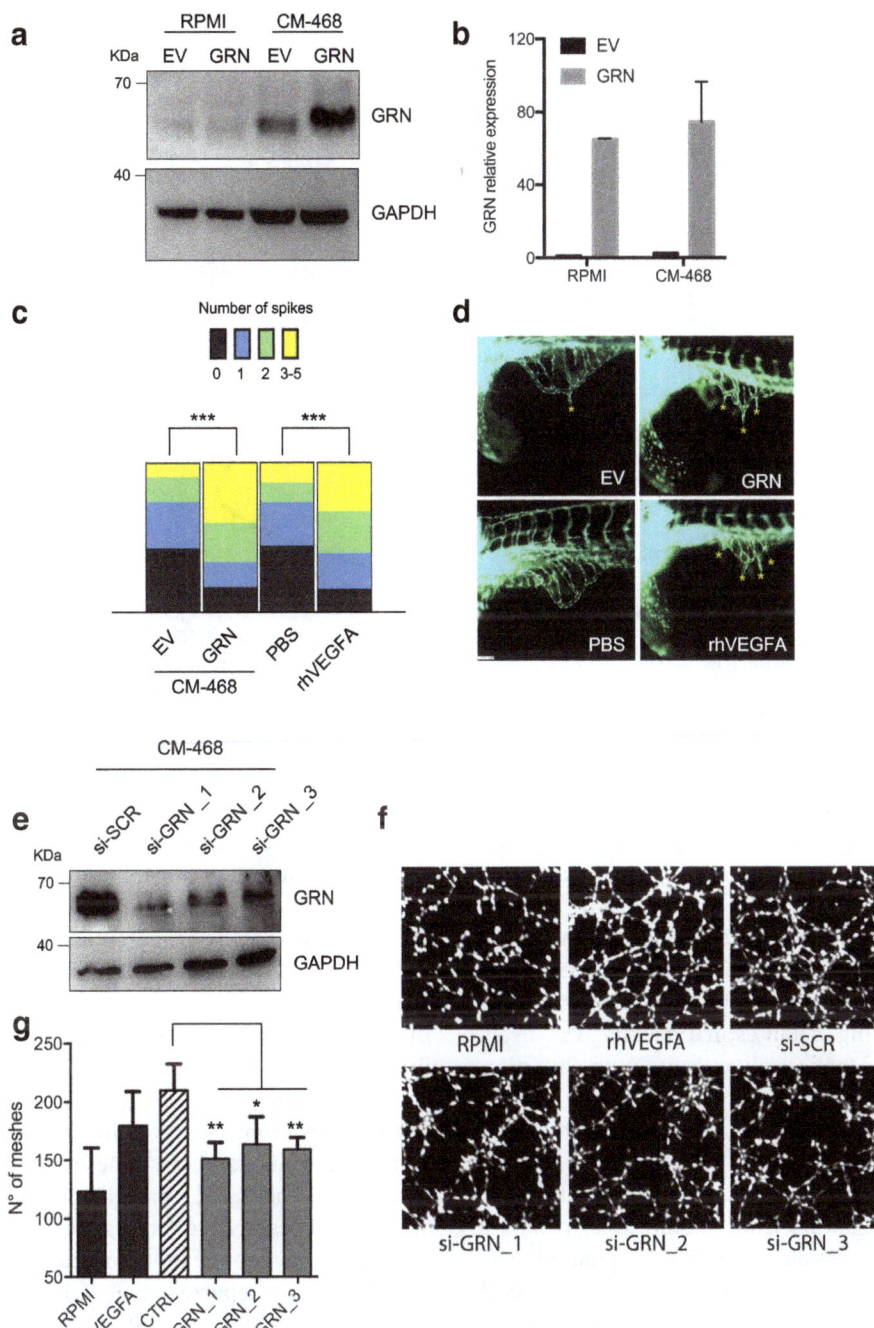

Fig. 5 Modulation of granulin (GRN) expression affects the angiogenic potential of macrophages. **a** Western blot analysis of GRN in U937 cells transfected with a GRN expression vector or an empty vector (EV) and cultured in the presence of RPMI medium or conditioned media (CM) from MDA-MB-468 cells. **b** RT-qPCR analysis of *GRN* messenger RNA levels in the same experimental conditions described in (**a**). **c** CM from the indicated experimental conditions were injected into the perivitelline space of zebrafish embryos, and neovascular response originating from the developing subintestinal plexus was evaluated. Injection of PBS alone or PBS supplemented with recombinant vascular endothelial growth factor A (rhVEGFA) was used, respectively, as negative and positive controls. Spikes sprouting from subintestinal plexus were counted in at least 42 embryos per condition. Graph shows the distribution of the population of embryos evaluated for each condition. Representative images are shown in (**d**). Significance was evaluated by one-way analysis of variance followed by Sidak's multiple comparisons test using GraphPad software (GraphPad, La Jolla, CA, USA). ***$P < 0.0005$. **e** Western blot analysis of GRN in U937 cells transfected for 8 hours with control small interfering RNA (si-SCR) or three different GRN-targeting siRNAs (si-GRN_#1,_#2,_#3) and subsequently cultured in the presence of CM from MDA-MB-468 cells for 72 hours. **f** and **g** Tube-formation assays involving EA.Hy926 endothelial cells performed in the presence of CM from the conditions indicated in (**e**). RPMI medium, supplemented (rhVEGFA) or not (RPMI) with recombinant VEGFA, was used as a positive or negative control, respectively. Data are presented as mean ± SEM. *$P < 0.05$, **$P < 0.005$ calculated by two-tailed *t* test

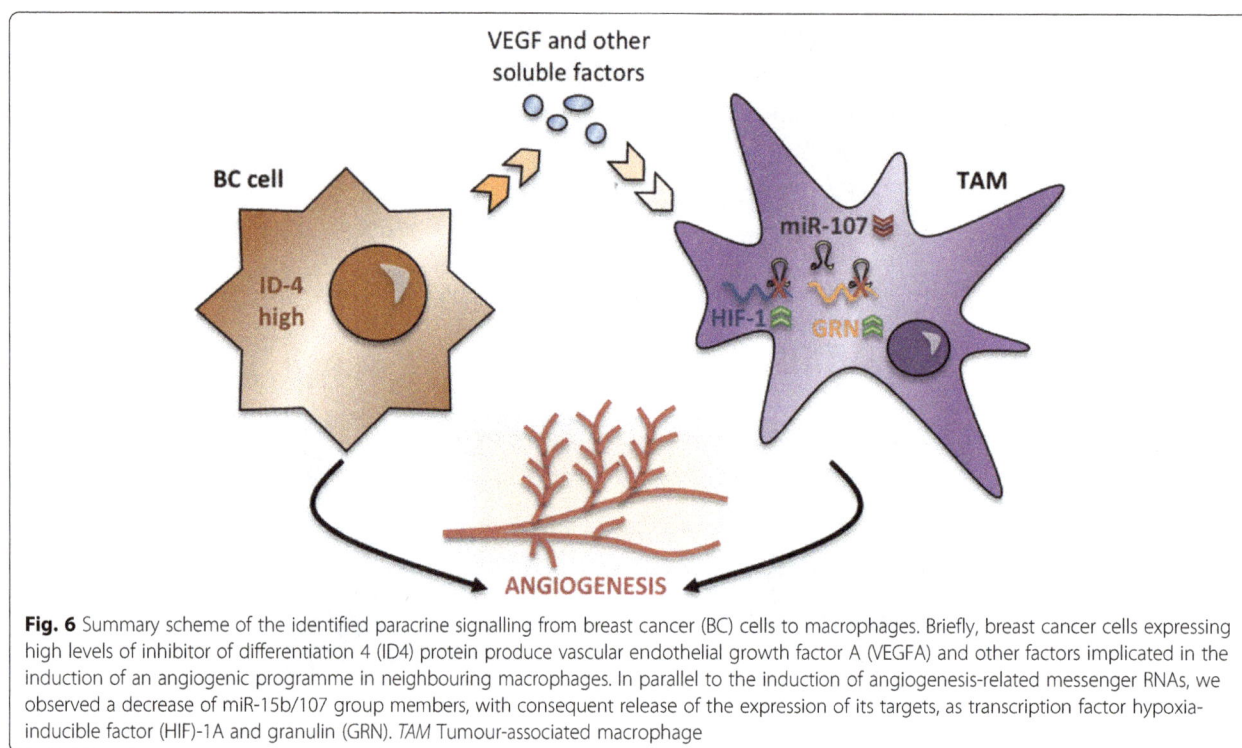

Fig. 6 Summary scheme of the identified paracrine signalling from breast cancer (BC) cells to macrophages. Briefly, breast cancer cells expressing high levels of inhibitor of differentiation 4 (ID4) protein produce vascular endothelial growth factor A (VEGFA) and other factors implicated in the induction of an angiogenic programme in neighbouring macrophages. In parallel to the induction of angiogenesis-related messenger RNAs, we observed a decrease of miR-15b/107 group members, with consequent release of the expression of its targets, as transcription factor hypoxia-inducible factor (HIF)-1A and granulin (GRN). *TAM* Tumour-associated macrophage

CM from MDA-MB-468 cells using transgenic zebrafish embryos expressing enhanced green fluorescent protein in the entire vasculature. Specifically, Matrigel plugs containing CM from each experimental condition were injected into the perivitelline space of zebrafish embryos, and neovascular response originating from the developing subintestinal plexus was evaluated. Injection of Matrigel plugs containing PBS alone or PBS supplemented with recombinant VEGFA (rhVEGFA) was used as a negative and positive control, respectively. As shown in Fig. 5c and d, we observed a greater number of embryos presenting two or more spikes sprouting from subintestinal plexus in the GRN overexpression condition compared with that in the EV condition. Accordingly, in the GRN overexpression condition, we also observed a reduced number of embryos showing one or no spikes (Fig. 5c and d). No effects on macrophage viability and differentiation were observed in the presence of GRN overexpression (Additional file 9: Figure S6).

Next, we evaluated the effect of GRN depletion on macrophage angiogenic potential. To this end, we transfected siRNAs directed to GRN or control siRNAs (si-SCR) in U937-derived macrophages, which were then cultured with CM from MDA-MB-468 cells (Fig. 5e). CM from each experimental condition was then evaluated in tube-formation assays involving the growth of endothelial cells. Conditions with RPMI medium

supplemented or not with rhVEGFA were included as positive and negative controls, respectively. As shown in Fig. 5f and g, GRN depletion led to the significant decrease of tube-formation potential.

Discussion

In this study, we demonstrated that expression of ID4 in BC cells is an important determinant of TAM behaviour. High ID4 expression in BC cells indeed is able to cause not only macrophage recruitment but also the reprogramming of macrophage gene expression (Fig. 6). Specifically, we observed that ID4 modulates a panel of angiogenesis-associated factors, among which there is an important regulator of inflammation, GRN [32, 52].

It has been reported that GRN directly binds to tumour necrosis factor (TNF) receptors and counteracts the TNF-mediated inflammatory signalling pathway. GRN also induces regulatory T-cell populations and IL-10 production and inhibits CXCL9 and CXCL10 chemokine release. It will be interesting to evaluate in further studies whether ID4-dependent GRN induction occurring in macrophages has an immunomodulatory effect in BC. Analysis of tumour tissues from a cohort of patients with BC revealed that high GRN expression correlated with the most aggressive triple-negative BLBC and reduced patient survival [50].

In addition to the angiogenesis-related factors induced in an ID4-dependent manner, we observed in macrophages a similar increase of transcription factor HIF-1. HIF-1 has previously been reported to be strongly involved in TAM pro-tumourigenic activities. Of note, the majority of the angiogenesis-related factors that we have identified present HIF-1 consensus sequences in their promoter regions and therefore could be subjected to HIF-1-dependent transactivation (Additional file 9: Table S3).

Another important aspect of this study is the identification of VEGF, whose isoform synthesis is controlled by ID4 in BC cells [30], as one of the soluble factors participating in the paracrine activation of the angiogenic programme in co-cultured macrophages. We have indeed recently identified that VEGFA isoform expression is controlled in BC cells by a ribonucleoprotein complex containing, in addition to ID4, the splicing factor SRSF1, the mutant p53 protein and the long non-coding RNA *MALAT1* [30]. This complex favours the production of VEGF121 and VEGF165 isoforms. Because the addition of blocking antibodies directed to VEGFA in CM from BC cells significantly reduced the angiogenic programme activation in macrophages, it is highly probable that this programme depends on the ribonucleoprotein complex controlling VEGFA expression in BC cells. Interestingly, we showed that blocking of VEGFA prevents CM-dependent activation of *EPHB2* and *NRP2*, among others. Of note, both these genes have been reported to participate in the enhancement of VEGFA signalling through VEGFR2 [53–55]. Activation of *EPHB2* and *NRP2* then could represent a mechanism for VEGFA signalling amplification in macrophages, because an increase of these molecules will probably lead to a more efficient response to the VEGFA present in the CM (in our experimental system) and in the in vivo tumour microenvironment.

Finally, we identified an additional layer of control of the angiogenesis-related genes in macrophages (i.e., the post-transcriptional layer). Indeed, among the identified angiogenesis-related factors, HIF-1 and GRN are interestingly controlled by miR-107, whose expression is downregulated in macrophages in an ID4-dependent manner. miR-107 and another miRNA of this family (miR-195) that we have found downregulated in an ID4-dependent manner in macrophages were previously shown to have tumour-suppressive properties in BC [56–59]. Our study elucidates a novel role for these miRNAs in the control of the angiogenic programme in TAMs.

Conclusion

Taken together, our results reveal that ID4 protein, previously shown to control the stem-like phenotype of normal and transformed mammary epithelial cells, also controls the angiogenic potential in breast cancer through the modulation of tumor-associated macrophage activity. The identified paracrine signaling may represent a promising basis for the development of therapies aimed at disrupting the cross-talk between cancer cells and tumor stroma.

Additional files

Additional file 1: Figure S3 Growth curve of MDA-MB-468 cells depleted (si-ID4) or not (si-SCR) of ID4 expression by siRNA transfection (**a**). Cells were transfected for 16 hours, and then equal numbers of cells were plated and counted at the indicated time points. Efficiency of ID4 depletion at 48 hours and 72 hours was evaluated by Western blotting (**b**). (PDF 4554 kb)

Additional file 2: Table S1 Characteristics of patients selected for the analysis of ID4 protein expression. (DOCX 17 kb)

Additional file 3: Figure S1. Comparison of ID4 mRNA expression in basal-like breast cancer (BLBC) and triple-negative breast cancer (TNBC) versus all other breast cancer subtypes (Others) in the indicated representative datasets [19, 22, 60]. (PDF 143 kb)

Additional file 4: Table S2 Predictive power of ID4, CD68 and the macrophage signature (MacSig) comprising eight widely used markers (CD14, CD105, CD11b, CD68, CD93, CD33, IL4R, CD163) for the mononuclear phagocyte system [37]. Analysis was performed using datasets deposited in the KMplot database [36]. *DMFS* Distant metastasis-free survival, *OS* Overall survival. (DOCX 21 kb)

Additional file 5: Table S3 mRNAs modulated in an ID4-dependent manner in differentiated HL60 cells cultured with conditioned medium from control (CM EV) or ID4-overexpressing (CM ID4) MDA-MB-468 cells. The presence of HIF-1 consensus sequences on promoters was evaluated using the LASAGNA-Search web tool (http://biogrid-lasagna.engr.uconn. edu/lasagna_search/). The presence of putative binding sites for miR-107, miR-15b and miR-195 on 3'-UTR or coding (CDS) sequences of mRNAs was evaluated using the miRWalk analysis tool (http://zmf.umm.uni-heidelberg.de/ apps/zmf/mirwalk2/) by selecting the following databases: (1) 3'-UTR analysis = miRWalk, miRanda, miRDB, miRNAMap, Pictar2, RNA22, RNAhybrid, TargetScan; and (2) CDS analysis = miRWalk, miRanda, RNA22, RNAhybrid, TargetScan. (DOCX 22 kb)

Additional file 6: Figure S2. Predictive power of *ID4* mRNA expression for overall survival (OS) was evaluated by Kaplan-Meier analysis on the TCGA cohort in BLBCs showing high or low CD68 (**a** and **b**) or macrophage signature (MacSig) (**c** and **d**) levels. Macrophage signature is composed of eight widely used markers for the mononuclear phagocyte system (CD14, CD105, CD11b, CD68, CD93, CD33, IL4R and CD163 [37]). **e** Evaluation of association between ID4 or CD68 and the pathological variables T, N, G and *TP53* status in the BLBCs from the TCGA cohort. (PDF 4464 kb)

Additional file 7: Figure S4 a Modulation of selected genes modulated in the TLDA was validated by RT-qPCR in differentiated HL60 cells cultured in CM from ID4-overexpressing (CM ID4-HA) or control (CM EV) MDA-MB-468 cells (left panel). The same transcripts were analysed in MDA-MB-468 cells transfected with ID4-HA expression vector (ID4-HA) or control empty vector (EV) (right panel). **b** Expression of EphB2, MDK and GRN protein evaluated by Western blotting on lysates from differentiated HL60 cells cultured as in (**a**); secreted GRN (sGRN) was evaluated on CM from differentiated HL60 cells in the same conditions. **c** HIF1A protein expression evaluated by Western blotting in differentiated U937 cells cultured in RPMI medium or in CM from SKBR3 cells stably interfered for ID4 expression (sh-ID4) or control cells (sh-CTR). (PDF 1320 kb)

Additional file 8: Figure S5 a Expression of miR-107, miR-15b and miR-195 in differentiated HL60 cells cultured with CM from control (CM EV) or ID4-overexpressing (CM ID4) MDA-MB-468 cells. **b–e** Expression of miR-15b and miR-195 in HL60 and U937 cells cultured with CM from control (si-SCR) or ID4-depleted (si-ID4) BC cells. **f** miR-107, miR-15b and miR-195 expression evaluated by RT-qPCR in differentiated U937 cells cultured with CM from MDA-MB-468 cells depleted or not of VEGFA expression. VEGFA interference efficiency is shown in Fig. 3i. **g** Expression levels of miR-15b and miR-195 in differentiated U937 cells cultivated in RPMI medium (CTR) or CM from MDA-MB-468 cells for the indicated time points. **h** and **i** HIF1A mRNA (**h**) and protein (**i**) expression evaluated, respectively, by RT-qPCR and immunofluorescence in differentiated U937 cells transfected with control mimic or miR-107 mimic and cultured in the presence of CM from MDA-MB-468 cells for 48 hours. (PDF 2150 kb)

Additional file 9: Figure S6 Differentiated U937 cells transfected with an empty vector (EV) or a granulin (GRN) expression vector and subsequently cultivated in the presence of CM from MDA-MB-468 cells were evaluated for their differentiation state (percentage of CD11b⁺ cells) (**a**) and for their viability (**b**) by, respectively, FACS analysis and ATPlite assay at the indicated time points after CM addition. **c** Overexpression of GRN evaluated by Western blotting. (PDF 141 kb)

Abbreviations
APC: Allophycocyanin; BC: Breast cancer; BLBC: Basal-like breast cancer; CM: Conditioned media; DAB: Diaminobenzidine; DMFS: Distant metastasis-free survival; EV: Empty vector; FACS: Fluorescence-activated cell sorting; GRN: Granulin; HA: Hemagglutinin; HIF: Hypoxia-inducible factor; ID: Inhibitors of differentiation; LNA: Locked nucleic acid; mAb: Monoclonal antibodies; MacSig: Macrophage signature; miRNA, miR: MicroRNA; mRNA: Messenger RNA; OS: Overall survival; RT: Room temperature; si-ID4: ID4-depleted breast cancer cells; siRNA: Small interfering RNA; si-SCR: Control breast cancer cells; TAM: Tumour-associated macrophage; TLDA: TaqMan Low Density Array; TNBC: Triple-negative breast cancer; TNF: Tumour necrosis factor; UTR: Untranslated region; VitD3: 1,25-dihydroxyvitamin D_3

Acknowledgements
The authors acknowledge Dr. Peter Nelson, who generously provided the full-length granulin expression vector.

Funding
This work was supported by the Italian Ministry of Health (GR-2011-02348567) and the Associazione Italiana per la Ricerca sul Cancro (AIRC) (MFAG10728) (to GF); the Italian Ministry of Education, University and Research (MIUR) Epigen (13/05/R/42) and the AIRC (IG14455) (to GB); and the National Science Centre under Maestro programme number 2012/06/A/NZ1/00089 (to MP, AZ and MZ).

Authors' contributions
GF designed the research study and wrote the manuscript. SD and EMi performed the majority of the experiments. AS performed bioinformatic analyses on breast cancer databases. II, SM and FF prepared primary cultures of macrophage precursors from mouse bone marrow and performed experiments in mice. EG, MM, EMe and IT evaluated and analysed IHC data from patients with breast cancer. MP, AZ and MZ evaluated angiogenic potential using tube-formation assays and an in vivo zebrafish embryo system. GF, FF and GB interpreted and discussed the research results. All authors read and approved the final manuscript.

Competing interests
The authors declare that they have no competing interests.

Author details
¹Oncogenomics and Epigenetics Unit, IRCCS Regina Elena National Cancer Institute, Via Elio Chianesi 53, 00144 Rome, Italy. ²Department of Molecular Biology, International Institute of Molecular and Cell Biology in Warsaw, Księcia Trojdena 4, 02-109 Warsaw, Poland. ³Department of Anatomical, Histological, Forensic & Orthopaedic Sciences, Section of Histology & Medical Embryology, Sapienza University of Rome, Via A. Scarpa, 16, 00161 Rome, Italy. ⁴Laboratory affiliated with Istituto Pasteur Italia-Fondazione Cenci Bolognetti, Rome, Italy. ⁵Pathology Department, IRCCS Regina Elena National Cancer Institute, Via Elio Chianesi 53, 00144 Rome, Italy. ⁶Biostatistics Unit, Scientific Direction, IRCCS Regina Elena National Cancer Institute, Via Elio Chianesi 53, 00144 Rome, Italy.

References
1. Ferlay J, Soerjomataram I, Dikshit R, Eser S, Mathers C, Rebelo M, et al. Cancer incidence and mortality worldwide: sources, methods and major patterns in GLOBOCAN 2012. Int J Cancer. 2015;136(5):E359–86.
2. Sorlie T, Perou CM, Tibshirani R, Aas T, Geisler S, Johnsen H, et al. Gene expression patterns of breast carcinomas distinguish tumor subclasses with clinical implications. Proc Natl Acad Sci U S A. 2001;98(19):10869–74.
3. McAllister SS, Weinberg RA. The tumour-induced systemic environment as a critical regulator of cancer progression and metastasis. Nat Cell Biol. 2014;16:717–27.
4. Kitamura T, Qian BZ, Pollard JW. Immune cell promotion of metastasis. Nat Rev Immunol. 2015;15:73–86.
5. Lin EY, Li JF, Gnatovskiy L, Deng Y, Zhu L, Grzesik DA, et al. Macrophages regulate the angiogenic switch in a mouse model of breast cancer. Cancer Res. 2006;66(23):11238–46.
6. Noy R, Pollard JW. Tumor-associated macrophages: from mechanisms to therapy. Immunity. 2014;41(1):49–61.
7. Franklin RA, Liao W, Sarkar A, Kim MV, Bivona MR, Liu K, et al. The cellular and molecular origin of tumor-associated macrophages. Science. 2014; 344(6186):921–5.
8. Campbell MJ, Wolf D, Mukhtar RA, Tandon V, Yau C, Au A, et al. The prognostic implications of macrophages expressing proliferating cell nuclear antigen in breast cancer depend on immune context. PLoS One. 2013;8(10):e79114.
9. Mukhtar RA, Moore AP, Tandon VJ, Nseyo O, Twomey P, Adisa CA, et al. Elevated levels of proliferating and recently migrated tumor-associated macrophages confer increased aggressiveness and worse outcomes in breast cancer. Ann Surg Oncol. 2012;19(12):3979–86.
10. Wynn TA, Chawla A, Pollard JW. Macrophage biology in development, homeostasis and disease. Nature. 2013;496:445–55.
11. Joyce JA, Pollard JW. Microenvironmental regulation of metastasis. Nat Rev Cancer. 2009;9(4):239–52.
12. Qian BZ, Pollard JW. Macrophage diversity enhances tumor progression and metastasis. Cell. 2010;141(1):39–51.
13. Pollard JW. Tumour-educated macrophages promote tumour progression and metastasis. Nat Rev Cancer. 2004;4:71–8.
14. Condeelis J, Pollard JW. Macrophages: obligate partners for tumor cell migration, invasion, and metastasis. Cell. 2006;124(2):263–6.
15. Bingle L, Brown NJ, Lewis CE. The role of tumour-associated macrophages in tumour progression: implications for new anticancer therapies. J Pathol. 2002;196:254–65.
16. Perk J, Iavarone A, Benezra R. Id family of helix-loop-helix proteins in cancer. Nat Rev Cancer. 2005;5(8):603–14.
17. Badve S, Dabbs DJ, Schnitt SJ, Baehner FL, Decker T, Eusebi V, et al. Basal-like and triple-negative breast cancers: a critical review with an emphasis on the implications for pathologists and oncologists. Mod Pathol. 2011;24(2):157–67.
18. Wen YH, Ho A, Patil S, Akram M, Catalano J, Eaton A, et al. Id4 protein is highly expressed in triple-negative breast carcinomas: possible implications for BRCA1 downregulation. Breast Cancer Res Treat. 2012;135(1):93–102.
19. Hu Z, Fan C, Oh DS, Marron JS, He X, Qaqish BF, et al. The molecular portraits of breast tumors are conserved across microarray platforms. BMC Genomics. 2006;7:96.
20. Thike AA, Tan PH, Ikeda M, Iqbal J. Increased ID4 expression, accompanied by mutant p53 accumulation and loss of BRCA1/2 proteins in triple-negative breast cancer, adversely affects survival. Histopathology. 2016;68(5):702–12.
21. Junankar S, Baker LA, Roden DL, Nair R, Elsworth B, Gallego-Ortega D, et al. ID4 controls mammary stem cells and marks breast cancers with a stem cell-like phenotype. Nat Commun. 2015;6:6548.
22. Cancer Genome Atlas Network. Comprehensive molecular portraits of human breast tumours. Nature. 2012;490(7418):61–70.

23. Baker LA, Holliday H, Swarbrick A. ID4 controls luminal lineage commitment in normal mammary epithelium and inhibits BRCA1 function in basal-like breast cancer. Endocr Relat Cancer. 2016;23(9):R381–92.

24. Beger C, Pierce LN, Kruger M, Marcusson EG, Robbins JM, Welcsh P, et al. Identification of *Id4* as a regulator of *BRCA1* expression by using a ribozyme-library-based inverse genomics approach. Proc Natl Acad Sci U S A. 2001; 98(1):130–5.

25. Roldán G, Delgado L, Musé IM. Tumoral expression of BRCA1, estrogen receptor α and ID4 protein in patients with sporadic breast cancer. Cancer Biol Ther. 2006;5(5):505–10.

26. Crippa E, Lusa L, De Cecco L, Marchesi E, Calin GA, Radice P, et al. miR-342 regulates BRCA1 expression through modulation of ID4 in breast cancer. PLoS One. 2014;9(1):e87039.

27. Prat A, Cruz C, Hoadley KA, Díez O, Perou CM, Balmaña J. Molecular features of the basal-like breast cancer subtype based on BRCA1 mutation status. Breast Cancer Res Treat. 2014;147:185–91.

28. Fontemaggi G, Dell'Orso S, Trisciuoglio D, Shay T, Melucci E, Fazi F, et al. The execution of the transcriptional axis mutant p53, E2F1 and ID4 promotes tumor neo-angiogenesis. Nat Struct Mol Biol. 2009;16(10):1086–93.

29. Dell'Orso S, Ganci F, Strano S, Blandino G, Fontemaggi G. ID4: a new player in the cancer arena. Oncotarget. 2010;1(1):48–58.

30. Pruszko M, Milano E, Forcato M, Donzelli S, Ganci F, Di Agostino S, et al. The mutant p53-ID4 complex controls VEGFA isoforms by recruiting lncRNA MALAT1. EMBO Rep. 2017;18(8):1331–51.

31. Doedens AL, Stockmann C, Rubinstein MP, Liao D, Zhang N, DeNardo DG, et al. Macrophage expression of hypoxia-inducible factor-1 α suppresses T-cell function and promotes tumor progression. Cancer Res. 2010;70(19):7465–75.

32. Jian J, Li G, Hettinghouse A, Progranulin LC. A key player in autoimmune diseases. Cytokine. 2016;101:48–55.

33. Fontemaggi G, Bellissimo T, Donzelli S, Iosue I, Benassi B, Bellotti G, et al. Identification of post-transcriptional regulatory networks during myeloblast-to-monocyte differentiation transition. RNA Biol. 2015;12(7):690–700.

34. Novelli F, Milella M, Melucci E, Di Benedetto A, Sperduti I, Perrone-Donnorso R, et al. A divergent role for estrogen receptor-β in node-positive and node-negative breast cancer classified according to molecular subtypes: an observational prospective study. Breast Cancer Res. 2008;10(5):R74.

35. Zhao X, Qu J, Sun Y, Wang J, Liu X, Wang F, et al. Prognostic significance of tumor-associated macrophages in breast cancer: a meta-analysis of the literature. Oncotarget. 2017;8(18):30576–86.

36. Gyorffy B, Lanczky A, Eklund AC, Denkert C, Budczies J, Li Q, et al. An online survival analysis tool to rapidly assess the effect of 22,277 genes on breast cancer prognosis using microarray data of 1809 patients. Breast Cancer Res Treat. 2010;123(3):725–31.

37. Murray PJ, Wynn TA. Protective and pathogenic functions of macrophage subsets. Nat Rev Immunol. 2011;11(11):723–37.

38. Montrucchio G, Lupia E, Battaglia E, Passerini G, Bussolino F, Emanuelli G, et al. Tumor necrosis factor α-induced angiogenesis depends on in situ platelet-activating factor biosynthesis. J Exp Med. 1994;180(1):377–82.

39. Anghelina M, Krishnan P, Moldovan L, Moldovan NI. Monocytes/macrophages cooperate with progenitor cells during neovascularization and tissue repair: conversion of cell columns into fibrovascular bundles. Am J Pathol. 2006;168(2):529–41.

40. Murao S, Gemmell MA, Callaham MF, Anderson NL, Huberman E. Control of macrophage cell differentiation in human promyelocytic HL-60 leukemia cells by 1,25-dihydroxyvitamin D_3 and phorbol-12-myristate-13-acetate. Cancer Res. 1983;43(10):4989–96.

41. Mangelsdorf DJ, Koeffler HP, Donaldson CA, Pike JW, Haussler MR. 1,25-Dihydroxyvitamin D_3-induced differentiation in a human promyelocytic leukemia cell line (HL-60): receptor-mediated maturation to macrophage-like cells. J Cell Biol. 1984;98(2):391–8.

42. Wang WX, Kyprianou N, Wang X, Nelson PT. Dysregulation of the mitogen granulin in human cancer through the miR-15/107 microRNA gene group. Cancer Res. 2010;70(22):9137–42.

43. Finnerty JR, Wang WX, Hébert SS, Wilfred BR, Mao G, Nelson PT. The miR-15/107 group of microRNA genes: evolutionary biology, cellular functions, and roles in human diseases. J Mol Biol. 2010;402(3):491–509.

44. Yamakuchi M, Lotterman CD, Bao C, Hruban RH, Karim B, Mendell JT, et al. P53-induced microRNA-107 inhibits HIF-1 and tumor angiogenesis. Proc Natl Acad Sci U S A. 2010;107(14):6334–9.

45. Chen L, Li ZY, Xu SY, Zhang XJ, Zhang Y, Luo K, et al. Upregulation of miR-107 inhibits glioma angiogenesis and VEGF expression. Cell Mol Neurobiol. 2016;36(1):113–20.

46. Wang R, Zhao N, Li S, Fang JH, Chen MX, Yang J, et al. MicroRNA-195 suppresses angiogenesis and metastasis of hepatocellular carcinoma by inhibiting the expression of VEGF, VAV2, and CDC42. Hepatology. 2013;58(2):642–53.

47. Wang Y, Zhang X, Zou C, Kung HF, Lin MC, Dress A, et al. miR-195 inhibits tumor growth and angiogenesis through modulating IRS1 in breast cancer. Biomed Pharmacother. 2016;80:95–101.

48. Shi Y, Zhao Y, Shao N, Ye R, Lin Y, Zhang N, et al. Overexpression of microRNA-96-5p inhibits autophagy and apoptosis and enhances the proliferation, migration and invasiveness of human breast cancer cells. Oncol Lett. 2017;13(6):4402–12.

49. Wang WX, Wilfred BR, Madathil SK, Tang G, Hu Y, Dimayuga J, et al. miR-107 regulates granulin/progranulin with implications for traumatic brain injury and neurodegenerative disease. Am J Pathol. 2010;177(1):334–45.

50. Elkabets M, Gifford AM, Scheel C, Nilsson B, Reinhardt F, Bray MA, et al. Human tumors instigate granulin-expressing hematopoietic cells that promote malignancy by activating stromal fibroblasts in mice. J Clin Invest. 2011;121(2):784–99.

51. Eguchi R, Nakano T, Wakabayashi I. Progranulin and granulin-like protein as novel VEGF-independent angiogenic factors derived from human mesothelioma cells. Oncogene. 2017;36(5):714–22.

52. Mundra JJ, Jian J, Bhagat P, Liu CJ. Progranulin inhibits expression and release of chemokines CXCL9 and CXCL10 in a TNFR1 dependent manner. Sci Rep. 2016;6:21115.

53. Sawamiphak S, Seidel S, Essmann CL, Wilkinson GA, Pitulescu ME, Acker T, et al. Ephrin-B2 regulates VEGFR2 function in developmental and tumour angiogenesis. Nature. 2010;465(7297):487–91.

54. Neufeld G, Kessler O, Herzog Y. The interaction of neuropilin-1 and neuropilin-2 with tyrosine-kinase receptors for VEGF. Adv Exp Med Biol. 2002;515:81–90.

55. Sulpice E, Plouët J, Bergé M, Allanic D, Tobelem G, Merkulova-Rainon T. Neuropilin-1 and neuropilin-2 act as coreceptors, potentiating proangiogenic activity. Blood. 2008;111:2036–45.

56. Gao B, Hao S, Tian W, Jiang Y, Zhang M, Guo L, et al. MicroRNA-107 is downregulated and having tumor suppressive effect in breast cancer by negatively regulating BDNF. J Gene Med. 2016;19(12):e2932.

57. Li XY, Luo QF, Wei CK, Li DF, Li J, Fang L. MiRNA-107 inhibits proliferation and migration by targeting CDK8 in breast cancer. Int J Clin Exp Med. 2014;7(1):32–40.

58. Polytarchou C, Iliopoulos D, Struhl K. An integrated transcriptional regulatory circuit that reinforces the breast cancer stem cell state. Proc Natl Acad Sci U S A. 2012;109(36):14470–5.

59. Thakur S, Grover RK, Gupta S, Yadav AK, Das BC. Identification of specific miRNA signature in paired sera and tissue samples of Indian women with triple negative breast cancer. PLoS One. 2016;11(7):e0158946.

60. Ven't Veer LJ, Dai H, van de Vijver MJ, He YD, Hart AA, Mao M, Peterse HL, van der Kooy K, Marton MJ, Witteveen AT: Gene expression profiling predicts clinical outcome of breast cancer. Nature. 2002, 415 (6871): 530-536. https://doi.org/10.1038/415530a.

11

A survey of microRNA single nucleotide polymorphisms identifies novel breast cancer susceptibility loci in a case-control, population-based study of African-American women

Jeannette T. Bensen[1*], Mariaelisa Graff[1], Kristin L. Young[1], Praveen Sethupathy[2], Joel Parker[3], Chad V. Pecot[4], Kevin Currin[3,5], Stephen A. Haddad[6], Edward A. Ruiz-Narváez[7], Christopher A. Haiman[8], Chi-Chen Hong[9], Lara E. Sucheston-Campbell[9], Qianqian Zhu[9], Song Liu[9], Song Yao[10], Elisa V. Bandera[11], Lynn Rosenberg[6], Kathryn L. Lunetta[12], Christine B. Ambrosone[9], Julie R. Palmer[6], Melissa A. Troester[1] and Andrew F. Olshan[1]

Abstract

Background: MicroRNAs (miRNAs) regulate gene expression and influence cancer. Primary transcripts of miRNAs (pri-miRNAs) are poorly annotated and little is known about the role of germline variation in miRNA genes and breast cancer (BC). We sought to identify germline miRNA variants associated with BC risk and tumor subtype among African-American (AA) women.

Methods: Under the African American Breast Cancer Epidemiology and Risk (AMBER) Consortium, genotyping and imputed data from four studies on BC in AA women were combined into a final dataset containing 224,188 miRNA gene single nucleotide polymorphisms (SNPs) for 8350 women: 3663 cases and 4687 controls. The primary miRNA sequence was identified for 566 miRNA genes expressed in Encyclopedia of DNA Elements (ENCODE) Tier 1 cell types and human pancreatic islets. Association analysis was conducted using logistic regression for BC status overall and by tumor subtype.

Results: A novel BC signal was localized to an 8.6-kb region of 17q25.3 by four SNPs (rs9913477, rs1428882938, rs28585511, and rs7502931) and remained statistically significant after multiple test correction (odds ratio (OR) = 1.44, 95% confidence interval (CI) = 1.26–1.65; $p = 3.15 \times 10^{-7}$; false discovery rate (FDR) = 0.03). These SNPs reside in a genomic location that includes both the predicted primary transcript of the noncoding miRNA gene *MIR3065* and the first intron of the gene for brain-specific angiogenesis inhibitor 1-associated protein 2 (*BAIAP2*). Furthermore, miRNA-associated SNPs on chromosomes 1p32.3, 5q32, and 3p25.1 were the strongest signals for hormone receptor, luminal versus basal-like, and HER2 enrichment status, respectively. A second phase of genotyping (1397 BC cases, 2418 controls) that included two SNPs in the 8.6-kb region was used for validation and meta-analysis. While neither rs4969239 nor rs9913477 was validated, when meta-analyzed with the original dataset their association with BC remained directionally consistent (OR = 1.29, 95% CI = 1.16–1.44 ($p = 4.18 \times 10^{-6}$) and OR = 1.33, 95% CI = 1.17–1.51 ($p = 1.6 \times 10^{-5}$), respectively).

(Continued on next page)

* Correspondence: jbensen@med.unc.edu
[1]Department of Epidemiology, Gillings School of Global Public Health, University of North Carolina at Chapel Hill, Chapel Hill, NC 27599, USA
Full list of author information is available at the end of the article

(Continued from previous page)

Conclusion: Germline genetic variation indicates that *MIR3065* may play an important role in BC development and heterogeneity among AA women. Further investigation to determine the potential functional effects of these SNPs is warranted. This study contributes to our understanding of BC risk in AA women and highlights the complexity in evaluating variation in gene-dense regions of the human genome.

Keywords: microRNA, miRNA, SNP, Breast cancer, African American, Case-control

Background

MicroRNAs (miRNAs) are small noncoding RNAs that were formally recognized in 2001 [1] as one of the largest classes of gene regulators in eukaryotes [2]. miRNAs undergo a complex, multistep process of biogenesis summarized by Lin and Gregory in 2015 [3]. Briefly, within the nucleus, a primary miRNA transcript (pri-miRNA)—usually several hundred nucleotides (nt) to greater than 1 megabase (Mb) in length—is cleaved to create a precursor miRNA (pre-miRNA) approximately 70 nt in length which folds to form a stem-loop intermediate. This intermediate is exported from the nucleus and further processed to a miRNA duplex, approximately 22 nt in length. One strand of the miRNA duplex is loaded onto the RNA-induced silencing complex (RISC) to form a functional mature miRNA. Cleavage and processing of the pri- and pre-miRNA require sequence and secondary structure recognition by several RNA-binding proteins and their partners. Approximately 30% of mature miRNAs are processed from introns or exons of coding genes, while the remaining miRNAs are intergenic and expressed from independent transcription units. Mature miRNAs bind to the 3' untranslated region (UTR) of target genes to silence them by either translational repression or messenger RNA (mRNA) degradation [4]. There are over 2500 identified human miRNAs [5] and each may bind to hundreds or even thousands of different target genes, coordinating expression of a large number of mRNAs; this makes them key players in gene regulatory networks [3].

miRNAs have been shown to influence numerous molecular pathways and pathological conditions, including cancer [3, 6–10], and can function as both oncogenes and tumor suppressors depending on the context. Furthermore, oncoproteins such as MYC bind to the promoters of key miRNAs, activating oncogenic miRNAs (oncomiRs) and downregulating tumor suppressor miRNAs [11–13]. In breast cancer (OMIM #114480), miRNAs have been implicated in the regulation of genes involved in pathways critically relevant to disease etiology and severity including apoptosis, cell cycle checkpoints, cell migration, invasion, and metastasis [14–17]. To a large extent, the miRNA repertoire that is present in normal and paired tumor tissue from the same organ is quite similar; however, specific miRNAs are often aberrantly elevated or suppressed in the tumor [18]. In 2011, Persson et al. performed one of the first comprehensive characterizations via next-generation

sequencing (NGS) of miRNAs in paired normal and tumor breast tissue and identified 361 new miRNAs [18]. While the functionality of some of the miRNAs identified by deep sequencing remains unknown, about two-thirds of these newly identified miRNAs were expressed in other tissues, and nearly half were associated with components of the RISC and were found in estrogen receptor-positive, invasive breast ductal carcinoma cells. Germline single nucleotide polymorphisms (SNPs) in critical regions of miRNA genes including the promoter and primary transcripts may contribute to the dysregulation in miRNA biogenesis and expression differences common in breast cancer.

Over the last decade there has been tremendous progress made in the field of miRNAs and cancer, particularly centered on miRNA expression patterns that are emerging as promising diagnostic tools and predictive markers because of their correlation with cancer progression and patient survival [3]. However, little is known about the role of germline variation in miRNAs and susceptibility to cancer.

Currently, known germline genetic variation primarily from studies of European women explains only 50% of the familial aggregation of breast cancer (BC), suggesting that numerous other susceptibility gene variants have yet to be uncovered [19]. Several molecular epidemiologic studies have assessed the association of common germline miRNA gene variation in mature and precursor miRNA sequences with disease risk, including BC [20–29]. Few epidemiologic studies have evaluated the association between a large number of germline genetic variants in the promoter and primary sequences of miRNAs and BC risk, particularly among African-American (AA) women. We sought to identify large numbers of germline miRNA gene variants associated with BC risk and subtype among women participating in a large AA BC consortium.

Methods

Study population

This research was conducted using data from the African American Breast Cancer Epidemiology and Risk (AMBER) Consortium, a collaboration of two case-control studies of BC in AA women (the Carolina Breast Cancer Study (CBCS) [30] and the Women's Circle of Health Study (WCHS) [31, 32]) and two cohort studies (the Black Women's Health Study (BWHS) [33] and the Multiethnic

Cohort (MEC) [34]). AMBER has been described previously [35]. All study participants provided written informed consent and all studies obtained Institutional Review Board approval.

This analysis utilizes data from 3663 cases and 4687 controls in AMBER who provided either blood or saliva for DNA analysis. For the case-control studies, controls were identified either through Division of Motor Vehicles lists (age < 65 years) and Health Care Financing Administration lists (age ≥ 65) (CBCS), or random digit dialing and community controls (WCHS). For BWHS and MEC, controls were chosen from among women without BC, and were frequency matched to cases on geographical region, sex, race, and 5-year age group. Eligible cases were AA women with incident invasive BC or ductal carcinoma in situ (DCIS). Estrogen receptor (ER), progesterone receptor (PR), epidermal growth factor receptor 2 (HER2) receptor, and invasive status for cases was determined using pathology data from hospital or cancer registry records.

Genotyping and quality control (QC)
Genotyping of DNA from participants in the BWHS, CBCS, and WCHS was performed by the Center for Inherited Disease Research (CIDR) using the Illumina Human Exome BeadChip v1.1. This array includes > 200,000 coding variants, as well as tag SNPs for genome-wide association study (GWAS) hits, a grid of common variants, and ancestry informative markers (AIMs). A description of the exome chip design is available from http://genome.sph.umich.edu/wiki/Exome_Chip_Design.
In addition to the standard BeadChip, the chip included approximately 159,000 SNPs of custom content focused on BC pathways (e.g., steroid hormone metabolism, insulin and insulin-like growth factors, inflammatory and immune factors, and vitamin D).

A total of 405,555 SNPs were genotyped, and 300,008 SNPs remained after excluding variants that failed technical filters imposed by CIDR, or QC filters recommended by the University of Washington. Briefly, genotypes with a GenCall score < 0.15 were classified as missing, and SNPs were removed if they were monomorphic, had poor cluster properties (ex. cluster separation < 0.2 or < 0.3 depending on allele frequency), call rates < 0.98, Hardy-Weinberg Equilibrium $p < 1 \times 10^{-4}$, > 1 Mendelian error in trios from HapMap, or > 2 discordant calls in duplicate samples. Mitochondrial and Y chromosome SNPs were also removed. Genotypes were attempted for 6936 participants from the BWHS, CBCS, and WCHS, and were completed with a call rate > 98% for 6828 participants, which included 3130 cases (963 ER negative, 1674 ER positive, 493 ER unknown) and 3698 controls. Imputation was performed by the University of Washington using the IMPUTE2

software [36] and the 1000 Genomes Phase I reference panel (5/21/2011 1000 Genomes data, December 2013 haplotype release).

Genetic data from 533 cases (135 ER negative, 309 ER positive, and 89 ER unknown) and 989 controls in the MEC were available from a previous GWAS on the Illumina Human 1 M-Duochip [37]. SNPs from MEC were imputed to the same release of 1000 Genomes and combined with the genotype data from the Illumina Human Exome BeadChip v1.1. Additional exclusion criteria applied to the four-study merged dataset were: variants with mismatching alleles or allele frequencies that were different by more than 0.15 in MEC when compared with the other three studies; variants with allele frequencies < 0.5%; and variants with imputation score INFO < 0.5 in either MEC or any of the other three studies. The final merged dataset included genotypes from 8350 women, 3663 cases (1983 ER positive, 1098 ER negative, 582 unknown), and 4687 controls.

miRNA annotation, SNP selection and QC
Among the genotyped and imputed SNPs, miRNA variants were defined as those within promoter, pri-miRNA, pre-miRNA, mature, or downstream regions of a known human miRNA. Mature and pre-miRNA sequence locations were identified from the miRNA database, miRBase release 21 [5, 38] . Pri-miRNAs were identified by integrative analysis of chromatin immunoprecipitation and massively parallel DNA sequencing (ChIP-seq) data from the Encyclopedia of DNA Elements (ENCODE) project using an algorithm described previously [39]. Five hundred and sixty six miRNA genes with pri-miRNA sequence expressed in six cell lines and tissue types (all ENCODE Tier 1 cell types plus human pancreatic islets) were the focus of this analysis. We extended the pri-miRNA 5 kilobases (kb) upstream of the 5′-end (putative promoter) and 1 kb downstream of the 3′-end (additional putative regulatory region). Variants that could be defined as having multiple miRNA locations were defined by their most unique location with the following priority: mature > precursor > primary > promoter > downstream. For example, a variant in the mature miRNA sequence is also by default in the pri-miRNA; however, according to our prioritization it would be defined as a mature miRNA sequence variant. SNPs were restricted to those variants with minor allele frequencies (MAF) ≥ 1%. Annotation defined a total of 224,188 miRNA gene SNPs, with MAF ≥ 1%, from the following miRNA gene regions: 10,435 promoter, 182,593 primary, 272 precursor, 158 mature, and 2150 downstream variants. The impact of genotype platform was evaluated by quantile-quantile plots both

with and without MEC genotypes, both yielding a lambda = 0.991.

Association analysis

Single variant analyses were conducted using logistic regression as implemented in PLINK version 1.07. Models were adjusted for age group (by ~ 10-year intervals), study site, geographic group of residence, DNA source, and ancestry by including principal components 5, 6, and 8 in the model given their association with BC at $p < 0.1$ [40]. Models were run for all cases versus all controls and for all hormone receptor subtyped (ER, PR, and HER2) cases versus controls, respectively. Additional models were run for case-only subtype analyses ($n = 3663$, eligible cases with biomarker and covariate information) using ER, PR, and HER2 receptor marker status. Specifically, the following three case-only subtype analyses were performed: 1) hormone receptor positive (ER positive or PR positive, $n = 2081$) versus hormone receptor negative (ER negative and PR negative, $n = 997$); 2) luminal (ER positive or PR positive, $n = 1613$) versus basal-like (ER negative, PR negative, and HER2 negative, $n = 405$) [41]; and 3) HER2 enriched ($n = 1356$) versus HER2 negative ($n = 344$). P values were corrected within subtype analyses for multiple comparisons using the false discovery rate (FDR) at 5% [42]. In all analyses, both invasive and in situ cases were combined.

Validation and meta-analysis

A second phase of genotyping (1397 BC cases, 2418 controls) conducted in three of the four studies within AMBER (CBCS, WCHS, and BWHS) on the Illumina's Infinium Multi-Ethnic Genotyping Array (MEGA) Chip that included study-specific content and SNPs rs4969239 and rs9913477 was used for validation and meta-analysis. Similar to the association analysis, logistic regression implemented in PLINK version 1.07 was used and models were adjusted for age group (by ~ 10-year intervals), study site, DNA source, and ancestry by including principal component 1 in the model given its association with BC at $p < 0.1$. Validation for each variant was evaluated for directional consistency and tested at the $p < 0.05$ level. In the meta-analysis, both the original and the second phase of genotyping were combined and the p value corrected for multiple comparisons using an FDR at 5% [42].

Power was calculated for detecting an odds ratio (OR) of 1.44 and an OR of 1.30 (a 10% reduction in effect estimate assuming the original OR is an overestimate of the actual effect) using a two-sided, $p = 0.05$ significance, log-additive mode of inheritance, allele frequency of 0.06 (the same as rs9913477 MAF in the study population), control to case ratio of 1.7 with 1397 cases, and prevalence of disease of 10%.

Results

Table 1 provides a distribution of key characteristics of the study population by case or control status and includes age at diagnosis, study site, DNA source, as well as clinical parameters (tumor stage and receptor status). The study population originates from a broad geographical region of the United States with most cases from the Northeast and South. Overall, the vast majority of the cases have known ER or PR receptor status; however, over half do not have known HER2 receptor status. Among cases with known receptor status for all three markers, approximately 20% are triple negative.

Genomic location of novel miRNA SNPs associated with BC in African-American women: case-control analysis

The main case-control association analysis identified seven SNPs (five imputed and two genotyped) in a 16.5-kb region on chromosome 17q25.3 (Fig. 1 and Table 2), with imputed rs9913477 (INFO $r^2 = 0.99$; MAF = 0.06; OR = 1.44, 95% confidence interval (CI) = 1.26–1.65; $p = 3.15 \times 10^{-7}$; FDR = 0.03) emerging as the top hit. Following FDR correction, four of the seven remained significantly associated with BC risk, spanning an 8.6-kb region (Table 2). All four SNPs reside in a genomic region that includes the first intron of the brain-specific angiogenesis inhibitor 1-associated protein 2 (BAIAP2), as well as the predicted primary transcript for MIR3065. Linkage disequilibrium (LD) between the top hit (rs9913477) and the other three statistically significant SNPs was high ($r^2 = 0.94$) for two (rs1428882938 and rs28585511) and perfect ($r^2 = 1.0$) for the third (rs7502931), suggesting they are all tagging the same signal in this population. Subsequently, ER/PR subtype analysis was conducted for all seven SNPs with $p < 5 \times 10^{-6}$ in the full analysis (Additional file 1: Table S1) and identified that the signal and pattern of association in this region was statistically significant based on FDR in ER+ versus controls, most likely because it had the largest sample size. While the other subtype analyses versus controls were not significant, the magnitude of the odds ratio was similar to that observed in ER+ versus controls. However, when we look at the case-only subtype analyses (e.g., ER+ versus ER−, PR+ versus PR−) we see a reduction in the magnitude of the odds ratio suggesting that this region is more likely to be associated generally with the development of breast cancer rather than a particular subtype. Additionally, in a subanalysis of ER positive cases ($n = 1983$) versus controls ($n = 4687$) and PR positive cases ($n = 1580$) versus controls ($n = 4687$) the same 17q25.3 locus top hit (rs9913477) emerged, but was statistically significantly associated with BC after FDR correction only for the largest subgroup of ER positive cases (INFO $r^2 = 0.99$, MAF = 0.58; OR = 1.53, 95% CI = 1.30–1.81; $p = 4.29 \times 10^{-7}$; FDR = 0.027). The variant rs9913477 was also the second most significant SNP in the ER positive plus PR-positive case group versus

Table 1 Characteristics of the study population

	Controls (n = 4687)		Cases (n = 3663)	
	Frequency	Mean (SD) or %	Frequency	Mean (SD) or %
Age at enrollment (years)	4687	55.62 (12.01)	3663	54.94 (11.74)
Age at enrollment (years)				
18–29	24	0.51	30	0.82
30–39	396	8.45	306	8.35
40–49	1107	23.62	945	25.8
50–59	1461	31.17	1087	29.68
60–69	986	21.04	819	22.36
70–79	609	12.99	433	11.82
80+	104	2.22	43	1.17
DNA source				
Blood	1817	38.77	1961	53.54
Mouthwash	2243	47.86	853	23.29
Saliva	627	13.38	849	23.18
Study				
BWHS	2249	48.98	901	24.6
WCHS	834	17.79	821	22.41
CBCS	615	13.12	1408	38.44
MEC	989	21.1	533	14.55
Location				
New Jersey (NJ)	573	12.23	613	16.73
Northeast (except NJ)	1245	26.56	441	12.04
South	1476	31.49	1720	46.96
Midwest	238	5.08	200	5.46
West	1155	24.64	689	18.81
Stage				
In situ	NA		376	10.26
Invasive	NA		2528	69.01
Unknown	NA		759	20.72
Tumor receptor status				
ER				
Positive	NA		1983	54.14
Negative	NA		1098	29.98
Unknown	NA		582	15.89
PR				
Positive	NA		1580	43.13
Negative	NA		1343	36.66
Unknown	NA		740	20.2
HER2				
Positive	NA		344	9.39
Negative	NA		1356	37.02
Unknown	NA		1963	53.59
Triple negative				
Yes	NA		405	11.06

Table 1 Characteristics of the study population (Continued)

	Controls (n = 4687)		Cases (n = 3663)	
	Frequency	Mean (SD) or %	Frequency	Mean (SD) or %
No	NA		1613	44.03
Unknown	NA		1645	44.91

BWHS, Black Women's Health Study; CBCS, Carolina Breast Cancer Study; ER, estrogen receptor; HER2, human epidermal growth factor receptor 2; MEC, Multiethnic Cohort; NA, not applicable; PR, progesterone receptor; SD, standard deviation; WCHS, Women's Circle of Health Study

control analysis but did not reach statistical significance after FDR correction (data not shown). In the ER negative, PR-negative, and ER negative plus PR-negative cases versus control analysis, rs80339298 located in the primary sequence of *MIR761* on chromosome 1 emerged as the top SNP but did not reach statistical significance after FDR correction (data not shown).

Case-only subtype analysis

Top SNPs identified in each of the three subtype analyses are provided in Table 3. These top SNPs were located on chromosomes 1p32.3 (rs80339298, *OSBPL9* intron 11, NT_032977.10), 5q32 (rs147821319, *PPARGC1B* intron 7, NM_001172698), and 3p25.1 (rs116367195, intergenic between *BTD* and *ANKRD2*, NM_001195099) from the GRCh38.p2 assembly for hormone receptor, luminal versus basal-like, and HER2 enrichment status, respectively. All three SNPs were low frequency (MAF < 5%) and none were statistically significant after FDR correction.

Validation and meta-analysis

A stage 2 analysis of rs4969239 (OR = 1.07, 95% CI = 0.83–1.39; p = 5.78×10^{-1} and rs9913477 (OR = 0.86, 95% CI = 0.62–1.18; p = 3.56×10^{-1}) failed to validate their association with BC at a nominal p value. However, when meta-analyzed with the original dataset, the association of rs4969239 (OR = 1.29, 95% CI = 1.16–1.44); p = 4.18×10^{-6}) and rs9913477 (OR = 1.33, 95% CI = 1.17–

1.51; p = 1.60×10^{-5}) with BC remained directionally consistent (Table 4).

Power calculations for the detection of a SNP associated with BC at ORs of 1.44 and 1.30 at a significance of $p \leq 0.05$ indicated that validation among the study set undergoing the second phase of genotyping was 97% and 77%, respectively.

Discussion

In a combined analysis of four large studies of BC in AA women, we identified and annotated a novel genomic region on chromosome 17q25.3 significantly associated with BC and extended its functional interpretation with a comprehensive evaluation of miRNA gene sequence. Specifically, we have localized the BC association signal to an 8.6-kb region on chromosome 17 marked by four tightly linked, significantly associated SNPs, with rs9913477 demonstrating the strongest association. Using a second phase of genotyping we were unable to validate the association of either rs4969239 or rs9913477 with BC; however, in a meta-analysis these SNPs remained directionally consistent (OR = 1.29 and 1.33, respectively). Power calculations indicate that the validation analysis was well powered (97%) at an OR of 1.44 (our original finding and likely an overestimate of effect size) and slightly underpowered (77%) at an OR of 1.3, which represents an effect estimate 10% less that the original OR. No statistically significant miRNA SNP associations were identified in the

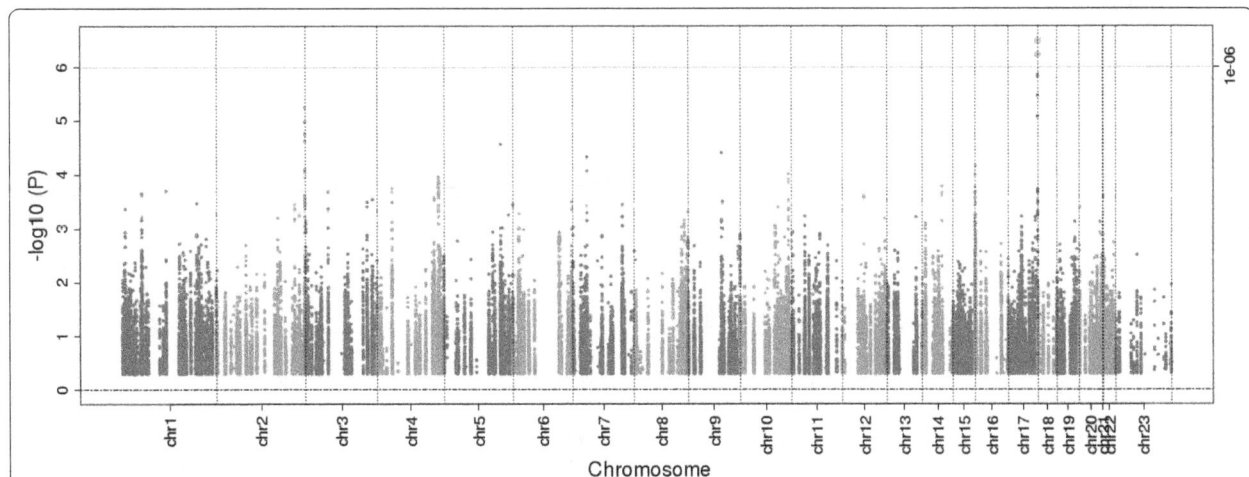

Fig. 1 Manhattan plot of miRNA SNP and breast cancer risk in the four-site AMBER Consortium (n = 8350, with 3663 cases and 4687 controls). The green line represents a significant p value threshold of 1×10^{-6} at a false discovery rate (FDR) of 5%

Table 2 Association of the top seven miRNA SNPs with $p < 5 \times 10^{-6}$ and breast cancer risk

SNP	Chromosome:position[a]	Effect/other allele	EAF	OR (95% CI)	p[b]	FDR p[c]	INFO (r^2)
rs142882938	17:79010031	C/CT	0.06	1.45 (1.24–1.70)	5.9×10^{-7}	**0.03**	0.97
rs4969239[d]	17:79010544	G/A	0.08	1.35 (1.20–1.52)	1.4×10^{-6}	0.06	–
rs28585511	17:79010609	T/A	0.06	1.45 (1.26–1.66)	5.8×10^{-7}	**0.03**	0.98
rs4969351	17:79011141	A/G	0.08	1.35 (1.20–1.52)	3.4×10^{-6}	0.11	0.99
rs9913477	17:79015698	G/A	0.06	1.44 (1.26–1.65)	3.2×10^{-7}	**0.03**	0.99
rs7502931	17:79018677	G/A	0.06	1.44 (1.26–1.65)	3.4×10^{-7}	**0.03**	0.99
rs4969366[d]	17:79026572	G/A	0.05	1.45 (1.24–1.70)	1.5×10^{-6}	0.06	–

The seven single nucleotide polymorphisms (SNPs) are intronic to BAIAP2 and located in the primary transcript of miR-3065
Significant FDR results are shown in bold
CI, confidence interval; EAF, effect allele frequency; FDR, false discovery rate; INFO, imputation quality score; OR, odds ratio
[a]Human Genome GRCh37/hg19 assembly, NT_010783.15
[b]Additive genetic models were adjusted for age group (by ~ 10-year intervals), study site, geographic region of residence, DNA source, and ancestry (PCs 5, 6, and 8 associated with cancer trait, $p < 0.1$). Sample size: 3663 cases and 4687 controls
[c]Adjustment for multiple comparisons using the FDR
[d]Genotyped SNPs, with the other SNPs having been imputed to 1000 Genome Project data

subanalyses of hormone receptor-negative tumors. Additionally, a case-only analysis that encompassed comparisons of hormone receptor status, luminal versus basal-like subtypes, and HER2 enrichment status did not identify any statistically significant associations with BC after FDR correction. The most strongly associated miRNA-associated SNPs for each subtype analysis identified regions on chromosomes 1p32.3, 5q32, and 3p25.1, respectively. None of these regions or SNPs have been previously implicated in BC GWAS according to the GWAS Catalog (release dated 12 June 2016) [43].

Given their genomic location within the intron of BAIAP2 and pri-MIR3065 sequence, these four SNPs have the potential to impact BAIAP2 expression, BAIAP2 gene intron 1 binding proteins, and/or MIR3065 biogenesis. Mature MIR3065 resides in a gene adjacent to BAIAP2 known as apoptosis-associated tyrosine kinase (AATK) where it is located in the seventh intron and is transcribed in the opposite direction from its host gene. In this gene (AATK)

and miRNA-rich region, mature MIR3065 and mature MIR338 share the same genomic location but are transcribed from opposite DNA strands (Fig. 2) [44]. This critical miRNA sequence region is highly conserved across species [44].

To better understand the implications of inherited susceptibility to BC that may involve BAIAP2, we examined expression of this gene in human tissues using data from the Genotype-Tissue Expression (GTEx) project portal version 6 [45]. Human brain-specific angiogenesis inhibitor 1-associated protein 2 (BAIAP2) demonstrates a range of expression across various human tissues including brain and breast [45] (Additional file 2: Figure S1). Using data from the Human Protein Atlas project that includes immunochemistry results on 83 different normal cell types from 44 tissue types, we note that moderate BAIAP2 protein expression is observed in human breast tissue when compared with other normal tissue types [46, 47]. Furthermore, when examining RNA

Table 3 Top SNP hits for breast cancer subtype analyses

Breast Cancer Subtype	Hormone Receptor +/−	Luminal / Basal-like	HER2 +/−
Sample size	2081/997	1613/405	1356/344
SNP ID	rs80339298	rs147821319	rs116367195
Chromosome:Position*	1:52244019	5:149217038	3:15693446
Effect/Other	A/G	A/G	G/A
Reference Sequence	NT_032977.10	NM_001172698	NM_001195099
OR (95%CI)	2.11 (1.54, 2.89)	2.20 (1.52, 3.19)	2.70 (1.72, 4.24)
EAF	0.02	0.04	0.97
p-value**	2.90×10^{-6}	2.34×10^{-5}	1.59×10^{-5}
FDR p-value***	0.16	0.37	0.84

Abbreviations: OR: odds ratio; 95% CI of the OR; EAF: effect allele frequency; FDR: false discovery rate
* Chromosome: position from GRCh37/hg19 Assembly
** Additive genetic model was adjusted for age group (by ~ 10 year intervals), study site, geographic region of residence, DNA source, and ancestry (PCs 5, 6 and 8 - associated with cancer trait, p-value< 0.1)
***Adjustment for multiple comparisons using the False Discovery Rate (FDR) within each subtype analysis

Table 4 Stages 1 and 2 and meta-analysis of rs9913477 and rs4969239 located in the primary transcript of miR-3065

SNP	Chromosome:Position[a]	Effect/other allele	Stage[b]	Sample size	EAF	OR (95% CI)	p
rs4969239	17:79010544	G/A	Stage 1	8350	0.08	1.35 (1.2–1.52)	1.40×10^{-6}
			Stage 2	3814	0.08	1.07 (0.83–1.39)	5.78×10^{-1}
			Meta-analysis	12,164	0.08	1.29 (1.16–1.44)	4.18×10^{-6}
rs9913477	17:79015698	G/A	Stage 1	8350	0.06	1.44 (1.30–1.58)	3.15×10^{-7}
			Stage 2	3815	0.06	0.86 (0.62–1.18)	3.56×10^{-1}
			Meta-analysis	12,165	0.06	1.33 (1.17–1.51)	1.60×10^{-5}

CI, confidence interval; EAF, effect allele frequency; OR, odds ratio; SNP, single nucleotide polymorphism

[a]Human Genome GRCh37/hg19 assembly, NT_010783.15

[b]Stage 1 model: Additive genetic models were adjusted for age group (by ~ 10-year intervals), WCHS study site, geographic region of residence, DNA source, and ancestry (PCs 5, 6 and 8 associated with cancer trait, $p < 0.1$); Stage 2 model: Additive genetic models were adjusted for age group (by ~ 10-year intervals), DNA source, and ancestry (PCs 1); Meta-analysis was performed in METAL [67]; heterogeneity $I^2 = 88.1$ for rs9913477 and 58.1 for rs4969239

sequencing gene expression of *BAIAP2* in 47 invasive breast carcinoma cell lines from the Cancer Cell Line Encyclopedia [48], we note differential expression with the highest levels (10-fold or more) of *BAIAP2* occurring in four cell lines: EFM-192A, HCC1937, HCC202, and ZR-75-30. Of these four cell lines, two are derived from metastatic sites, with one of these from an African-American woman, the other Caucasian. Of the remaining two cell lines (HCC1937, HCC202), both are from Caucasian women, from primary ductal carcinoma, are ER and PR negative, p53 mutation negative, and positive for EFP2 and CK19 expression; however, they differed in BRCA1 mutation and HER2 status.

The 17q25.3 region containing the top four BC-associated SNPs is extensively marked in the human mammary epithelial cell (HMEC) line by regulatory chromatin states from DNase and histones H3K27ac and H3K4me1, reflecting a number of active promoter and enhancer sequences in the region [44, 49–54].

Furthermore, a number of regulatory sequence motifs (e.g. , sequence-specific binding sites for transcription factors) located within intron 1 of *BAIAP2* are altered by these SNPs. Specifically rs9913477 alters regulatory motifs for CDP1 and SOX3 binding while rs7502931 alters a regulatory motif for *ZNF143* [55]. No expression quantitative trait loci (eQTL) were identified in GTEx for any of the four top SNPs [45].

Several epidemiological studies, including both admixture mapping and association analysis of the insulin-related pathway, have examined the 17q region for association with BC in AMBER. A recently published genome-wide case-only admixture scan using 2624 AIMs in the AMBER consortium identified a novel region of excess African ancestry associated with BC risk at 17q25.1 (confirmed in a case-control admixture analysis in the same consortium) [56]. In this admixture scan, AIM rs496948172 provided the largest Z score and marked a wide 17q25.1 region of approximately 4.6 Mb where Z scores remained above 3.7

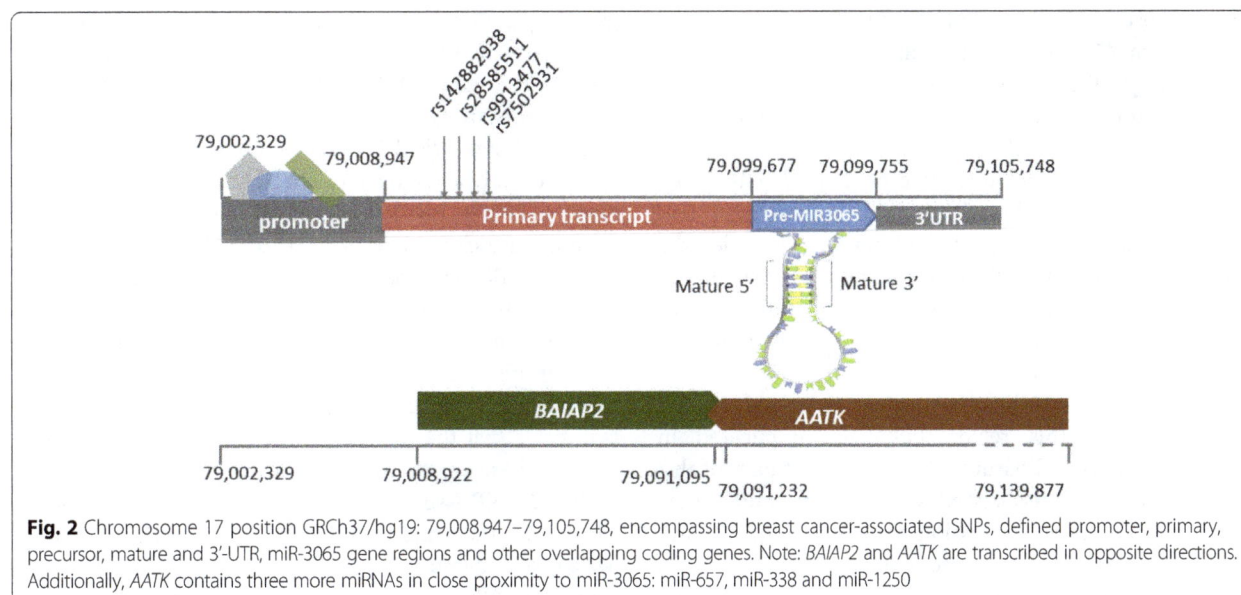

Fig. 2 Chromosome 17 position GRCh37/hg19: 79,008,947–79,105,748, encompassing breast cancer-associated SNPs, defined promoter, primary, precursor, mature and 3'-UTR, miR-3065 gene regions and other overlapping coding genes. Note: *BAIAP2* and *AATK* are transcribed in opposite directions. Additionally, *AATK* contains three more miRNAs in close proximity to miR-3065: miR-657, miR-338 and miR-1250

indicating excess African ancestry associated with BC. Elevated Z scores of 2.4 for this case analysis extend into the 17q25.3 region, where the top hit for the current association analysis (rs9913477) is approximately 1 Mb from the top admixture hit (rs4969481), although LD between these variants is limited (D' = 0.19, r^2 = 0.0009) based on AFR 1000 Genomes reference panel [57]. Thus, the region of excess African ancestry associated with BC marked by an AIM at 17q25.1 could include the more distal 17q25.3 region as well, providing evidence that variation in this genomic region associated with BC may contribute to disparity in risk. A second AMBER gene-based analysis of 184 genes in the insulin/insulin-like growth factor, leptin, and growth hormone pathways identified BAIP2 and CALM2, and AIAP2 and CSNK2A1 as the most significant gene associations (gene-based $p \leq 0.01$) with both overall and ER positive BC, respectively [58]. Thus, both admixture and insulin pathway-specific association analyses in AMBER provide suggestive evidence of an association with overall and ER-positive BC in the 17q21–25 region. However, due to the relatively less dense SNP set used to evaluate this genomic region in the admixture scan and the less granular nature of the gene-based insulin pathway analysis, neither identified the specific set of four miRNA-associated SNPs localizing a statistically significant association with BC reported here. Additionally, each study strategy for multiple test correction varied in accordance with its statistical methods, with the admixture analysis using a more conservative Bonferroni correction, the gene-based method utilizing a gene-level correction factor, and our current study using a false discovery rate.

A recently published epidemiological study examining miRNA genes and BC among women of African ancestry found fourteen miRNA SNPs associated with overall BC risk at the significance level of 0.05 [29]. Included among these SNPs was rs73410309 within the precursor sequence of MIR4739 located on chromosome 17q25.3 (OR = 1.1; p = 0.039), which is approximately 1.5 Mb from our top hit in MIR3065 (rs9913477) and not in high LD with this SNP (D' = 0.007 and R^2 = 0.0) based on AFR 1000 Genomes reference panel [57]. This study was restricted to SNPs within miRNA precursor and mature sequences and thus would not have included the SNP in the primary miRNA sequence identified in our study, but highlights the potential role for miRNA SNPs in BC risk among women of African ancestry in this genomic region.

While no GWAS hits have been reported in the 17q25.3 region, this region has been implicated in several studies of BC tissues where recurrent gain of this genomic region is associated with subtype and recurrence [59, 60]. Gene expression studies of 17q25.3 have identified significant overexpression of 17q25.3 genes in BRCA1 mutated triple-negative breast cancer (TNBC)

as compared with BRCA1 nonmutated TNBC [59], highlighting the important role that overexpressed sets of genes in this region may play in BC. Given the major role that miRNAs play in global gene regulation it is possible that, even in the absence of a copy number gain, abnormal expression of miRNA genes intended to suppress expression across multiple oncogenes could lead to similar upregulation of sets of genes in this region with similar BC effect. Studies of higher-order chromatin organization have identified regional epigenetic regulation (RER) in breast tumors and BC cell lines that are independent of copy number [61], where 26 regions of coordinate expression were identified between breast tumors and BC cell lines with nine RER showing upregulated gene expression relative to normal breast tissue. Included among these upregulated regions was a 0.9-Mb 17q25.1 region with correlated expression of KCTD2, GGA3, MRPS7, and GRB2, and a 0.58-Mb 17q25.3 region (approximately 900 kb from the four associated SNPs reported here) with correlated expression of STRA13, RFNG, CSNK1D, and SECTM1.

Perhaps the most compelling support implicating MIR3065 and BC comes from a recent study by Perrson et al. in which NGS expression analysis in paired normal and breast tumor tissue demonstrates a strikingly disparate expression pattern for MIR3065 [18]. Among the 361 newly NGS identified miRNA precursors, tumor identity was defined by differences in expression level of a large and common set of miRNAs rather than tissue specific expression [18]. While tissue MIR3065 expression was highest in breast tumors in a panel of nine human tissues, both lung and placenta demonstrated the next highest expression levels. Similar to previous studies, through BAC array comparative genomic hybridization (CGH), MIR3065 was also identified as a gene encoded in a region with high-level genomic amplification in luminal B, ERBB2/HER2-positive, ER positive, and ER negative subtypes. Among TargetScan's (release 6.2, June 2012) MIR3065 gene top 15 predicted gene targets are the top hit AT-rich interaction domain 4B, ARID4B (alias BRCAA1, breast cancer antigen epitope-1) and RAB22A, a member of the RAS oncogene family of small GTPases involved in signal transduction [62–65]. Immunohistochemically, ARID4B/BRCAA1 was expressed in 65% of BC specimens but not in noncancerous tissues. and expression was closely associated with ER- and PR-positive status [66]. BC patients also had significantly higher titers of this epitope than healthy donors ($p < 0.001$). Given that two of the top predicted targets are likely oncogenes, it is possible that the role of MIR3065 is to suppress expression of these oncogenes. It is also possible that the primary MIR3065 SNP associated with BC (or a SNP in LD) impairs MIR3065 processing, leading to lower levels of mature MIR3065 and reduced inhibition of these oncogenes. Of course, specific gene targets of this new miRNA are not yet fully known and new information may emerge as target prediction algorithms improve and functional data become available. For example, in addition to supporting the potential role of *MIR3065* in BC, Perrson et al. also uncovered a new miRNA in a very well-studied region within the intron of *ERBB2/HER2*, a major predictive marker in BC [18]. This discovery highlights the importance of evaluating genomic regulation beyond the protein coding gene level to examine the major role that noncoding genes, such as miRNAs, may play in cancer development and heterogeneity. These insights will prove invaluable in our understanding of disease development, identifying at-risk populations and providing targets for cancer treatment.

Although this study was limited in scope to miRNAs with SNPs represented or imputed from the Illumina Human Exome BeadChip v1.1 and AMBER custom content (and thus only surveys one-third of all SNPS in the miRBase), as well as by miRNAs with predicted primary sequence from six cell lines, this study is one of the largest evaluations of miRNAs for association with BC. Moreover, it is the largest investigation among African-American women with BC annotated for subtype. Furthermore, predicted boundaries of primary transcripts at both 5′ and 3′ ends were extended from the start of the H3K4me3 peak at the 5′ end (which is often upstream from the actual transcription start site (TSS)) and through the end of the H3K79me2 or H3K36me3 signal (which may or may not be downstream of the transcription termination site). Thus, SNPs defined as retained within the primary transcript may reside just upstream in the miRNA promoter region or may reside just downstream beyond the 3′ end of the primary transcript, thus potentially altering our interpretation of function. Specifically, we predicted that the BC-associated SNPs identified may affect miRNA processing; however, if in fact they reside in the promoter regions, they may influence miRNA expression through other mechanisms. More experimental validation of discrete TSS and end sites is needed for the majority of known miRNAs. Additionally, while this is one of the largest populations of African-Americans with BC examined for miRNA gene association, the subtype analyses remain underpowered for the genetic effect sizes anticipated.

Despite these limitations, this study provides valuable new information about the relationship between numerous miRNA genes and BC in an understudied population, African-American women. It emphasizes the complexity of SNP association analyses and interpretation of function in gene-dense regions, and also the complex interplay of evidence from studies of coding genes, copy number variation, epigenetic regulation, and admixture mapping in an important chromosomal region associated with BC. Functional assessment of the BC-associated SNPs in *BAIAP2* and *MIR3065* are needed to identify the potential molecular mechanism behind their association with BC

risk, in particular the risk of ER positive BC, the most common subtype. Larger studies of African-American women are needed to address subtype-specific biology and genetics, including those related to miRNAs.

Conclusions

This study reports a novel BC signal within an 8.6-kb locus on chromosome 17q25.3, where germline genetic variation is associated with overall and ER positive BC risk among African-American women. This complex and gene-dense region contains *BAIAP2*, a protein-coding gene, and *MIR3065*, an important nonprotein coding regulatory gene, which may play key roles in BC development and heterogeneity among AA women. An understanding of the potentially functional implications of variation in these genes is necessary and may uncover important genetic risk factors and mechanisms for BC in general and, more specifically, for ER positive BC, the most common subtype. Understanding risk factors and mechanisms for BC may lead to improved screening, risk stratification, and novel treatments.

Abbreviations
AA: African-American; AIM: Ancestry informative marker; AMBER: African American Breast Cancer Epidemiology and Risk; BC: Breast cancer; BWHS: Black Women's Health Study; CBCS: Carolina Breast Cancer Study; CGH: Comparative genomic hybridization; ChIP-seq: Chromatin immunoprecipitation and massively parallel DNA sequencing; CI: Confidence interval; CIDR: Center for Inherited Disease Research; DCIS: Ductal carcinoma in situ; ENCODE: Encyclopedia of DNA Elements; eQTL: Expression quantitative trait loci; ER: Estrogen receptor; FDR: False discovery rate; GTEx: Genotype-Tissue Expression; GWAS: Genome-wide association study; HER2: Human epidermal growth factor receptor 2; HMEC: Human mammary epithelial cell; kb: Kilobase; LD: Linkage disequilibrium; MAF: Minor allele frequencies; Mb: Megabase; MEC: Multiethnic Cohort; MEGA: Multi-Ethnic Genotyping Array; miRNA: MicroRNA; mRNA: Messenger RNA; NGS: Next-generation sequencing; nt: Nucleotide; oncomiR: Oncogenic miRNA; OR: Odds ratio; PR: Progesterone receptor; pre-miRNA: Precursor microRNA; pri-miRNA: Primary microRNA transcript; QC: Quality control; RER: Regional epigenetic regulation; RISC: RNA-induced silencing complex; SNPs: Single nucleotide polymorphisms; TNBC: Triple-negative breast cancer; TSS: Transcription start site; UTR: untranslated region; WCHS: Women's Circle of Health Study

Acknowledgements
We thank the participants and staff of the contributing studies. We wish also to acknowledge the late Robert Millikan, DVM, MPH, PhD, who was instrumental in the creation of this consortium. Pathology data were obtained from numerous state cancer registries (Arizona, California, Colorado, Connecticut, Delaware, District of Columbia, Florida, Georgia, Hawaii, Illinois, Indiana, Kentucky, Louisiana, Maryland, Massachusetts, Michigan, New Jersey, New York, North Carolina, Oklahoma, Pennsylvania, South Carolina, Tennessee, Texas, and Virginia). The results reported do not necessarily represent their views or the views of the National Institutes of Health.

Funding
This research was funded by the National Institutes of Health: P01 CA151135 (CBA, JRP, and AFO), R01 CA058420 (LR), UM1 CA164974 (JRP and LR), R01

CA098663 (JRP), R01 CA100598 (CBA), UM1 CA164973 (CAH), R01 CA54281 (CAH), P50 CA58223 (MAT and AO), U01 CA179715 (MAT and AO),

KL2TR001109 (KLY), R01CA185623 (EVB and CCH), R25 5R25GM089569 (KC), the Komen for the Cure Foundation, the Breast Cancer Research Foundation (CBA), and the University Cancer Research Fund of North Carolina (JTB, AFO, and MAT).

Authors' contributions

JTB played a central role in the study design and data interpretation and made a major contribution to the manuscript as the primary author. MG made a major contribution to the analysis and interpretation of genetic association data and provided supportive details from public genetic and expression databases. KLY analyzed and interpreted genetic association data. PS provided miRNA promoter annotation using six cell lines and tissue types (all ENCODE Tier 1 cell types plus human pancreatic islets) and integrative analysis of ChIP-seq data from the NIH ENCODE project and algorithm described previously. Provided input on functional interpretation of miRNA SNPs associated with breast cancer. JP provided extensive bioinformatics support for gene annotation and SNP identification and selection. CVP provided clinical input and functional interpretation of miRNA SNPs associated with breast cancer. KC provided miRNA promoter annotation using six cell lines and tissue types (all ENCODE Tier 1 cell types plus human pancreatic islets) and integrative analysis of ChIP-seq data from the NIH ENCODE project and algorithm described previously. CAH facilitated access to MEC biospecimens and data and provided input regarding genetic data interpretation in AMBER. SAH, ERA-N, C-CH, LES-C, QZ, SL, SY, EVB, and LR provided input regarding genetic data interpretation in AMBER. KLL made a major contribution to the evaluation, quality control, coordination and management, and interpretation of the genetic data for AMBER and linkage with other study-specific clinical and demographic variables. CBA facilitated access to WCHS biospecimens and data and provided input regarding genetic data interpretation in AMBER. JRP facilitated access to BWHS biospecimens and data and provided input regarding genetic data interpretation in AMBER. MAT and AFO facilitated access to CBCS biospecimens and data and provided input regarding genetic data interpretation in AMBER. All authors read and approved the final manuscript.

Competing interests

The authors declare that they have no competing interests.

Author details

[1]Department of Epidemiology, Gillings School of Global Public Health, University of North Carolina at Chapel Hill, Chapel Hill, NC 27599, USA. [2]Department of Biomedical Sciences, College of Veterinary Medicine, Cornell University, Ithaca, NY 14853, USA. [3]Department of Genetics, University of North Carolina at Chapel Hill, Chapel Hill, NC 27599, USA. [4]Department of Medicine, Division of Oncology, School of Medicine, University of North Carolina at Chapel Hill, Chapel Hill, NC 27599, USA. [5]Biological and Biomedical Sciences Program, University of North Carolina at Chapel Hill, Chapel Hill, NC 27599, USA. [6]Slone Epidemiology Center at Boston University, Boston, MA 02215, USA. [7]Department of Nutritional Sciences, University of Michigan School of Public Health, Ann Arbor, MI 48109, USA. [8]Department of Preventive Medicine, Keck School of Medicine, University of Southern California/Norris Comprehensive Cancer Center, Los Angeles, CA 90033, USA. [9]Department of Cancer Prevention and Control, Roswell Park Cancer Institute, Buffalo, NY 14263, USA. [10]Department of Biostatistics and Bioinformatics, Roswell Park Cancer Institute, Buffalo, NY 14263, USA. [11]Cancer Prevention and Control, Rutgers Cancer Institute of New Jersey, New Brunswick, NJ 08903, USA. [12]Department of Biostatistics, Boston University School of Public Health, Boston, MA 02118, USA.

References

1. Lee RC, Ambros V. An extensive class of small RNAs in Caenorhabditis elegans. Science. 2001;294(5543):862–4.
2. Bentwich I, Avniel A, Karov Y, Aharonov R, Gilad S, Barad O, Barzilai A, Einat P, Einav U, Meiri E, et al. Identification of hundreds of conserved and nonconserved human microRNAs. Nat Genet. 2005;37(7):766–70.
3. Lin S, Gregory RI. MicroRNA biogenesis pathways in cancer. Nat Rev Cancer. 2015;15(6):321–33.
4. Hausser J, Zavolan M. Identification and consequences of miRNA-target interactions—beyond repression of gene expression. Nat Rev Genet. 2014; 15(9):599–612.
5. Griffiths-Jones S. The microRNA Registry. Nucleic Acids Res. 2004; 32(Database issue):D109–11.
6. Sethupathy P, Borel C, Gagnebin M, Grant GR, Deutsch S, Elton TS, Hatzigeorgiou AG, Antonarakis SE. Human microRNA-155 on chromosome 21 differentially interacts with its polymorphic target in the AGTR1 3′ untranslated region: a mechanism for functional single-nucleotide polymorphisms related to phenotypes. Am J Hum Genet. 2007;81(2):405–13.
7. Mishra PJ, Humeniuk R, Longo-Sorbello GS, Banerjee D, Bertino JR. A miR-24 microRNA binding-site polymorphism in dihydrofolate reductase gene leads to methotrexate resistance. Proc Natl Acad Sci U S A. 2007;104(33): 13513–8.
8. Landi D, Gemignani F, Naccarati A, Pardini B, Vodicka P, Vodickova L, Novotny J, Försti A, Hemminki K, Canzian F, et al. Polymorphisms within micro-RNA-binding sites and risk of sporadic colorectal cancer. Carcinogenesis. 2008;29(3):579–84.
9. Brendle A, Lei H, Brandt A, Johansson R, Enquist K, Henriksson R, Hemminki K, Lenner P, Försti A. Polymorphisms in predicted microRNA-binding sites in integrin genes and breast cancer: ITGB4 as prognostic marker. Carcinogenesis. 2008;29(7):1394–9.
10. Larrea E, Sole C, Manterola L, Goicoechea I, Armesto M, Arestin M, Caffarel MM, Araujo AM, Araiz M, Fernandez-Mercado M, et al. New concepts in cancer biomarkers: circulating miRNAs in liquid biopsies. Int J Mol Sci. 2016;17(5)627. doi:https://doi.org/10.3390/ijms17050627.
11. O'Donnell KA, Wentzel EA, Zeller KI, Dang CV, Mendell JT. c-Myc-regulated microRNAs modulate E2F1 expression. Nature. 2005;435(7043):839–43.
12. Dews M, Homayouni A, Yu D, Murphy D, Sevignani C, Wentzel E, Furth EE, Lee WM, Enders GH, Mendell JT, et al. Augmentation of tumor angiogenesis by a Myc-activated microRNA cluster. Nat Genet. 2006;38(9):1060–5.
13. Chang TC, Yu D, Lee YS, Wentzel EA, Arking DE, West KM, Dang CV, Thomas-Tikhonenko A, Mendell JT. Widespread microRNA repression by Myc contributes to tumorigenesis. Nat Genet. 2008;40(1):43–50.
14. Heneghan HM, Miller N, Lowery AJ, Sweeney KJ, Kerin MJ. MicroRNAs as novel biomarkers for breast cancer. J Oncol. 2009;2009:950201.
15. O'Day E, Lal A. MicroRNAs and their target gene networks in breast cancer. Breast Cancer Res. 2010;12(2):201.
16. Yu Z, Baserga R, Chen L, Wang C, Lisanti MP, Pestell RG. microRNA, cell cycle, and human breast cancer. Am J Pathol. 2010;176(3):1058–64.
17. Tang J, Ahmad A, Sarkar FH. The role of microRNAs in breast cancer migration, invasion and metastasis. Int J Mol Sci. 2012;13(10):13414–37.
18. Persson H, Kvist A, Rego N, Staaf J, Vallon-Christersson J, Luts L, Loman N, Jonsson G, Naya H, Hoglund M, et al. Identification of new microRNAs in paired normal and tumor breast tissue suggests a dual role for the ERBB2/Her2 gene. Cancer Res. 2011;71(1):78–86.
19. Aloraifi F, Boland MR, Green AJ, Geraghty JG. Gene analysis techniques and susceptibility gene discovery in non-BRCA1/BRCA2 familial breast cancer. Surg Oncol. 2015;24(2):100–9.
20. Duan S, Mi S, Zhang W, Dolan ME. Comprehensive analysis of the impact of SNPs and CNVs on human microRNAs and their regulatory genes. RNA Biol. 2009;6(4):412–25.
21. Hoffman AE, Zheng T, Yi C, Leaderer D, Weidhaas J, Slack F, Zhang Y, Paranjape T, Zhu Y. microRNA miR-196a-2 and breast cancer: a genetic and epigenetic association study and functional analysis. Cancer Res. 2009; 69(14):5970–7.
22. Hu Z, Liang J, Wang Z, Tian T, Zhou X, Chen J, Miao R, Wang Y, Wang X, Shen H. Common genetic variants in pre-microRNAs were associated with increased risk of breast cancer in Chinese women. Hum Mutat. 2009;30(1):79–84.

23. Kontorovich T, Levy A, Korostishevsky M, Nir U, Friedman E. Single nucleotide polymorphisms in miRNA binding sites and miRNA genes as breast/ovarian cancer risk modifiers in Jewish high-risk women. Int J Cancer. 2010;127(3):589–97.

24. Akkız H, Bayram S, Bekar A, Akgöllü E, Ulger Y. A functional polymorphism in pre-microRNA-196a-2 contributes to the susceptibility of hepatocellular carcinoma in a Turkish population: a case-control study. J Viral Hepat. 2011; 18(7):e399–407.

25. Mittal RD, Gangwar R, George GP, Mittal T, Kapoor R. Investigative role of pre-microRNAs in bladder cancer patients: a case-control study in North India. DNA Cell Biol. 2011;30(6):401–6.

26. Okubo M, Tahara T, Shibata T, Yamashita H, Nakamura M, Yoshioka D, Yonemura J, Ishizuka T, Arisawa T, Hirata I. Association between common genetic variants in pre-microRNAs and gastric cancer risk in Japanese population. Helicobacter. 2010;15(6):524–31.

27. Jedlinski DJ, Gabrovska PN, Weinstein SR, Smith RA, Griffiths LR. Single nucleotide polymorphism in hsa-mir-196a-2 and breast cancer risk: a case control study. Twin Res Hum Genet. 2011;14(5):417–21.

28. Bensen JT, Tse CK, Nyante SJ, Barnholtz-Sloan JS, Cole SR, Millikan RC. Association of germline microRNA SNPs in pre-miRNA flanking region and breast cancer risk and survival: the Carolina Breast Cancer Study. Cancer Causes Control. 2013;24(6):1099–109.

29. Qian F, Feng Y, Zheng Y, Ogundiran TO, Ojengbede O, Zheng W, Blot W, Ambrosone CB, John EM, Bernstein L, et al. Genetic variants in microRNA and microRNA biogenesis pathway genes and breast cancer risk among women of African ancestry. Hum Genet. 2016;135(10):1145–59.

30. Newman B, Moorman PG, Millikan R, Qaqish BF, Geradts J, Aldrich TE, Liu ET. The Carolina Breast Cancer Study: integrating population-based epidemiology and molecular biology. Breast Cancer Res Treat. 1995;35(1):51–60.

31. Ambrosone CB, Ciupak GL, Bandera EV, Jandorf L, Bovbjerg DH, Zirpoli G, Pawlish K, Godbold J, Furberg H, Fatone A, et al. Conducting molecular epidemiological research in the age of HIPAA: a multi-institutional case-control study of breast cancer in African-American and European-American women. J Oncol. 2009;2009:871250.

32. Bandera EV, Chandran U, Zirpoli G, McCann SE, Ciupak G, Ambrosone CB. Rethinking sources of representative controls for the conduct of case-control studies in minority populations. BMC Med Res Methodol. 2013;13:71.

33. Rosenberg L, Adams-Campbell L, Palmer JR. The Black Women's Health Study: a follow-up study for causes and preventions of illness. J Am Med Womens Assoc. 1995;50(2):56–8.

34. Kolonel LN, Henderson BE, Hankin JH, Nomura AM, Wilkens LR, Pike MC, Stram DO, Monroe KR, Earle ME, Nagamine FS. A multiethnic cohort in Hawaii and Los Angeles: baseline characteristics. Am J Epidemiol. 2000; 151(4):346–57.

35. Palmer JR, Ambrosone CB, Olshan AF. A collaborative study of the etiology of breast cancer subtypes in African American women: the AMBER consortium. Cancer Causes Control. 2014;25(3):309–19.

36. Howie BN, Donnelly P, Marchini J. A flexible and accurate genotype imputation method for the next generation of genome-wide association studies. PLoS Genet. 2009;5(6):e1000529.

37. Chen F, Chen GK, Stram DO, Millikan RC, Ambrosone CB, John EM, Bernstein L, Zheng W, Palmer JR, Hu JJ, et al. A genome-wide association study of breast cancer in women of African ancestry. Hum Genet. 2013;132(1):39–48.

38. Ambros V, Bartel B, Bartel DP, Burge CB, Carrington JC, Chen X, Dreyfuss G, Eddy SR, Griffiths-Jones S, Marshall M, et al. A uniform system for microRNA annotation. RNA. 2003;9(3):277–9.

39. Sethupathy P. Illuminating microRNA transcription from the epigenome. Curr Genomics. 2013;14(1):68–77.

40. Haddad SA, Ruiz-Narváez EA, Haiman CA, Sucheston-Campbell LE, Bensen JT, Zhu Q, Liu S, Yao S, Bandera EV, Rosenberg L, et al. An exome-wide analysis of low frequency and rare variants in relation to risk of breast cancer in African American Women: the AMBER Consortium. Carcinogenesis. 2016;37(9):870-877. doi: https://doi.org/10.1093/carcin/bgw067. Epub 2016 Jun 7.

41. Allott EH, Cohen SM, Geradts J, Sun X, Khoury T, Bshara W, Zirpoli GR, Miller CR, Hwang H, Thorne LB, et al. Performance of three-biomarker immunohistochemistry for intrinsic breast cancer subtyping in the AMBER consortium. Cancer Epidemiol Biomark Prev. 2016;25(3):470–8.

42. Benjamini Y, Hochberg Y. Controlling the false discovery rate: a practical and powerful approach to multiple testing. J R Stat Soc Ser B Methodol. 1995;57(1):289–300.

43. Welter D, MacArthur J, Morales J, Burdett T, Hall P, Junkins H, Klemm A, Flicek P, Manolio T, Hindorff L, et al. The NHGRI GWAS Catalog, a curated resource of SNP-trait associations. Nucleic Acids Res. 2014;42(Database issue):D1001–6.

44. Kent WJ, Sugnet CW, Furey TS, Roskin KM, Pringle TH, Zahler AM, Haussler D. The human genome browser at UCSC. Genome Res. 2002;12(6):996–1006.

45. The GTEx Consortium, Lonsdale JTJ, Salvatore M, Phillips R, Lo E, Shad S, Hasz R, Walters G, Garcia F, Young N, Foster B, Moser M, Karasik E, Gillard B, Ramsey K, Sullivan S, Bridge J, Magazine H, Syron J, Fleming J, Siminoff L, Traino H, Mosavel M, Barker L, Jewell S, Rohrer D, Maxim D, Filkins D, Harbach P, Cortadillo E, Berghuis B, Turner L, Hudson E, Feenstra K, Sobin L, Robb J, Branton P, Korzeniewski G, Shive C, Tabor D, Qi L, Groch K, Nampally S, Buia S, Zimmerman A, Smith A, Burges R, Robinson K, Valentino K, Bradbury D, Cosentino M, Diaz-Mayoral N, Kennedy M, Engel T, Williams P, Erickson K, Ardlie K, Winckler W, Getz G, DeLuca D, MacArthur D, Kellis M, Thomson A, Young T, Gelfand E, Donovan M, Grant G, Mash D, Marcus Y, Basile M, Liu J, Zhu J, Tu Z, Cox NJ, Nicolae DL, Gamazon ER, Kyung H, Konkashbaev A, Pritchard J, Stevens M, Flutre T, Wen X, Dermitzakis T, Lappalainen T, Guigo R, Monlong J, Sammeth M, Koller D, Battle A, Mostafavi S, McCarthy M, Rivas M, Maller J, Rusyn I, Nobel A, Wright F, Shabalin A, Feolo M, Sharopova N, Sturcke A, Paschal J, Anderson JM, Wilder EL, Derr LK, Green ED, Struewing JP, Temple G, Volpi S, Boyer JT, Thomson EJ, Guyer MS, Ng C, Abdallah A, Colantuoni D, Insel TR, Koester SE, Little AR, Bender PK, Lehner T, Yao Y, Compton CC, Vaught JB, Sawyer S, Lockhart NC, Demchok J, Moore HF. The Genotype-Tissue Expression (GTEx) project. Nat Genet. 2013;45(6):580–5.

46. Petryszak R, Burdett T, Fiorelli B, Fonseca NA, Gonzalez-Porta M, Hastings E, Huber W, Jupp S, Keays M, Kryvych N, et al. Expression Atlas update—a database of gene and transcript expression from microarray- and sequencing-based functional genomics experiments. Nucleic Acids Res. 2014;42(Database issue):D926–32.

47. Kapushesky M, Adamusiak T, Burdett T, Culhane A, Farne A, Filippov A, Holloway E, Klebanov A, Kryvych N, Kurbatova N, et al. Gene Expression Atlas update—a value-added database of microarray and sequencing-based functional genomics experiments. Nucleic Acids Res. 2012;40(Database issue):D1077–81.

48. Barretina J, Caponigro G, Stransky N, Venkatesan K, Margolin AA, Kim S, Wilson CJ, Lehár J, Kryukov GV, Sonkin D, et al. The Cancer Cell Line Encyclopedia enables predictive modelling of anticancer drug sensitivity. Nature. 2012;483(7391):603–7.

49. Kent WJ. BLAT—the BLAST-like alignment tool. Genome Res. 2002;12(4):656–64.

50. Karolchik D, Hinrichs AS, Furey TS, Roskin KM, Sugnet CW, Haussler D, Kent WJ. The UCSC Table Browser data retrieval tool. Nucleic Acids Res. 2004; 32(Database issue):D493–6.

51. Kent WJ, Zweig AS, Barber G, Hinrichs AS, Karolchik D. BigWig and BigBed: enabling browsing of large distributed datasets. Bioinformatics. 2010;26(17):2204–7.

52. Raney BJ, Dreszer TR, Barber GP, Clawson H, Fujita PA, Wang T, Nguyen N, Paten B, Zweig AS, Karolchik D, et al. Track data hubs enable visualization of user-defined genome-wide annotations on the UCSC Genome Browser. Bioinformatics. 2014;30(7):1003–5.

53. Kent WJ, Hsu F, Karolchik D, Kuhn RM, Clawson H, Trumbower H, Haussler D. Exploring relationships and mining data with the UCSC Gene Sorter. Genome Res. 2005;15(5):737–41.

54. Ward LD, Kellis M. HaploReg: a resource for exploring chromatin states, conservation, and regulatory motif alterations within sets of genetically linked variants. Nucleic Acids Res. 2012;40(Database issue):D930–4.

55. Kheradpour P, Ernst J, Melnikov A, Rogov P, Wang L, Zhang X, Alston J, Mikkelsen TS, Kellis M. Systematic dissection of regulatory motifs in 2000 predicted human enhancers using a massively parallel reporter assay. Genome Res. 2013;23(5):800–11.

56. Ruiz-Narváez EA, Sucheston-Campbell L, Bensen JT, Yao S, Haddad S, Haiman CA, Bandera EV, John EM, Bernstein L, Hu JJ, et al. Admixture mapping of African-American women in the AMBER consortium identifies new loci for breast cancer and estrogen-receptor subtypes. Front Genet. 2016;7:170.

57. Machiela MJ, Chanock SJ. LDlink: a web-based application for exploring population-specific haplotype structure and linking correlated alleles of possible functional variants. Bioinformatics. 2015;31(21):3555–7.

58. Ruiz-Narváez EA, Lunetta KL, Hong CC, Haddad S, Yao S, Cheng TD, Bensen JT, Bandera EV, Haiman CA, Troester MA, et al. Genetic variation in the insulin, insulin-like growth factor, growth hormone, and leptin pathways in relation to breast cancer in African-American women: the AMBER consortium. NPJ Breast Cancer. 2016;2:16034.

59. Toffoli S, Bar I, Abdel-Sater F, Delrée P, Hilbert P, Cavallin F, Moreau F, Van Criekinge W, Lacroix-Triki M, Campone M, et al. Identification by array comparative genomic hybridization of a new amplicon on chromosome 17q highly recurrent in BRCA1 mutated triple negative breast cancer. Breast Cancer Res. 2014;16(6):466.

60. Hwang KT, Han W, Cho J, Lee JW, Ko E, Kim EK, Jung SY, Jeong EM, Bae JY, Kang JJ, et al. Genomic copy number alterations as predictive markers of systemic recurrence in breast cancer. Int J Cancer. 2008;123(8):1807–15.

61. Rafique S, Thomas JS, Sproul D, Bickmore WA. Estrogen-induced chromatin decondensation and nuclear re-organization linked to regional epigenetic regulation in breast cancer. Genome Biol. 2015;16:145.

62. Lewis BP, Burge CB, Bartel DP. Conserved seed pairing, often flanked by adenosines, indicates that thousands of human genes are microRNA targets. Cell. 2005;120(1):15–20.

63. Grimson A, Farh KK, Johnston WK, Garrett-Engele P, Lim LP, Bartel DP. MicroRNA targeting specificity in mammals: determinants beyond seed pairing. Mol Cell. 2007;27(1):91–105.

64. Friedman RC, Farh KK, Burge CB, Bartel DP. Most mammalian mRNAs are conserved targets of microRNAs. Genome Res. 2009;19(1):92–105.

65. Garcia DM, Baek D, Shin C, Bell GW, Grimson A, Bartel DP. Weak seed-pairing stability and high target-site abundance decrease the proficiency of lsy-6 and other microRNAs. Nat Struct Mol Biol. 2011;18(10):1139–46.

66. Cui D, Jin G, Gao T, Sun T, Tian F, Estrada GG, Gao H, Sarai A. Characterization of BRCAA1 and its novel antigen epitope identification. Cancer Epidemiol Biomark Prev. 2004;13(7):1136–45.

67. Willer CJ, Li Y, Abecasis GR. METAL: fast and efficient meta-analysis of genome-wide association scans. Bioinformatics. 2010;26(17):2190–1.

BHLHE40 confers a pro-survival and pro-metastatic phenotype to breast cancer cells by modulating HBEGF secretion

Aarti Sethuraman, Martin Brown, Raya Krutilina, Zhao-Hui Wu, Tiffany N. Seagroves, Lawrence M. Pfeffer and Meiyun Fan*

Abstract

Background: Metastasis is responsible for a significant number of breast cancer-related deaths. Hypoxia, a primary driving force of cancer metastasis, induces the expression of BHLHE40, a transcription regulator. This study aimed to elucidate the function of BHLHE40 in the metastatic process of breast cancer cells.

Methods: To define the role of BHLHE40 in breast cancer, BHLHE40 expression was knocked down by a lentiviral construct expressing a short hairpin RNA against BHLHE40 or knocked out by the CRISPR/Cas9 editing system. Orthotopic xenograft and experimental metastasis (tail vein injection) mouse models were used to analyze the role of BHLHE40 in lung metastasis of breast cancer. Global gene expression analysis and public database mining were performed to identify signaling pathways regulated by BHLHE40 in breast cancer. The action mechanism of BHLHE40 was examined by chromatin immunoprecipitation (ChIP), co-immunoprecipitation (CoIP), exosome analysis, and cell-based assays for metastatic potential.

Results: BHLHE40 knockdown significantly reduced primary tumor growth and lung metastasis in orthotopic xenograft and experimental metastasis models of breast cancer. Gene expression analysis implicated a role of BHLHE40 in transcriptional activation of heparin-binding epidermal growth factor (HBEGF). ChIP and CoIP assays revealed that BHLHE40 induces HBEGF transcription by blocking DNA binding of histone deacetylases (HDAC)1 and HDAC2. Cell-based assays showed that HBEGF is secreted through exosomes and acts to promote cell survival and migration. Public databases provided evidence linking high expression of BHLHE40 and HBEGF to poor prognosis of triple-negative breast cancer.

Conclusion: This study reveals a novel role of BHLHE40 in promoting tumor cell survival and migration by regulating HBEGF secretion.

Keywords: BHLHE40, Hypoxia, Breast cancer, Metastasis, Exosomes, HBEGF

Background

One in every eight women in the USA will be diagnosed with breast cancer over the course of her lifetime [1]. An estimated 266,120 new cases are expected, and 40,920 women are expected to die from breast cancer in 2018 in the USA [1]. Distant metastasis is the major cause of breast cancer-related deaths. Hypoxia has been recognized as a primary driving force of distant metastasis of breast cancer [2–7]. Among hypoxia-responsive genes are both promoting and suppressive factors for malignant progression. It is unclear how the expression and activities of metastasis-promoting factors are preferentially augmented in metastatic tumors. A large body of studies have focused on elucidating the molecular mechanisms by which hypoxia enables cancer cells to survive a variety of stresses imposed by the metastatic process, including nutrient depletion, loss of attachment, and deprivation of growth factors.

Hypoxia-induced exosomic secretion of cytokines and growth factors plays a key role in promoting metastasis through both tumor autonomous and non-autonomous

* Correspondence: mfan2@uthsc.edu
Department of Pathology and Laboratory Medicine, and the Center for Cancer Research, University of Tennessee Health Science Center, 19 South Manassas Street, Memphis, TN 38163, USA

mechanisms [8, 9]. Exosomes are microvesicles (40–130 nm) constitutively released by a variety of cells into the extracellular environment to promote cell-to-cell communication [10]. Tumor cells have been reported to utilize exosomes to transfer nucleotides, lipids, and proteins into surrounding cells or cells in distant metastatic niches [10, 11]. Hypoxia is known to markedly increase the number of secreted exosomes, as well as alter the contents of exosomes [12]. However, our understanding of the regulation of exosome secretion is rudimentary.

Although the cellular response to hypoxia is mainly controlled by two basic helix-loop-helix transcription factors, hypoxia inducible factor (HIF)1A and EPAS1/HIF2A, the outcomes of the hypoxia response are modified by other transcription regulators that are regulated by hypoxia or interact with HIF1A or EPAS1 [13, 14]. This study focuses on the role of a basic helix-loop-helix transcription factor BHLHE40 (also known as DEC1/BHLHB2/SHARP2/STRA13) in metastasis of breast cancer. BHLHE40 expression is directly activated by HIF1A in a variety of tumor cells under hypoxia [15, 16]. High BHLHE40 expression has been linked to activation of a hypoxia-response pathway, elevated metastatic potentials, and poor prognosis of various types of tumors, including hepatocellular carcinoma, pancreatic cancer, and invasive breast cancer [17–19]. It was reported that BHLHE40 binds to the E-box elements and regulates the expression of genes associated with circadian rhythm, cell differentiation, cell senescence, lipid metabolism, DNA damage response, and immune response [20–23]. However, the mechanism of action and downstream targets of BHLHE40 in breast cancer cells is largely unknown. In this study, we provide evidence which suggests that BHLHE40 is a pro-metastasis factor in breast cancer cells which promotes tumor cell survival and migration by modulating exosomic secretion of heparin-binding epidermal growth factor (HBEGF).

Methods
Cell culture
Breast cancer MDA-MB-231 and MCF7 cells were obtained from ATCC (Manassas, VA, USA) and maintained in minimal essential medium (ThermoFisher Scientific, Rockford, IL, USA) supplemented with 10% fetal bovine serum (FBS), 200 U/ml penicillin-streptomycin, and 0.5 µg/ml amphotericin B (Cellgro, Manassa, VA, USA). A lung metastatic derivative of MDA-MB-231 (LM) and a tamoxifen-resistant derivative of MCF7 (TR) were established as described previously [24, 25]. A stable line (BHLHE40-KD) expressing a short hairpin RNA (shRNA) against BHLHE40 (TRCN0000232187, Sigma-Aldrich, St. Louis, MO, USA) was generated by lentiviral transduction and selected in medium containing 2 µg/ml puromycin (Sigma-Aldrich). A colony of BHLHE40 knockout variant (BHLHE40-KO) of MDA-MB-231 was generated by using the CRISPR/Cas9 all-in-one expression system (HCP221270-CG01–1, GeneCopoeia) and selected in medium supplemented with 500 µg/ml gentamicin. Elimination of BHLHE40 expression was examined by immunoblotting and quantitative polymerase chain reaction (qPCR) with a forward primer designed to cover the CRISPR editing site (forward 5′GACGGGGAATAAAG CGGAGC and reverse 5′CCGGTCACGTCTCTTTTTC TC). To knockout HIF1A and EPAS1 by CRISPR/Cas9 editing, gRNA targeting exon 1 of HIF1A or EPAS1 was individually cloned into the pX462-puromycin and pX462-hygromycin vectors (expressing Cas9n, AddGene), respectively. MDA-MB-231 cells were transfected with pX462-puro-HIF1A gRNAs using FuGene HD followed by selection in puromycin. A clonal line that had no HIF1A protein detected by immunoblotting was transfected with pX462-hygromycin-EPAS1 gRNA and selected by hygromycin. Hygromycin-resistant colonies that had no EPAS1 detected by immunoblotting were pooled to generate a HIF1A/EPAS1 double-knockout (HIF-dKO) subline. For all knockdown (KD) or KO sublines, control cells were transfected with corresponding empty vectors (EV) and selected in antibiotics in parallel with cells transfected with shRNAs or gRNAs. Pooled drug-resistant colonies of control cells were used as EV control lines. Cells were exposed to different conditions relevant to solid tumors, including loss of attachment (suspension culture), hypoxia (1% O₂), hypoxia in combination with low (1 mg/ml) glucose (1%O₂/LG), and hypoxia in combination with glucose depletion (1%O₂/GF, a condition that induces rapid apoptosis of tumor cells).

Orthotropic xenograft and experimental lung metastasis models
All in-vivo studies were performed in accordance with the protocols approved by the Institutional Animal Care and Use Committee (IACUC) of the University of Tennessee Health Science Center. NOD.Cg-PrkdcscidIl2rgtm1Wjl/SzJ (NSG) mice were purchased from Jackson Laboratories (Bar Harbor, ME, USA). Orthotropic xenograft and experimental lung metastasis (tail vein injection) models were established using fluorescence-labeled tumor cells, as previously described [24, 26]. Tumor size was monitored and measured weekly using digital calipers. Tumor volume was calculated as: volume = (width² × length)/2. Lung metastasis was quantified by fluorescent imaging of lungs and qPCR of human Alu DNA repeats (forward primer: 5′: GTCAGGAGATCGAGACCATCCC 3′; reverse primer: 5′: TCCTGCCTCAGCCTCCCAAG 3′). Circulating tumor cells in whole blood collected by cardiac puncture were isolated using the Ficoll-Paque PLUS medium (GE Healthcare Life Sciences, Piscataway, NJ, USA) and counted under fluorescent microscope.

Migration, invasion, and wound healing assays

Transwell membrane inserts with 8-μm pores (BD Biosciences, Bedford, MA, USA), uncoated or coated with Matrigel, were used to determine the migratory and invasive activities of cancer cells, respectively. Cells undergoing migration and invasion were expressed as: percent migration = mean number of cells migrating through the uncoated transwell × 100/mean number of seeded cells; percent invasion = mean number of cells migrating through the Matrigel-coated transwell × 100/mean number of migrating cells through the uncoated pores. Real-time assessment of migratory activity during scratch wound healing was performed using the IncuCyte ZOOM-ImageLock plate system (Essen Bioscience, Michigan, USA). To examine the expression levels of proteins in response to scratch wounds, the EMD Millipore Chemicon Cell Comb Scratch assay kit (Millipore) was used to generate a high-density field of scratches in a confluent cell monolayer to maximize the area of wound edges. To examine the effect of HBEGF on cell migration and invasion, a neutralizing antibody to HBEGF (10 μg/ml; AF-259-NA, R&D systems, Minneapolis, MN, USA) or a HBEGF peptide (20 μg/ml) was added to the medium.

Suspension culture, viable cell counting, and caspase assays

To mimic the loss of attachment, cells were cultured in PolyHEMA (Sigma-Aldrich)-coated plates to prevent adherence. Methylcellulose (1%) was added to the medium to prevent formation of large cell aggregates to accurately measure tumor cell proliferation in the suspension. Viable cells were counted by the Trypan blue exclusion method. Cell apoptosis was determined using the caspase Glo 3/7 assay kit (Promega, Madison, WI, USA) or immunoblotting of cleaved Caspase 9.

Luciferase reporter assay for HIF activity

Luciferase reporter constructs driven by hypoxia responsive elements of LDHA (LDHA-Luc, S721613) and ITGA6 (ITGA6-Luc, S708174) were purchased from SwitchGear Genomics (Carlsbad, CA, USA). Cells (3×10^5) were transfected with 500 ng LDHA-Luc or ITGA6-Luc and 10 ng CMV-β-galactosidase (a control for transfection efficiency), along with 250 ng of an empty vector or a HIF1A-expressing construct (HsCD00444875, DNASU plasmid repository), using Fugene6 (Promega). Forty-eight hours after transfection, the cells were exposed to hypoxia (1% O_2) for 6 h. Luciferase and β-galactosidase (β-gal) activities were measured using the LightSwitch Luciferase Assay System and Promega Beta-Glo Assay System, respectively. Relative luciferase activities normalized to β-gal were presented as mean ± SD, $n = 6$.

Exosome isolation and analysis

To isolate exosomes, 5×10^6 cells were cultured in medium supplemented with exosome-free serum (SystemBio, Palo Alto, CA, USA). Exosomes in the conditioned medium were purified using the ExoQuick-TC solution (SystemBio) and quantified under a fluorescent microscope after being labeled with carboxyfluorescein diacetate succinimidyl ester (CFSE) using the Exo-Glow labeling kit (SystemBio) that is designed to exclude background particles. To analyze the protein content, isolated exosomes were lysed in RIPA buffer (Pierce, ThermoScientific) containing protease inhibitor cocktail (Sigma-Aldrich) and subjected to immunoblot analysis. To examine the effect of purified exosomes on cell migration, exosomes were re-suspended in exosome-free medium and added to cells seeded in transwells.

Gene expression microarray and qPCR analysis

Total RNA from cells exposed to hypoxia (1% O_2 for 6 and 48 h) was purified using the RNeasy kit (Qiagen) and submitted to the Molecular Resource Center at the University of Tennessee Health Science Center for labeling and hybridization to the HT-12 expression BeadChips (Illumina, Chicago, IL, USA). Hybridization signals were processed for annotation, background subtraction, quantile normalization, and presence call filtering using the Gene Expression Module of the Genome Studio Software (Illumina). The microarray data can be found in the Gene Expression Omnibus database with accession number GSE107300. Hypoxia-responsive genes were defined as genes whose expression was altered ≥ 1.5-fold (hypoxia versus control) in two independent experiments. BHLHE40 target genes were defined as genes whose expression was altered ≥ 1.5-fold (BHLHE40-KD versus EV) in two independent experiments. To examine the effect of BHLHE40-KD on gene expression in cells exposed to hypoxia (1% O_2) in combination with low glucose (1 mM; 1%O_2/LG), a condition frequently encountered by cells in solid tumors, total RNA of cells exposed to 1%O_2/LG for 4 h from three independent experiments were pooled and analyzed using the GeneChip Human Gene 1.0 ST array (Affymetrix, Santa Clara, CA, USA). The Affymetrix data were extracted, normalized, and summarized with the robust multi-average (RMA) method implemented in the Affymetrix Expression Console. To validate microarray data by qPCR, total RNA from cells in three independent experiments with duplicates was prepared using trizol (Life Technologies, Grand Island, NY, USA). cDNAs were synthesized using iScript cDNA Synthesis kits (Bio-Rad, Hercules, CA, USA) and qPCR was performed on the CFX96TM Real-Time PCR detection system using SYBR green supermix (Bio-Rad). Expression data of mRNA were normalized by the $2^{-\Delta\Delta CT}$ method to RPL13A and presented as mean ± SD. Primers for qPCR were obtained from the Primerbank [27].

Protein extraction, co-immunoprecipitation, and immunoblotting

For immunoblotting (IB) analysis, whole cell lysates and nuclear proteins were prepared using RIPA buffer supplemented with protease inhibitor cocktails (Sigma-Aldrich) and the NE-PER Nuclear and Cytoplasmic Extraction Reagents (Thermo Scientific), respectively. To detect protein-protein interaction, soluble proteins were extracted using the Pierce IP Lysis Buffer (Thermo Scientific) supplemented with protease inhibitor cocktails and co-immunoprecipitation (CoIP) was performed using the TrueBlot Immunoprecipitation and Western Blot Kit (Rockland Immunochemicals Inc., Limerick, PA, USA). IB signals were developed using the SuperSignal West Dura Extended Duration Substrate and the CL-XPosure Film (Thermo Scientific). Antibodies used in this study were: anti-EGFR-Tyr1110P, anti-EGFR, anti-ERK1/2-Thr202/Tyr204P, anti-ERK1/2, anti-AKT-Tyr416P, anti-AKT, anti-Caspase9, anti-HDAC1, and anti-HDAC2 from Cell Signaling Technologies (Boston, MA, USA), anti-GAPDH from Millipore (Merck, Darmstadt, Germany), anti-TBP from Abcam (Cambridge, MA, USA), anti-CTGF from Abgent (San Diego, CA, USA), anti-HBEGF and anti-CD9 from R&D Biosystems (Minneapolis, MN, USA), anti-BHLHE40, anti-HIF1A, and anti-EPAS1 from Novus Biologicals (Littleton, CO, USA), and anti-ALIX, anti-TSG101, and anti-CD81 from Santa Cruz (Dallas, TX, USA).

Chromatin immunoprecipitation (ChIP)

Protein-DNA crosslink, nuclear fraction extraction, and chromatin fragmentation were performed as described previously [26]. The soluble fraction of sheared chromatin (200–500 bp in length) was pre-cleaned with Magnabind Goat anti-Rabbit IgG (for anti-BHLHE40 and anti-HDAC1) or Magnabind Goat anti-Mouse (for anti-HDAC2) (Life Technologies), followed by immunoprecipitation with control IgG or antibodies against BHLHE40, histone deacetylases (HDAC)1 or HDAC2, and Magnabind beads conjugated with a secondary antibody. DNA in the de-crosslinked immunocomplexes was isolated with the MiniElute PCR purification kit (Qiagen, Germantown, MD, USA). qPCR was performed to detect the presence of the proximal promoter region of HBEGF (−529 to −372 from the transcription start site) using the following primers: forward 5'TGCCTGCAACTTCAACT CTG3' and reverse 5'CCATCCCTGTCACCCTCTAA3'.

Statistical analysis

Student's t tests, one-way analysis of variance (ANOVA) with post-hoc Tukey test and correlation significance analyses were performed using the GraphPad Prism 5 software (GraphPad, San Diego, CA, USA); p values < 0.05 were considered statistically significant.

Results

BHLHE40 knockdown leads to decreased primary tumor growth and lung metastases

To define the role of BHLHE40 in breast cancer metastasis, we examined the effect of its knockdown (KD) by a shRNA lentiviral construct on spontaneous lung metastasis of orthotopic xenograft tumors derived from a lung metastasis-enriched subline (LM) of breast cancer MDA-MB-231 cells [28]. The protein levels of BHLHE40 is low in cells under normal growth conditions but is significantly induced by hypoxia (1% O_2, 16 h). BHLHE40-shRNA expression effectively reduced both baseline and hypoxia-induced levels of BHLHE40 in LM cells (Fig. 1a). In NSG mice inoculated with 2×10^5 control LM-EV (empty vector) cells in the inguinal mammary gland fat pads, palpable tumors were detected at 2 weeks (Fig. 1b) and lung metastasis became evident at 5 weeks (Fig. 1c) post-inoculation. BHLHE40-KD delayed the onset of primary tumors, which became palpable 3 weeks after inoculation, and reduced the growth rate of primary tumors, coincident with decreased lung metastases (Fig. 1a–c). To further investigate the effect of BHLHE40-KD on lung metastases, primary tumors of EV and BHLHE40-KD cells were surgically removed at 3 and 5 weeks post-inoculation, respectively, when they reached similar size with a diameter of 4–5 mm. Lung metastasis was examined 4 weeks after primary tumor resection (Fig. 1d). BHLHE40-KD substantially reduced lung metastasis in mice with similar primary tumor burdens. Taken together, these results suggest that BHLHE40 plays a role in promoting primary tumor growth and spontaneous distant metastasis of breast cancer cells.

BHLHE40 knockdown reduces lung colonization of tumor cells inoculated through tail vein

To determine whether BHLHE40 regulates late metastatic events after entry of tumor cells into the blood stream, we examined the effect of BHLHE40-KD on the ability of tumor cells to survive circulation and colonize in the lungs using an experimental metastasis model, in which tumor cells were delivered into the blood stream through tail vein injection to bypass the initial steps of metastasis such as migration and intravasation. LM-EV and LM-BHLHE40-KD cells (5×10^5) were injected into the left lateral tail veins of 5-week-old female NSG mice, and tumor cells in the bloodstream and lung tissues were examined at various times post-injection (Fig. 2). Compared with control LM-EV cells, LM-BHLHE40-KD cells were more rapidly eliminated from the bloodstream (Fig. 2a). LM-EV cells were observed in lung tissues at 72 h and formed large metastatic foci at 4 weeks after tail vein injection (Fig. 2b, c). In contrast, BHLHE40-KD cells were not detected in lung tissue at 72 h and formed less metastatic foci in lungs than EV cells at various time points (Fig. 2b, c). No fluorescent loci of EV or BHLHE40-KD cells were found in other organs (i.e., livers,

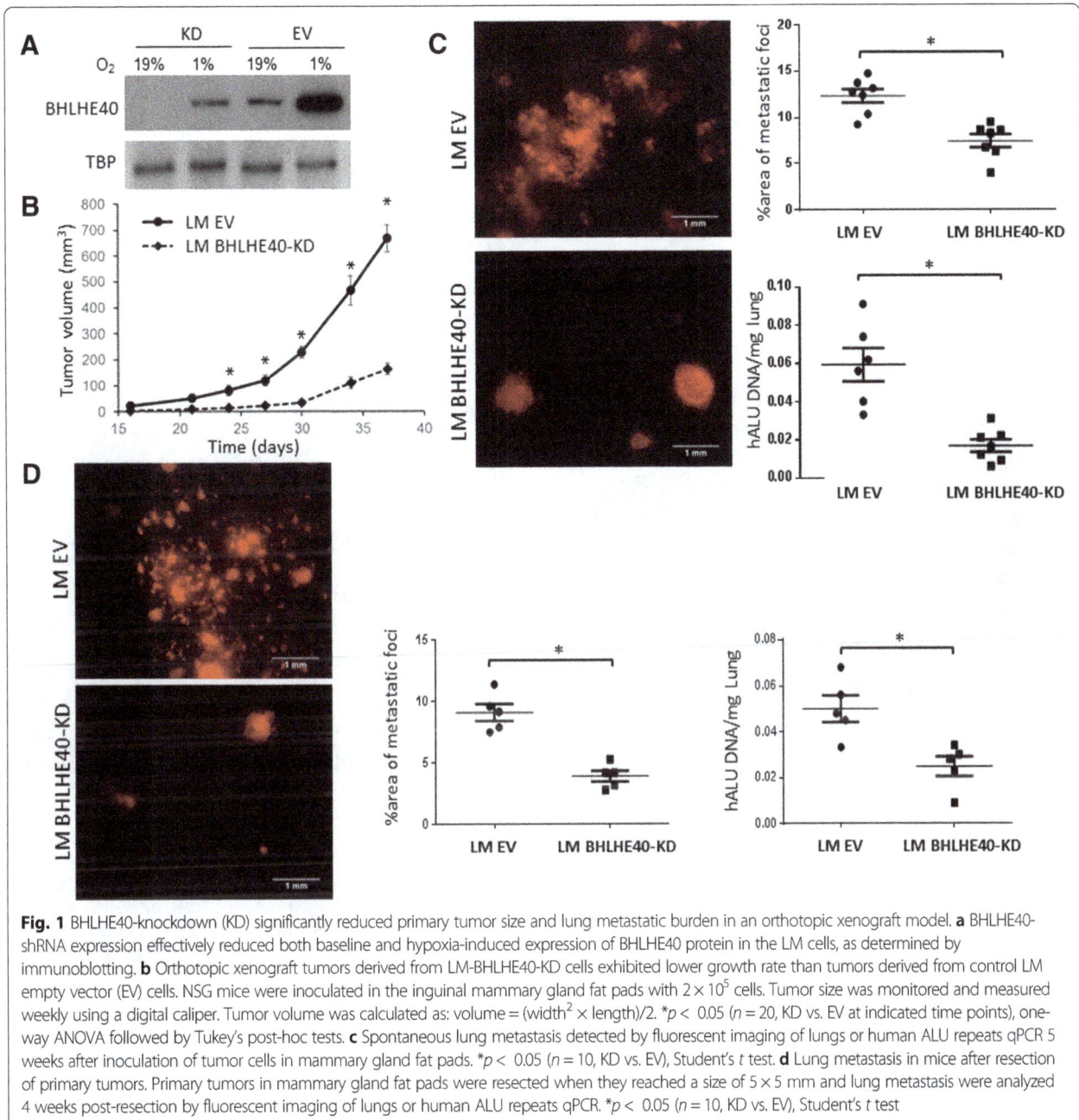

Fig. 1 BHLHE40-knockdown (KD) significantly reduced primary tumor size and lung metastatic burden in an orthotopic xenograft model. **a** BHLHE40-shRNA expression effectively reduced both baseline and hypoxia-induced expression of BHLHE40 protein in the LM cells, as determined by immunoblotting. **b** Orthotopic xenograft tumors derived from LM-BHLHE40-KD cells exhibited lower growth rate than tumors derived from control LM empty vector (EV) cells. NSG mice were inoculated in the inguinal mammary gland fat pads with 2×10^5 cells. Tumor size was monitored and measured weekly using a digital caliper. Tumor volume was calculated as: volume = (width^2 × length)/2. *$p < 0.05$ ($n = 20$, KD vs. EV at indicated time points), one-way ANOVA followed by Tukey's post-hoc tests. **c** Spontaneous lung metastasis detected by fluorescent imaging of lungs or human ALU repeats qPCR 5 weeks after inoculation of tumor cells in mammary gland fat pads. *$p < 0.05$ ($n = 10$, KD vs. EV), Student's t test. **d** Lung metastasis in mice after resection of primary tumors. Primary tumors in mammary gland fat pads were resected when they reached a size of 5×5 mm and lung metastasis were analyzed 4 weeks post-resection by fluorescent imaging of lungs or human ALU repeats qPCR. *$p < 0.05$ ($n = 10$, KD vs. EV), Student's t test

spleens, and kidneys) within 5 weeks after tail vein inoculation. Together, these results suggest that BHLHE40 is required for tumor cells to survive in the circulation and establish metastatic foci in the lungs.

BHLHE40 acts to promote cell migration, invasion and survival

Having established a role for BHLHE40 in distant metastasis of breast cancer cells in vivo, we sought to identify the specific cellular processes that require BHLHE40 activity. Despite the significant effect of BHLHE40-KD on

primary tumor growth and lung metastasis of LM cells in vivo, BHLHE40-KD showed no significant effect on proliferation of LM cells under normal two-dimensional growth conditions in vitro. The doubling times, determined by Trypan blue exclusion-based cell counting (daily for 7 days), of LM-EV and LM-BHLHE40-KD cells were 36.37 ± 0.49 h ($n = 6$) and 38.95 ± 3.61 h ($n = 6$), respectively. Therefore, we focused on investigating whether BHLHE40 is a downstream effector of HIF1A activation by hypoxia or loss of attachment. Detached breast cells were reported to rely on HIF1A activation to survive

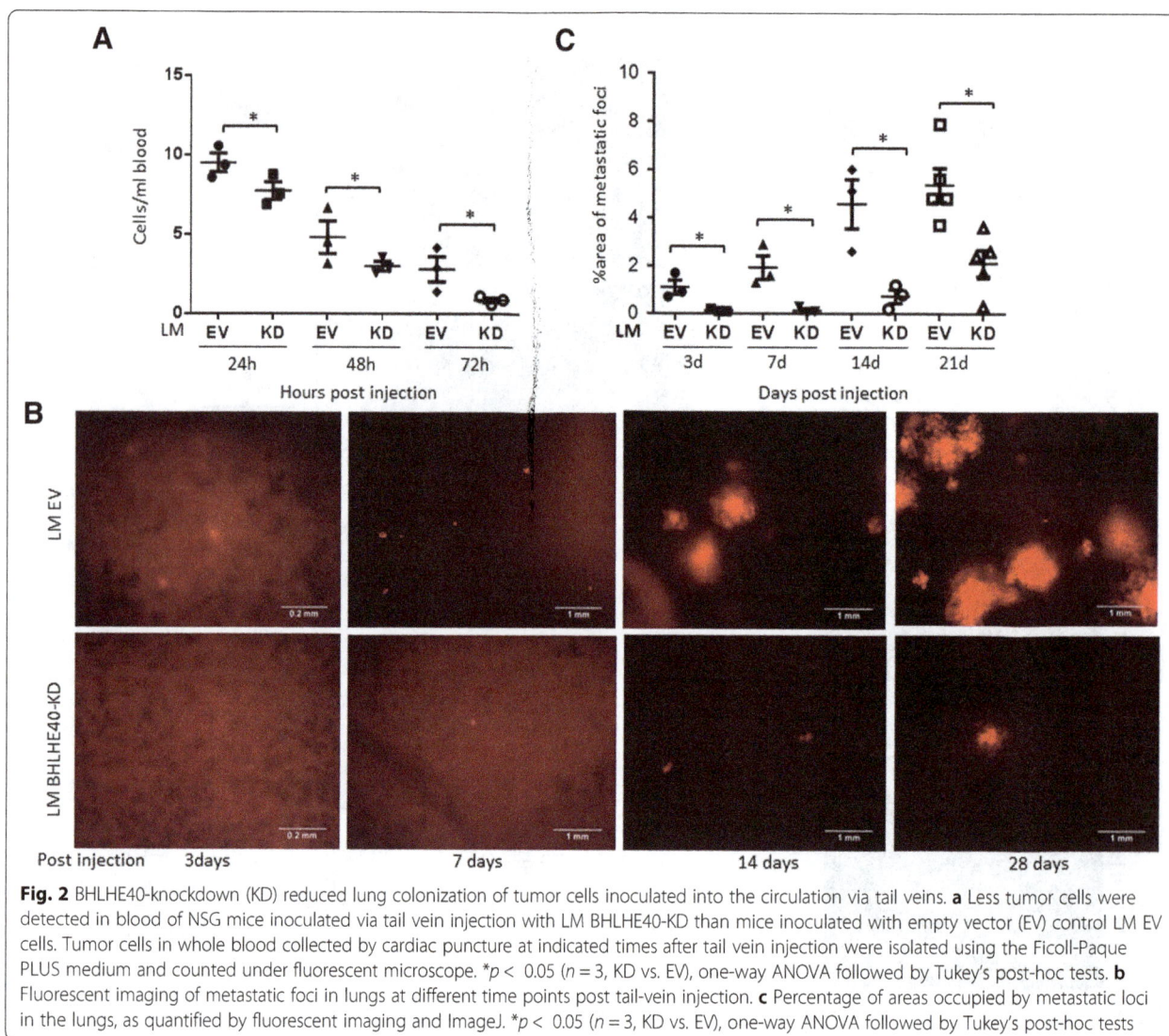

Fig. 2 BHLHE40-knockdown (KD) reduced lung colonization of tumor cells inoculated into the circulation via tail veins. **a** Less tumor cells were detected in blood of NSG mice inoculated via tail vein injection with LM BHLHE40-KD than mice inoculated with empty vector (EV) control LM EV cells. Tumor cells in whole blood collected by cardiac puncture at indicated times after tail vein injection were isolated using the Ficoll-Paque PLUS medium and counted under fluorescent microscope. *$p <$ 0.05 ($n = 3$, KD vs. EV), one-way ANOVA followed by Tukey's post-hoc tests. **b** Fluorescent imaging of metastatic foci in lungs at different time points post tail-vein injection. **c** Percentage of areas occupied by metastatic loci in the lungs, as quantified by fluorescent imaging and ImageJ. *$p <$ 0.05 ($n = 3$, KD vs. EV), one-way ANOVA followed by Tukey's post-hoc tests

under normoxia [29]. In-vitro cell migration and invasion assays showed that BHLHE40-KD reduced the ability of cells to penetrate either uncoated or Matrigel-coated transwells under hypoxia conditions (1% O_2; Fig. 3a). Under the nonadherent culture condition for 15 days, in which cells were mixed with growth medium supplemented with 1% methylcellulose to prevent cell aggregation and then seeded in plates coated with poly-HEMA to prevent adherence, the number of viable LM BHLHE40-KD cells was significantly lower than LM EV cells (Fig. 3a, lower panel). To examine whether the effects exerted by BHLHE40-KD on LM cells can be extended to the parent MDA-MB-231 cells, we established a BHLHE40 knockout (KO) subline using the CRISPR/Cas9 editing system. BHLHE40 protein depletion in the KO subline under normoxia or hypoxia was confirmed by im-munoblotting (Fig. 3b, upper panel). Although residue

BHLHE40 protein was detected in the KO subline by im-munoblotting, no wild-type mRNA was detected by qPCR with a forward primer designed to cover the CRISPR edit-ing site. BHLHE40-KO resulted in a reduced number of viable cells after a 15-day suspension culture in plates coated with polyHEMA to prevent attachment (Fig. 3b, middle panel), while it showed no significant effect on the number of viable cells after a 5-day adherence culture. In addition, BHLHE40-KO significantly sensitized MDA-MB-231 cells to apoptosis induced by hypoxia in combination with glucose depletion (1%O_2/GF, 6 h), as ev-idenced by the appearance of apoptotic morphology and activation of caspase3/7 (Fig. 3b, lower panel).

We further examined the function of BHLHE40 in breast tumor cells with elevated baseline activation of HIF1A and BHLHE40 using the tamoxifen-resistant (TR) and fulvestrant-resistant (FR) variants of MCF7 cells [25]. As

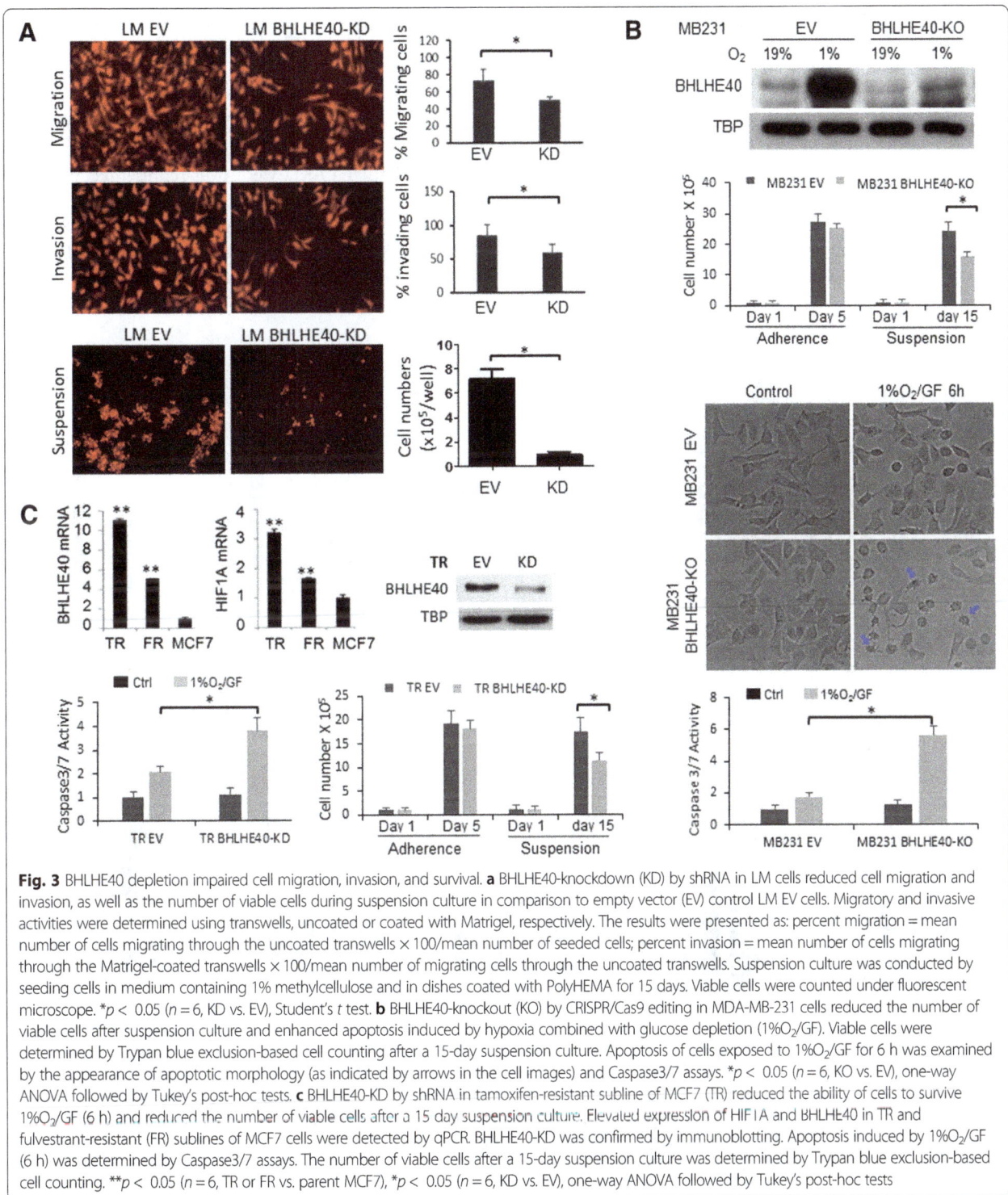

Fig. 3 BHLHE40 depletion impaired cell migration, invasion, and survival. **a** BHLHE40-knockdown (KD) by shRNA in LM cells reduced cell migration and invasion, as well as the number of viable cells during suspension culture in comparison to empty vector (EV) control LM EV cells. Migratory and invasive activities were determined using transwells, uncoated or coated with Matrigel, respectively. The results were presented as: percent migration = mean number of cells migrating through the uncoated transwells × 100/mean number of seeded cells; percent invasion = mean number of cells migrating through the Matrigel-coated transwells × 100/mean number of migrating cells through the uncoated transwells. Suspension culture was conducted by seeding cells in medium containing 1% methylcellulose and in dishes coated with PolyHEMA for 15 days. Viable cells were counted under fluorescent microscope. *$p <$ 0.05 ($n = 6$, KD vs. EV), Student's t test. **b** BHLHE40-knockout (KO) by CRISPR/Cas9 editing in MDA-MB-231 cells reduced the number of viable cells after suspension culture and enhanced apoptosis induced by hypoxia combined with glucose depletion (1%O$_2$/GF). Viable cells were determined by Trypan blue exclusion-based cell counting after a 15-day suspension culture. Apoptosis of cells exposed to 1%O$_2$/GF for 6 h was examined by the appearance of apoptotic morphology (as indicated by arrows in the cell images) and Caspase3/7 assays. *$p <$ 0.05 ($n = 6$, KO vs. EV), one-way ANOVA followed by Tukey's post-hoc tests. **c** BHLHE40-KD by shRNA in tamoxifen-resistant subline of MCF7 (TR) reduced the ability of cells to survive 1%O$_2$/GF (6 h) and reduced the number of viable cells after a 15 day suspension culture. Elevated expression of HIF1A and BHLHE40 in TR and fulvestrant-resistant (FR) sublines of MCF7 cells were detected by qPCR. BHLHE40-KD was confirmed by immunoblotting. Apoptosis induced by 1%O$_2$/GF (6 h) was determined by Caspase3/7 assays. The number of viable cells after a 15-day suspension culture was determined by Trypan blue exclusion-based cell counting. **$p <$ 0.05 ($n = 6$, TR or FR vs. parent MCF7), *$p <$ 0.05 ($n = 6$, KD vs. EV), one-way ANOVA followed by Tukey's post-hoc tests

shown in Fig. 3c, mRNA expression levels of BHLHE40 and HIF1A are significantly elevated in TR and FR cells in comparison with parent MCF7 cells. BHLHE40-KD in TR cells substantially increased apoptosis induced by glucose depletion, under both normoxia and hypoxia conditions, as well as reducing the number of viable cells after a 15-day

suspension culture in polyHEMA-coated plates (Fig. 3c). Similarly, BHLHE40-KD reduced the number of viable cells in suspension culture and the ability of FR cells to survive glucose depletion (data not shown). Collectively, these observations provide evidence supporting a role for BHLHE40 in promoting survival and migration.

BHLHE40 is required for transcription activation of a set of cytokines and growth factors

To delineate the molecular pathways regulated by BHLHE40, we performed global gene expression analysis of LM-EV and LM BHLHE40-KD cells exposed to hypoxia (1% O_2, 6 h or 48 h). The microarray data can be found in the Gene Expression Omnibus database with accession number GSE107300. Overall, the expression levels of 521 and 646 genes in LM-EV cells were altered (fold-change ≥ 1.5 in two independent experiments) by hypoxia at 6 h and 48 h, respectively. BHLHE40-KD abolished the hypoxia-mediated upregulation of 45 (out of 261, 17.2%) and 98 (out of 361, 27.1%) genes at 6 h and 48 h, respectively. In addition, BHLHE40-KD abolished the hypoxia-mediated downregulation of 30 (out of 260, 10.5%) and 44 (out of 285, 15.4%) genes at 6 h and 48 h, respectively. The hypoxia-induced genes that were affected by BHLHE40-KD were over-represented by genes that encode proteins with cytokine or growth factor activities as defined by Gene Ontology annotation GO:0005125 and GO:0008083 (Fisher's exact test, $p < 0.0001$; Fig. 4a). The expression of a subset of these genes was also reduced

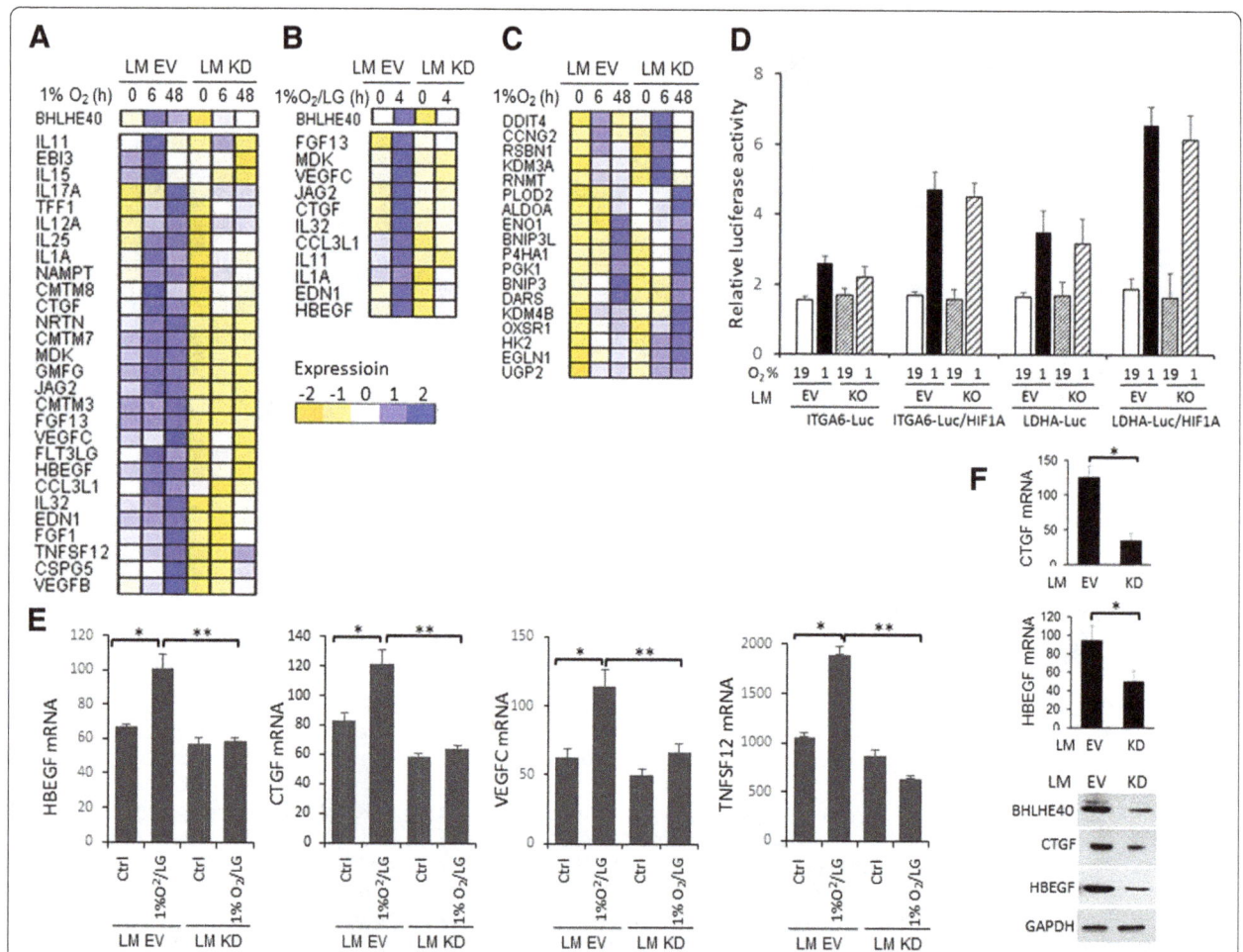

Fig. 4 BHLHE40-knockdown reduced hypoxia-induced expression of a panel of cytokines and growth factors. **a** Heatmaps of cytokines and growth factors whose hypoxia-induced expression (1% O_2 at 6 h or 48 h, fold-change ≥ 1.5 in two independent experiments) was diminished by BHLHE40-knockdown (KD) in LM cells. The gene expression levels were determined using the Illumina Human HT-12 expression BeadChips. Normalized (quantile normalization) hybridization signals were log2 transformed and standardized by genes across experiment conditions to generate the heatmap. **b** Heatmaps of a subset of genes list in **a** whose expression was affected by BHLHE40-KD in LM cells exposed to hypoxia combined with low (1 mM) glucose (1%O_2/LG, 4 h). The gene expression levels were determined using the Affymetrix Human Gene 1.0 ST array. **c** Heatmaps of hypoxia-induced genes whose expression was not significantly affected by BHLHE40-KD in LM cells as determined by the Illumina Human HT-12 expression BeadChips. **d** Expression of luciferase reporters driven by hypoxia-responsive elements of ITGA6 or LDHA was not affected by BHLHE40 knockout (KO) by CRISPR/Cas9 editing in MDA-MB-231 cells, in the absence or presence of exogenous HIF1A. Luciferase activities were normalized to co-transfected CMV-β-galactosidase and presented as mean ± SD ($n = 6$). **e** Expression of genes in control LM empty vector (EV) and LM BHLHE40-KD cells exposed to 1%O_2/LG (4 h). mRNA expression levels were determined by qPCR, normalized to RPL13A, and presented as mean ± SD ($n = 6$). *$p < 0.05$ ($n = 6$, 1%O_2/LG vs. untreated control), **$p < 0.05$ ($n = 6$, KD vs. EV), one-way ANOVA followed by Tukey's post-hoc tests. **f** mRNA and protein expression levels of HBEGF and CTGF in primary xenograft tumors, determined by qPCR and immunoblotting, respectively. *$p < 0.05$ ($n = 6$, KD vs. EV), Student's *t* test. Representative immunoblotting images of three tumors of KD or EV cells are presented

Table 1 Correlated expression of BHLHE40 and its putative targets in breast tumors (The Cancer Genome Atlas)

Gene	BL ($n = 230$)		Her2 ($n = 162$)		LA ($n = 315$)		LB ($n = 300$)	
	Pearson r	p value	Pearson r	p value	Pearson r	p value	Pearson r	p value
CCL3L1	0.1210	0.0694	−0.2045	0.0095	0.0504	0.3792	0.0480	0.4136
CMTM3	−0.0042	0.9494	0.0358	0.6510	0.5065	< 0.0001	−0.0521	0.3687
CMTM7	−0.2761	< 0.0001	−0.0697	0.3780	0.2516	< 0.0001	0.0635	0.2729
CMTM8	−0.1580	0.0165	−0.0886	0.2624	0.1034	0.0670	−0.0013	0.9817
CSPG5	−0.1333	0.0435	−0.0309	0.6961	−0.0351	0.5345	−0.0504	0.3850
CTGF	0.0203	0.7593	0.3087	< 0.0001	0.4876	< 0.0001	0.0631	0.2760
EBI3	0.2135	0.0011	−0.2060	0.0085	0.0805	0.1543	−0.0271	0.6402
EDN1	0.0705	0.2867	0.0928	0.2401	0.3805	< 0.0001	0.0273	0.6379
FGF1	0.1666	0.0114	0.2470	0.0015	0.4225	< 0.0001	0.0357	0.5384
FGF13	−0.1105	0.0946	−0.1782	0.0233	0.1393	0.0134	−0.1276	0.0271
FLT3LG	0.2436	0.0002	−0.0588	0.4573	0.2878	< 0.0001	−0.0264	0.6487
GMFG	0.2593	< 0.0001	−0.1764	0.0247	0.3367	< 0.0001	−0.1271	0.0277
HBEGF	0.3871	< 0.0001	0.2873	0.0002	0.3254	< 0.0001	0.1577	0.0062
IL11	0.1413	0.0322	0.1762	0.0249	0.2053	0.0002	0.0328	0.5710
IL12A	0.0325	0.6207	−0.0582	0.4618	−0.1035	0.0649	−0.1543	0.0069
IL15	0.3407	< 0.0001	0.0628	0.4273	0.1632	0.0037	−0.0913	0.1146
IL17A	0.1036	0.1139	0.0845	0.2850	−0.0221	0.6942	−0.0919	0.1094
IL1A	0.2140	0.0013	−0.0057	0.9440	0.0399	0.4960	−0.0720	0.2359
IL25	−0.1011	0.3633	0.0560	0.6578	−0.1569	0.0293	0.1617	0.0661
IL32	0.1597	0.0153	−0.0571	0.4704	0.3242	< 0.0001	−0.0473	0.4141
JAG2	−0.0418	0.5287	0.0387	0.6250	0.0880	0.1190	−0.0167	0.7729
MDK	−0.0837	0.2057	−0.0947	0.2305	0.1107	0.0496	0.0066	0.9099
NAMPT	0.2678	< 0.0001	0.0873	0.2691	0.1667	0.0030	−0.1819	0.0016
NRTN	−0.4457	< 0.0001	−0.0350	0.6596	0.0672	0.2411	−0.0288	0.6220
TFF1	0.2156	0.0009	−0.0148	0.8516	0.0221	0.6936	−0.1243	0.0300
TNFSF12	0.1690	0.0102	−0.0271	0.7323	0.1482	0.0084	0.0565	0.3296
VEGFB	−0.0460	0.4879	0.0811	0.3049	0.2028	0.0003	0.0443	0.4449
VEGFC	0.3664	< 0.0001	0.1760	0.0251	1.0000	< 0.0001	−0.0922	0.1110

The correlation analysis was performed using the mRNA expression z scores (RNA Seq V2 RSEM, The Cancer Genome Atlas)

BL basal-like, *Her2* ERBB2-enriched, *LA* luminal A, *LB* luminal B

in BHLHE40-KD cells exposed to $1\%O_2$/LG for 4 h compared with EV cell (Fig. 4b). In contrast, hypoxia-induced expression of a panel of the core hypoxia-responsive genes that are known to be directly targeted by HIF1A [14] was not significantly affected by BHLHE40-KD (Fig. 4c). These observations suggest that BHLHE40-KD preferentially reduced the hypoxia-induced expression of a set of cytokines and growth factors but did not cause a global defect in HIF1A-mediated transcription activation. To confirm this notion, we examined the effect of BHLHE40-KO on HIF-mediated expression of reporter luciferase driven by well-characterized HIF1A-binding sites in the promoter regions of LDHA and ITGA6 [26–28]. As shown in Fig. 4d, BHLHE40-KD exhibited no significant effect on

hypoxia-induced luciferase activities, in the absence or presence of exogenous HIF1A protein. The effect of BHLHE40-KD on the expression of cytokines and growth factors in cells exposed to $1\%O_2$/LG (4 h) was validated by qPCR (Fig. 4e). Consistent with results in BHLHE40-KD cells cultured in vitro, we detected reduced expression of CTGF and HBEGF, at both the mRNA and protein levels, in the LM-BHLHE40-KD primary tumors in comparison with LM-EV tumors established in mouse mammary gland fat pads (Fig. 4f).

To determine whether BHLHE40-mediated expression of genes encoding cytokine or growth factors is relevant to clinical samples, we analyzed the mRNA expression data of breast tumors in The Cancer Genome Atlas

(TCGA) database [30, 31]. The expression of 71.4% (20 out of 28) of these BHLHE40-dependent genes (as shown in Fig. 4a) was found to be positively correlated with BHLHE40 expression, with statistical significance ($p < 0.05$) in at least one of the four major subtypes of breast tumors (Table 1). This observation provides supporting evidence of a role for BHLHE40 in the expression of these genes in human breast tumors.

Since hypoxia-induced cytokines and growth factors are commonly exported to the extracellular space by exosomes [32], we sought to determine whether BHLHE40-KD could affect exosome secretion. As shown in Fig. 5, the number of isolated exosomes was significantly reduced in the conditioned medium from MDA-MB-231 BHLHE40-KO and TR-BHLHE40-KD cells in comparison with the corresponding control cells cultured under both normal conditions or exposed to $1\%O_2/LG$ for 6 h. The presence of exosomic markers (i.e., CD9, CD81, ALIX, and TSG101) [33, 34]) in the isolated exosomes was confirmed by immunoblotting (Fig. 5). BHLHE40 depletion reduced the protein levels of HBEGF in the purified exosomes (Fig. 5), reflecting the reduced levels of HBEGF mRNA and HBEGF protein in whole cell extracts of BHLHE40-KD or KO cells (Figs. 4e and 5). These observations suggest that BHLHE40 depletion reduced overall exosome secretion and sorting of HBEGF into exosomes.

BHLHE40 activates HBEGF transcription by sequestering HDAC1 and HDAC2 from promoter binding

Among the cytokines and growth factors affected by BHLHE40-KD in LM cells, the expression level of HBEGF mRNA is positively correlated with the expression level of BHLHE40 mRNA in all four major subtypes of breast tumors in the TCGA database (Figs. 4 and 5 and Table 1). HBEGF is a heparin-binding epidermal growth factor (EGF)-like growth factor that promotes cell proliferation and invasion through EGF receptor (EGFR) activation [35]. To examine the molecular mechanism underlying BHLHE40-mediated HBEGF transcription, we performed ChIP analysis. BHLHE40 binding to the proximal promoter region of HBEGF was not affected by $1\%O_2/LG$ (data not shown), indicating that HBEGF transcription activation was not caused by increased BHLHE40-DNA binding. However, $1\%O_2/LG$ treatment reduced binding of HDAC1 and HDAC2 to the HBEGF promoter (Fig. 6a), which is coincident with increased BHLHE40-HDAC1/2 interaction in the soluble cellular fraction, as detected by reciprocal CoIP followed by IB (Fig. 6b). In cells lacking BHLHE40, HDAC1/HDAC2 remained bound to the promoter region of HBEGF after $1\%O_2/LG$ treatment (Fig. 6a). This result suggests that BHLHE40 plays a role in facilitating the dissociation of HDAC1/2 from promoters through protein-protein interaction. To examine whether HDAC1/2-DNA binding plays a key role in suppressing

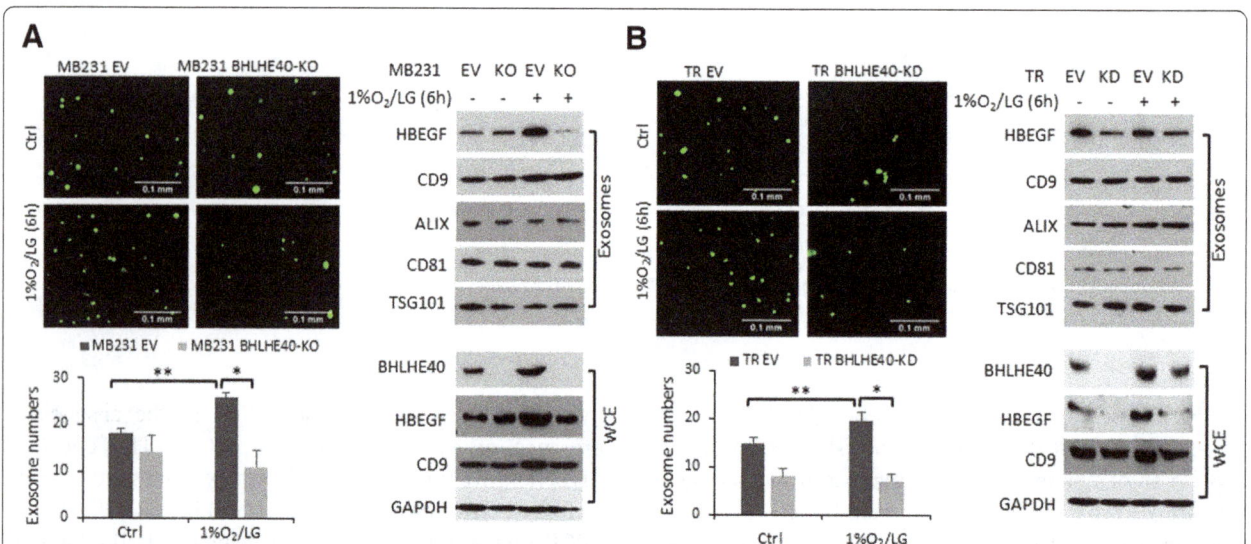

Fig. 5 Exosomic secretion of HBEGF was reduced by BHLHE40 depletion in MDA-MB231 or TR cells. a BHLHE40-knockout (KO) by CRISPR/Cas9 editing in MDA-MB-231 cells reduced the total number of exosomes and the amount of HBEGF protein in exosomes in comparison with empty vector (EV) control cells. b BHLHE40-knockdown (KD) by shRNA in tamoxifen-resistant (TR) cells reduced the total number of exosomes and the amount of HBEGF protein in exosomes in comparison with TR EV cells. Exosomes were purified from conditioned medium of 5×10^6 cells cultured in medium supplemented with exosome-free serum, either under normal culture condition or exposed to 1% O_2/low glucose (LG) for 6 h. Exosomes were purified using the ExoQuick-TC solution and quantified under a fluorescent microscope after being labeled with carboxyfluorescein diacetate succinimidyl ester (CFSE) using the Exo-Glow labeling kit, which is designed to exclude background particles. Exosome number in the bar graph is presented as mean number of exosomes per field ± SD (total of nine fields from three independent experiments were examined). The presence of HBEGF and exosome markers in purified exosomes (3 μg protein/lane) or whole cell extracts (WCE; 30 μg protein/lane) were detected by immunoblotting. **$p < 0.05$ ($n = 9$, $1\%O_2/LG$ vs. control), *$p < 0.05$ ($n = 9$, KO or KD vs. EV), one-way ANOVA followed by Tukey's post-hoc tests

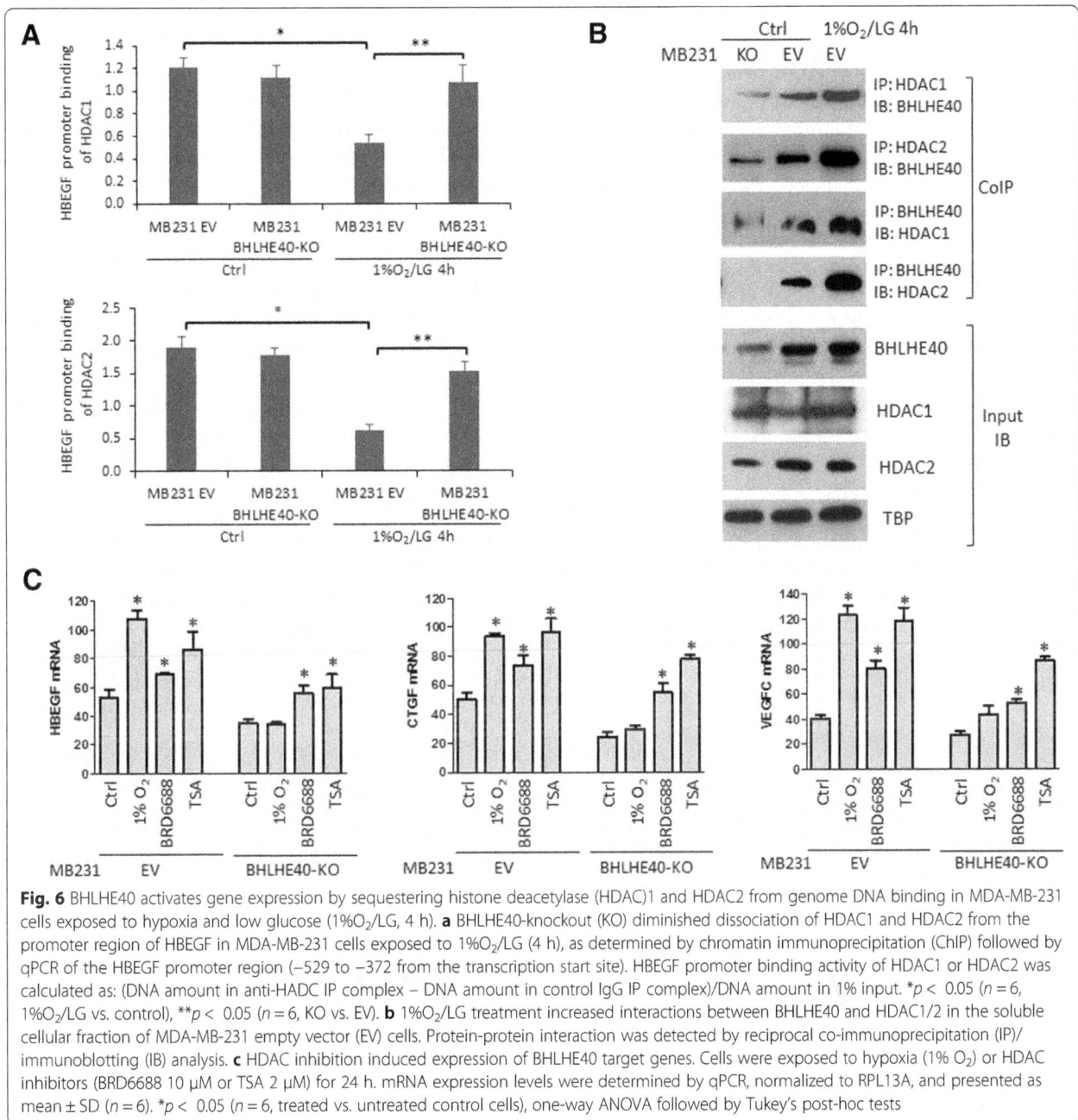

Fig. 6 BHLHE40 activates gene expression by sequestering histone deacetylase (HDAC)1 and HDAC2 from genome DNA binding in MDA-MB-231 cells exposed to hypoxia and low glucose (1%O$_2$/LG, 4 h). **a** BHLHE40-knockout (KO) diminished dissociation of HDAC1 and HDAC2 from the promoter region of HBEGF in MDA-MB-231 cells exposed to 1%O$_2$/LG (4 h), as determined by chromatin immunoprecipitation (ChIP) followed by qPCR of the HBEGF promoter region (−529 to −372 from the transcription start site). HBEGF promoter binding activity of HDAC1 or HDAC2 was calculated as: (DNA amount in anti-HADC IP complex − DNA amount in control IgG IP complex)/DNA amount in 1% input. *$p < 0.05$ ($n = 6$, 1%O$_2$/LG vs. control), **$p < 0.05$ ($n = 6$, KO vs. EV). **b** 1%O$_2$/LG treatment increased interactions between BHLHE40 and HDAC1/2 in the soluble cellular fraction of MDA-MB-231 empty vector (EV) cells. Protein-protein interaction was detected by reciprocal co-immunoprecipitation (IP)/immunoblotting (IB) analysis. **c** HDAC inhibition induced expression of BHLHE40 target genes. Cells were exposed to hypoxia (1% O$_2$) or HDAC inhibitors (BRD6688 10 μM or TSA 2 μM) for 24 h. mRNA expression levels were determined by qPCR, normalized to RPL13A, and presented as mean ± SD ($n = 6$). *$p < 0.05$ ($n = 6$, treated vs. untreated control cells), one-way ANOVA followed by Tukey's post-hoc tests

transcription of BHLHE40 target genes, we examined the effect of HDAC inhibitors on the mRNA expression of HBEGF, CTGF, and VEGFC. As shown in Fig. 6c, both HDAC2-specific (BRD6688, 10 μM) and pan-HDAC inhibitor (TSA, 2 μM) increased the expression of BHLHE40 target genes in MDA-MB-231 EV and BHLHE40-KD cells, supporting a role for HDAC1/2 in suppressing transcription of BHLHE40 target genes. Taken together, these observations suggest that sequestering HDAC1/2 from DNA binding contributes to BHLHE40-mediated transcription activation.

HBEGF acts to promote cell survival and migration

To examine whether BHLHE40-driven HBEGF expression plays a role in EGFR activation to promote cell survival, we examined the phosphorylation status of EGFR and its downstream targets in MDA-MB-231 and TR sublines exposed to 1%O$_2$/GF for 6 h, a condition known to induce apoptosis as shown in Fig. 3. Compared with cells with intact BHLHE40 activity, MDA-MB-231-BHLHE40-KO and TR-BHLHE40-KD cells expressed lower levels of HBEGF mRNA and protein, which was coincident with reduced levels of phosphorylation of EGFR, AKT, and ERK, and increased caspase 9 cleavage (Fig. 7a, b). Next, we examined whether active HBEGF peptide could rescue MDA-MB-231-BHLHE40-KO cells from apoptosis. As shown in Fig. 7c, the addition of HBEGF peptide into the culture medium of cells exposed to 1%O$_2$/GF significantly reduced activation of caspase 3/7. These observations provide evidence supporting a role of HBEGF in promoting cell survival.

Monolayer scratch was found to induce the expression of HIF1A, BHLHE40, and HBEGF in MDA-MB-231-EV cells (Fig. 8a), implicating a role for the HIF1A-BHLHE40-HBEGF axis in cell migration during wound healing. Using the IncuCyte ZOOM-ImageLock plate system, we demonstrated that BHLHE40-KO substantially diminished the ability of MDA-MB-231 cells to close the wound gaps, which was restored by the addition of HBEGF peptide (Fig. 8b, c). In contrast, a HBEGF-neutralizing antibody [36] inhibited wound healing of LM-EV cells (Fig. 8b, c). To confirm that exosomic HBEGF plays a key role in promoting cell migration, we examined the migratory activities of MDA-MB-231 BHLHE40-KO cells in the presence of conditioned medium or purified exosomes which were collected from the MDA-MB-231 EV cells at 24 h after extensive wound scratch. The transwell migration assay showed that both conditioned medium and purified exosomes from the wounded EV cells increased the migratory activity of BHLHE40-KO cells (Fig. 8d). Together, these observations suggest that HBEGF act downstream of BHLHE40 to promote cell migration.

To confirm that BHLHE40 and HBEGF are key downstream effectors of HIFs in promoting cell migration, we examined the effect of BHLHE40 overexpression on a MDA-MB-231 subline (HIF-dKO) in which both HIF isoforms (HIF1A and EPAS1) were knocked out by using the CRISPR/Cas9 editing system. Although the HIF1A mRNA expression level is approximately sixfold higher than EPAS1 mRNA in MDA-MB-231 cells according to reported RNAseq data (GSE73526), compensatory activation of EPAS1 could compromise the effect of HIF1A knockout. Therefore, we used HIF-dKO cells to examine whether BHLHE40 overexpression can rescue molecular and phenotypic changes caused by complete elimination of HIF activities. Gene expression analysis by qPCR showed that HIF-dKO reduced baseline and 1%O$_2$/LG-induced expression of BHLHE40, HBEGF, CTGF, and VEGFC mRNA, which was restored by BHLHE40 overexpression (Fig. 9a). In addition, BHLHE40 overexpression reduced cell-cell contact, as shown by cell

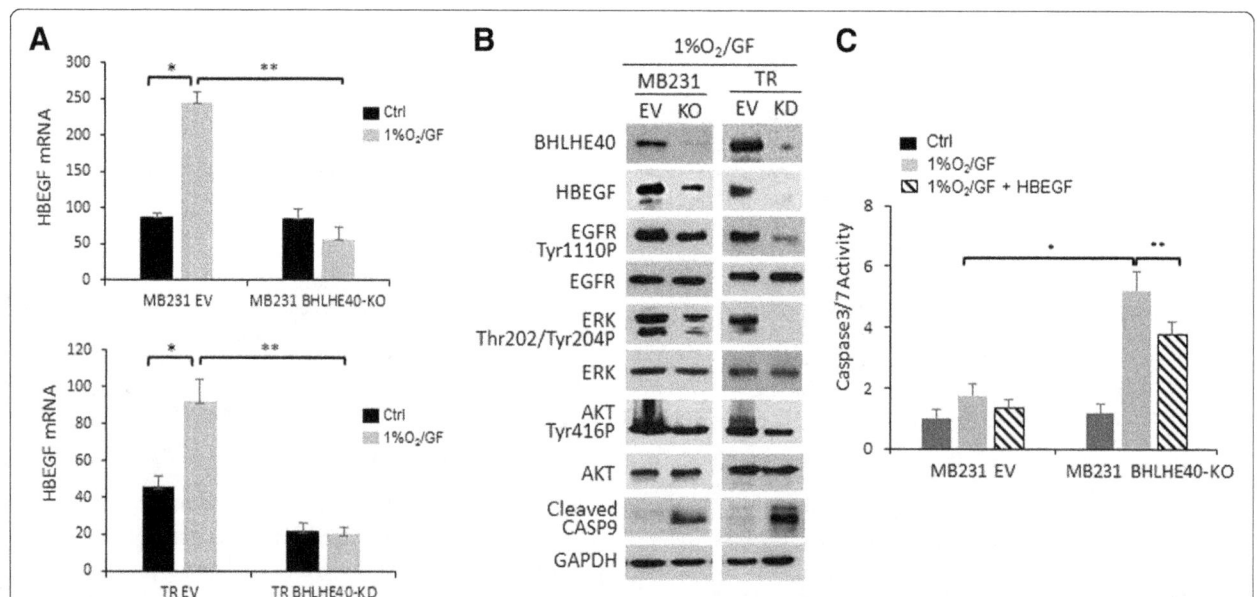

Fig. 7 BHLHE40 depletion reduced phosphorylation of epidermal growth factor receptor (EGFR), while it increased Caspase 9 cleavage, in cells exposed to glucose depletion and hypoxia (1%O$_2$/GF). **a** BHLHE40-knockout (KO) by CRISPR/Cas9 editing in MDA-MB-231 and BHLHE40-knockdown (KD) by shRNA in tamoxifen resistant (TR) cells diminished HBEGF induction by 1%O$_2$/GF (6 h). mRNA expression levels were determined by qPCR, normalized to RPL13A, and presented as mean ± SD ($n = 6$). *$p < 0.05$ ($n = 6$, 1%O$_2$/GF vs. control), **$p < 0.05$ ($n = 6$, KO vs. EV), one-way ANOVA followed by Tukey's post-hoc tests. **b** BHLHE40 depletion reduced EGFR activation, as indicated by reduced phosphorylation of EGFR and its downstream targets (ERK and AKT), while increasing apoptosis, as indicated by detection of cleaved caspase 9. Data from three independent immunoblotting analyses are presented. **c** HBEGF peptide (10 μg/ml) reduced apoptosis induced by 1%O$_2$/GF (6 h) in MDA-MB-231 BHLHE40-KO cells. Apoptosis was determined by Caspase 3/7 assays. *$p < 0.05$ ($n = 6$, 1%O$_2$/GF vs. control), **$p < 0.05$ ($n = 6$, HBEGF vs. untreated with HBEGF), one-way ANOVA followed by Tukey's post-hoc tests

BHLHE40 confers a pro-survival and pro-metastatic phenotype to breast cancer cells by modulating...

153

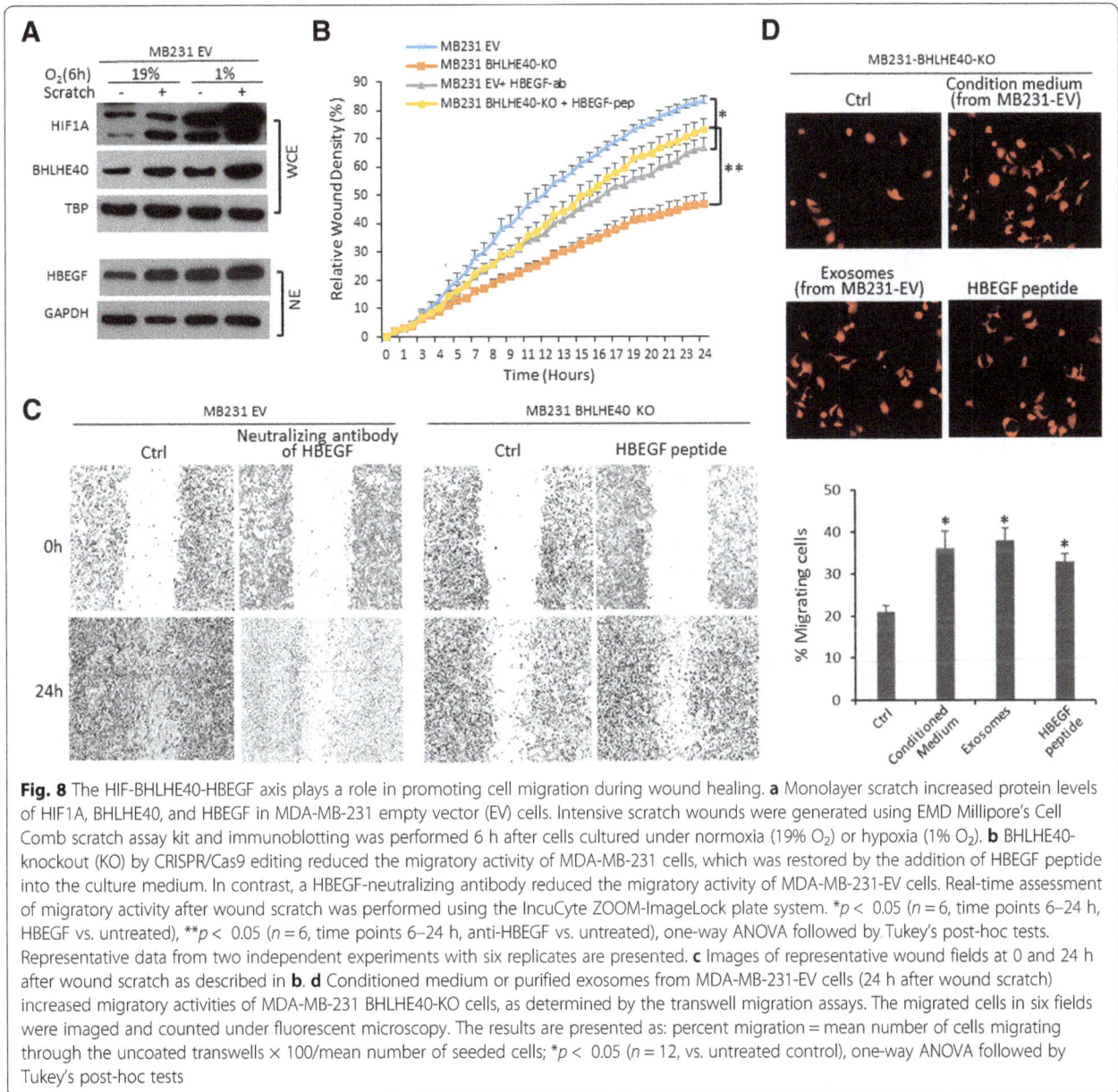

Fig. 8 The HIF-BHLHE40-HBEGF axis plays a role in promoting cell migration during wound healing. **a** Monolayer scratch increased protein levels of HIF1A, BHLHE40, and HBEGF in MDA-MB-231 empty vector (EV) cells. Intensive scratch wounds were generated using EMD Millipore's Cell Comb scratch assay kit and immunoblotting was performed 6 h after cells cultured under normoxia (19% O_2) or hypoxia (1% O_2). **b** BHLHE40-knockout (KO) by CRISPR/Cas9 editing reduced the migratory activity of MDA-MB-231 cells, which was restored by the addition of HBEGF peptide into the culture medium. In contrast, a HBEGF-neutralizing antibody reduced the migratory activity of MDA-MB-231-EV cells. Real-time assessment of migratory activity after wound scratch was performed using the IncuCyte ZOOM-ImageLock plate system. *$p < 0.05$ ($n = 6$, time points 6–24 h, HBEGF vs. untreated), **$p < 0.05$ ($n = 6$, time points 6–24 h, anti-HBEGF vs. untreated), one-way ANOVA followed by Tukey's post-hoc tests. Representative data from two independent experiments with six replicates are presented. **c** Images of representative wound fields at 0 and 24 h after wound scratch as described in **b**. **d** Conditioned medium or purified exosomes from MDA-MB-231-EV cells (24 h after wound scratch) increased migratory activities of MDA-MB-231 BHLHE40-KO cells, as determined by the transwell migration assays. The migrated cells in six fields were imaged and counted under fluorescent microscopy. The results are presented as: percent migration = mean number of cells migrating through the uncoated transwells × 100/mean number of seeded cells; *$p < 0.05$ ($n = 12$, vs. untreated control), one-way ANOVA followed by Tukey's post-hoc tests

imaging, and increased the migratory activity of HIF-dKO cells, as determined by transwell assays (Fig. 9b). Immunoblotting analysis confirmed that BHLHE40 overexpression restored expression levels of HBEGF protein in HIF-dKO cells exposed to 1%O_2/LG (Fig. 9c). Together, these observations support the notion that BHLHE40 and HBEGF act as key downstream effectors of HIFs to promote cell migration.

High expression of BHLHE40 and HBEGF is associated with poor prognosis of breast cancer

Having established a role of the BHLHE40-HBEGF axis in enhancing cell survival and migration, we sought to examine the association of BHLHE40 and HBEGF with clinical characteristics of breast tumors using the gene expression data in the Kaplan-Meier plotter database, which contains the Affymetrix microarray expression data of 2178 breast cancer patients [37]. We found that high expression of BHLHE40 or HBEGF is significantly associated with shorter interval of relapse-free survival (RFS) among patients diagnosed with triple-negative breast cancer (TNBC; $n = 255$) and patients treated with chemotherapy ($n = 602$) (Fig. 10). However, BHLHE40 and HBEGF are not poor prognostic markers for patients with estrogen receptor-positive tumors or patients treated with endocrine therapy. In addition, we analyzed the

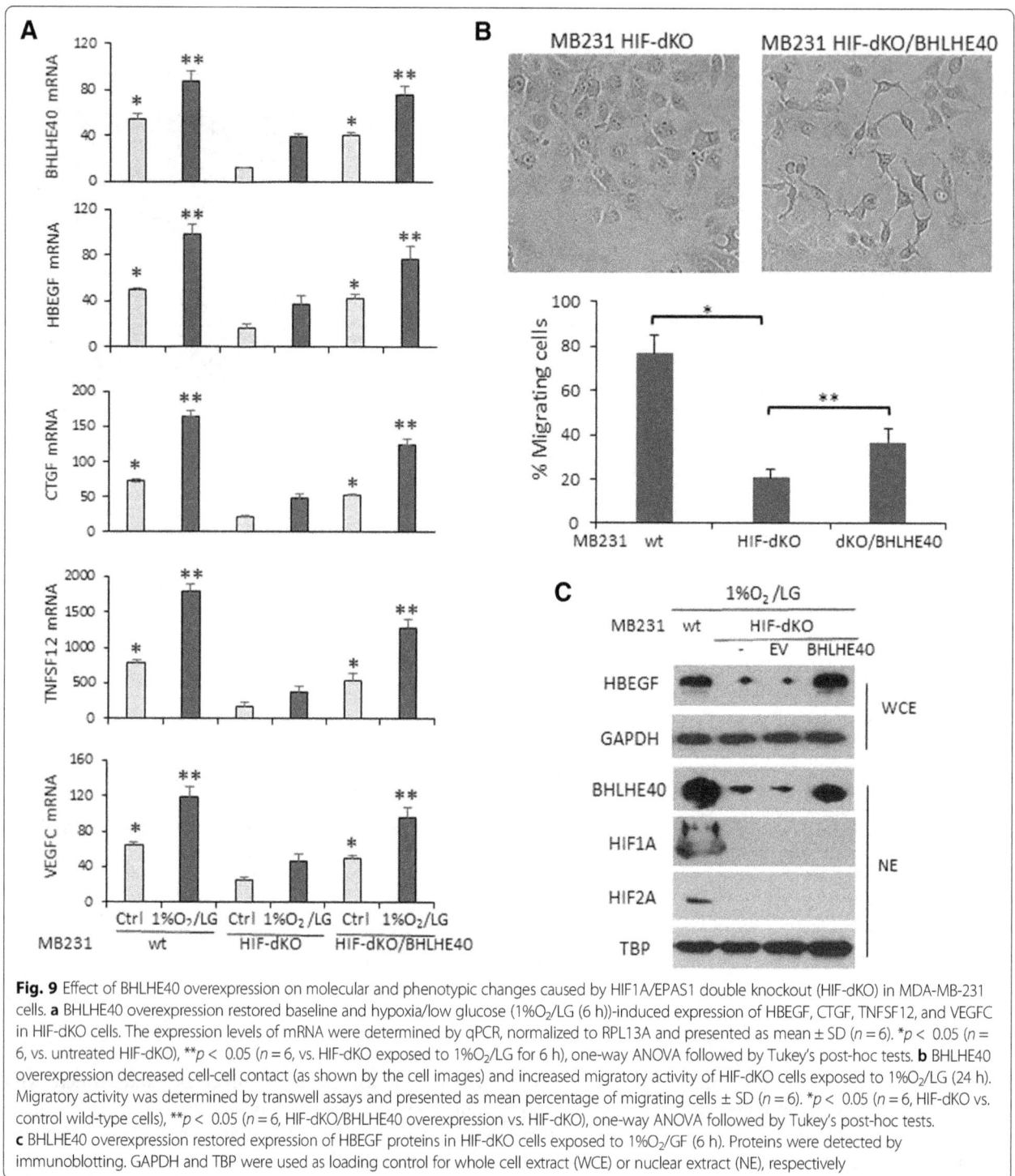

Fig. 9 Effect of BHLHE40 overexpression on molecular and phenotypic changes caused by HIF1A/EPAS1 double knockout (HIF-dKO) in MDA-MB-231 cells. **a** BHLHE40 overexpression restored baseline and hypoxia/low glucose (1%O$_2$/LG (6 h))-induced expression of HBEGF, CTGF, TNFSF12, and VEGFC in HIF-dKO cells. The expression levels of mRNA were determined by qPCR, normalized to RPL13A and presented as mean ± SD ($n = 6$). *$p < 0.05$ ($n = 6$, vs. untreated HIF-dKO), **$p < 0.05$ ($n = 6$, vs. HIF-dKO exposed to 1%O$_2$/LG for 6 h), one-way ANOVA followed by Tukey's post-hoc tests. **b** BHLHE40 overexpression decreased cell-cell contact (as shown by the cell images) and increased migratory activity of HIF-dKO cells exposed to 1%O$_2$/LG (24 h). Migratory activity was determined by transwell assays and presented as mean percentage of migrating cells ± SD ($n = 6$). *$p < 0.05$ ($n = 6$, HIF-dKO vs. control wild-type cells), **$p < 0.05$ ($n = 6$, HIF-dKO/BHLHE40 overexpression vs. HIF-dKO), one-way ANOVA followed by Tukey's post-hoc tests. **c** BHLHE40 overexpression restored expression of HBEGF proteins in HIF-dKO cells exposed to 1%O$_2$/GF (6 h). Proteins were detected by immunoblotting. GAPDH and TBP were used as loading control for whole cell extract (WCE) or nuclear extract (NE), respectively

association of BHLHE40 and HBEGF with overall survival (OS) of TNBC using the METABRIC dataset in the cBioPortal for Cancer Genomics. High HBEGF expression was found to be associated with a short interval of OS (Fig. 10c). Although TNBC with higher expression of BHLHE40 tends to have a shorter interval of OS, this correlation did not reach statistical significance (Fig. 10c).

These findings suggest that activation of the BHLHE40-HBEGF pathway contributes to aggressive behaviors of TNBC and chemoresistance.

Discussion

Breast cancer metastasis is the major cause of death in breast cancer patients. Adaptation to hypoxia is a driving

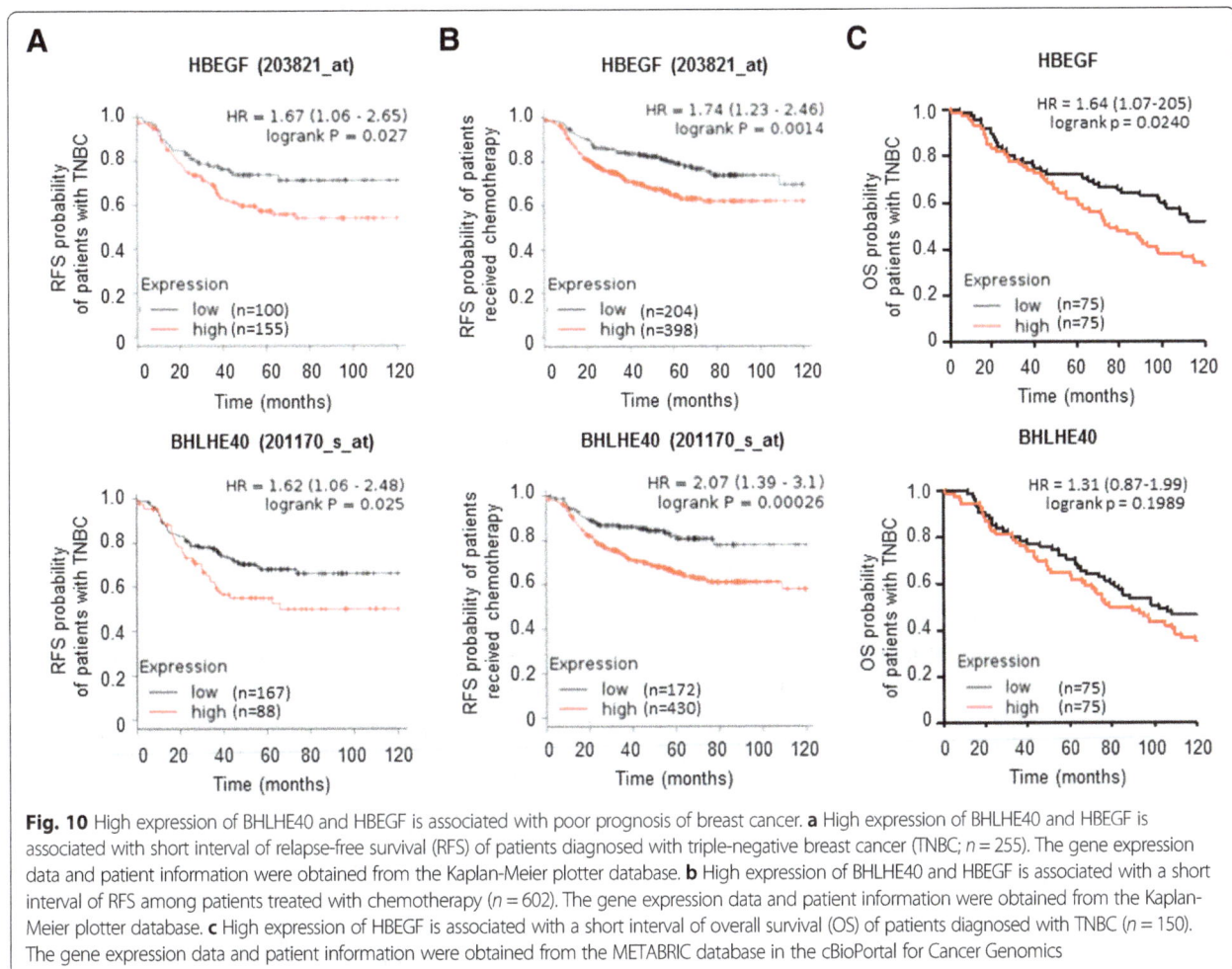

Fig. 10 High expression of BHLHE40 and HBEGF is associated with poor prognosis of breast cancer. **a** High expression of BHLHE40 and HBEGF is associated with short interval of relapse-free survival (RFS) of patients diagnosed with triple-negative breast cancer (TNBC; $n = 255$). The gene expression data and patient information were obtained from the Kaplan-Meier plotter database. **b** High expression of BHLHE40 and HBEGF is associated with a short interval of RFS among patients treated with chemotherapy ($n = 602$). The gene expression data and patient information were obtained from the Kaplan-Meier plotter database. **c** High expression of HBEGF is associated with a short interval of overall survival (OS) of patients diagnosed with TNBC ($n = 150$). The gene expression data and patient information were obtained from the METABRIC database in the cBioPortal for Cancer Genomics

force of metastatic progression and drug resistance [3]. Proteins secreted by tumor cells under hypoxia promote metastasis by altering tumor cell behaviors and modifying the tumor microenvironment [2]. Therefore, the regulation of hypoxia-driven protein secretion is currently under intense investigation. In this study, we report a novel role of BHLHE40, a transcription factor directly targeted by HIF1A, in regulating exosomic release of HBEGF. Our results suggest that the HIF-BHLHE40-HBEGF axis constitutes an important signaling mechanism to promote metastasis of breast tumors.

Exosomes are 40- to 100-nm vesicles that originate from the endocytic compartment. Exosomes contain a wide range of proteins, lipids, mRNAs, and microRNAs (miR-NAs) that reflect the molecular contents of the parental cells [32]. Compared with normal cells, cancer cells exhibit higher activity of exosome secretion, which is further augmented by stress conditions including TP53 activation, alteration of intracellular calcium levels, senescence, hypoxia, and acidosis [38]. Exosomes released by tumor cells have been reported to contain cytokines and growth factors that promote metastasis and chemoresistance [38–40].

However, the precise molecular mechanism governing the release of exosomes remains elusive. This study suggests that BHLHE40 acts as a key downstream effector of HIFs to activate transcription and subsequent exosome secretion of a set of cytokines and growth factors.

BHLHE40 was previously described as a transcriptional repressor that binds to the class B E-box (CACGTG) and recruits HDAC1 and HDAC2 to block transcription [41]. BHLHE40 activation has been linked to cell cycle arrest, senescence, differentiation, and apoptosis [42–44]. On the other hand, emerging evidence supports a role for BHLHE40 in transcription activation and promoting cell survival. For instance, BHLHE40 was reported to activate transcription of pro-survival factors in tumor cells, including BIRC5 and DeltaNp63 [45, 46]. In addition, BHLHE40 was reported to activate the transcription of a panel of cytokines required for activation of murine CD4$^+$ T cells [47, 48]. Which factors determine the selectivity of BHLHE40 to suppress or activate transcription remains undefined. The BHLHE40-mediated transcription activation of Del-taNp63 was shown to depend on its direct interaction with HDAC2 [45]. In agreement with this observation, our results suggest that BHLHE40 activates HBEGF transcription by sequestering HDAC1/2 from DNA binding. It remains to be determined whether interfering with HDAC1/2-DNA binding is a general mechanism responsible for BHLHE40-mediated transcription activation.

Elevated EGFR activation is known to promote survival, proliferation, and invasion of tumor cells under hypoxia, and multiple mechanisms have been linked to hypoxia-induced EGFR activation [49]. For example, EPAS1 activation by hypoxia was shown to increase EGFR mRNA translation [50]. Hypoxia-mediated activation of metalloproteases (e.g., ADAM12 and ADAM17) was reported to activate EGFR by increasing ectodomain shedding of HBEGF [51, 52]. Our study provides a novel aspect of EGFR activation through the BHLHE40-HBEGF axis. In addition to autocrine or paracrine effects within tumor cells, exosomic release of HBEGF might exert paracrine effects to remodel tumor stroma or endocrine effects to prime distant metastatic niches [53].

In conclusion, this study provides evidence supporting an essential role of BHLHE40 in exosomic release of HBEGF, a critical pro-survival and pro-metastasis factor. The clinical relevance of our findings is evidenced by the fact that the elevated expression of BHLHE40 and HBEGF in breast tumors is associated with poor prognosis of patients with TNBC and chemoresistance. Therapeutic intervention targeting the BHLHE40-HBEGF axis may represent an effective approach to combat hypoxia-driven drug resistance and metastasis.

Conclusion

Hypoxia-induced activation of BHLHE40 plays a key role in promoting cell survival and metastasis by modulating exosomic secretion of HBEGF.

Abbreviations

BHLHE40: Basic helix-loop-helix family member E40; ChIP: Chromatin immunoprecipitation; CoIP: Co-immunoprecipitation; EGF: Epidermal growth factor; EGFR: Epidermal growth factor receptor; EV: Empty vectors; FR: Fulvestrant-resistant; GF: Glucose depletion; HBEGF: Heparin-binding epidermal growth factor; HDAC: Histone deacetylases; HIF: Hypoxia inducible factor; HIF-dKO: HIF1A and EPAS1 double knockout; IB: Immunoblotting; KD: Knockdown; KO: Knockout; LG: Low glucose; LM: Lung metastatic cell line derived from MDA-MB-231; NSG: NOD.Cg-Prkdcscid Il2rgtm1Wjl/SzJ; OS: Overall survival; qPCR: Quantitative polymerase chain reaction; RFS: Relapse-free survival; shRNA: Short hairpin RNA; TCGA: The Cancer Genome Atlas; TNBC: Triple-negative breast cancer; TR: Tamoxifen-resistant

Funding

This work was supported by a National Institutes of Health grant (CA197206 to MF).

Authors' contributions

AS carried out the majority of the experiments and drafted the manuscript. MB and RK participated in the cell-based assays and manuscript preparation. TNS, Z-HW, and LMP participated in experiment design and manuscript preparation. MF is responsible for the overall experiment design and manuscript preparation. All authors read and approved the final manuscript.

Competing interests

The authors declare that they have no competing interests.

References

1. Siegel RL, Miller KD, Jemal A. Cancer statistics, 2018. CA Cancer J Clin. 2018; 68(1):7–30.
2. Gilkes DM, Semenza GL, Wirtz D. Hypoxia and the extracellular matrix: drivers of tumour metastasis. Nat Rev Cancer. 2014;14(6):430–9.
3. Rankin EB, Giaccia AJ. Hypoxic control of metastasis. Science. 2016; 352(6282):175–80.
4. Petrova V, Annicchiarico-Petruzzelli M, Melino G, Amelio I. The hypoxic tumour microenvironment. Oncogenesis. 2018;7(1):10.
5. Sormendi S, Wielockx B. Hypoxia pathway proteins as central mediators of metabolism in the tumor cells and their microenvironment. Front Immunol. 2018;9:40.
6. Muz B, de la Puente P, Azab F, Azab AK. The role of hypoxia in cancer progression, angiogenesis, metastasis, and resistance to therapy. Hypoxia. 2015;3:83–92.
7. Semenza GL. The hypoxic tumor microenvironment: a driving force for breast cancer progression. Biochim Biophys Acta. 2016;1863(3):382–91.
8. Weidle HU, Birzele F, Kollmorgen G, RÜGer R. The multiple roles of exosomes in metastasis. Cancer Genomics Proteomics. 2017;14(1):1–16.
9. Harris DA, Patel SH, Gucek M, Hendrix A, Westbroek W, Taraska JW. Exosomes released from breast cancer carcinomas stimulate cell movement. PLoS One. 2015;10(3):e0117495.
10. O'Driscoll L. Expanding on exosomes and ectosomes in cancer. N Engl J Med. 2015;372(24):2359–62.
11. Melo SA, Sugimoto H, O'Connell JT, Kato N, Villanueva A, Vidal A, Qiu L, Vitkin E, Perelman LT, Melo CA, et al. Cancer exosomes perform cell-independent microRNA biogenesis and promote tumorigenesis. Cancer Cell. 2014;26(5):707–21.
12. King HW, Michael MZ, Gleadle JM. Hypoxic enhancement of exosome release by breast cancer cells. BMC Cancer. 2012;12:421.
13. Pawlus MR, Wang L, Hu CJ. STAT3 and HIF1alpha cooperatively activate HIF1 target genes in MDA-MB-231 and RCC4 cells. Oncogene. 2014;33(13):1670–9.
14. Villar D, Ortiz-Barahona A, Gomez-Maldonado L, Pescador N, Sanchez-Cabo F, Hackl H, Rodriguez BA, Trajanoski Z, Dopazo A, Huang TH, et al. Cooperativity of stress-responsive transcription factors in core hypoxia-inducible factor binding regions. PLoS One. 2012;7(9):e45708.
15. Miyazaki K, Kawamoto T, Tanimoto K, Nishiyama M, Honda H, Kato Y. Identification of functional hypoxia response elements in the promoter region of the DEC1 and DEC2 genes. J Biol Chem. 2002;277(49):47014–21.
16. Khurana P, Sugadev R, Jain J, Singh SB. HypoxiaDB: a database of hypoxia-regulated proteins. Database (Oxford). 2013;2013:bat074.
17. Xiong J, Yang H, Luo W, Shan E, Liu J, Zhang F, Xi T, Yang J. The anti-metastatic effect of 8-MOP on hepatocellular carcinoma is potentiated by the down-regulation of bHLH transcription factor DEC1. Pharmacol Res. 2016;105:121–33.
18. Wu Y, Sato F, Yamada T, Bhawal UK, Kawamoto T, Fujimoto K, Noshiro M, Seino H, Morohashi S, Hakamada K, et al. The BHLH transcription factor DEC1 plays an important role in the epithelial-mesenchymal transition of pancreatic cancer. Int J Oncol. 2012;41(4):1337–46.
19. Chakrabarti J, Turley H, Campo L, Han C, Harris AL, Gatter KC, Fox SB. The transcription factor DEC1 (stra13, SHARP2) is associated with the hypoxic response and high tumour grade in human breast cancers. Br J Cancer. 2004;91(5):954–8.

20. Nakashima A, Kawamoto T, Honda KK, Ueshima T, Noshiro M, Iwata T, Fujimoto K, Kubo H, Honma S, Yorioka N, et al. DEC1 modulates the circadian phase of clock gene expression. Mol Cell Biol. 2008;28(12):4080–92.

21. Nishiyama Y, Goda N, Kanai M, Niwa D, Osanai K, Yamamoto Y, Senoo-Matsuda N, Johnson RS, Miura S, Kabe Y, et al. HIF-1alpha induction suppresses excessive lipid accumulation in alcoholic fatty liver in mice. J Hepatol. 2012;56(2):441–7.

22. Chung SY, Kao CH, Villarroya F, Chang HY, Chang HC, Hsiao SP, Liou GG, Chen SL. Bhlhe40 represses PGC-1alpha activity on metabolic gene promoters in myogenic cells. Mol Cell Biol. 2015;35(14):2518–29.

23. Kanda M, Yamanaka H, Kojo S, Usui Y, Honda H, Sotomaru Y, Harada M, Taniguchi M, Suzuki N, Atsumi T, et al. Transcriptional regulator Bhlhe40 works as a cofactor of T-bet in the regulation of IFN-gamma production in iNKT cells. Proc Natl Acad Sci U S A. 2016;113(24):E3394–402.

24. Fan M, Krutilina R, Sun J, Sethuraman A, Yang CH. Wu Z-h, Yue J, Pfeffer LM: comprehensive analysis of microRNA (miRNA) targets in breast cancer cells. J Biol Chem. 2013;288(38):27480–93.

25. Fan M, Yan PS, Hartman-Frey C, Chen L, Paik H, Oyer SL, Salisbury JD, Cheng AS, Li L, Abbosh PH, et al. Diverse gene expression and DNA methylation profiles correlate with differential adaptation of breast cancer cells to the antiestrogens tamoxifen and fulvestrant. Cancer Res. 2006;66(24):11954–66.

26. Sethuraman A, Brown M, Seagroves TN, Wu ZH, Pfeffer LM, Fan M. SMARCE1 regulates metastatic potential of breast cancer cells through the HIF1A/PTK2 pathway. Breast Cancer Res. 2016;18(1):81.

27. Patsialou A, Wang Y, Lin J, Whitney K, Goswami S, Kenny PA, Condeelis JS. Selective gene-expression profiling of migratory tumor cells in vivo predicts clinical outcome in breast cancer patients. Breast Cancer Res. 2012;14(5):R139.

28. Krutilina R, Sun W, Sethuraman A, Brown M, Seagroves TN, Pfeffer LM, Ignatova T, Fan M. MicroRNA-18a inhibits hypoxia-inducible factor 1alpha activity and lung metastasis in basal breast cancers. Breast Cancer Res. 2014;16(4):R78.

29. Whelan KA, Schwab LP, Karakashev SV, Franchetti L, Johannes GJ, Seagroves TN, Reginato MJ. The oncogene HER2/neu (ERBB2) requires the hypoxia-inducible factor HIF-1 for mammary tumor growth and anoikis resistance. J Biol Chem. 2013;288(22):15865–77.

30. Cancer Genome Atlas N. Comprehensive molecular portraits of human breast tumours. Nature. 2012;490(7418):61–70.

31. Ciriello G, Gatza ML, Beck AH, Wilkerson MD, Rhie SK, Pastore A, Zhang H, McLellan M, Yau C, Kandoth C, et al. Comprehensive molecular portraits of invasive lobular breast cancer. Cell. 2015;163(2):506–19.

32. Keerthikumar S, Chisanga D, Ariyaratne D, Al Saffar H, Anand S, Zhao K, Samuel M, Pathan M, Jois M, Chilamkurti N, et al. ExoCarta: a web-based compendium of exosomal cargo. J Mol Biol. 2016;428(4):688–92.

33. Yáñez-Mó M, Siljander PRM, Andreu Z, Zavec AB, Borràs FE, Buzas EI, Buzas K, Casal E, Cappello F, Carvalho J, et al. Biological properties of extracellular vesicles and their physiological functions. J Extracellular Vesicles. 2015;4. https://doi.org/10.3402/jev.v3404.27066.

34. Yáñez-Mó M, Siljander PR, Andreu Z, Zavec AB, Borràs FE, Buzas EI, Buzas K, Casal E, Cappello F, Carvalho J, et al. Biological properties of extracellular vesicles and their physiological functions. J Extracell Vesicles. 2015;4:27066.

35. Prenzel N, Zwick E, Daub H, Leserer M, Abraham R, Wallasch C, Ullrich A. EGF receptor transactivation by G-protein-coupled receptors requires metalloproteinase cleavage of proHB-EGF. Nature. 1999;402(6764):884–8.

36. Rubin JS, Chan AM, Bottaro DP, Burgess WH, Taylor WG, Cech AC, Hirschfield DW, Wong J, Miki T, Finch PW, et al. A broad-spectrum human lung fibroblast-derived mitogen is a variant of hepatocyte growth factor. Proc Natl Acad Sci U S A. 1991;88(2):415–9.

37. Gyorffy B, Lanczky A, Eklund AC, Denkert C, Budczies J, Li Q, Szallasi Z. An online survival analysis tool to rapidly assess the effect of 22,277 genes on breast cancer prognosis using microarray data of 1,809 patients. Breast Cancer Res Treat. 2010;123(3):725–31.

38. Atretkhany KSN, Drutskaya MS, Nedospasov SA, Grivennikov SI, Kuprash DV. Chemokines, cytokines and exosomes help tumors to shape inflammatory microenvironment. Pharmacol Ther. 2016;168:98–112.

39. Kucharzewska P, Christianson HC, Welch JE, Svensson KJ, Fredlund E, Ringner M, Morgelin M, Bourseau-Guilmain E, Bengzon J, Belting M. Exosomes reflect the hypoxic status of glioma cells and mediate hypoxia-dependent activation of vascular cells during tumor development. Proc Natl Acad Sci U S A. 2013;110(18):7312–7.

40. Keerthikumar S, Gangoda L, Liem M, Fonseka P, Atukorala I, Ozcitti C, Mechler A, Adda CG, Ang CS, Mathivanan S. Proteogenomic analysis reveals exosomes are more oncogenic than ectosomes. Oncotarget. 2015;6(17):15375–96.

41. St-Pierre B, Flock G, Zacksenhaus E, Egan SE. Stra13 homodimers repress transcription through class B E-box elements. J Biol Chem. 2002;277(48):46544–51.

42. Bhawal UK, Sato F, Arakawa Y, Fujimoto K, Kawamoto T, Tanimoto K, Ito Y, Sasahira T, Sakurai T, Kobayashi M, et al. Basic helix-loop-helix transcription factor DEC1 negatively regulates cyclin D1. J Pathol. 2011;224(3):420–9.

43. Seino H, Wu Y, Morohashi S, Kawamoto T, Fujimoto K, Kato Y, Takai Y, Kijima H. Basic helix-loop-helix transcription factor DEC1 regulates the cisplatin-induced apoptotic pathway of human esophageal cancer cells. Biomed Res. 2015;36(2):89–96.

44. Bi H, Li S, Qu X, Wang M, Bai X, Xu Z, Ao X, Jia Z, Jiang X, Yang Y, et al. DEC1 regulates breast cancer cell proliferation by stabilizing cyclin E protein and delays the progression of cell cycle S phase. Cell Death Dis. 2015;6:e1891.

45. Qian Y, Jung YS, Chen X. DeltaNp63, a target of DEC1 and histone deacetylase 2, modulates the efficacy of histone deacetylase inhibitors in growth suppression and keratinocyte differentiation. J Biol Chem. 2011;286(14):12033–41.

46. Li Y, Xie M, Yang J, Yang D, Deng R, Wan Y, Yan B. The expression of antiapoptotic protein survivin is transcriptionally upregulated by DEC1 primarily through multiple sp1 binding sites in the proximal promoter. Oncogene. 2006;25(23):3296–306.

47. Martinez-Llordella M, Esensten JH, Bailey-Bucktrout SL, Lipsky RH, Marini A, Chen J, Mughal M, Mattson MP, Taub DD, Bluestone JA. CD28-inducible transcription factor DEC1 is required for efficient autoreactive CD4+ T cell response. J Exp Med. 2013;210(8):1603–19.

48. Cowley GS, Weir BA, Vazquez F, Tamayo P, Scott JA, Rusin S, East-Seletsky A, Ali LD, Gerath WF, Pantel SE, et al. Parallel genome-scale loss of function screens in 216 cancer cell lines for the identification of context-specific genetic dependencies. Sci Data. 2014;1:140035.

49. Chen Y, Henson ES, Xiao W, Huang D, McMillan-Ward EM, Israels SJ, Gibson SB. Tyrosine kinase receptor EGFR regulates the switch in cancer cells between cell survival and cell death induced by autophagy in hypoxia. Autophagy. 2016;12(6):1029–46.

50. Franovic A, Gunaratnam L, Smith K, Robert I, Patten D, Lee S. Translational up-regulation of the EGFR by tumor hypoxia provides a nonmutational explanation for its overexpression in human cancer. Proc Natl Acad Sci U S A. 2007;104(32):13092–7.

51. Diaz B, Yuen A, Iizuka S, Higashiyama S, Courtneidge SA. Notch increases the shedding of HB-EGF by ADAM12 to potentiate invadopodia formation in hypoxia. J Cell Biol. 2013;201(2):279–92.

52. Wang XJ, Feng CW, Li M. ADAM17 mediates hypoxia-induced drug resistance in hepatocellular carcinoma cells through activation of EGFR/PI3K/Akt pathway. Mol Cell Biochem. 2013;380(1–2):57–66.

53. Yotsumoto F, Tokunaga E, Oki E, Maehara Y, Yamada H, Nakajima K, Nam SO, Miyata K, Koyanagi M, Doi K, et al. Molecular hierarchy of heparin-binding EGF-like growth factor-regulated angiogenesis in triple-negative breast cancer. Mol Cancer Res. 2013;11(5):506–17.

13

Evaluation of α-tubulin, detyrosinated α-tubulin, and vimentin in CTCs: identification of the interaction between CTCs and blood cells through cytoskeletal elements

G. Kallergi[1,2]* ⓘ, D. Aggouraki[1], N. Zacharopoulou[2], C. Stournaras[2], V. Georgoulias[1] and S. S. Martin[3]

Abstract

Background: Circulating tumor cells (CTCs) are the major players in the metastatic process. A potential mechanism of cell migration and invasion is the formation of microtentacles in tumor cells. These structures are supported by α-tubulin (TUB), detyrosinated α-tubulin (GLU), and vimentin (VIM). In the current study, we evaluated the expression of those cytoskeletal proteins in CTCs.

Methods: Forty patients with breast cancer (BC) (16 early and 24 metastatic) were enrolled in the study. CTCs were isolated using the ISET platform and stained with the following combinations of antibodies: pancytokeratin (CK)/VIM/TUB and CK/VIM/GLU. Samples were analyzed with the ARIOL platform and confocal laser scanning microscopy.

Results: Fluorescence quantification revealed that the ratios CK/TUB, CK/VIM, and CK/GLU were statistically increased in MCF7 compared with more aggressive cell lines (SKBR3 and MDA-MB-231). In addition, all of these ratios were statistically increased in MCF7 cells compared with metastatic BC patients' CTCs ($p = 0.0001$, $p = 0.0001$, and $p = 0.003$, respectively). Interestingly, intercellular connections among CTCs and between CTCs and blood cells through cytoskeleton bridges were revealed, whereas microtentacles were increased in patients with CTC clusters. These intercellular connections were supported by TUB, VIM, and GLU. Quantification of the examined molecules revealed that the median intensity of TUB, GLU, and VIM was significantly increased in patients with metastatic BC compared with those with early disease (TUB, 62.27 vs 11.5, $p = 0.0001$; GLU, 6.99 vs 5.29, $p = 0.029$; and VIM, 8.24 vs 5.38, $p = 0.0001$, respectively).

Conclusions: CTCs from patients with BC aggregate to each other and to blood cells through cytoskeletal protrusions, supported by VIM, TUB, and GLU. Quantification of these molecules could potentially identify CTCs related to more aggressive disease.

Keywords: CTCs, Microtentacles, α-Tubulin, Detyrosinated α-tubulin, Vimentin, Breast cancer, Cytoskeleton, Metastasis

Background

Metastasis, rather than the primary tumor, is mainly responsible for cancer-related death. The metastatic process is associated with the presence of circulating tumor cells (CTCs) and disseminated tumor cells in peripheral blood and bone marrow, respectively [1, 2]. CTCs hold stem and epithelial-to-mesenchymal transition (EMT) properties,

which are difficult to target with common chemotherapeutic agents [3–5]. The malignant nature of CTCs is supported by the presence of chromosomal alterations and by xenograft mouse models [6–9]. However, some of them are dormant or apoptotic [10, 11], and it seems that only a small proportion of CTCs are capable of forming overt tumor deposits [12].

CTCs are an extremely heterogeneous population; therefore, it is crucial to isolate and effectively characterize CTCs according to their tumorigenic capacity [12]. We have reported that CTCs express growth factor receptors and activated signaling kinases such as epidermal growth

* Correspondence: kalergi@med.uoc.gr
[1]Laboratory of Tumor Cell Biology, School of Medicine, University of Crete, Heraklion, Greece
[2]Department of Biochemistry, University of Crete, Greece Medical School, Heraklion, Greece
Full list of author information is available at the end of the article

factor receptor, human epidermal growth factor receptor 2 (HER2), phosphorylated phosphatidylinositol 3-kinase, p-AKT, and p-FAK [13, 14]. However, it has been shown that there are important phenotypic and biological discrepancies between CTCs and patients' primary tumors, implying that it is crucial to characterize these cells and use them as potential targets for cancer treatment [13, 15–17]. To this end, we have reported that it is possible to improve patients' outcomes by targeting CTCs rather than primary tumors and prevent tumor cell spreading [18].

A mechanism for metastatic dissemination is the formation of microtentacles. These cytoskeletal structures are supported by α-tubulin (TUB) and associated with the EMT pathways [19, 20]. Vimentin (VIM), Twist, and Snail are particularly upregulated in microtentacle-expressing cells. Furthermore, cancer cells with the capacity for cell migration and invasion are characterized by stem cell phenotype and microtentacle protrusions [19–24]. Detyrosinated α-tubulin (GLU) is another interesting characteristic of these cytoskeletal structures, considering the fact that GLU is a poor prognostic factor for patients with positive primary tumors [25].

Recent evidence indicates that common chemotherapeutic agents such as taxanes cause shedding of CTCs into the bloodstream, which can dramatically increase cancer spread and relapse [26, 27]. Taxanes can also increase microtentacles, promoting tumor cell reattachment [28]. However, other drugs such as kinesin inhibitors or curcumin can diminish microtentacles and inhibit tumor cell dissemination [22, 29].

The characterization of the microtentacles' structural proteins in isolated CTCs from patients with breast cancer (BC) has not been extensively addressed so far. The goal of the current study was to identify these molecules on isolated CTCs and to explore their potential interference with the metastatic process. Finally, we investigated possible implications of microtentacles in inter-CTC communication and in CTC-to-blood cell crosstalk.

Methods
Cell cultures
Three different BC cell lines, representative of distinct subtypes, were used to create an expression pattern of the assessed molecules: MCF7 (hormone receptor-positive [HR$^+$]), SKBR3 (HER2$^+$), and MDA-MB-231 (basal-like). All cell lines were obtained from the American Type Culture Collection (Manassas, VA, USA). The MCF7 cells were cultured in 1:1 (vol/vol) DMEM/Ham's F-12 medium (Life Technologies, Carlsbad, CA, USA) supplemented with 10% FBS (Life Technologies), 2 mM L-glutamine (Life Technologies) 30 mM NaHCOB$_{3B}$, 16 ng/ml insulin, and 50 mg/ml penicillin/streptomycin (Life Technologies). SKBR3 cells were cultured in McCoy's medium (Life Technologies)

enriched with 10% FBS and 2 mM L-glutamine supplemented with 50 mg/ml penicillin/streptomycin. MDA-MB-231 cells were cultured in high-glucose DMEM (Life Technologies) with 10% FBS and 2 mM L-glutamine supplemented with 50 mg/ml penicillin/streptomycin. Cells were maintained in a humidified atmosphere of 5% CO_2/95% air. Subcultivation for all cell lines was performed with 0.25% trypsin and 5 mM ethylenediaminetetraacetic acid (EDTA). All experiments were performed during the logarithmic growth phase. For spiking experiments, various dilutions (10 cells/ml, 100 cells/ml, and 1000 cells/ml of blood) of cells from three cell lines were spiked in 10 ml of blood obtained from healthy blood volunteers.

Patients' blood samples
Peripheral blood (10 ml in EDTA) was obtained from 16 chemotherapy-naïve patients with early BC and 24 patients with metastatic disease, before the initiation of any line of treatment, according to the design of a previous study [30]. Patients without evidence of metastatic disease (stages I–II) were considered to have early BC, whereas patients with stage IV disease were included in the metastatic group. Most of the patients were postmenopausal (62.5% early and 58.3% metastatic) in both cohorts. The HR$^+$ type comprised 75% of adjuvant and 62.5% of metastatic subjects. Triple-negative tumors (HR$^-$HER2$^-$) were represented in 6.3% of the patients with early disease and in 25% with metastatic disease. Sixteen patients from the metastatic group were initially diagnosed with early and operable disease, and seven other patients were diagnosed with metastatic disease from the beginning of the study. All the patients' characteristics are shown in Table 1.

Blood samples were collected at the middle of vein puncture after the first 5 ml of blood were discarded in order to avoid contamination of the blood sample with epithelial cells from the skin during sample collection. This protocol was approved by the ethics and scientific committees of our institution, and all patients and healthy blood donors gave their informed consent to participate in the study.

ISET system isolation of circulating tumor cells
CTCs were isolated using the ISET (Isolation by SizE of Tumor cells) platform (Rarecells Diagnostics, Paris, France) according to the manufacturer's instructions. This isolation system was chosen because in a previous study it was shown that the ISET platform has a high recovery rate of tumor cells, regardless of the BC subtype [31]. Briefly, 10 ml of peripheral blood were diluted in 1:10 ISET buffer (Rarecells Diagnostics) for 10 min at room temperature (RT), and 100 ml of the diluted sample was filtered using a depression tab adjusted at −10 kPa. The membrane was dried for 2 h at RT and

Table 1 Patients' characteristics

Early disease (16 patients)		Metastatic disease (24 patients)	
Age, yr, median (range)	53 (33–77)	Age, yr, median (range)	58 (39–70)
	No. (%)		No. (%)
Menopausal status		Menopausal status	
Premenopausal	4 (25%)	Premenopausal	7 (29.2%)
Postmenopausal	10 (62.5%)	Postmenopausal	14 (58.3%)
Unknown	2 (12.5%)	Unknown	3 (12.5%)
Tumor size		Tumor size	
pT1	9 (56.3%)	pT1	4 (16.7%)
pT2	5 (31.3%)	pT2	12 (50%)
pT3	0 (0%)	pT3	4 (16.7%)
Unknown	2 (12.5%)	Unknown	4 (16.7%)
Lymph node status		Lymph node status	
Node-negative	4 (25%)	Node-negative	9 (37.5%)
Node-positive	11 (68.8%)	Node-positive	10 (41.7%)
Unknown	1 (6.3%)	Unknown	5 (20.8%)
Histologic grade		Histologic grade	
Grade 1	0 (0%)	Grade 1	0 (0%)
Grade 2	10 (62.5%)	Grade 2	12 (50%)
Grade 3	3 (18.8%)	Grade 3	9 (37.5%)
Grade 4		Grade 4	3 (12.5%)
Unknown	3 (18.8%)	Unknown	0 (0%)
Histologic subtype		Histologic subtype	
Ductal	12 (75%)	Ductal	17 (70.8)
Lobular	1 (6.3%)	Lobular	2 (8.3%)
Other	3 (18.8%)	Other	5 (20.8%)
ER/PR tumor status		ER/PR tumor status	
Positive	12 (75%)	Positive	15 (62.5%)
Negative	2 (12.5%)	Negative	6 (25%)
Unknown	2 (12.5%)	Unknown	3 (12.5%)
HER2 tumor status		HER2 tumor status	
Positive[a]	7 (43.8%)	Positive[a]	3 (12.5%)
Negative	6 (37.5%)	Negative	18 (75%)
Unknown	3 (18.8%)	Unknown	3 (12.5%)
$HR^+/HER2^-$	5 (31.3%)	$HR^+/HER2^-$	12 (50%)
$HR^+/HER2^+$	6 (37.5%)	$HR^+/HER2^+$	3 (12.5%)
$HR^-/HER2^+$	1 (6.3%)	$HR^-/HER2+$	0 (0%)
$HR^-/HER2^-$	1 (6.3%)	$HR^-/HER2^-$	6 (25%)
Unknown combination	3 (18.8%)	Unknown combination	3 (12.5%)
		Disease sites	
		1	8 (33.3%)
		2	11 (45.8%)
		≥ 3	4 (16.6%)
		Unknown	1 (4.2%)
		Predominantly visceral disease	

Table 1 Patients' characteristics *(Continued)*

Early disease (16 patients)	Metastatic disease (24 patients)	
	Yes	15 (62.5%)
	No	7 (29.1%)
	Unknown	2 (8.3%)
	Primary breast cancer	
	Adjuvant	16 (66.7%)
	Metastatic	7 (29.2%)
	Unknown	1 (4.2%)
	Line of treatment	
	First	8 (33.3%)
	Second	8 (33.3%)
	Third	3 (12.5%)
	Fourth or later	5 (20.8%)

Abbreviations: ER Estrogen receptor, *PR* Progesterone receptor, *HR* Hormone receptor, *HER2* Human epidermal growth factor receptor 2
[a]positive were considered all the patients with HER2 score +3 in immunohistochemistry staining or +2 with positive FISH

stored at −20 °C. Each membrane spot was used for identification of CTCs after immunostaining and fluorescence microscopy analysis.

Confocal laser scanning and Ariol system microscopy

The presence of CTCs on ISET spots was evaluated using A45-B/B3 mouse antibody (Micromet, Munich, Germany) detecting CK8, CK18, and CK19, along with CD45 antibody (common leukocyte antigen), in order to exclude possible ectopic expression of cytokeratins by hematopoietic cells. A patient was considered as CTC-positive only if she harvested CK$^+$/CD45$^-$ cells (Fig. 2d). In addition, the cytomorphological criteria followed by Meng et al. were also used in order to characterize a cell as CTCs [9].

Consequently, patients were analyzed for the expression of TUB, GLU, and VIM. Triple-staining experiments were performed with the following combinations of antibodies: CK/TUB/VIM and CK/GLU/VIM. The samples were subsequently evaluated using the Ariol system (Leica Biosystems, Buffalo Grove, IL, USA) and confocal laser scanning microscopy.

For CK/TUB/VIM immunofluorescence staining, spots were incubated with PBS for 5 min, and then cells were permeabilized with 2% Triton X-100 for 10 min. After 1 h blocking with PBS/10% FBS, cells were incubated with VIM antirabbit antibody (Santa Cruz Biotechnology, Santa Cruz, CA, USA), followed by Alexa Fluor 633 antirabbit secondary antibody (Life Technologies). Subsequently, samples were stained with TUB antimouse antibody (Sigma-Aldrich, Taufkirchen, Germany) and Alexa Fluor 555 antimouse secondary antibody (Life Technologies) for 45 min Zenon technology (fluorescein

isothiocyanate-conjugated immunoglobulin G1 [IgG1] antibody; Molecular Probes, Eugene, OR, USA) was used for CK detection with the A45-B/B3 antibody. Zenon antibodies were prepared within 30 min before use [16].

For triple-staining of CK/GLU/VIM, the same blocking and permeabilization procedures were followed, and the membranes were incubated with A45-B/B3 mouse antibody for 1 h. Consequently, after incubation for 45 min with the secondary antibody (Alexa Fluor 488 antimouse; Life Technologies), cells were stained with GLU antirabbit antibody (Abcam, Cambridge, MA, USA) overnight. Subsequently, cells were incubated with Alexa Fluor 633 antirabbit antibody. Finally, Zenon technology (Alexa Fluor 555-conjugated IgG1 antibody) was used for VIM staining (Santa Cruz Biotechnology). Positive controls were also included in each experiment, using the aforementioned cell lines spiked in healthy volunteers' blood, whereas negative controls were prepared by omitting the corresponding primary antibodies and incubating the cells with the matching IgG isotype bound to the corresponding fluorochrome. Each patient with at least one CTC belonging to a distinct phenotype was considered as positive for this phenotype.

Statistical analysis

The criteria for the evaluation of objective response rate (ORR) were according to RECIST 1.1 (Response Evaluation Criteria In Solid Tumors): tumor size, lymph node status, lesion number, and so forth [32]. Overall survival (OS) was defined as the time from entrance into the study until death from any cause. Progression-free survival (PFS) was defined as extending from study enrollment until disease relapse or death, whichever occurred first. Kaplan-Meier curves and Cox regression analysis for PFS and OS were compared using the log-rank test to provide a univariate assessment of the prognostic value of selected clinical risk factors. Variables that were found to be significant in univariate analysis were then entered in a stepwise multivariate Cox proportional hazards regression model to identify those with independent prognostic value. All statistical tests were performed at the 5% level of significance. IBM SPSS Statistics version 22 software (IBM, Armonk, NY, USA) was used for the analysis.

Results
Evaluation of TUB, GLU, and VIM in BC cell lines
The expression of TUB, GLU, and VIM in MCF7, SKBR3, and MDA-MB-231 cell lines was initially assessed with spiking experiments followed by ISET system isolation. Triple-staining experiments revealed that the ratios CK/TUB, CK/GLU, and CK/VIM were significantly increased in the well-differentiated HR$^+$ MCF7 cells compared with the more aggressive cell lines, such as SKBR3 and MDA-MB-231 (Table 2).

TUB intensity did not differ significantly among the cell lines. The highest GLU expression was observed in SKBR3 cells, where it was significantly different from MCF7 and MDA-MB-231 cells. VIM was extremely high in MDA-MB-231 cells compared with MCF7 and SKBR3 cells.

Microtentacles were observed mainly in MDA-MB-231 cells. We also noticed that coincubation of cancer cells with blood samples resulted in the appearance of cytoskeletal bridges between cancer and blood cells. This communication was observed mainly in SKBR3 and MDA-MB-231 spiked samples (Additional file 1: Figure S1).

Evaluation of TUB and CK/TUB ratio in CTCs isolated from patients with early and metastatic BC
CTCs were detected in 11 of 16 (68.8%) and 16 of 24 (66.7%) patients with early and metastatic BC, respectively. The mean and median numbers of CTCs per patient were 4.6 and 1 (range, 0–37), respectively, for early BC, whereas in metastatic subjects, the corresponding numbers were 59.5 and 1.5 (range, 0–1062). Triple-staining experiments (TUB/VIM/CK) and confocal laser scanning analysis revealed that CTCs contacted each other through cytoskeletal bridges (Fig. 1a–d, white arrows). In addition, they communicated with microtentacle connections with nearby blood cells. These inter-CTC bridges supported by TUB, VIM, and cytokeratin (Fig. 1a–d). However, microtentacles that connected CTCs to blood cells (Fig. 1e–h, white arrows) were mostly supported by TUB and VIM. Each patient with at least one TUB$^+$VIM$^+$CK$^+$ cell is considered as positive for this phenotype.

Ariol system analysis revealed that the phenotype (TUB$^+$VIM$^+$CK$^+$) prevailed in CTCs from patients with metastatic disease (8 of 16 CK$^+$ patients; 50%) compared with patients with early disease (2 of 11 CK$^+$ patients; 18.2%) (p = 0.058) (Fig. 2a). Conversely, the incidence of the TUB$^+$VIM$^-$CK$^+$ phenotype was not changed between the two groups (18.75% and 18.2%, respectively). The

Table 2 Expression of α-tubulin, detyrosinated α-tubulin, and vimentin in cell lines and circulating tumor cells

	Ratio CK/TUB	Tubulin	Ratio CK/GLU	GLU	Ratio CK/VIM	Vimentin
MCF7	5.46 ± 0.7	30.8 ± 3.5	20.41 ± 0.6	9.08 ± 0.3	42.22 ± 2.8	4.27 ± 0.5
SKBR3	1.49 ± 0.7	29.37 ± 6.6	12.49 ± 0.9	12.89 ± 0.7	31.34 ± 2.4	4.94 ± 0.4
MDA-MB 231	3.09 ± 0.4	26.19 ± 3.1	11.225 ± 0.7	8.045 ± 0.2	3.46 ± 0.8	28.87 ± 3.7
CTCs in patients with early breast cancer	4.58 ± 0.4	11.50 ± 0.4	15.5 ± 0.6	5.29 ± 0.6	14.33 ± 0.6	5.38 ± 0.3
CTCs in patients with metastatic breast cancer	1.75 ± 0.4	62.27 ± 18.7	15.28 ± 2.8	6.99 ± 0.4	8.05 ± 1.9	8.24 ± 1
t tests	p values					
MCF7 vs MD-MB231	0.002	0.307	0.0001	0.0001	0.002	0.001
MCF7 vs SKBR3	0.0001	0.463	0.0001	0.005	0.011	0.235
MCF7 vs CTCs early	0.038	0.0001	0.185	0.0001	0.002	0.022
MCF7 vs CTCs metastatic	0.0001	0.0001	0.0001	0.0001	0.003	0.000
MDA-MB231 vs SKBR3	0.032	0.344	0.446	0.001	0.0001	0.0001
MDA-MB231 vs CTCs early	0.332	0.0001	0.001	0.0001	0.0001	0.0001
MDA-MB231 vs CTCs metastatic	0.0001	0.0001	0.000	0.124	0.000	0.0001
SKBR3 vs CTCs early	0.036	0.010	0.001	0.0001	0.001	0.429
SKBR3 vs CTCs metastatic	0.282	0.0001	0.002	0.0001	0.0001	0.0001
CTCs early vs CTCs metastatic	0.0001	0.0001	0.937	0.029	0.007	0.0001

Abbreviations: CK Cytokeratin, *TUB* α-Tubulin, *GLU* Detyrosinated α-tubulin, *VIM* Vimentin, *CTCs* Circulating tumor cells

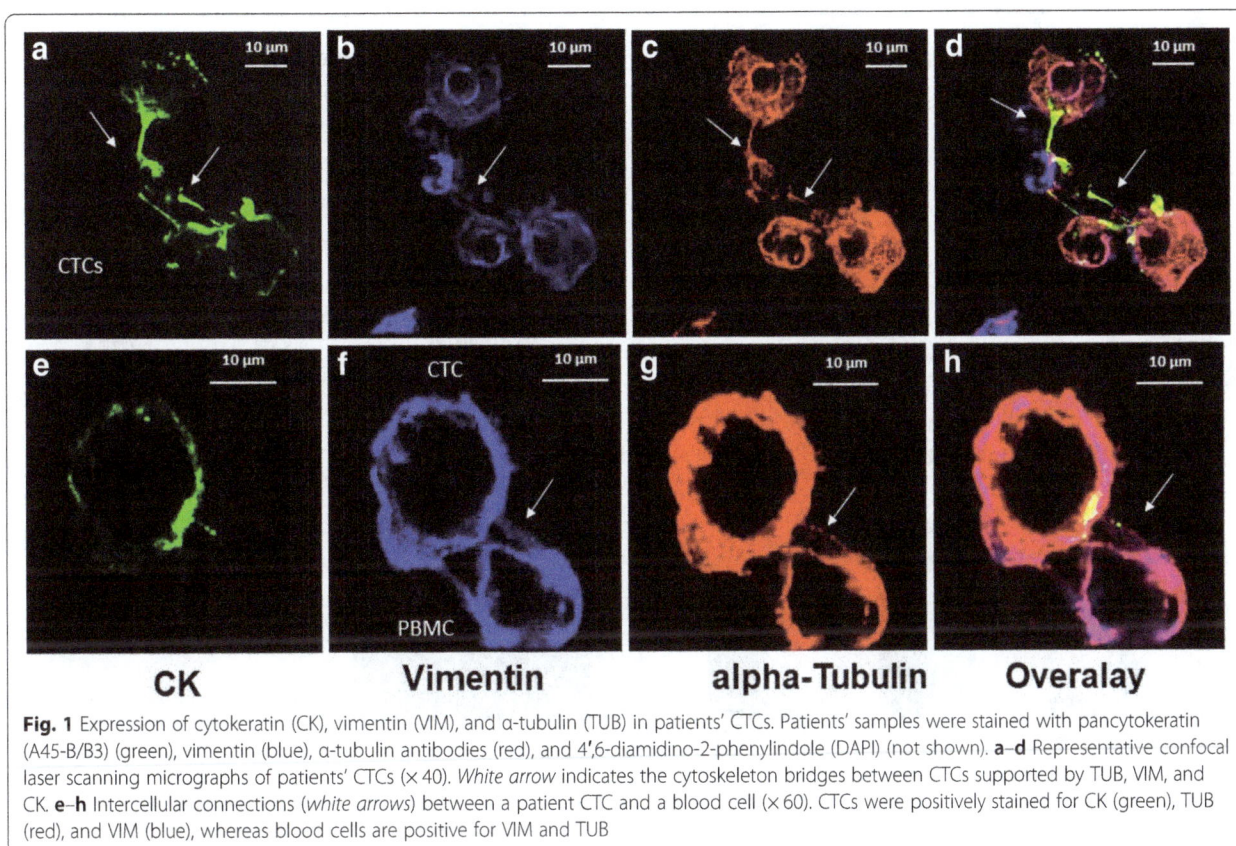

Fig. 1 Expression of cytokeratin (CK), vimentin (VIM), and α-tubulin (TUB) in patients' CTCs. Patients' samples were stained with pancytokeratin (A45-B/B3) (green), vimentin (blue), α-tubulin antibodies (red), and 4',6-diamidino-2-phenylindole (DAPI) (not shown). **a–d** Representative confocal laser scanning micrographs of patients' CTCs (× 40). *White arrow* indicates the cytoskeleton bridges between CTCs supported by TUB, VIM, and CK. **e–h** Intercellular connections (*white arrows*) between a patient CTC and a blood cell (× 60). CTCs were positively stained for CK (green), TUB (red), and VIM (blue), whereas blood cells are positive for VIM and TUB

absolute number of CTCs per patient for each distinct phenotype is shown in Table 3.

Quantification of TUB expression revealed statistically increased intensity in CTCs derived from patients with metastatic BC compared with all the examined cell lines (Table 2). Moreover, the intensity of TUB was statistically ($p = 0.0001$) lower in CTCs from patients with early BC (11.5 ± 0.4) compared with that observed in patients with metastatic disease (62.27 ± 18.7) (Table 2, Fig. 2b). Furthermore, the ratio CK/TUB was statistically lower ($p = 0.0001$) in metastatic patients' samples (1.75 ± 0.4) compared with the MCF7 (5.46 ± 0.7) and MDA-MB-231 (3.09 ± 0.4) cell lines (Table 2).

The ratio of CK/TUB was significantly higher in CTCs detected in patients with early BC compared with that observed in CTCs from patients with metastatic disease (4.58 ± 0.4 vs 1.75 ± 0.4; $p = 0.0001$) (Table 2; Fig. 2c).

The distribution of all the CTCs regarding TUB intensity and CK/TUB ratio in both groups compared with MCF7, SKBR3, and MDA-MB-231 is shown in Additional files 2 and 3: Figures S2a, b and S3a, b, respectively.

Evaluation of GLU and CK/GLU ratio in patients with early and metastatic BC

Our results revealed that GLU participates in intercellular connections among patients' CTCs (Fig. 3).

GLU was expressed in a high percentages of patients with early and metastatic BC. The GLU⁺VIM⁺CK⁺ phenotype could be identified in 54.5% (6 of 11) of patients with early BC and in 62.5% of patients with metastatic disease (10 of 16) (Fig. 2a). In addition, GLU⁺VIM⁻CK⁺) CTCs could be detected in both patients with early BC (2 of 11 patients; 18.2%) and patients with metastatic disease (6 of 16 patients; 37.5%) ($p = 0.69$). Conversely, the phenotypes without GLU expression prevailed in an adjuvant setting compared with metastatic BC (GLU⁻VIM⁺CK⁺) (27.3% [3 of 11] vs 13% [2 of 16; $p = 0.357$]). In addition, the GLU⁻VIM⁻CK⁺ phenotype was detected in 36.36% (4 of 11) of patients with early BC and in 13.33% (2 of 16) with metastatic disease ($p = 0.357$) (Fig. 2a).

The ratio CK/GLU was significantly higher in MCF7 cells (20.41 ± 0.6; $p = 0.0001$) than in CTCs from patients with metastatic BC (15.28 ± 2.8) (Table 2). Median intensity of GLU per patient was significantly increased in patients with metastatic BC compared with patients with early disease (5.29 ± 0.6 in early vs 6.99 ± 0.4 in metastatic setting; $p = 0.029$) (Fig. 2b); however, the ratio of CK/GLU (Fig. 2c) did not reach statistical significance (15.5 ± 0.6 vs 15.28 ± 2.8; $p = 0.937$). The distribution of all the CTCs regarding GLU intensity and CK/GLU

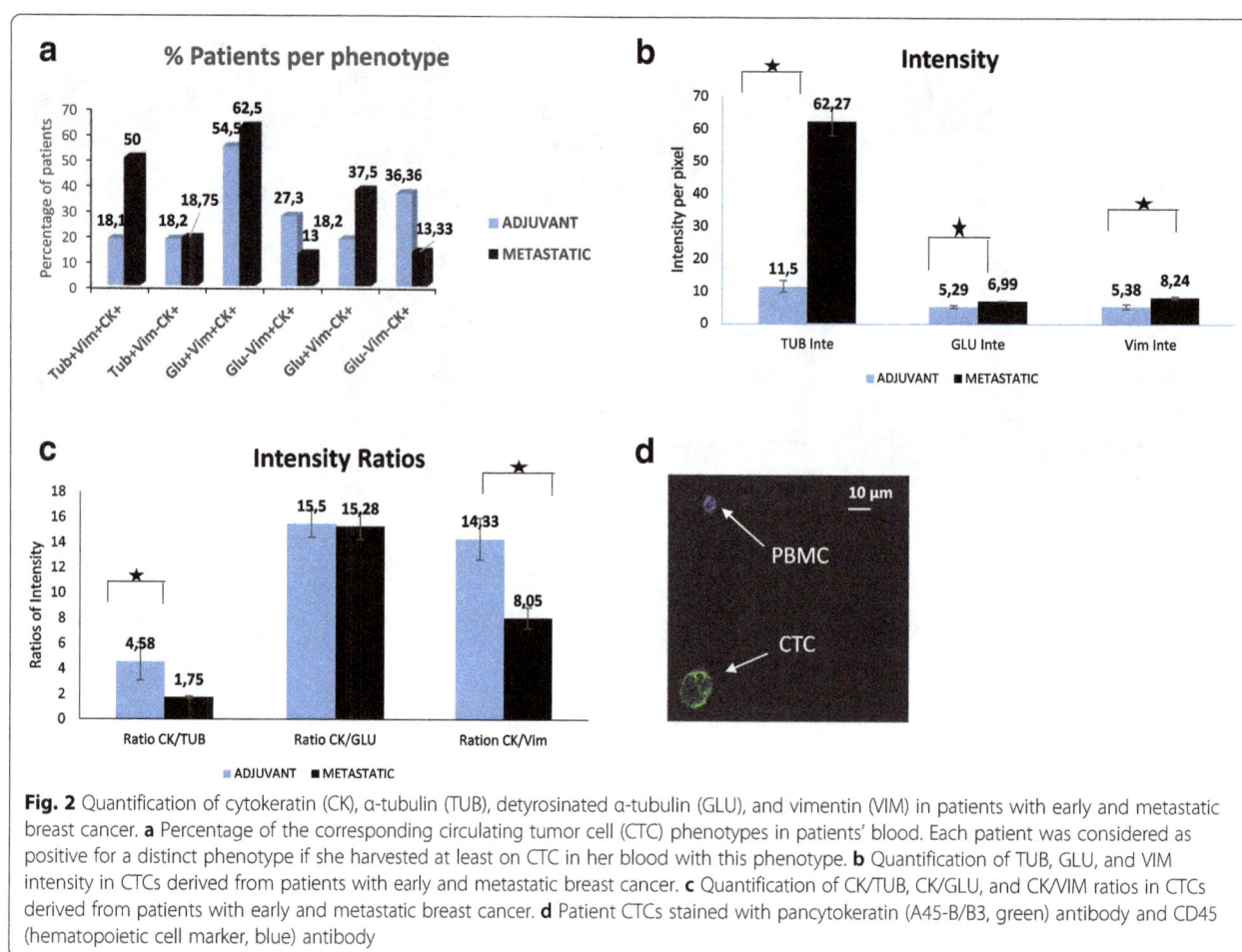

Fig. 2 Quantification of cytokeratin (CK), α-tubulin (TUB), detyrosinated α-tubulin (GLU), and vimentin (VIM) in patients with early and metastatic breast cancer. **a** Percentage of the corresponding circulating tumor cell (CTC) phenotypes in patients' blood. Each patient was considered as positive for a distinct phenotype if she harvested at least on CTC in her blood with this phenotype. **b** Quantification of TUB, GLU, and VIM intensity in CTCs derived from patients with early and metastatic breast cancer. **c** Quantification of CK/TUB, CK/GLU, and CK/VIM ratios in CTCs derived from patients with early and metastatic breast cancer. **d** Patient CTCs stained with pancytokeratin (A45-B/B3, green) antibody and CD45 (hematopoietic cell marker, blue) antibody

ratio is shown in Additional files 2 and 3: Figures S2c, d and S3c, d.

Evaluation of VIM and CK/VIM ratio in patients with early and metastatic BC

The intensity of VIM in CTCs detected in patients with metastatic BC (8.24 ± 1) was statistically higher than in MCF7 (4.27 ± 0.5; $p = 0.0001$) and SKBR3 (4.94 ± 0.4; $p = 0.0001$) cells (Table 2). In addition, the intensity of VIM in patients with early (5.38 ± 0.3; $p = 0.022$) and metastatic disease (8.24 ± 1; $p = 0.0001$) was also significantly higher than in MCF7 cells (Table 2). Mann-Whitney analysis also revealed significantly increased VIM expression in CTCs from patients with metastatic BC (8.24 ± 1) compared with early disease (5.38 ± 0.3) ($p = 0.0001$) (Fig. 2b).

CK/VIM ratio was lower in CTCs, regardless of disease stage, than in MCF7 cells (Table 2). In addition, the CK/VIM ratio was significantly lower (Fig. 2c) in patients with metastatic BC (8.05 ± 1.9) than in those with early disease (14.33 ± 0.6, $p = 0.007$).

There was also a positive correlation between the CK/TUB and CK/GLU ratios in CTCs (Spearman's correlation analysis; $p = 0.011$). In addition, there was a positive correlation between CTC phenotypes TUB+VIM+CK+ and GLU+VIM+CK+ ($p = 0.001$) in patients with metastatic BC. Moreover, as shown in Table 3, only one patient with metastatic BC and one in the early BC group harvested both GLU+VIM+CK+ and GLU−VIM+CK+ CTCs in their blood. Conversely, in the rest of the patients, all the CTCs were either positive or negative for these phenotypes. The distribution of all the CTCs regarding VIM intensity and CK/VIM ratio identified in both settings is shown in Additional file 2: Figure S2e and f and Figure S4e and f).

Evaluation of TUB, GLU, and VIM in sequential samples from a patient with BC

During this study, one patient with early BC relapsed and developed metastatic disease. Therefore, it was possible to analyze two different blood draws during the course of the disease. The first blood sample was obtained before any clinical or imaging evidence of relapse, whereas the second corresponded to the time of documentation of metastatic disease. In accordance with our previous observations, TUB's intensity in CTCs was statistically increased in the metastatic sample ($p = 0.002$)

Table 3 Number of circulating tumor cells per phenotype in each patient

Patients	TUB$^+$VIM$^+$CK$^+$	TUB$^+$VIM$^-$CK$^+$	GLU$^+$VIM$^+$CK$^+$	GLU$^-$VIM$^+$CK$^+$	GLU$^+$VIM$^-$CK$^+$	GLU$^-$VIM$^-$CK$^+$
Patients with early breast cancer						
1	0	13	8	0	16	0
2	0	0	0	0	0	0
3	0	0	0	0	0	0
4	1	0	12	0	4	0
5	1	0	1	0	0	0
6	0	0	0	2	0	0
7	0	0	1	0	0	3
8	0	1	0	0	0	1
9	0	0	0	1	0	0
10	0	0	0	0	0	1
11	0	0	0	0	0	0
12	0	0	0	0	0	0
13	0	0	0	0	0	1
14	0	0	1	0	0	0
15	0	0	0	0	0	0
16	0	0	1	5	0	0
Patients with metastatic breast cancer						
1	531		531	0	0	0
2	3	2	2	9	0	0
3	193	0	35	0	19	0
4	0	5	0	0	0	8
5	0	0	0	0	0	0
6	0	3	7	0	3	0
7	0	0	0	0	0	0
8	0	0	0	0	0	0
9	0	0	0	0	0	0
10	0	0	0	0	1	0
11	1	0	0	0	0	0
12	0	0	6	0	0	0
13	1	0	2	0	0	0
14	7	0	7	0	0	
15	0	0	0	0	0	0
16	0	0	0	0	0	0
17	16	0	7	0	7	
18	0	0	0	0	1	0
19	0	0	0	0	0	0
20	0	0	0	1	0	0
21	0	0	0	0	0	0
22	0	0	3	0	0	0
23	0	0	13	0	2	0
24	1	0	0	0	0	1

Abbreviations: CK Cytokeratin, *TUB* α-Tubulin, *GLU* Detyrosinated α-tubulin, *VIM* Vimentin

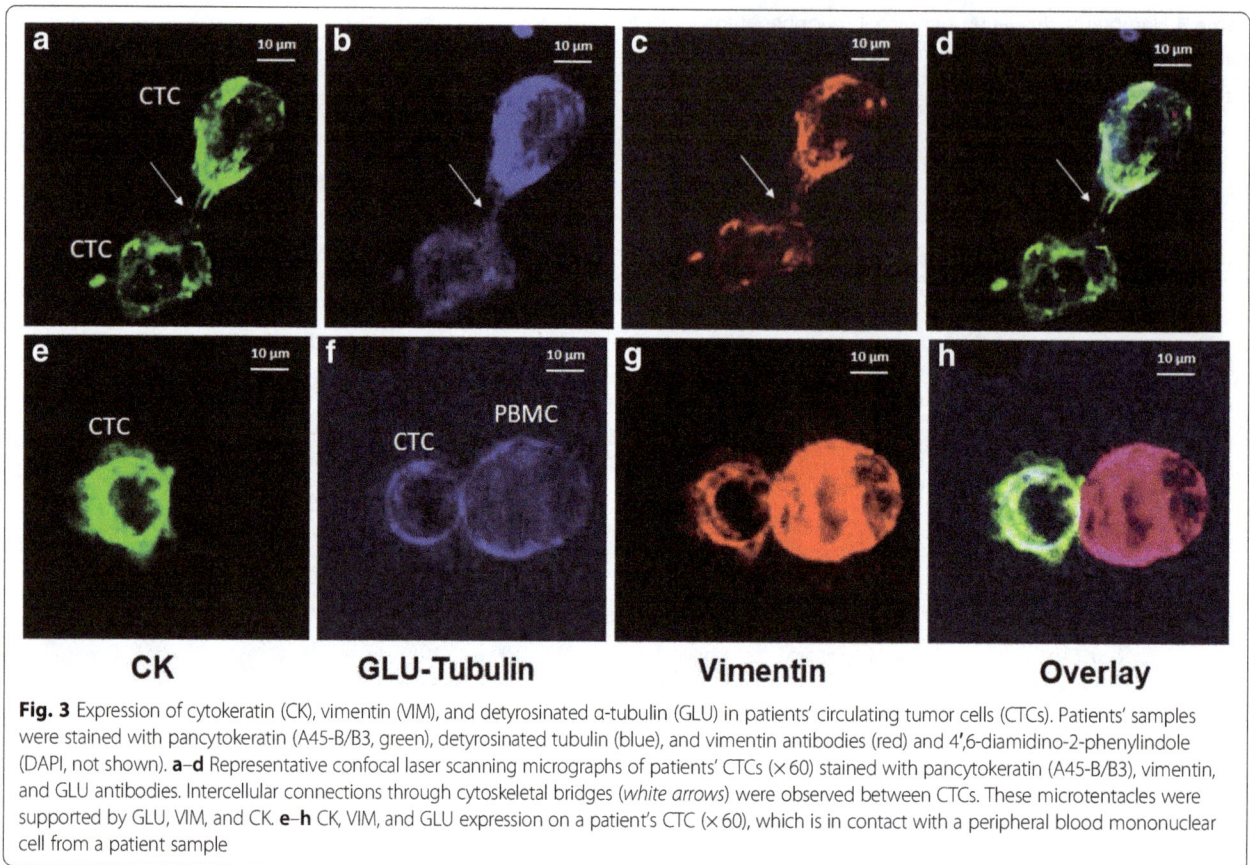

Fig. 3 Expression of cytokeratin (CK), vimentin (VIM), and detyrosinated α-tubulin (GLU) in patients' circulating tumor cells (CTCs). Patients' samples were stained with pancytokeratin (A45-B/B3, green), detyrosinated tubulin (blue), and vimentin antibodies (red) and 4',6-diamidino-2-phenylindole (DAPI, not shown). **a–d** Representative confocal laser scanning micrographs of patients' CTCs (×60) stained with pancytokeratin (A45-B/B3), vimentin, and GLU antibodies. Intercellular connections through cytoskeletal bridges (*white arrows*) were observed between CTCs. These microtentacles were supported by GLU, VIM, and CK. **e–h** CK, VIM, and GLU expression on a patient's CTC (×60), which is in contact with a peripheral blood mononuclear cell from a patient sample

(Fig. 4Ia). In addition, the CK/TUB ratio was progressively statistically reduced ($p = 0.003$) (Fig. 4Id). Similarly, the intensity of GLU expression in CTCs was statistically increased ($p = 0.002$) between baseline and the time of relapse (Fig. 4Ib). The ratio CK/GLU was not significantly altered ($p = 0.076$) (Fig. 4Ie). Finally, there was also a statistical increase in VIM expression in CTCs ($p = 0.011$) when the patient's BC became metastatic (Fig. 4Ic). The CK/VIM ratio was also statistically decreased ($p = 0.01$), between the first and the second sample draws (Fig. 4If).

CTC phenotypic profile and clinical outcome

Although this study was a small pilot study and the results regarding clinical outcome are only exploratory, we analyzed the available clinical data from 22 of 24 patients with metastatic BC enrolled in this study. After a median follow-up of 8 months (range, 0–21), six patients (25%) had died. Three of them presented with overt metastasis at the time of initial diagnosis, whereas the rest presented with early BC. Patients who died during the follow-up harbored more CTCs (mean, 15; median, 9.5; range, 0–54) than survivors (mean, 2.31; median, 1; range, 0–15); however, survival analysis for total CTCs per patient (Cox regression $p = 0.142$, Kaplan-Meier $p = 0.124$) did not show statistical differences in patient outcomes. On the other hand, survival analysis regarding distinct phenotypes revealed that median PFS was 3.0 months for the patients with detectable GLU+VIM+CK+-expressing CTCs compared with 7.5 months for patients who did not have detectable CTCs with this phenotype ($p = 0.004$) (Fig. 4IIa). Similarly, patients with detectable GLU−VIM+CK+-expressing CTCs had a median PFS of 1.0 month compared with 7.0 months for patients who did not have detectable CTCs with this phenotype ($p = 0.007$) (Fig. 4IIb).

Finally, the ORR was significantly lower in patients with TUB+VIM+CK+-expressing CTCs compared with patients without CTCs bearing this phenotype ($p = 0.046$). Moreover, the ORR was significantly lower in patients with metastatic disease who had CTCs with high numbers of microtentacles (5 of 16 patients with CK+) ($p = 0.019$). The criteria for the evaluation of ORR were according to RECIST 1.1: tumor size, lymph node status, lesion number, and so forth [32].

Discussion

It is widely accepted that although CTCs hold a crucial role in the metastatic process, the changes occurring during disease evolution on these cells are not fully characterized yet. CTCs hold significant prognostic value for patients with both early and metastatic BC [33–35]. It is also well known that microtentacles are increased in

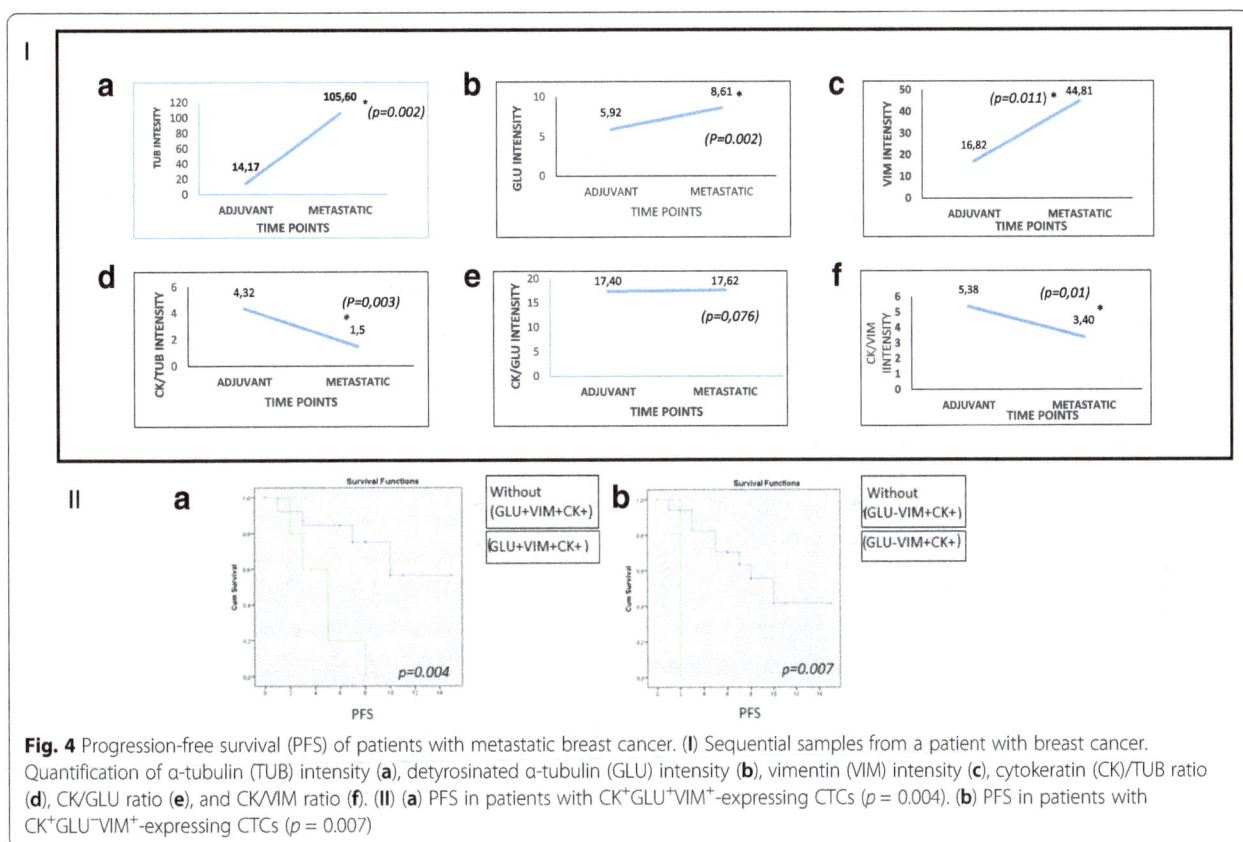

Fig. 4 Progression-free survival (PFS) of patients with metastatic breast cancer. (**I**) Sequential samples from a patient with breast cancer. Quantification of α-tubulin (TUB) intensity (**a**), detyrosinated α-tubulin (GLU) intensity (**b**), vimentin (VIM) intensity (**c**), cytokeratin (CK)/TUB ratio (**d**), CK/GLU ratio (**e**), and CK/VIM ratio (**f**). (**II**) (**a**) PFS in patients with CK⁺GLU⁺VIM⁺-expressing CTCs ($p = 0.004$). (**b**) PFS in patients with CK⁺GLU⁻VIM⁺-expressing CTCs ($p = 0.007$)

aggressive BC cells compared with less invasive phenotypes [19]. Microtentacles are supported by TUB, GLU, and VIM [19, 20]. In the current study, we investigated the presence of those filamentous protrusions in CTCs isolated from early and metastatic patients with BC. Moreover, the expression of the implicated molecules was quantified, and their association with the patients' clinical outcomes was assessed.

Our experiments revealed that microtentacles supported by TUB could be detected in patients early BC but mainly in those with metastatic BC. Interestingly, patients with increased numbers of microtentacle-presenting CTCs experienced a significantly lower ORR than patients with a low number of microtentacles ($p = 0.019$), suggesting that their tumors were more resistant to treatment. Furthermore, the results of the current study demonstrated that CTCs could contact each other (Figs. 1 and 3, white arrows) with filamentous protrusions supported by TUB, VIM, and GLU. These protrusions were also observed to connect CTCs with blood cells; however, in such junctions, only TUB and VIM were present, whereas CK expression was limited (Figs. 1 and 3). These findings are in agreement with previous observations in two other studies in which researchers reported that CTCs could be accompanied in the vessels by blood cells (giant macrophages) that seem to be associated

with an unfavorable clinical outcome [36, 37]. Therefore, our results could potentially explain how CTCs may travel in the bloodstream next to blood cells.

In our quantification of the ratios CK/TUB, CK/GLU, and CK/VIM in three representative subtypes of BC (MCF7 [HR⁺], SKBR3 [HER2⁺], and MDA-MB-231 [basal-like]), we observed that these ratios were statistically increased in MCF7 compared with SKBR3 and MDA-MB-231 cells. This suggests that they can be used as distinct markers to characterize less aggressive tumor cells, such as the HR⁺ subtype from more invasive phenotypes. In addition, microtentacles were observed mostly in MDA-MB-231 cells (Additional file 1: Figure S1). These findings support previous studies in that basal-like cell lines have increased numbers of microtentacles [38]. Furthermore, MDA-MB-231 cells have significantly higher levels of VIM intensity (28.87 ± 3.7) than other cell lines (Additional file 2: Figure S2, Table 2), in accordance with previously published data [39].

Characterization of CTCs on the basis of these markers clearly indicated that CK/TUB and TUB intensity were statistically different in early BC compared with the metastatic setting (Table 2), implying that during disease evolution, the level of TUB increases relative to cytokeratin intensity. This observation could be a useful tool for the characterization of CTCs with more aggressive features, mostly in patients with early BC, where the cells are very heterogeneous [12]. The analysis of sequential samples from a patient with BC during the early and metastatic stages of the disease confirmed the previous observations. Indeed, during the course of the disease, the expression of TUB was significantly increased (Fig. 4a), whereas the CK/TUB ratio was decreased (Fig. 4d). These results strongly suggest that follow-up samples regarding TUB expression in CTCs could potentially give useful information about disease relapse before the appearance of clinical and laboratory findings of overt metastasis.

VIM intensity was also statistically increased in the basal-like cell line MDA-MB-231 compared with HR$^+$ MCF7 cells (Table 2). Consequently, the ratio of CK/VIM was also decreased in the aggressive cell line compared with HR$^+$ cells (Table 2). These results imply that VIM is also characteristic of more aggressive phenotypes, in accordance with previous studies [39]. These observations were confirmed in patients' samples, indicating that VIM intensity was statistically increased in metastatic ($p = 0.0001$) compared with early disease, whereas the CK/VIM ratio was significantly decreased ($p = 0.007$) in patients with advanced BC (Table 2).

Furthermore, although the CK/GLU ratio did not reach statistical significance between early and metastatic disease (Table 2), the intensity of GLU was significantly higher ($p = 0.029$) in patients with metastatic BC than in those with early BC (Table 2). These findings strongly suggest that GLU can also be a marker characterizing invasive subpopulations. In accordance with this, the presence of the CK$^+$GLU$^+$VIM$^+$ phenotype in patients' blood was associated with worse PFS ($p = 0.004$), suggesting that both markers (GLU and VIM) could represent poor prognosis factors when coexpressed in patients' CTCs. Interestingly, the total number of CTCs did not correlate with prognosis in patients with metastatic BC, implying that the characterization of distinct phenotypes is critical for disease outcome, as we have previously shown [16]. This assumption is in line with previous studies regarding GLU expression in primary tumors [25]. However, this is a pilot study with a small number of patients; therefore, our results are only exploratory. A larger study with an increased number of patients is needed to confirm our observations.

It was also interesting that Spearman's correlation analysis revealed a correlation between CK/TUB and CK/GLU ratios ($p = 0.005$) in CTCs. In addition, CK/GLU ratio was also significantly correlated to CK/VIM ratio ($p = 0.011$), implying that all these markers can be used concomitantly to underline an aggressive signature of CTCs in patients with BC. Finally, it is noteworthy that all these molecules were present in the junctions among CTCs, mostly in patients with CTC clusters, and it is of interest that these patients have a 50-fold increased risk of relapse [40].

Conclusions

Microtentacles observed in CTCs isolated from patients with BC participate in the communication among CTCs and the interaction between CTCs and blood cells. The proteins that support these protrusions (TUB, VIM, and GLU) potentially represent markers for the identification of CTCs with a more aggressive phenotype in patients with BC; however, a study with a larger group of patients is necessary to further confirm the clinical relevance of these findings.

Additional files

Additional file 1: Figure S1. Expression of cytokeratin, vimentin, and α-tubulin on MCF7, SKBR3, and MDA-MB 231 cells spiked in normal blood and isolated with the ISET system. Representative confocal laser scanning micrographs of MCF7 (× 60), SKBR3 (× 40), and MDA-MB 231 (× 40) cells, triple-stained with pancytokeratin (A45-B/B3), vimentin, and α-tubulin antibodies. (JPG 117 kb)

Additional file 2: Figure S2. Single CTC distribution regarding TUB, VIM, and GLU intensity. TUB expression in CTCs obtained from patients with (**a**) early and (**b**) metastatic breast cancer. Each dot represents the intensity of one CTC. GLU expression in CTCs obtained from patients with (**c**) early and (**d**) metastatic breast cancer. Each dot represents the intensity of one CTC. VIM expression in CTCs obtained from patients with (**e**) early and (**f**) metastatic breast cancer. Each dot represents the intensity of one CTC. (JPG 122 kb)

Additional file 3: Single CTC distribution regarding CK/TUB, CK/VIM, and CK/GLU ratios. CK/TUB ratio in CTCs obtained from patients with (**a**) early and (**b**) metastatic breast cancer. Each dot represents the intensity of one CTC. CK/GLU ratio in CTCs obtained from patients with (**c**) early and (**d**) metastatic breast cancer. Each dot represents the intensity of one CTC. CK/VIM ratio in CTCs obtained from patients with (**e**) early and (**f**) metastatic breast cancer. Each dot represents the intensity of one CTC. (JPG 130 kb)

Abbreviations

CTC: Circulating tumor cell; EDTA: Ethylenediaminetetraacetic acid; EMT: Epithelial-to-mesenchymal transition; ER: Estrogen receptor; GLU: Detyrosinated α-tubulin; HER: Human epidermal growth factor receptor 2; HR: Hormone receptor; IgG1: Immunoglobulin G1; ORR: Objective response rate; OS: Overall survival; PFS: Progression-free survival; PR: Progesterone receptor; RT: Room temperature; TUB: α-Tubulin; VIM: Vimentin

Acknowledgements

The authors acknowledge the partial support of this work by the Hellenic Oncology Research Group (HORG).

Authors' contributions

GK participated in the design, coordination and supervision of the study and in the preparation of the manuscript. DA performed staining experiments and ISET isolations. NZ performed immunofluorescence experiments. CS provided general support and participated in study design and manuscript preparation. VG provided general support, participated in study design, and provided the clinical samples. SSM participated in study design and manuscript preparation. All authors read and approved the final manuscript.

Competing interests
The authors declare that they have no competing interests.

Author details
[1]Laboratory of Tumor Cell Biology, School of Medicine, University of Crete, Heraklion, Greece. [2]Department of Biochemistry, University of Crete, Greece Medical School, Heraklion, Greece. [3]Department of Physiology, Marlene and Stewart Greenebaum Comprehensive Cancer Center, University of Maryland School of Medicine, 655 W. Baltimore Street, Baltimore, MD, USA.

References
1. Braun S, Harbeck N. Molecular markers of metastasis in breast cancer: current understanding and prospects for novel diagnosis and prevention. Expert Rev Mol Med. 2001;3(22):1–14.
2. Pantel K, Muller V, Auer M, Nusser N, Harbeck N, Braun S. Detection and clinical implications of early systemic tumor cell dissemination in breast cancer. Clin Cancer Res. 2003;9(17):6326–34.
3. Kallergi G, Papadaki MA, Politaki E, Mavroudis D, Georgoulias V, Agelaki S. Epithelial to mesenchymal transition markers expressed in circulating tumour cells of early and metastatic breast cancer patients. Breast Cancer Res. 2011;13(3):R59.
4. Papadaki MA, Kallergi G, Zafeiriou Z, Manouras L, Theodoropoulos PA, Mavroudis D, Georgoulias V, Agelaki S. Co-expression of putative stemness and epithelial-to-mesenchymal transition markers on single circulating tumour cells from patients with early and metastatic breast cancer. BMC Cancer. 2014;14:651.
5. Aktas B, Tewes M, Fehm T, Hauch S, Kimmig R, Kasimir-Bauer S. Stem cell and epithelial-mesenchymal transition markers are frequently overexpressed in circulating tumor cells of metastatic breast cancer patients. Breast Cancer Res. 2009;11(4):R46.
6. Bozionellou V, Mavroudis D, Perraki M, Papadopoulos S, Apostolaki S, Stathopoulos E, Stathopoulou A, Lianidou E, Georgoulias V. Trastuzumab administration can effectively target chemotherapy-resistant cytokeratin-19 messenger RNA-positive tumor cells in the peripheral blood and bone marrow of patients with breast cancer. Clin Cancer Res. 2004;10(24):8185–94.
7. Fehm T, Sagalowsky A, Clifford E, Beitsch P, Saboorian H, Euhus D, Meng S, Morrison L, Tucker T, Lane N, et al. Cytogenetic evidence that circulating epithelial cells in patients with carcinoma are malignant. Clin Cancer Res. 2002;8(7):2073–84.
8. Hodgkinson CL, Morrow CJ, Li Y, Metcalf RL, Rothwell DG, Trapani F, Polanski R, Burt DJ, Simpson KL, Morris K, et al. Tumorigenicity and genetic profiling of circulating tumor cells in small-cell lung cancer. Nat Med. 2014;20(8):897–903.
9. Meng S, Tripathy D, Frenkel EP, Shete S, Naftalis EZ, Huth JF, Beitsch PD, Leitch M, Hoover S, Euhus D, et al. Circulating tumor cells in patients with breast cancer dormancy. Clin Cancer Res. 2004;10(24):8152–62.
10. Kallergi G, Konstantinidis G, Markomanolaki H, Papadaki MA, Mavroudis D, Stournaras C, Georgoulias V, Agelaki S. Apoptotic circulating tumor cells in early and metastatic breast cancer patients. Mol Cancer Ther. 2013;12(9):1886–95.
11. Spiliotaki M, Mavroudis D, Kapranou K, Markomanolaki H, Kallergi G, Koinis F, Kalbakis K, Georgoulias V, Agelaki S. Evaluation of proliferation and apoptosis markers in circulating tumor cells of women with early breast cancer who are candidates for tumor dormancy. Breast Cancer Res. 2014;16(6):485.
12. Klein CA, Blankenstein TJ, Schmidt-Kittler O, Petronio M, Polzer B, Stoecklein NH, Riethmuller G. Genetic heterogeneity of single disseminated tumour cells in minimal residual cancer. Lancet. 2002;360(9334):683–9.
13. Kallergi G, Mavroudis D, Georgoulias V, Stournaras C. Phosphorylation of FAK, PI-3K, and impaired actin organization in CK-positive micrometastatic breast cancer cells. Mol Med. 2007;13(1–2):79–88.
14. Kallergi G, Agelaki S, Kalykaki A, Stournaras C, Mavroudis D, Georgoulias V. Phosphorylated EGFR and PI3K/Akt signaling kinases are expressed in circulating tumor cells of breast cancer patients. Breast Cancer Res. 2008; 10(5):R80.
15. Agelaki S, Dragolia M, Markonanolaki H, Alkahtani S, Stournaras C, Georgoulias V, Kallergi G. Phenotypic characterization of circulating tumor cells in triple negative breast cancer patients. Oncotarget. 2017; 8(3):5309–22.
16. Kallergi G, Agelaki S, Papadaki MA, Nasias D, Matikas A, Mavroudis D, Georgoulias V. Expression of truncated human epidermal growth factor receptor 2 on circulating tumor cells of breast cancer patients. Breast Cancer Res. 2015;17:113.
17. Kalykaki A, Agelaki S, Kallergi G, Xyrafas A, Mavroudis D, Georgoulias V. Elimination of EGFR-expressing circulating tumor cells in patients with metastatic breast cancer treated with gefitinib. Cancer Chemother Pharmacol. 2014;73(4):685–93.
18. Georgoulias V, Bozionelou V, Agelaki S, Perraki M, Apostolaki S, Kallergi G, Kalbakis K, Xyrafas A, Mavroudis D. Trastuzumab decreases the incidence of clinical relapses in patients with early breast cancer presenting chemotherapy-resistant CK-19 mRNA-positive circulating tumor cells: results of a randomized phase II study. Ann Oncol. 2012;23(7):1744–50.
19. Whipple RA, Balzer EM, Cho EH, Matrone MA, Yoon JR, Martin SS. Vimentin filaments support extension of tubulin-based microtentacles in detached breast tumor cells. Cancer Res. 2008;68(14):5678–88.
20. Whipple RA, Matrone MA, Cho EH, Balzer EM, Vitolo MI, Yoon JR, Ioffe OB, Tuttle KC, Yang J, Martin SS. Epithelial-to-mesenchymal transition promotes tubulin detyrosination and microtentacles that enhance endothelial engagement. Cancer Res. 2010;70(20):8127–37.
21. Balzer EM, Whipple RA, Thompson K, Boggs AE, Slovic J, Cho EH, Matrone MA, Yoneda T, Mueller SC, Martin SS. C-Src differentially regulates the functions of microtentacles and invadopodia. Oncogene. 2010;29(48):6402–8.
22. Charpentier MS, Whipple RA, Vitolo MI, Boggs AE, Slovic J, Thompson KN, Bhandary L, Martin SS. Curcumin targets breast cancer stem-like cells with microtentacles that persist in mammospheres and promote reattachment. Cancer Res. 2014;74(4):1250–60.
23. Matrone MA, Whipple RA, Thompson K, Cho EH, Vitolo MI, Balzer EM, Yoon JR, Ioffe OB, Tuttle KC, Tan M, et al. Metastatic breast tumors express increased tau, which promotes microtentacle formation and the reattachment of detached breast tumor cells. Oncogene. 2010;29(22):3217–27.
24. Perry NA, Vitolo MI, Martin SS, Kontrogianni-Konstantopoulos A. Loss of the obscurin-RhoGEF downregulates RhoA signaling and increases microtentacle formation and attachment of breast epithelial cells. Oncotarget. 2014;5(18):8558–68.
25. Mialhe A, Lafanechere L, Treilleux I, Peloux N, Dumontet C, Bremond A, Panh MH, Payan R, Wehland J, Margolis RL, et al. Tubulin detyrosination is a frequent occurrence in breast cancers of poor prognosis. Cancer Res. 2001; 61(13):5024–7.
26. Hekimian K, Meisezahl S, Trompelt K, Rabenstein C, Pachmann K. Epithelial cell dissemination and readhesion: analysis of factors contributing to metastasis formation in breast cancer. ISRN Oncol. 2012;2012:601810.
27. Karagiannis GS, Pastoriza JM, Wang Y, Harney AS, Entenberg D, Pignatelli J, Sharma VP, Xue EA, Cheng E, D'Alfonso TM, et al. Neoadjuvant chemotherapy induces breast cancer metastasis through a TMEM-mediated mechanism. Sci Transl Med. 2017;9(397):eaan0026.
28. Balzer EM, Whipple RA, Cho EH, Matrone MA, Martin SS. Antimitotic chemotherapeutics promote adhesive responses in detached and circulating tumor cells. Breast Cancer Res Treat. 2010;121(1):65–78.
29. Yoon JR, Whipple RA, Balzer EM, Cho EH, Matrone MA, Peckham M, Martin SS. Local anesthetics inhibit kinesin motility and microtentacle protrusions in human epithelial and breast tumor cells. Breast Cancer Res Treat. 2011; 129(3):691–701.
30. Cristofanilli M, Budd GT, Ellis MJ, Stopeck A, Matera J, Miller MC, Reuben JM, Doyle GV, Allard WJ, Terstappen LW, et al. Circulating tumor cells, disease

progression, and survival in metastatic breast cancer. N Engl J Med. 2004; 351(8):781–91.

31. Kallergi G, Politaki E, Alkahtani S, Stournaras C, Georgoulias V. Evaluation of isolation methods for circulating tumor cells (CTCs). Cell Physiol Biochem. 2016;40(3–4):411–9.

32. Eisenhauer EA, Therasse P, Bogaerts J, Schwartz LH, Sargent D, Ford R, Dancey J, Arbuck S, Gwyther S, Mooney M, et al. New response evaluation criteria in solid tumours: revised RECIST guideline (version 1.1). Eur J Cancer. 2009;45(2):228–47.

33. Cristofanilli M, Hayes DF, Budd GT, Ellis MJ, Stopeck A, Reuben JM, Doyle GV, Matera J, Allard WJ, Miller MC, et al. Circulating tumor cells: a novel prognostic factor for newly diagnosed metastatic breast cancer. J Clin Oncol. 2005;23(7):1420–30.

34. Stathopoulou A, Vlachonikolis I, Mavroudis D, Perraki M, Kouroussis C, Apostolaki S, Malamos N, Kakolyris S, Kotsakis A, Xenidis N, et al. Molecular detection of cytokeratin-19-positive cells in the peripheral blood of patients with operable breast cancer: evaluation of their prognostic significance. J Clin Oncol. 2002;20(16):3404–12.

35. Xenidis N, Perraki M, Kafousi M, Apostolaki S, Bolonaki I, Stathopoulou A, Kalbakis K, Androulakis N, Kouroussis C, Pallis T, et al. Predictive and prognostic value of peripheral blood cytokeratin-19 mRNA-positive cells detected by real-time polymerase chain reaction in node-negative breast cancer patients. J Clin Oncol. 2006;24(23):3756–62.

36. Adams DL, Martin SS, Alpaugh RK, Charpentier M, Tsai S, Bergan RC, Ogden IM, Catalona W, Chumsri S, Tang CM, et al. Circulating giant macrophages as a potential biomarker of solid tumors. Proc Natl Acad Sci U S A. 2014; 111(9):3514–9.

37. Adams DL, Adams DK, Alpaugh RK, Cristofanilli M, Martin SS, Chumsri S, Tang CM, Marks JR. Circulating cancer-associated macrophage-like cells differentiate malignant breast Cancer and benign breast conditions. Cancer Epidemiol Biomarkers Prev. 2016;25(7):1037–42.

38. Boggs AE, Vitolo MI, Whipple RA, Charpentier MS, Goloubeva OG, Ioffe OB, Tuttle KC, Slovic J, Lu Y, Mills GB, et al. Alpha-tubulin acetylation elevated in metastatic and basal-like breast cancer cells promotes microtentacle formation, adhesion, and invasive migration. Cancer Res. 2015;75(1):203–15.

39. Flodrova D, Toporova L, Macejova D, Lastovickova M, Brtko J, Bobalova J. A comparative study of protein patterns of human estrogen receptor positive (MCF-7) and negative (MDA-MB-231) breast cancer cell lines. Gen Physiol Biophys. 2016;35(3):387–92.

40. Aceto N, Bardia A, Miyamoto DT, Donaldson MC, Wittner BS, Spencer JA, Yu M, Pely A, Engstrom A, Zhu H, et al. Circulating tumor cell clusters are oligoclonal precursors of breast cancer metastasis. Cell. 2014;158(5):1110–22.

14

Metformin inhibits stromal aromatase expression and tumor progression in a rodent model of postmenopausal breast cancer

Erin D. Giles[1]*[iD], Sonali Jindal[6], Elizabeth A. Wellberg[5], Troy Schedin[4], Steven M. Anderson[5], Ann D. Thor[5], Dean P. Edwards[8], Paul S. MacLean[2,3,5†] and Pepper Schedin[6,7†]

Abstract

Background: Obesity and type II diabetes are linked to increased breast cancer risk in postmenopausal women. Patients treated with the antidiabetic drug metformin for diabetes or metabolic syndrome have reduced breast cancer risk, a greater pathologic complete response to neoadjuvant therapy, and improved breast cancer survival. We hypothesized that metformin may be especially effective when targeted to the menopausal transition, as this is a lifecycle window when weight gain and metabolic syndrome increase, and is also when the risk for obesity-related breast cancer increases.

Methods: Here, we used an 1-methyl-1-nitrosourea (MNU)-induced mammary tumor rat model of estrogen receptor (ER)-positive postmenopausal breast cancer to evaluate the long-term effects of metformin administration on metabolic and tumor endpoints. In this model, ovariectomy (OVX) induces rapid weight gain, and an impaired whole-body response to excess calories contributes to increased tumor glucose uptake and increased tumor proliferation. Metformin treatment was initiated in tumor-bearing animals immediately prior to OVX and maintained for the duration of the study.

Results: Metformin decreased the size of existing mammary tumors and inhibited new tumor formation without changing body weight or adiposity. Decreased lipid accumulation in the livers of metformin-treated animals supports the ability of metformin to improve overall metabolic health. We also found a decrease in the number of aromatase-positive, CD68-positive macrophages within the tumor microenvironment, suggesting that metformin targets the immune microenvironment in addition to improving whole-body metabolism.

Conclusions: These findings suggest that peri-menopause/menopause represents a unique window of time during which metformin may be highly effective in women with established, or at high risk for developing, breast cancer.

Keywords: Obesity, Macrophage, Metabolism, Adipose, Tumor microenvironment, Liver

* Correspondence: egiles@tamu.edu
†Paul S. MacLean and Pepper Schedin contributed equally to this work.
[1]Department of Nutrition & Food Science, Texas A&M University, 373 Olsen Blvd; 2253 TAMU, College Station, TX 77843, USA
Full list of author information is available at the end of the article

Background

Obesity and type II diabetes are associated with an increased risk of breast cancer and poorer clinical prognosis, particularly in postmenopausal women. Over the past several years, many studies have reported decreased breast cancer incidence and/or mortality in diabetics receiving the widely prescribed antidiabetic drug metformin relative to those receiving other diabetic drugs [1–3]. Furthermore, these studies have found a dose-response relationship whereby women receiving the highest metformin dose for the longest duration show the most benefit [4, 5]. Despite the routine use of this drug, the anticancer mechanisms of metformin are not well understood. Additionally, some studies have failed to show a beneficial effect of metformin as an antitumor agent [6, 7]. Thus, there is ongoing interest in identifying patient populations who may benefit from metformin treatment, and the mechanisms by which metformin decreases cancer risk and/or improves tumor outcomes.

As a diabetic agent, metformin stabilizes glucose flux and reduces insulin resistance. It is used worldwide because of its low toxicity profile and low cost. Metformin activates AMP-dependent kinase (AMPK) to stimulate glucose uptake and glycogen synthesis, while suppressing gluconeogenesis, thereby improving whole-body insulin sensitivity. Beyond this, however, the exact mechanisms of action of metformin, even in diabetic patients, are not fully understood.

The antitumor activity of metformin has generally been attributed to its ability to decrease circulating insulin levels and improve whole-body metabolic health, as hyperinsulinemia has been associated with increased risk for breast cancer development, recurrence, and even death [8, 9]. There is also a growing body of literature to suggest that metformin may directly target both tumor cells and tumor stem cells [10–14]. These direct and indirect effects are not mutually exclusive, and it is possible that the effects of metformin involve a combination of the two.

Additional questions also remain regarding the patients and/or tumor subtypes for which metformin may be most effective. Preclinical studies suggest that at least some underlying whole-body metabolic dysfunction is needed to see beneficial effects of metformin, at least for breast cancer prevention [15, 16]. Clinical data to date are primarily derived from diabetic patients receiving metformin and, from the few clinical trials completed to date, it is unclear which patients benefit most [17–19]. The results of an ongoing clinical study are anticipated to shed light on this issue [20]. In-vitro studies have demonstrated potential therapeutic utility against all breast cancer cell lines tested, but there is emerging preclinical and clinical data suggesting that metformin may be more effective in treating specific tumor subtypes (reviewed in [21]). In cell lines, estrogen receptor (ER+) and tamoxifen-resistant breast cancers have been identified as a therapeutic target since metformin has been shown to inhibit the expression and function of ERα [12, 13]. Consistent with these in-vitro studies, a recent clinical study reported that metformin specifically benefits women with ER+ as well as human epidermal growth factor receptor 2 (HER2)-positive breast tumors [14]. Finally, we recently reported that tumor expression of organic cation transporter-2, which regulates metformin uptake, correlates with tumor responsiveness to metformin [22]. Thus, evidence suggests both host- and tumor-specific targets, and while understanding of the anti-cancer mechanisms of metformin are emerging, there are still many questions that remain unanswered. Here we focus on host biology, namely the metabolic dysregulation that occurs during the menopausal transition, as a potential window of increased metformin efficacy.

In a rodent model of ER+ postmenopausal breast cancer we have shown that, during ovariectomy (OVX)-induced weight gain, an impaired ability to clear excess nutrients from the circulation and store them in mammary adipose tissue correlated with tumor glucose uptake, markers of proliferation, and tumor progression [23]. Given these findings, we hypothesized that improving the whole-body metabolic response to excess calories during the window of weight gain that follows loss of ovarian function would decrease tumor growth and lead to improved tumor outcomes. We further hypothesized that both lean and obese animals would benefit from this treatment because they both experience overfeeding, rapid weight gain, and a decline in metabolic health in response to OVX [23, 24].

Here, we report that metformin effectively decreased mammary tumor burden in both obese and lean animals, and also prevented the formation of new tumors in the postmenopausal period. In addition to improving overall metabolic health, metformin also decreased the number of aromatase-positive, CD68-positive macrophages within the tumor microenvironment, suggesting a new role for metformin in targeting immune cells. We therefore propose that the menopause and the peri-menopausal window represent a unique opportunity for metformin therapy, specifically for women with existing ER+ tumors and/or those who may be at risk for the development of postmenopausal breast cancer.

Methods

Animal care and treatment

Female Wistar rats (100–125 g, 5 weeks of age) were purchased from Charles River Laboratories (Wilmington, MA) and housed at the University of Colorado Anschutz Medical Campus Center for Comparative Medicine (22–24 °C; 12-h/12-h light-dark cycle) with free access to water. All procedures were approved by the Institutional Animal Care and Use Committee.

Animal model

Our OP-OR/OVX model of obesity and postmenopausal breast cancer was used as previously described [25]. We and others have shown that tumors that develop using this method are similar to human breast tumors with regard to: 1) the percentage of tumors that are intraductal; 2) the progression of histologic stages from hyperplasia, to carcinoma in situ, to invasive cancer; and 3) steroid receptor status [23, 25–27].

To induce obesity in these genetically susceptible rats, animals were individually housed in wire-bottomed metabolic cages to limit physical activity, and were given ad libitum access to a purified high-fat diet (HF; 46% kcal fat; Research Diets, New Brunswick, NJ; RD# D12344) for the duration of the study. Animals were ranked by their rate of weight gain from 5 to 15 weeks of age. Rats in the top and bottom tertiles of weight gain were matured to produce obese and lean animals, respectively. Rats from the middle tertile were removed from the study.

To induced mammary tumor formation, 55-day-old female rats (± 1 day) were given a single injection of the carcinogen 1-methyl-1-nitrosourea (MNU; 50 mg/kg; #ASI-701, Ash Stevens, Detroit, MI). Tumors were monitored by manual palpation at weekly intervals for the duration of the study and measured in three dimensions using digital calipers.

Body weight and food intake were monitored weekly, as previously described [24, 28]. Body composition was determined on the day of OVX, 5 weeks post-OVX, and again at the time of sacrifice by quantitative magnetic resonance (qMR; EchoMRI Whole Body Composition Analyzer; Echo Medical Systems, Houston, TX).

Metformin treatment

In a rolling study design, animals were randomly assigned to either metformin treatment (2 mg/mL in the drinking water, $n = 7$ lean and $n = 10$ obese) or control group (water only, $n = 8$ lean and $n = 9$ obese) after at least one tumor in the animal reached a volume > 1 cm^3. Rats were maintained on their respective treatments for the duration of the study. This dose was chosen based on results of pilot studies that produced plasma metformin levels similar to those used clinically, and because this dose demonstrated antitumor efficacy in obese rats in our previous short-term studies, with no observable negative side effects [22, 23]. Metformin treatment was initiated 1 week prior to OVX surgery to assure drug bioavailability during the critical window of rapid weight gain that immediately follows OVX. One week following the initiation of metformin treatment, the animals underwent surgical ovariectomy (OVX) under isoflurane anesthesia to mimic the postmenopausal state. At the time of OVX, biopsies of mammary tumors were obtained via fine needle aspiration (FNA).

Plasma measurements

Tail vein blood was collected on the second diestrus day of the estrous cycle [24] during the week prior to OVX, at 5 weeks post-OVX, and again at the time of sacrifice. Blood was drawn during the latter part of the light cycle; plasma was isolated and stored at –80 °C until analyzed. Concentrations of insulin, leptin, amylin, and glucagon were simultaneously measured using the Rat Endocrine LINCOplex Kit 96 Well Plate Assay (RENDO-85 K; Millipore, St Charles, MO). Colorimetric assays were used to measure plasma free fatty acids (Wako Chemicals USA, Richmond, VA), glucose, triglycerides (TG), and total cholesterol (#TR15421, TR22321, and TR13521, respectively; Thermo Fisher Scientific, Waltham, MA).

Histological staining and imaging

Sections of formalin-fixed paraffin-embedded tissue (4 µm) were stained with hematoxylin and eosin (H&E) using a Sakura autostainer (Sakura Finetek, Torrance, CA). Mammary tumors were classified histologically by the criteria of Young and Hallowes [29], and only adenocarcinomas were included in subsequent analyses. For immunohistochemical detection of progesterone (PR)-positive cells, 4 µm mammary tissue sections were stained with mouse monoclonal αPR, clone 6F11 at 1:100 (Vector Laboratories, Burlingame, CA). The dual localization of CD68 and aromatase was performed by staining for CD68 (Ab4059, Serotec, 1:200 dilution) sequentially followed by a mouse monoclonal aromatase antibody (clone 677) at a 1:100 dilution. The 677 monoclonal antibody was generated in one of the author's laboratories (DPE) and has been validated extensively for specificity by immunohistochemistry (IHC) [30–33]. For CD68, mouse on rat secondary antibody (MRT621H, Biocare) for 30 mins was used followed by 3,3'-diaminobenzidine chromogen (DAB; K3467, Dako, Carpinteria, CA). The slides were sequentially stained with aromatase primary followed by Rat on mouse AP polymer (MALP521, Biocare) followed by Permanent red chromogen (K0640, Dako, Carpinteria, CA). The adipophilin primary antibody (LS-C348703, Lifespan Biosciences) was incubated on rat livers at 1:300 dilution for 60 min followed by mouse on rat secondary antibody (MRT621H, Biocare) for 30 min and DAB chromogen. Livers from lean and obese pre-OVX animals were obtained from a separate cohort of rats in which animals were terminated with the ovaries intact. All slides were counterstained with hematoxylin (S330130, Dako, Carpinteria, CA).

For mammary tumor ER and PR analysis, at least 11 tumors per group, and 8–10 fields/section (40× objective) were evaluated. Given the effectiveness of metformin in shrinking tumors in this study, the number of samples from metformin-treated rats with sufficient tissue to perform IHC analysis was limited; thus, for the

CD68 and aromatase IHC in tumors and adjacent tumor border, our analysis was restricted to tumors from obese control and metformin-treated rats. CD68 and aromatase stained slides were scanned using an Aperio Scanscope3 system (Aperio, Vista, CA) at 20× magnification, corresponding to 0.43 μm per pixel which enables high-resolution access to the entire tissue section via a virtual image. Images were evaluated using Imagescope software and the signal captured and quantitated using Aperio algorithms. For tumor border analysis, the tumor boundary was outlined on H&E stained slides using the Aperio Annotation tool within Leica Image Scope (Leica Technologies, CA) by an MD pathologist (SJ). The tumor boundary images were then exported and overlaid (imported) onto an adjacent serial section dual stained for CD68 and aromatase using the Export/Import tool within Leica Image Scope. The tumor border was then defined as 100 μm external to the tumor boundary and captured using the Aperio Ruler tool. The Aperio system was also used for liver adipophilin quantitation, where a minimum of nine livers per group were evaluated.

In-vitro macrophage differentiation

Rat macrophages were derived from a pooled bone marrow stock aspirated from femurs and tibias of 7-week-old female Wistar rats. Once isolated, marrow was cultured in vitro in Dulbecco's Modified Eagle's medium (DMEM) low glucose with 30% L929-cell conditioned media (as a source of macrophage colony-stimulating factor (M-CSF)) containing either 5 ng/mL lipopolysaccharide and 12 ng/mL interferon (IFN)-gamma to promote differentiation to an M1 phenotype, or 10 ng/mL interleukin (IL)-4 to promote an M2 phenotype. Following 48 h in differentiation medium, cells were rinsed twice with phosphate-buffered saline (PBS) and harvested in cell lysis buffer (50 mM Tris pH 7.4, 150 mM NaCl, 2.0 mM EDTA, 50 mM NaF, 5. 0 mM sodium orthovanadate, 1% Triton X-100, 1% deoxycholate, 0.1% SDS) supplemented with Halt™ Protease and Phosphatase Inhibitor cocktail (Thermo Scientific). Lysates were centrifuged for 20 min at 14,000 g, and total protein concentration of the supernatant was determined by BioRad protein assay according to the manufacturer's instructions.

ProteinSimple© Western blotting and analysis

Protein levels of aromatase in M1 and M2 macrophages were measured using the Simple Western size-based capillary electrophoresis system (WES, ProteinSimple, San Jose, CA). Two different anti-aromatase primary antibodies were used, including Novus NB100-1596 (1:50 dilution) and clone #677 used for the previously described IHC (1:25 dilution). All procedures were performed according to the manufacturer's protocol and immunodetection was conducted with default settings. Data were

analyzed with ProteinSimple Compass software. Additional controls included the use of a blocking peptide against aromatase antibody #1 (Novus NB100-1596PEP) to verify the band size and specificity using this antibody on the WES system, and the use of forskolin-treated steroidogenic human granulosa-like tumor cells (KGN cells) to induced aromatase expression as a positive control with aromatase antibody #2.

Statistical analysis

Data were examined with SPSS 24.0 software by ANOVA or χ^2 analysis for nominal and ordinal data, respectively. Relationships between variables were assessed with the Spearman correlation coefficient. In some cases, data were analyzed by analysis of covariance with a specified covariate in the model.

Results

Baseline rat characteristics

Body weights and adiposity

Body weight and adiposity were measured pre-OVX, during OVX-induced weight gain, and bi-weekly until the study end. As we have shown previously [23–25, 34, 35], at the time of OVX surgery, mature obese rats had higher body weight (434 ± 19 g vs 338 ± 7 g) due to both higher lean mass (253 ± 5 g vs 215 ± 4 g) and percent body fat ($31.9 \pm 1.8\%$ vs $25.9 \pm 1.4\%$) when compared with their lean counterparts (Fig. 1a, b). In response to OVX, all animals, independent of pre-OVX obesogenic status, experienced a transient surgery-induced weight loss, followed by a significant amount of weight gain, as previously reported for female rats (Fig. 1c) [23–25]. Metformin did not significantly affect food intake during either the early (first 4 weeks) or late (weeks 5–8) post-OVX period (Fig. 1d); thus, it was not surprising that we found no differences in weight gain between the metformin-treated and control groups (Fig. 1c). Finally, at the study end, obese rats remained heavier than their lean counterparts, with higher fat and lean mass, with no statistical differences between the metformin-treated and control animals (Fig. 1e).

Plasmas measures

Blood samples were obtained at several time points throughout the study to measure both metabolic factors (1 week prior to OVX and again at the end of the study) and plasma levels of metformin (at the time of OVX, and 6 weeks post-OVX). Prior to OVX, obese animals had higher circulating TG than lean animals (Table 1; $p < 0.05$). By the study end, at 8 weeks post-OVX, we found no differences in plasma glucose, free fatty acids, or cholesterol between the lean and obese groups, likely because all animals were consuming a HF diet, gaining weight, and had developed metabolic disease. After 1 week of metformin treatment (at the time of OVX), plasma metformin averaged 1.15 ± 0.

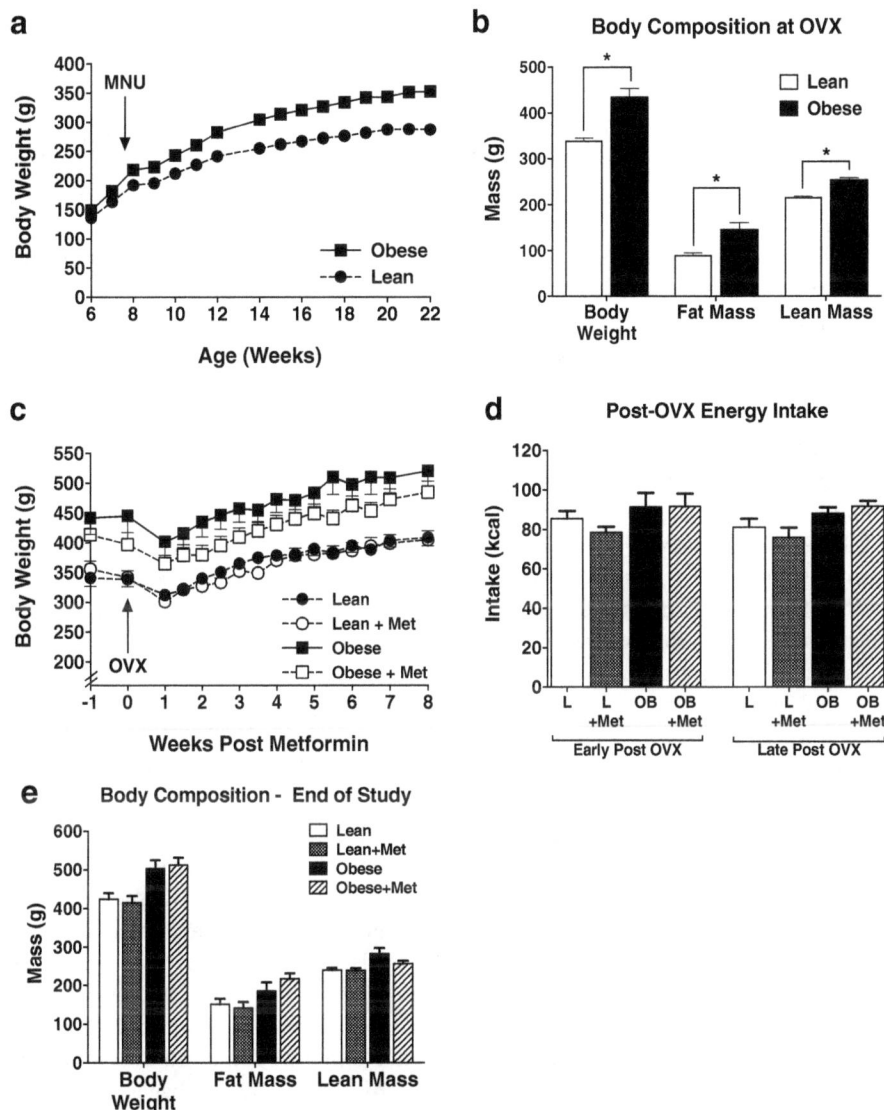

Fig. 1 Body weight, composition, and food intake. **a** Body weights across the pre-ovariectomy (OVX) period for rats selected as lean or obese. **b** At the time of OVX (when animals had at least 1 tumor > 1cm³), obese (OB) rats were significantly heavier than the lean (L) group, and this was due to both higher fat and lean mass. **c** Body weights for lean and obese rats, with and without metformin (Met) treatment (2 mg/mL in drinking water), across the post-OVX period. Metformin was started at time −1 week; OVX occurred at week 0. Body weight was measured twice per week for the first 6 weeks following OVX, then weekly for weeks 7–8. A brief surgery-induced weight loss was followed by OVX-induced weight gain in both lean and obese animals, with no difference between metformin-treated and untreated animals. **d** Food intake is reported as the mean intake measured over the early (first 4 weeks) and late (weeks 5–8) post-OVX period. Metformin had no significant effect on food intake. **e** Body weight, fat mass, and lean mass measured by qMR at the end of the study. Obese rats had significantly higher body weight, fat mass, and lean mass than lean rats ($p < 0.05$), but metformin had no significant effect on these measures. *$p < 0.05$. MNU, 1-methyl-1-nitrosourea

Table 1 Plasma characteristics prior to ovariectomy

	Lean	Obese
n	14	15
Glucose (mM)	5.74 ± 0.51	7.42 ± 0.51
Triglycerides (mM)	0.40 ± 0.05	0.78 ± 0.12*
Nonesterified fatty acids (µM)	536.8 ± 30.3	572.1 ± 42.0
Cholesterol (mM)	2.14 ± 0.09	2.33 ± 0.11

*$p < 0.05$

50 mg/mL, and this increased to 1.57 ± 0.47 mg/mL by 6 weeks. These levels are within the range reported in humans receiving daily metformin treatment [36, 37].

Host responses
Metformin modestly improves markers of metabolic function

Despite achieving clinically relevant levels of metformin in the circulation, the impact of metformin on plasma metabolites was minimal in this study. One week of metformin treatment (the week prior to OVX) did not significantly alter glucose, insulin, leptin, glucagon, cholesterol, or nonesterified fatty acid (NEFA) levels (Table 2). A caveat of these metabolic analyses is that the animals were not fasted when plasma samples were taken, and this, combined with the ad libitum consumption of a diet high in fat, may have masked our ability to detect metformin-induced changes in levels of these metabolic markers. Metformin treatment tended to decrease two markers suggestive of improved metabolic health, namely TG ($p = 0.058$) and amylin ($p = 0.095$), which works synergistically with insulin to contribute to glycemic control (Table 2).

Since accumulation of lipid in the liver reflects an overall decline in metabolic health, we assessed the impact of metformin treatment on hepatic lipid accumulation. To quantify hepatic lipid accumulation, two independent measures were used: 1) semi-quantitative IHC staining for adipophilin, a marker of lipid droplet accumulation; and 2) qMR analysis of the liver, which measures the gross lipid content of the tissue. Figure 2 shows representative images of adipophilin-stained livers from lean and obese rats, prior to OVX and following 8 weeks of OVX-induced weight gain with or without metformin treatment. Prior to OVX, both lean and obese rats have low to moderate hepatic adipophilin staining, data consistent with overall normal or healthy livers (Fig. 2a). However, adipophilin is significantly increased in the post-OVX livers, regardless of pre-OVX adiposity (Fig. 2b). Quantitative assessment of these IHC-based data support minimal differences in hepatic lipid accumulation between lean and obese rats prior to OVX (Fig. 2d), followed by an extensive increase in lipid deposition in the livers of all animals following OVX. These observations highlight the role OVX plays in metabolic dysregulation independent of pre-existing adiposity status. In support of improved metabolic health in metformin-treated animals, adipophilin staining decreased significantly with metformin treatment (Fig. 2c, e; $p < 0.05$). qMR analysis further supports this finding as the percent fat in the liver decreased by

Table 2 Plasma characteristics at ovariectomy (after 1 week of metformin treatment)

	Control	Metformin	p value
Glucose (mM)	7.65 ± 0.82	6.91 ± 0.50	
Insulin (mM)	5.74 ± 2.59	3.31 ± 2.11	
Leptin (mM)	4.22 ± 1.82	5.32 ± 2.26	
Glucagon (mM)	3.71 ± 0.91	2.03 ± 0.54	
Cholesterol (mM)	1.81 ± 0.09	1.73 ± 0.09	
Nonesterified fatty acids (µM)	650 ± 64	658 ± 49	
Triglycerides (mM)	0.79 ± 0.14	0.51 ± 0.05**	0.058
Amylin (mM)	1.80 ± 0.69	0.65 ± 0.19**	0.095

**$p < 0.10$

21% in metformin-treated animals compared to untreated controls (Fig. 2f). Together, these data show that OVX is associated with weight gain and hepatic lipid accumulation reflective of impaired metabolic health irrespective of pre-OVX obesity status. Treatment with metformin improves this marker of metabolic health when administered continuously across the menopausal (post-OVX) period.

Metformin decreases adipose tissue inflammation in post-OVX animals

The link between whole-body metabolic dysfunction and adipose tissue inflammation has been well established [38, 39], and work from our laboratory and others has suggested that inflammation induced by weight gain plays a role in promoting tumor growth [25, 40]. Thus, based on our finding that metformin decreased hepatic lipid accumulation, data consistent with improved whole-body metabolic health, we hypothesized that metformin may similarly alter mammary adipose tissue inflammation.

Crown-like structures, comprised of macrophages in close proximity to adipocytes, are a hallmark of chronic adipose tissue inflammation, and their presence in the mammary gland or breast has been associated with insulin resistance in both rodent and human studies [41]. In the breast, the macrophage marker CD68 has been used to identify crown-like structures that may otherwise be missed using H&E staining [42]. Thus, we quantified the number of CD68-positive (CD68+) cells in IHC-stained sections of mammary tissue from nontumor bearing mammary glands taken at the study end. We stratified animals into those with high versus low rates of weight gain during the post-OVX period, which are predicted to have high versus low inflammatory milieus, respectively. While we found no overall differences in the number of CD68+ macrophages associated with mammary ducts, alveoli, stroma, or blood vessels (Fig. 3a), metformin treatment in the high-weight-gain animals significantly decreased the number of adipose-associated macrophages forming crown-like structures (CLS) (Fig. 3b, c). Furthermore, in animals with low post-OVX weight gain, metformin had no effect on the number of adipose-associated CD68+ cells (36.8 ± 10.8 vs 25.7 ± 4.8, metformin vs control; $p = 0.321$), suggesting that metformin may be specifically effective at decreasing the inflammation induced by weight gain following OVX. The decrease in crown-like structures in metformin-treated high-weight-gain animals suggests that, in addition to improving whole-body metabolic function (liver data above), metformin also contributes to adipose-specific metabolic improvements. Combined, these studies support beneficial effects of metformin on both whole-body metabolic health and mammary adipose tissue inflammation, which we anticipated may underlie the antitumor effects of metformin.

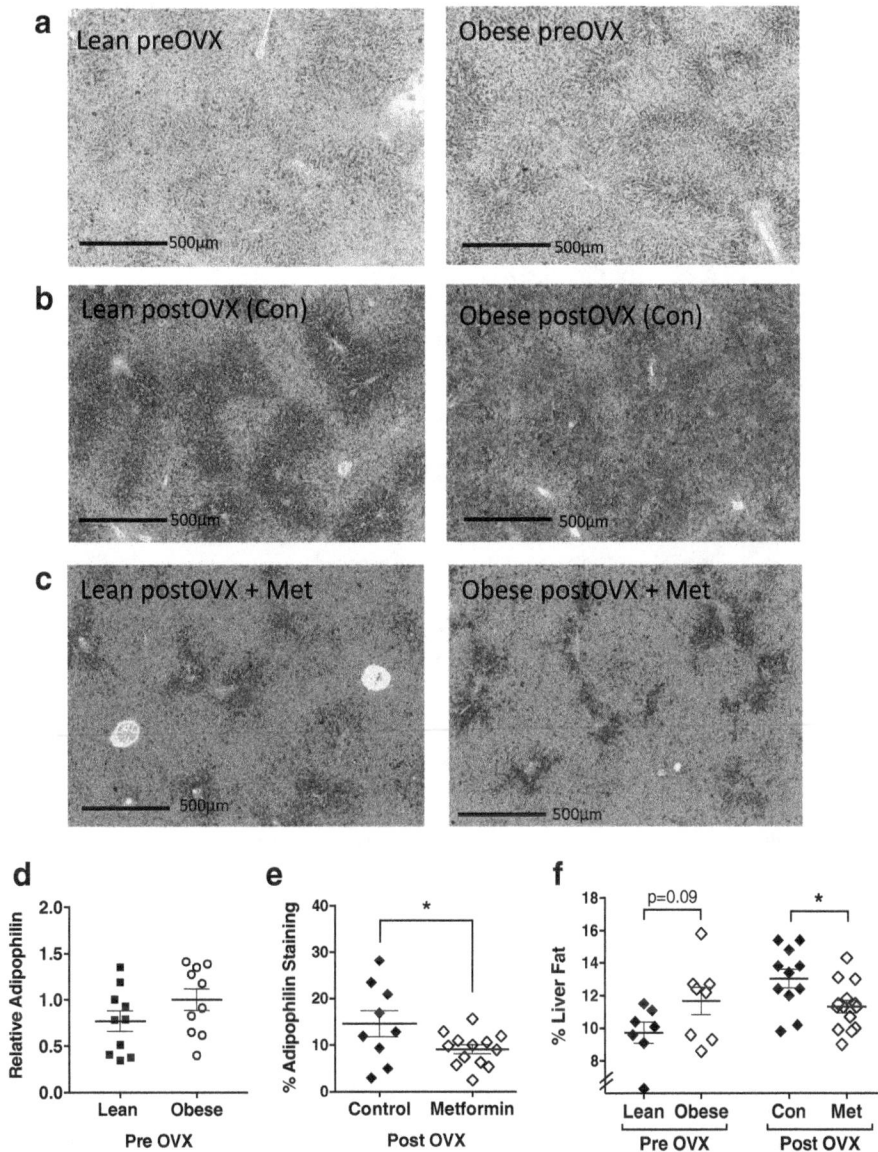

Fig. 2 Hepatic lipid accumulation is increased with ovariectomy (OVX) and reduced with metformin (Met). Representative images are shown for adipophilin staining in livers from lean and obese rats **a** prior to OVX, **b** after OVX-induced weight gain, and **c** after OVX-induced weight gain with concurrent metformin treatment. Scale bars = 500 μm. **d** In pre-OVX rats, adipophilin levels are not significantly different between lean and obese rats. **e** Metformin treatment significantly decreased hepatic adipophilin staining when compared with controls. **f** qMR analysis of the percent fat in livers shows that absolute lipid content was not different between lean and obese rats pre-OVX, but post-OVX hepatic lipid accumulation was significantly decreased in metformin-treated rats compared with controls (Con). *$p < 0.05$

Tumor response to metformin

Epidemiological data have, for the most part, focused on the beneficial role of metformin in improving tumor outcomes in individuals with type 2 diabetes, who are also commonly overweight and/or obese [43]. However, based on the knowledge that rapid weight gain occurs following OVX, regardless of adiposity phenotype, as well as the beneficial effects of metformin after OVX described above, we hypothesized that metformin would be effective in animals when administered during the period of OVX-induced weight gain, regardless of their pre-OVX obesogenic status.

As previously reported in this rodent model, lean and obese animals did not differ in the number of tumors prior to OVX (1.89 ± 0.34 vs 1.90 ± 0.42, lean vs obese), consistent with epidemiologic data showing minimal impact of obesity on breast cancer risk in premenopausal women [44]. Also, we found that pre-OVX adiposity (lean vs obese) did not affect post-OVX tumor response to metformin, with both groups

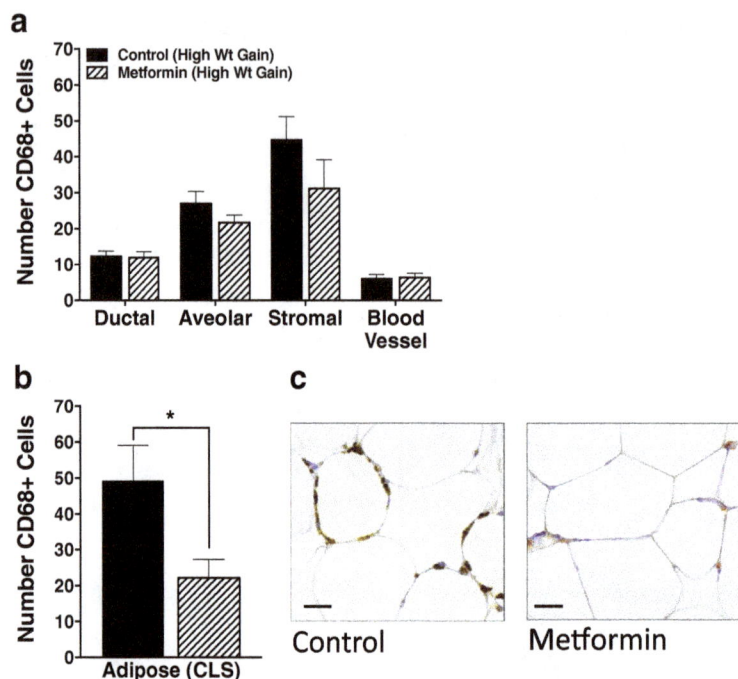

Fig. 3 Metformin decreases the number of adipose-associated mammary macrophages. Quantification and representative images of CD68[+] macrophages in normal mammary adipose tissue from metformin-treated and control rats experiencing high weight (Wt) gain in the post-OVX period. Rate of weight gain during the first 4 weeks after OVX was measured and those above the median were classified as high weight gainers and those below the median as low weight gainers. Mammary adipose was stained for CD68 as a macrophage marker. **a** Metformin did not affect the number of ductal, alveolar, stromal, or blood vessel-associated CD68[+] cells, but **b** metformin decreased the number of CD68[+] cells associated with adipocytes and crown-like structures (CLS) in rats rapidly gaining weight following OVX. **c** Representative images from control and metformin-treated adipose tissue are shown. Scale bars = 20 μm

experiencing similar OVX-induced weight gain and reduction in tumor burden with metformin treatment. Thus, for tumor burden and for subsequent analyses, data from lean and obese groups were combined and data are presented as control versus metformin-treated, unless indicated otherwise.

In the first 2 weeks following OVX, tumor burden decreased slightly in all animals regardless of metformin treatment, as predicted, based on the estrogen dependence of MNU-induced tumors. Beginning at 3 weeks post-OVX, in untreated rats, tumor growth increased significantly and continued to increase in size for the duration of the 8-week study (Fig. 4a). Conversely, treatment with metformin prevented this post-OVX tumor growth and also resulted in tumor regression such that many tumors present at the time of OVX were no longer palpable at 8 weeks post-OVX (Fig. 4a). Specifically, mean tumor burden in the metformin-treated rats was 86% lower than in their untreated counterparts. This decrease in tumor burden is primarily due to the fact that metformin prevented tumor progression after OVX, rather than directly causing tumor regression per se. At the study end, overall, metformin-treated animals had

significantly fewer tumors per rat that progressed (0.8 ± 0.3 vs 0.3 ± 0.1), no new tumors that emerged (0.4 ± 0.2 vs 0), and fewer tumors remaining (1.7 ± 0.4 vs 0.8 ± 0.1), irrespective of pre-OVX obesogenic status (Fig. 4b).

Metformin-induced changes in the tumor microenvironment

To explore potential mechanism(s) by which metformin exerted its antitumor effects, we returned to the demonstrable links between obesity, local estrogen production, and ER[+] breast cancers. In the postmenopausal setting, aromatase is the key enzyme responsible for estrogen production, as it converts testosterones to estrogens. Importantly, increased expression of aromatase in stromal adipocytes and associated vascular cells has been linked to inflamed adipose tissue in obese and overweight rodents and women [42, 45], and is thought to be the local source of growth promotion for breast cancers in the postmenopausal setting. Thus, one potential mechanism of action proposed for the antitumor effects of metformin in our postmenopausal breast cancer model is through the inhibition of stromal-derived aromatase.

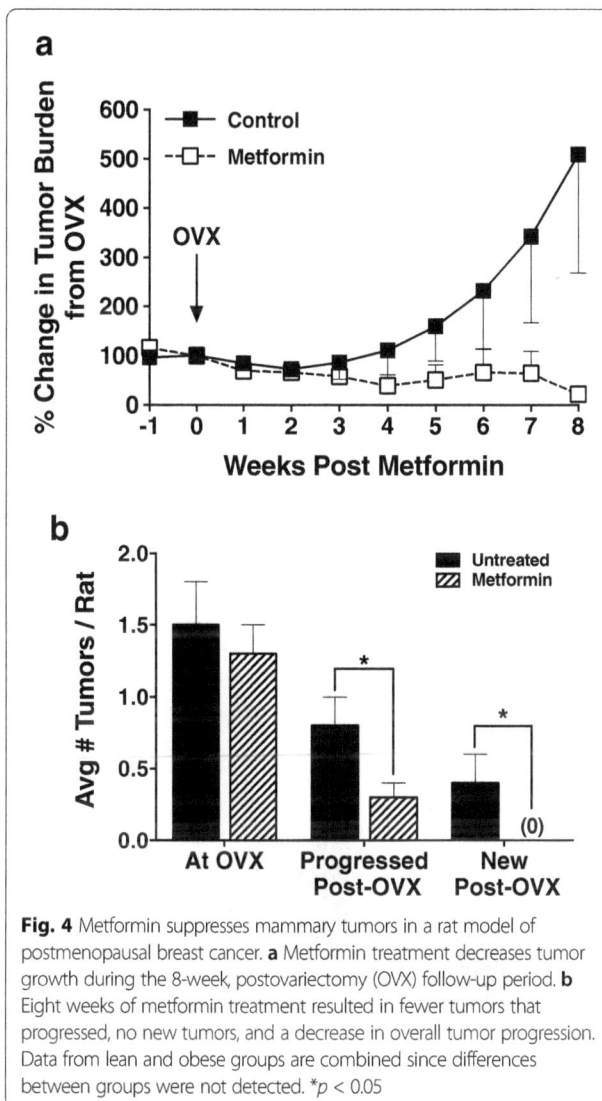

Fig. 4 Metformin suppresses mammary tumors in a rat model of postmenopausal breast cancer. **a** Metformin treatment decreases tumor growth during the 8-week, postovariectomy (OVX) follow-up period. **b** Eight weeks of metformin treatment resulted in fewer tumors that progressed, no new tumors, and a decrease in overall tumor progression. Data from lean and obese groups are combined since differences between groups were not detected. *$p < 0.05$

Metformin decreases aromatase-positive, CD68+ macrophages in the tumor border

To investigate if metformin exerted an antitumor effect by modulating aromatase expression in inflamed tissues, we returned to our observation that metformin reduced the number of CD68+ macrophages present within the mammary adipose compartment. While several studies have reported that aromatase expression/production occurs in mammary stromal vascular cells, there is only one other known report of CD68+ macrophages expressing aromatase [46]. Using a quantitative IHC approach with an IHC-validated antibody [30–33], we first evaluated whether metformin decreased aromatase levels in either mammary tumors or the surrounding tumor microenvironment. While metformin did not affect aromatase levels within the mammary tumor cells, we did find a significant decrease in the number of aromatase-positive stromal cells in the tumor border of metformin-treated animals compared with

controls (Fig. 5a). Dual staining for aromatase and the macrophage marker CD68+ revealed the aromatase-positive stromal cells to be heterogeneous, comprising CD68+ macrophages and additional unidentified stromal cell population(s). Furthermore, metformin specifically decreased the number of CD68+, aromatase-positive macrophages (Fig. 5b, c). This effect was specific to the tumor border since differences within the tumors themselves were not detected. This confirms the work of Mor and colleagues [46] identifying CD68+ macrophages as a cell type responsible for aromatase production, and the first report that macrophage expression of aromatase is metformin responsive.

Metformin targets a subset of M2-like macrophages

Because macrophages exhibit a wide range of antitumor abilities, which are determined in part by their polarization state, we next assessed if aromatase expression is influenced by macrophage phenotype. M1, or proinflammatory macrophages, are involved in antigen presentation, immune surveillance and killing of cells with foreign antigens, including tumor cells, and thus are considered tumor suppressive [47–49]. M2, or alternatively activated macrophages, represent the other end of the polarization spectrum, and are considered immunosuppressive and can promote tumor progression [50–52]. Using in vitro activated rat M1 and M2 macrophages, we found higher levels of aromatase protein in M2 compared to M1 polarized rat macrophages, as assessed by Western blot (Fig. 5c). Data were confirmed using three distinct sources of M1 and M2 polarized rat macrophages, and two different aromatase antibodies. Antibody specificity was also verified using a commercially available aromatase blocking peptide (Fig. 5d). Similar results have been obtained using murine macrophages (data not shown). In summary, we interpret these data to suggest that a specific subtype of aromatase-positive M2 polarized macrophages are elevated with OVX-induced weight gain, associate with increased tumor burden in our postmenopausal breast cancer rat model, and are suppressed by metformin.

Metformin decreases local estrogen levels and reduces ER signaling in tumors

One prediction of reduced macrophage-derived aromatase expression within the tumor-bearing mammary glands would be decreased ER signaling in the tumors. As a read out of ER signaling, we measured expression of the well-established ER response gene, the progesterone receptor (PR), by IHC. As expected, PR expression was decreased in metformin-treated tumors relative to controls (Fig. 5e). This observation is consistent with metformin acting, in part, by reducing ligand-dependent estrogen signaling within the mammary tumor microenvironment.

Breast Cancer: A Growing Concern

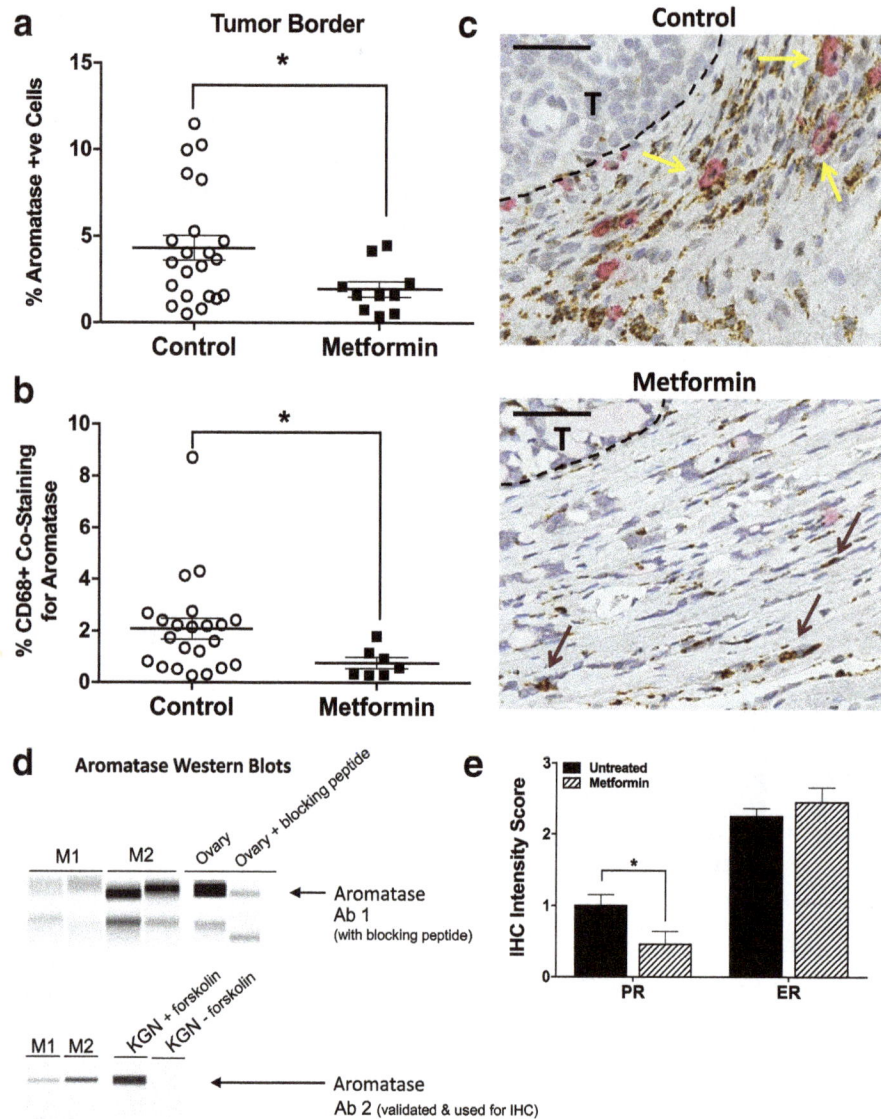

Fig. 5 Metformin decreases aromatase-positive, tumor-associated macrophages. **a** Quantification of aromatase-positive cells and **b** CD68-positive (CD68[+]) macrophages costaining for aromatase in the tumor border of tissues from control or metformin-treated rats. **c** Representative control and metformin-treated IHC images of CD68 and aromatase dual staining in tissue bordering mammary tumors (T) (arrows: yellow = CD68[+]aromatase[+], brown = CD68[+]; scale bar = 50um). **d** Aromatase expression by Western blotting (WES system) from in vitro activated M1 and M2 rat macrophages using two different primary antibodies (Ab #1: Novus NB100-1596; Ab #2: clone 677, Baylor College of Medicine). Controls include ovary (positive control) and ovary in which the primary antibody was preincubated with an aromatase blocking peptide for 1 h, as well as KGN cells with (positive control) and without (negative control) forskolin treatment. **e** IHC intensity score for ER and PR (0 = no stain; 1 = weak; 2 = moderate; 3 = strong staining). *$p < 0.05$

Importantly, we found no difference in ER levels (Fig. 5e), likely because ER levels are high in these tumors after OVX. Thus, our data suggest that through actions on mammary macrophages, metformin decreases local aromatase levels, leading to lower levels of estrogens and decreased ER activation within the tumors, which could ultimately decrease tumor growth.

Discussion

Menopause represents a lifecycle window of breast cancer risk that may be highly amenable to interventions that decrease risk. During menopause, energy balance, circulating hormones, chemokines and cytokines, and body fat distribution are in flux, and this is also the critical time when the tumor-promoting effects of obesity emerge [53–55]. Thus, interventions targeting the metabolic flux of menopause may effectively reduce breast cancer incidence and/or lethality. Using a rat model of postmenopausal breast cancer, our goal was to determine if targeting metformin treatment to the window of 'menopause'-induced weight gain could decrease tumor growth and improve tumor outcomes. Similar to menopause in women, OVX in this model induced weight gain and increased adiposity in all animals, regardless of their lean/obese status prior to OVX. Weight gain was associated with a decline in metabolic health, as demonstrated by increased liver fat deposition and adipose-tissue inflammation. Specifically, we identified a subtype of aromatase-positive, M2-like macrophages to be elevated in mammary adipose tissue post-OVX. Within this context of OVX-induced metabolic dysfunction, metformin decreased the size of existing tumors and prevented formation of new tumors. The antitumor effects of metformin were associated with a decrease in adipose inflammation, measured by a reduction in the number of aromatase expressing CD68$^+$ macrophages. Overall, our data suggest that a subtype of aromatase-positive, M2-like macrophages are elevated with OVX-induced weight gain, providing a growth advantage to ER$^+$ tumors in the absence of ovarian hormones. These macrophages are targeted by treatment with metformin, possibly mitigating the protumorigenic effects of OVX-induced weight gain through estrogen deprivation. While nonaromatase-dependent mechanisms of metformin most certainly also contribute to tumor reduction in this model, this newly identified mechanism of action warrants further investigation.

This study further supports our 'dual requirement' hypothesis of obesity and postmenopausal breast cancer. Our early work in this model established that both impaired metabolic regulation that underlies obesity and a positive energy imbalance are required for the emergence of obesity-associated tumor promotion after menopause. This combination of impaired metabolism and postmenopausal weight gain has direct effects on mammary tumors, specifically increasing tumor expression of PR, promoting a glycolytic/lipogenic gene expression profile, and promoting tumor glucose uptake [23]. More recently, we have also shown that this combination of obesity and OVX-induced overfeeding leads to nuclear localization of the androgen receptor, which promotes the growth of ER+ tumors under conditions of low estrogen availability after OVX [35]. Importantly, in that study we found a role for the inflammatory cytokine IL-6 in sensitizing breast cancer cells to low testosterone levels. Our current study now extends this work to suggest that rapid weight gain following OVX/menopause is associated with increased aromatase expression in mammary macrophages. Work in endometrial cancer has demonstrated that tumor cell production of IL-6 leads to upregulation of aromatase in stromal cells, creating a

cycle that drives tumor proliferation [56]. A similar IL-6-mediated increase in aromatase gene expression has been demonstrated in murine macrophages [57]. The existence of a similar paracrine mechanism in the context of postmenopausal breast cancer warrants further investigation.

The combination of impaired metabolic health and menopause-induced weight gain were likely critical to the anticancer effects of metformin observed in this study. A review of the literature would suggest that metformin is most effective when one or more of the following are present: 1) consumption of a moderate to high-fat diet; 2) poor metabolic health (insulin insensitivity, metabolic disease, etc.); 3) weight gain; and/or 4) increased adiposity (overweight or obesity). Our previous work demonstrating beneficial effects of metformin have all been conducted in animals consuming a high-fat diet [22, 23]. There are several examples where metformin had minimal or no impact on mammary tumor outcomes in the context of a low-fat diet [15, 58, 59]; however, in studies where medium [60] or high-fat [61] diets were used, metformin improved tumor outcome. Beneficial effects of metformin have also been reported in a study where 5% sucrose was added to the water of the animals [62], suggesting that this may have been sufficient to impair the metabolic health of these animals to an extent where the effects of metformin could be realized.

While the role of tumor-associated macrophages in breast cancer development and progression has been studied extensively over the past decade (reviewed in [63]), there are only a limited number of studies that have focused specifically on macrophage production of aromatase. Using IHC staining on serial sections, Mor and colleagues [46] demonstrated the presence of CD68$^+$, aromatase-positive macrophages both around and within human breast cancers. Using in vitro assays, they extended this work to show that aromatase expression and activity is acquired by tissue-activated macrophages but not by their circulating monocyte precursors. Furthermore, conditioned medium from activated macrophages was sufficient to stimulate the growth of estrogen-responsive MCF-7 cells—an effect blocked by the aromatase inhibitor letrazol. This demonstrates that, at least in vitro, macrophages can produce sufficient levels of estrogens to stimulate the growth of estrogen-responsive breast cancer cells. Our findings are the first, to our knowledge, to identify aromatase expression as a feature of a subpopulation of protumorigenic M2-like mammary macrophages that arise in the context of obesity. We speculate that, in our in-vivo model, locally produced estrogens reach sufficient levels to activate ER in mammary tumors, and the ability for metformin to decrease this local production of estrogen contributes to its antitumor effects. The question whether inflammatory cytokines such as IL-6 cooperate with stromal-derived estrogen and sensitize breast cancer cells to ER, as we observe for testosterone signaling through the androgen receptor [35], remains to be determined.

Our data build upon the work of Dannenberg's group who have demonstrated a causal link between obesity-induced inflammation and aromatase expression in the mammary gland. Their work shows that, in obese mice, release of free fatty acids from adipocytes activates NF-kB in the stromal vascular fraction of adipose tissue, which increases proinflammatory cytokine production [45]. In cell culture models, they have demonstrated that that these proinflammatory mediators (tumor necrosis factor (TNF)α, IL-1β, and prostaglandin E_2(PGE$_2$)) produced by cells in the stromal fraction of mammary glands from obese mice stimulate aromatase in preadipocytes [45]. They have further extended these findings to demonstrate increased inflammation, aromatase expression, and aromatase activity in the breast of overweight and obese women [42] and in a subset of nonoverweight women (body mass index (BMI) < 25 kg/m^2) who had underlying systemic metabolic dysfunction [41]. Our work extends these pioneering studies and indicates that M2-like macrophages themselves can produce aromatase. In our rat model, mature mammary adipocytes do not appear aromatase-positive, and estradiol in rat mammary adipose tissue was below the level of detection by mass spectrometry [35]. It is possible that the role of adipocytes in aromatase production could be model- or context-dependent. However, combined, these data highlight the fact that many stromal cell populations may contribute to local aromatase production under different conditions.

Conclusions

In conclusion, our work from preclinical models demonstrates that metformin specifically targets macrophage production of aromatase in the mammary adipose depot, identifying a potential novel antitumor mechanism of action for metformin. Additional studies are needed to confirm the relevance in women. Nonetheless, our findings provide the rationale for testing the efficacy of metformin in higher-risk populations, such as peri-menopausal or menopausal women with underlying metabolic disease. The menopause transition represents a lifecycle window of opportunity that may be specifically sensitive to the beneficial effects of metformin, and use of this agent during this time could improve outcomes for many women at risk for or those with established postmenopausal breast cancer.

Abbreviations
AMPK: AMP-dependent kinase; BMI: Body mass index; CD68+: CD68 positive; CLS: Crown like structure; ER: Estrogen receptor; ER+: Estrogen receptor positive; FNA: Fine needle aspiration; H&E: Hematoxylin and eosin;

HER2: Human epidermal growth factor receptor 2; HF: High fat; IHC: Immunohistochemistry; MNU: 1-methyl-1-nitrosourea; NEFA: Nonesterified fatty acid; OVX: Ovariectomy; PGE2: Prostaglandin E2; PR: Progesterone receptor; qMR: Quantitative magnetic resonance; TG: Triglycerides; TNFα: Tumor necrosis factor alpha

Acknowledgements
We would like to thank J. Higgins and M. Jackman for their helpful discussions throughout this study. We are also grateful for the technical assistance provided by S. Edgerton, K. Hedman, G. Johnson, D. Landrock, A. Lewis, J. Lopez, C. Mahan, R. Oljira, and V. Wessells.

Funding
This work was supported by NIH/NCI CA169430 (EDG) and CA164166 (PSM and PS), the Komen for the Cure Grant KG081323 (SMA), the Cancer League of Colorado (EAW), the University of Colorado Nutrition and Obesity Research Center Pilot Awards P30-DK048520 (EDG and EAW), and EDG was supported by a junior faculty award from the University of Colorado's Center for Women's Health Research. We also appreciate the generous support from both the Colorado Obesity Research Institute, and the Energy Balance and Metabolic Core Laboratories within the Colorado Nutrition Obesity Research Center.

Authors' contributions
EDG participated in the design and execution of the study, conducted data analysis and interpretation, and drafted the manuscript; SJ was responsible for all immunohistochemistry and related analyses in the study; EAW participated in execution of the study and data analysis and interpretation; TS contributed to the immunohistochemistry data and analysis; DPE developed the antibodies for the aromatase immunohistochemistry; SMA and ADT contributed to the design and data interpretation; PSM and PS oversaw all aspects of study design, execution, data analysis/interpretation, and writing of the manuscript. All authors read and approved the final manuscript.

Competing interests
The authors declare they have no competing interests.

Author details
[1]Department of Nutrition & Food Science, Texas A&M University, 373 Olsen Blvd; 2253 TAMU, College Station, TX 77843, USA. [2]Anschutz Health & Wellness Center, University of Colorado Anschutz Medical Campus, Aurora, CO 80045, USA. [3]Department of Medicine, Divisions of Endocrinology, Metabolism, and Diabetes, University of Colorado Anschutz Medical Campus, Aurora, CO 80045, USA. [4]Department of Medical Oncology, University of Colorado Anschutz Medical Campus, Aurora, CO 80045, USA. [5]Department of Pathology, University of Colorado Anschutz Medical Campus, Aurora, CO 80045, USA. [6]Department of Cell, Developmental and Cancer Biology, Oregon Health & Science University, 3181 S.W. Sam Jackson Park Rd, Mailing Code: L215, Portland, OR 97239, USA. [7]Knight Cancer Institute, Oregon Health & Science University, 1130 NW 22nd Ave #100, Portland, OR 97239, USA. [8]Departments of Molecular & Cellular Biology and Pathology Immunology, Baylor College of Medicine, Houston, TX 77030, USA.

References
1. Soranna D, Scotti L, Zambon A, Bosetti C, Grassi G, Catapano A, La Vecchia C, Mancia G, Corrao G. Cancer risk associated with use of metformin and sulfonylurea in type 2 diabetes: a meta-analysis. Oncologist. 2012;17(6):813–22.

2. Gong Z, Aragaki AK, Chlebowski RT, Manson JE, Rohan TE, Chen C, Vitolins MZ, Tinker LF, LeBlanc ES, Kuller LH, et al. Diabetes, metformin and incidence of and death from invasive cancer in postmenopausal women: results from the women's health initiative. Int J Cancer. 2016;138(8):1915–27.

3. Calip GS, Yu O, Elmore JG, Boudreau DM. Comparative safety of diabetes medications and risk of incident invasive breast cancer: a population-based cohort study. Cancer Causes Control. 2016;27(5):709–20.

4. Evans JM, Donnelly LA, Emslie-Smith AM, Alessi DR, Morris AD. Metformin and reduced risk of cancer in diabetic patients. BMJ. 2005;330(7503):1304–5.

5. Bodmer M, Meier C, Krahenbuhl S, Jick SS, Meier CR. Long-term metformin use is associated with decreased risk of breast cancer. Diabetes Care. 2010;33(6):1304–8.

6. Currie CJ, Poole CD, Gale EA. The influence of glucose-lowering therapies on cancer risk in type 2 diabetes. Diabetologia. 2009;52(9):1766–77.

7. Soffer D, Shi J, Chung J, Schottinger JE, Wallner LP, Chlebowski RT, Lentz SE, Haque R. Metformin and breast and gynecological cancer risk among women with diabetes. BMJ Open Diabetes Res Care. 2015;3(1):e000049.

8. Formica V, Tesauro M, Cardillo C, Roselli M. Insulinemia and the risk of breast cancer and its relapse. Diabetes Obes Metab. 2012;14(12):1073–80.

9. Goodwin PJ, Ennis M, Pritchard KI, Trudeau ME, Koo J, Taylor SK, Hood N. Insulin- and obesity-related variables in early-stage breast cancer: correlations and time course of prognostic associations. J Clin Oncol. 2012;30(2):164–71.

10. Alimova IN, Liu B, Fan Z, Edgerton SM, Dillon T, Lind SE, Thor AD. Metformin inhibits breast cancer cell growth, colony formation and induces cell cycle arrest in vitro. Cell Cycle. 2009;8(6):909–15.

11. Liu B, Fan Z, Edgerton SM, Deng XS, Alimova IN, Lind SE, Thor AD. Metformin induces unique biological and molecular responses in triple negative breast cancer cells. Cell Cycle. 2009;8(13):2031–40.

12. Kim J, Lee J, Jang SY, Kim C, Choi Y, Kim A. Anticancer effect of metformin on estrogen receptor-positive and tamoxifen-resistant breast cancer cell lines. Oncol Rep. 2016;35(5):2553–60.

13. Fuentes-Mattei E, Velazquez-Torres G, Phan L, Zhang F, Chou PC, Shin JH, Choi HH, Chen JS, Zhao R, Chen J et al. Effects of obesity on transcriptomic changes and cancer hallmarks in estrogen receptor-positive breast cancer. J Natl Cancer Inst. 2014;106(7). https://academic.oup.com/jnci/article/106/7/dju158/1010206. Accessed 1 July 2014.

14. Kim HJ, Kwon H, Lee JW, Kim HJ, Lee SB, Park HS, Sohn G, Lee Y, Koh BS, Yu JH, et al. Metformin increases survival in hormone receptor-positive, HER2-positive breast cancer patients with diabetes. Breast Cancer Res. 2015;17:64.

15. Thompson MD, Grubbs CJ, Bode AM, Reid JM, McGovern R, Bernard PS, Stijleman IJ, Green JE, Bennett C, Juliana MM, et al. Lack of effect of metformin on mammary carcinogenesis in nondiabetic rat and mouse models. Cancer Prev Res (Phila). 2015;8(3):231–9.

16. Zhu Z, Jiang W, Thompson MD, Echeverria D, McGinley JN, Thompson HJ. Effects of metformin, buformin, and phenformin on the post-initiation stage of chemically induced mammary carcinogenesis in the rat. Cancer Prev Res (Phila). 2015;8(6):518–27.

17. Bonanni B, Puntoni M, Cazzaniga M, Pruneri G, Serrano D, Guerrieri-Gonzaga A, Gennari A, Trabacca MS, Galimberti V, Veronesi P, et al. Dual effect of metformin on breast cancer proliferation in a randomized presurgical trial. J Clin Oncol. 2012;30(21):2593–600.

18. Niraula S, Dowling RJ, Ennis M, Chang MC, Done SJ, Hood N, Escallon J, Leong WL, McCready DR, Reedijk M, et al. Metformin in early breast cancer: a prospective window of opportunity neoadjuvant study. Breast Cancer Res Treat. 2012;135(3):821–30.

19. Dowling RJ, Niraula S, Chang MC, Done SJ, Ennis M, McCready DR, Leong WL, Escallon JM, Reedijk M, Goodwin PJ, et al. Changes in insulin receptor signaling underlie neoadjuvant metformin administration in breast cancer: a prospective window of opportunity neoadjuvant study. Breast Cancer Res. 2015;17:32.

20. Goodwin PJ, Stambolic V, Lemieux J, Chen BE, Parulekar WR, Gelmon KA, Hershman DL, Hobday TJ, Ligibel JA, Mayer IA, et al. Evaluation of metformin in early breast cancer: a modification of the traditional paradigm for clinical testing of anti-cancer agents. Breast Cancer Res Treat. 2011;126(1):215–20.

21. Grossmann ME, Yang DQ, Guo Z, Potter DA, Cleary MP. Metformin treatment for the prevention and/or treatment of breast/mammary tumorigenesis. Curr Pharmacol Rep. 2015;1(5):312–23.

22. Checkley LA, Rudolph MC, Wellberg EA, Giles ED, Wahdan-Alaswad RS, Houck JA, Edgerton SM, Thor AD, Schedin P, Anderson SM, et al. Metformin accumulation correlates with organic cation transporter 2 protein expression and predicts mammary tumor regression in vivo. Cancer Prev Res (Phila). 2017;10(3):198–207.

23. Giles ED, Wellberg EA, Astling DP, Anderson SM, Thor AD, Jindal S, Tan AC, Schedin PS, Maclean PS. Obesity and overfeeding affecting both tumor and systemic metabolism activates the progesterone receptor to contribute to postmenopausal breast cancer. Cancer Res. 2012;72(24):6490–501.

24. Giles ED, Jackman MR, Johnson GC, Schedin PJ, Houser JL, MacLean PS. Effect of the estrous cycle and surgical ovariectomy on energy balance, fuel utilization, and physical activity in lean and obese female rats. Am J Physiol Regul Integr Comp Physiol. 2010;299(6):R1634–42.

25. MacLean PS, Giles ED, Johnson GC, McDaniel SM, Fleming-Elder BK, Gilman KA, Andrianakos AG, Jackman MR, Shroyer KR, Schedin PJ. A surprising link between the energetics of ovariectomy-induced weight gain and mammary tumor progression in obese rats. Obesity (Silver Spring). 2010;18(4):696–703.

26. Thompson HJ, Adlakha H, Singh M. Effect of carcinogen dose and age at administration on induction of mammary carcinogenesis by 1-methyl-1-nitrosourea. Carcinogenesis. 1992;13(9):1535–9.

27. Thompson HJ, McGinley JN, Wolfe P, Singh M, Steele VE, Kelloff GJ. Temporal sequence of mammary intraductal proliferations, ductal carcinomas in situ and adenocarcinomas induced by 1-methyl-1-nitrosourea in rats. Carcinogenesis. 1998;19(12):2181–5.

28. MacLean PS, Higgins JA, Johnson GC, Fleming-Elder BK, Peters JC, Hill JO. Metabolic adjustments with the development, treatment, and recurrence of obesity in obesity-prone rats. Am J Physiol Regul Integr Comp Physiol. 2004;287(2):R288–97.

29. Young S, Hallowes RC. Tumours of the mammary gland. IARC Sci Publ. 1973;5:31–73.

30. Sasano H, Edwards DP, Anderson TJ, Silverberg SG, Evans DB, Santen RJ, Ramage P, Simpson ER, Bhatnagar AS, Miller WR. Validation of new aromatase monoclonal antibodies for immunohistochemistry: progress report. J Steroid Biochem Mol Biol. 2003;86(3-5):239–44.

31. Sasano H, Anderson TJ, Silverberg SG, Santen RJ, Conway M, Edwards DP, Krause A, Bhatnagar AS, Evans DB, Miller WR. The validation of new aromatase monoclonal antibodies for immunohistochemistry—a correlation with biochemical activities in 46 cases of breast cancer. J Steroid Biochem Mol Biol. 2005;95(1-5):35–9.

32. Geisler J, Suzuki T, Helle H, Miki Y, Nagasaki S, Duong NK, Ekse D, Aas T, Evans DB, Lonning PE, et al. Breast cancer aromatase expression evaluated by the novel antibody 677: correlations to intra-tumor estrogen levels and hormone receptor status. J Steroid Biochem Mol Biol. 2010;118(4-5):237–41.

33. Hong Y, Li H, Ye J, Miki Y, Yuan YC, Sasano H, Evans DB, Chen S. Epitope characterization of an aromatase monoclonal antibody suitable for the assessment of intratumoral aromatase activity. PLoS One. 2009;4(11):e8050.

34. Giles ED, Jackman MR, MacLean PS. Modeling diet-Induced obesity with obesity-prone rats: implications for studies in females. Front Nutr. 2016;3:50.

35. Wellberg EA, Checkley LA, Giles ED, Johnson SJ, Oljira R, Wahdan-Alaswad R, Foright RM, Dooley G, Edgerton SM, Jindal S, et al. The Androgen Receptor Supports Tumor Progression After the Loss of Ovarian Function in a Preclinical Model of Obesity and Breast Cancer. Horm Cancer. 2017;8(5-6):269–285.

36. Christensen MM, Brasch-Andersen C, Green H, Nielsen F, Damkier P, Beck-Nielsen H, Brosen K. The pharmacogenetics of metformin and its impact on plasma metformin steady-state levels and glycosylated hemoglobin A1c. Pharmacogenet Genomics. 2011;21(12):837–50.

37. Boule NG, Robert C, Bell GJ, Johnson ST, Bell RC, Lewanczuk RZ, Gabr RQ, Brocks DR. Metformin and exercise in type 2 diabetes: examining treatment modality interactions. Diabetes Care. 2011;34(7):1469–74.

38. Kanda H, Tateya S, Tamori Y, Kotani K, Hiasa K, Kitazawa R, Kitazawa S, Miyachi H, Maeda S, Egashira K, et al. MCP-1 contributes to macrophage infiltration into adipose tissue, insulin resistance, and hepatic steatosis in obesity. J Clin Invest. 2006;116(6):1494–505.

39. Weisberg SP, Hunter D, Huber R, Lemieux J, Slaymaker S, Vaddi K, Charo I, Leibel RL, Ferrante AW Jr. CCR2 modulates inflammatory and metabolic effects of high-fat feeding. J Clin Invest. 2006;116(1):115–24.

40. Doerstling SS, O'Flanagan CH, Hursting SD. Obesity and cancer metabolism: a perspective on interacting tumor-intrinsic and extrinsic factors. Front Oncol. 2017;7:216.

41. Iyengar NM, Brown KA, Zhou XK, Gucalp A, Subbaramaiah K, Giri DD, Zahid H, Bhardwaj P, Wendel NK, Falcone DJ, et al. Metabolic obesity, adipose inflammation and elevated breast aromatase in women with normal body mass index. Cancer Prev Res (Phila). 2017;10(4):235–43.

42. Morris PG, Hudis CA, Giri D, Morrow M, Falcone DJ, Zhou XK, Du B, Brogi E, Crawford CB, Kopelovich L, et al. Inflammation and increased aromatase expression occur in the breast tissue of obese women with breast cancer. Cancer Prev Res (Phila). 2011;4(7):1021–9.

43. Age-Adjusted Percentage of Adults with Diabetes Aged 18+ years With Overweight or Obesity; 1994 - 2015; United States. US Diabetes Surveillance System; Division of Diabetes Translation - Centers for Disease Control and Prevention. www.cdc.gov/diabetes/data. Accessed 1 Nov 2017.

44. Suzuki R, Orsini N, Saji S, Key TJ, Wolk A. Body weight and incidence of breast cancer defined by estrogen and progesterone receptor status—a meta-analysis. Int J Cancer. 2009;124(3):698–712.

45. Subbaramaiah K, Howe LR, Bhardwaj P, Du B, Gravaghi C, Yantiss RK, Zhou XK, Blaho VA, Hla T, Yang P, et al. Obesity is associated with inflammation and elevated aromatase expression in the mouse mammary gland. Cancer Prev Res (Phila). 2011;4(3):329–46.

46. Mor G, Yue W, Santen RJ, Gutierrez L, Eliza M, Berstein LM, Harada N, Wang J, Lysiak J, Diano S, et al. Macrophages, estrogen and the microenvironment of breast cancer. J Steroid Biochem Mol Biol. 1998;67(5-6):403–11.

47. Van Ginderachter JA, Movahedi K, Hassanzadeh Ghassabeh G, Meerschaut S, Beschin A, Raes G, De Baetselier P. Classical and alternative activation of mononuclear phagocytes: picking the best of both worlds for tumor promotion. Immunobiology. 2006;211(6-8):487–501.

48. Gordon S. Alternative activation of macrophages. Nat Rev. 2003;3(1):23–35.

49. Mantovani A, Sica A, Sozzani S, Allavena P, Vecchi A, Locati M. The chemokine system in diverse forms of macrophage activation and polarization. Trends Immunol. 2004;25(12):677–86.

50. De Wever O, Mareel M. Role of tissue stroma in cancer cell invasion. J Pathol. 2003;200(4):429–47.

51. Mueller MM, Fusenig NE. Friends or foes—bipolar effects of the tumour stroma in cancer. Nat Rev Cancer. 2004;4(11):839–49.

52. Mantovani A, Marchesi F, Porta C, Sica A, Allavena P. Inflammation and cancer: breast cancer as a prototype. Breast (Edinburgh, Scotland). 2007; 16(Suppl 2):S27–33.

53. Gambacciani M, Ciaponi M, Cappagli B, De Simone L, Orlandi R, Genazzani AR. Prospective evaluation of body weight and body fat distribution in early postmenopausal women with and without hormonal replacement therapy. Maturitas. 2001;39(2):125–32.

54. Kohrt WM, Ehsani AA, Birge SJ Jr. HRT preserves increases in bone mineral density and reductions in body fat after a supervised exercise program. J Appl Physiol (1985). 1998;84(5):1506–12.

55. Mattiasson I, Rendell M, Tornquist C, Jeppsson S, Hulthen UL. Effects of estrogen replacement therapy on abdominal fat compartments as related to glucose and lipid metabolism in early postmenopausal women. Horm Metab Res. 2002;34(10):583–8.

56. Che Q, Liu BY, Liao Y, Zhang HJ, Yang TT, He YY, Xia YH, Lu W, He XY, Chen Z, et al. Activation of a positive feedback loop involving IL-6 and aromatase promotes intratumoral 17beta-estradiol biosynthesis in endometrial carcinoma microenvironment. Int J Cancer. 2014;135(2):282–94.

57. Brady NJ, Farrar MA, Schwertfeger KL. STAT5 deletion in macrophages alters ductal elongation and branching during mammary gland development. Dev Biol. 2017;428(1):232–44.

58. Bojkova B, Orendas P, Garajova M, Kassayova M, Kutna V, Ahlersova E, Ahlers I. Metformin in chemically induced mammary carcinogenesis in rats. Neoplasma. 2009;56(3):269–74.

59. Anisimov VN, Berstein LM, Egormin PA, Piskunova TS, Popovich IG, Zabezhinski MA, Tyndyk ML, Yurova MV, Kovalenko IG, Poroshina TE, et al. Metformin slows down aging and extends life span of female SHR mice. Cell Cycle. 2008;7(17):2769–73.

60. Zhu P, Davis M, Blackwelder AJ, Bachman N, Liu B, Edgerton S, Williams LL, Thor AD, Yang X. Metformin selectively targets tumor-initiating cells in ErbB2-overexpressing breast cancer models. Cancer Prev Res (Phila). 2014; 7(2):199–210.

61. Bojkova B, Kajo K, Kiskova T, Kubatka P, Zubor P, Solar P, Pec M, Adamkov M. Metformin and melatonin inhibit DMBA-induced mammary tumorigenesis in rats fed a high-fat diet. Anti-Cancer Drugs. 2017;

62. Orecchioni S, Reggiani F, Talarico G, Mancuso P, Calleri A, Gregato G, Labanca V, Noonan DM, Dallaglio K, Albini A, et al. The biguanides metformin and phenformin inhibit angiogenesis, local and metastatic growth of breast cancer by targeting both neoplastic and microenvironment cells. Int J Cancer. 2015;136(6):E534–44.

63. Brady NJ, Chuntova P, Schwertfeger KL. Macrophages: regulators of the inflammatory microenvironment during mammary gland development and breast cancer. Mediat Inflamm. 2016;2016:4549676.

15

Long-term exposure to insulin and volumetric mammographic density: observational and genetic associations in the Karma study

Signe Borgquist[1,2]* , Ann H. Rosendahl[1], Kamila Czene[3], Nirmala Bhoo-Pathy[4], Mozhgan Dorkhan[5,6], Per Hall[3,7] and Judith S. Brand[3,8]

Abstract

Background: Long-term insulin exposure has been implicated in breast cancer etiology, but epidemiological evidence remains inconclusive. The aims of this study were to investigate the association of insulin therapy with mammographic density (MD) as an intermediate phenotype for breast cancer and to assess associations with long-term elevated circulating insulin levels using a genetic score comprising 18 insulin-associated variants.

Methods: We used data from the KARolinska MAmmography (Karma) project, a Swedish mammography screening cohort. Insulin-treated patients with type 1 (T1D, $n = 122$) and type 2 (T2D, $n = 237$) diabetes were identified through linkage with the Prescribed Drug Register and age-matched to 1771 women without diabetes. We assessed associations with treatment duration and insulin glargine use, and we further examined MD differences using non-insulin-treated T2D patients as an active comparator. MD was measured using a fully automated volumetric method, and analyses were adjusted for multiple potential confounders. Associations with the insulin genetic score were assessed in 9437 study participants without diabetes.

Results: Compared with age-matched women without diabetes, insulin-treated T1D patients had greater percent dense (8.7% vs. 11.4%) and absolute dense volumes (59.7 vs. 64.7 cm^3), and a smaller absolute nondense volume (615 vs. 491 cm^3). Similar associations were observed for insulin-treated T2D, and estimates were not materially different in analyses comparing insulin-treated T2D patients with T2D patients receiving noninsulin glucose-lowering medication. In both T1D and T2D, the magnitude of the association with the absolute dense volume was highest for long-term insulin therapy ($\geq$ 5 years) and the long-acting insulin analog glargine. No consistent evidence of differential associations by insulin treatment duration or type was found for percent dense and absolute nondense volumes. Genetically predicted insulin levels were positively associated with percent dense and absolute dense volumes, but not with the absolute nondense volume (percentage difference [95% CI] per 1-SD increase in insulin genetic score = 0.8 [0.0; 1.6], 0.9 [0.1; 1.8], and 0.1 [− 0.8; 0.9], respectively).

Conclusions: The consistency in direction of association for insulin treatment and the insulin genetic score with the absolute dense volume suggest a causal influence of long-term increased insulin exposure on mammographic dense breast tissue.

Keywords: Breast cancer, Insulin, Mammographic density, Diabetes, Insulin genetic score

* Correspondence: signe.borgquist@med.lu.se
[1]Division of Oncology and Pathology, Clinical Sciences, Lund University, SE-221 85 Lund, Sweden
[2]Clinical Trial Unit, Skåne University Hospital, Lund, Sweden
Full list of author information is available at the end of the article

Background

The role of insulin in breast cancer etiology has received growing attention in recent years [1]. Basic research suggests that long-term exposure to elevated exogenous and endogenous insulins promotes breast tumor growth, either directly by signaling mitogenic effects through the insulin receptor isoform A and the insulin-like growth factor 1 (IGF-1) receptor [2, 3] or indirectly by altering the levels of circulating estrogens [4]. The potential carcinogenic effect of insulin has been demonstrated in vitro in terms of increased proliferation in human breast epithelial cells and breast cancer cell lines [2, 3]. Whether these in vitro observations are relevant to humans and concerns surrounding risks of long-term exogenous insulin use and elevated circulating insulin levels are justified remains uncertain [5–8].

Thus far, observational studies [6, 9] and randomized clinical trials [10–12] have found no compelling evidence of an increased breast cancer incidence in insulin-treated diabetes patients, although recently some studies have suggested a possible elevated risk with long-term insulin glargine use [5, 13, 14], which might be related to the more constant pharmacokinetic profile and enhanced IGF-1 receptor affinity of this insulin analog [15, 16]. However, because of methodological limitations including short-term follow-up and confounding by indication, definitive conclusions cannot be drawn. Many agents affecting carcinogenesis have long latencies and require a minimum length of exposure. Most studies addressing recency or duration effects had limited control for confounding factors or were insufficiently powered to assess associations with long-term insulin therapy [6]. While randomized clinical trials are limited in size and follow-up to study cancer-specific outcomes, confounding by indication is a concern in observational studies, and the use of different comparators is necessary to disentangle treatment effects from their underlying indications. Studies investigating associations of circulating insulin levels with breast cancer risk have also yielded conflicting results, with either positive [17–19] or null associations [20]. Most of these findings, however, were based on small numbers of breast cancer patients and a single insulin measurement, which is not an ideal proxy for long-term insulin exposure 18].

Mammographic density (MD) refers to the amount of radiologically dense fibroglandular tissue in the breast, and high MD levels are a strong and independent predictor of breast cancer risk [21, 22]. Both traits also have several reproductive and lifestyle determinants in common, and MD is viewed as an intermediate phenotype in breast cancer etiology [23]. Because many insulin-treated diabetes patients are below the age at which breast cancer is usually diagnosed, and given the long latency of breast cancer,

MD serves as an attractive intermediate endpoint for identifying potential carcinogenic effects.

In the present study, we aimed to investigate the association of long-term insulin exposure with MD in a mammography screening cohort using different methodological approaches. First, we assessed associations of insulin therapy with MD by comparing insulin-treated type 1 (T1D) and type 2 (T2D) diabetes patients with age-matched individuals without diabetes, overall and stratified by duration of insulin treatment and insulin glargine use. Potential confounding by indication was addressed in case-only analyses and additional analyses comparing insulin-treated diabetes patients with patients receiving other glucose-lowering medication. Second, as an alternative means of overcoming confounding, we explored associations with an insulin genetic score in nondiabetic women. This score comprising 18 insulin-associated variants represents genetic predisposition to elevated circulating insulin levels over the life course. Because genotypes sort randomly at conception, genetic association analyses are less likely affected by confounding and hence can provide additional evidence of the likelihood of a causal effect of long-term increased insulin exposure [24].

Methods
Study populations

This study was nested within the KARolinska MAmmography Project for Risk Prediction of Breast Cancer (Karma), a prospective cohort of 70,877 women attending mammography screening or clinical mammography at one of four mammography units in Sweden between January 2011 and March 2013 [25]. All participants responded to a web-based questionnaire and ~ 55,000 women without a history of cancer, breast enlargement, reduction, or surgery had raw digital mammograms collected and stored at study entry, representing the study base for the present analysis. Information on diabetes diagnoses and insulin prescriptions was retrieved through linkage with the Swedish Patient Register [26] and Prescribed Drug Register [27]. The Patient Register has nationwide coverage and includes inpatient hospitalizations since 1987 and outpatient physician visits since 2001. The Prescribed Drug Register covers all drugs sold and dispensed by prescription since July 1, 2005.

Associations between insulin therapy and MD were analyzed in a matched cohort design including all insulin-treated T1D and T2D patients and a sample of age-matched individuals without diabetes. Insulin-treated diabetes patients were identified through the Prescribed Drug Register, with current insulin use defined as at least one dispensed prescription for insulin or insulin analogs (Anatomical Therapeutic Chemical Classification System [ATC] code A10A, including A10AE04 for insulin glargine) in the year prior to study entry (see Additional file 1:

Table S1 for all identified insulin prescriptions). Diabetes diagnoses were retrieved from the Karma questionnaire and Patient Register. All register-based diagnoses were based on International Classification of Diseases (ICD) code 250 (ICD-8 and ICD-9) until 1996 and unique codes for T1D and T2D as introduced from 1997 onward (ICD-10 codes E10 and E11, respectively). Because no distinction between T1D and T2D was made in the Karma questionnaire and earlier ICD versions (ICD-8 and ICD-9), T1D and T2D patients were differentiated on the basis of previously established cutoffs of diagnosis age (T1D, ≤ 30 years; T2D, ≥ 40 years) [28, 29] when diabetes-specific codes were missing. Using these prescription and diagnostic criteria, 359 insulin-treated diabetes patients were identified, including 122 T1D and 237 T2D patients (of whom 97 T1D [79.5%] and 76 T2D [32.1%] patients were differentiated on the basis of diagnosis age). For each patient, we randomly sampled up to five individuals without a diabetes diagnosis from the study base, matched on birth year. In total, 21 T2D patients could not be matched to a maximum of 5 individuals, leaving 1771 age-matched individuals without diabetes for analyses (i.e., 610 and 1161 for insulin-treated T1D and T2D, respectively).

We further evaluated insulin treatment effects in an analysis comparing T2D patients treated with insulin only ($n = 112$) with T2D patients receiving other noninsulin glucose-lowering medication ($n = 407$). This active comparator group comprised all T2D patients with at least one dispensed prescription for glucose-lowering medication (ATC code A10B), excluding insulins in the year prior to study entry (see Additional file 1: Table S2 for all identified noninsulin glucose-lowering prescriptions). Because insulin is the mainstay of therapy for T1D, we were unable to do a similar analysis for this group of patients.

Finally, we examined associations with an insulin genetic score comprising 18 insulin-associated variants (see details below) as an instrument to proxy long-term exposure to circulating insulin levels. Associations with the insulin genetic score were assessed in a subcohort of 9437 participants with available genotyping data. All women in the subcohort had no history of cancer or diabetes at the time of study entry when blood samples were obtained. The Karma study was approved by the ethical review committee at Karolinska Institutet, and all participants provided written informed consent.

Volumetric mammographic density
MD was estimated from raw digital mammograms collected at study entry using Volpara ™ version 1.5.0 (Volpara Solutions, Wellington, New Zealand) [30]. Volpara volumetric MD measures show good agreement with breast magnetic resonance imaging data [31] and have been validated as being predictive of breast cancer risk

[30, 32]. The Volpara algorithm estimates the thickness of dense tissue at each pixel using the X-ray attenuation of an entirely fatty region as an internal reference. The absolute dense volume (cm^3) is computed by integrating the dense thickness at each pixel over the whole mammogram, and the total breast volume (cm^3) is derived by multiplying the breast area by the recorded breast thickness, with an appropriate correction for the breast edge. From these measures, the absolute nondense volume (cm^3) and percentage of the breast covered by dense tissue (%) can be obtained. The average measurement of the left and right breasts of the mediolateral oblique view was taken for all analyses.

Covariates
The following potential confounders known to be associated with MD were extracted from the baseline questionnaire: education level, body mass index (BMI, based on self-reported height and weight), lifestyle measures (smoking, alcohol intake, and physical activity), reproductive and hormonal factors (age at menarche, number of births/age at first birth, menopausal status, use of oral contraceptives and hormone replacement therapy), and personal history of previous benign breast disease and breast cancer heredity. We also extracted information on prescriptions of comedication through linkage with the Prescribed Drug Register using the ATC coding system (including low-dose aspirin [ATC code B01AC06], statins [ATC codes C10AA01, C10AA03, C10AA04, C10AA05, C10AA07, C10AA08], and metformin [ATC code A10BA02]) and summarized data on comorbid conditions derived from the Patient Register into the Charlson comorbidity index score [33].

Insulin genetic score
Associations with the insulin genetic score were assessed in the Karma subcohort with genotyping data. Whole-blood samples of 9437 study participants were genotyped using Illumina iSelect arrays (iCOGS [$n = 3909$] and OncoArray [$n = 5528$], details of which have been described elsewhere [34, 35], and missing genotypes for common variants across the genome were imputed using the 1000 Genomes Project March 2012 release as a reference. The insulin genetic score was constructed using 18 independent single nucleotide polymorphisms (SNPs) shown to be robustly associated with circulating log insulin levels at $P < 5.0 \times 10^{-8}$ [36] (Additional file 1: Table S3). The score was calculated on the basis of a weighted method according to each SNP's effect size (β) obtained from the literature [24]:

$$\text{Insulin genetic score} = \beta_1 x_1 + \beta_2 x_2 + \dots \beta_k x_k + \beta_n x_n,$$

where β is the per-allele beta value for log-transformed fasting insulin levels associated with the effect allele for SNP k and x_k is the number of alleles for the same SNP

(0, 1, 2) and n is the total number of SNPs included in the score ($n = 18$).

Statistical analyses

To approximate the normal distribution, all mammographic measures were log-transformed prior to analyses, and geometric means and percentage (%) differences were calculated [37]. Differences in MD by insulin therapy were analyzed using generalized linear models, including a basic model with adjustment for age and BMI and a multivariable model with inclusion of other potential confounders (education level, age at menarche, parity and age at first birth, oral contraceptives, menopausal status, hormone replacement therapy, alcohol intake, smoking status, statins, low-dose aspirin, Charlson comorbidity index, history of benign breast disease, and family history of breast cancer). Analyses were additionally adjusted for metformin comedication to account for potential antiproliferative effects of this diabetes drug [6]. Differences in MD were assessed overall and by insulin glargine use and treatment duration. In T2D patients, treatment duration was defined from the first dispensed insulin prescription encountered in the Prescribed Drug Register. Because age at T1D onset is well below the age at which women undergo mammography screening, and with prescription data being available only from July 2005 onward, insulin treatment duration in T1D patients was calculated from the age at T1D diagnosis to study entry.

To address possible residual confounding by underlying disease, we also examined MD differences comparing insulin-treated with non-insulin-treated T2D patients. This active comparator analysis was adjusted for the same covariates as listed above and additionally for diabetes duration to account for differences in disease onset between the two patient groups.

Associations with the insulin genetic score were assessed using linear regression, with beta values representing percentage differences in MD per 1-SD increment in the score. Because there was no evidence of heterogeneity by genotyping array (iCOGS vs. OncoArray), a one-sample approach was undertaken. Genetic score analyses were adjusted for age, BMI, menopausal status, genotyping array, and six principal components to account for population stratification. To investigate the independence of genetic effects of other potential confounders, we also examined associations of the score with covariates entered in the insulin treatment analysis.

All analyses were undertaken using STATA version 14 (StataCorp, College Station, TX, USA) and PLINK version 1.9 [38]. Missing values on covariates were imputed using multivariate multiple imputation with chained equations, and ten imputed datasets were generated [39]. Imputation models included the outcome (MD), exposure (insulin treatment/insulin genetic score), and all covariates included in any of the analysis models (see Additional file 2: Supplementary Methods).

Results

Descriptive characteristics of the study populations are summarized in Table 1. Mean ages at diagnosis were 20 and 55 years for the insulin-treated T1D and T2D patients, respectively. Insulin glargine was prescribed to 53% of T1D patients and 31% of T2D patients, and combined therapy with metformin was given in 4% and 53% of T1D and T2D patients, respectively. Compared with age-matched individuals without diabetes, insulin-treated T1D and T2D patients were younger at first child's birth, less often used oral contraceptives in the past, more frequently reported a family history of breast cancer, and were more often alcohol abstainers and less physically active at study entry. As expected, insulin-treated T1D and T2D patients also presented with more comorbid conditions and were more often on statin and low-dose aspirin medications. Univariate associations with other participant characteristics were comparable for the two patient groups, except for BMI and age at menarche. Study participants of the subcohort for genetic analysis had characteristics similar to those of the age-matched individuals without T2D, except for a larger proportion being premenopausal. Descriptive characteristics of insulin-treated and non-insulin-treated T2D patients are summarized in Additional file 1: Table S4. Compared with T2D patients receiving other glucose-lowering medication, insulin-treated T2D patients were younger, had a lower BMI, and were more likely to have comorbid conditions and a history of benign breast disease. They also had a longer disease duration (8.3 vs. 4.8 years), as reflected by the younger age at diagnosis.

A summary plot of MD percentage differences estimated in each observational analysis is presented in Additional file 3: Figure S1 to facilitate comparison across the different analyses. Geometric means of MD in insulin-treated diabetics and age-matched individuals without diabetes are listed in Table 2 together with corresponding percentage differences. Compared with age-matched women without diabetes, T1D patients had a greater percent dense (11.3% vs. 8.7%) and absolute dense (65.7 vs. 59.6 cm^3) volume and a smaller absolute nondense volume (510 vs. 610 cm^3). These associations were not materially different after multivariable adjustment (percent dense volume [11.4 vs. 8.7%], absolute dense volume [64.7 vs. 59.7 cm^3], and absolute nondense volume [491 vs. 615 cm^3]). Compared with women without diabetes, the largest difference in absolute dense volume was found for current use of insulin glargine, whereas for percent dense and absolute nondense volumes, no notable difference in magnitude of association was observed by insulin type. Overall, similar associations were found for insulin-treated T2D. Compared with age-matched individuals without diabetes, insulin-treated T2D patients had

Table 1 Descriptive characteristics of the study population

Characteristic	Matched cohort analysis insulin-treated diabetes						Insulin genetic score analysis
	Insulin-treated T1D (n = 122)	Non-diabetics (n = 610)	P value	Insulin-treated T2D (n = 237)	Nondiabetics (n = 1161)	P value	Nondiabetics (n = 9437)
Age, years, mean (SD)	49.6 (8.6)	49.6 (8.5)	1.00	62.5 (8.0)	62.3 (7.9)	0.82	57.3 (9.8)
BMI, kg/m², mean (SD)	25.7 (4.3)	25.1 (4.3)	0.17	29.5 (5.7)	25.3 (3.9)	< 0.001	25.3 (4.1)
Education level, % (n)			0.09			0.09	
Compulsory	8.5 (10)	8.3 (49)		27.9 (62)	22.7 (250)		16.9 (1376)
Gymnasium	40.2 (47)	30.2 (178)		29.7 (66)	27.2 (300)		31.2 (2544)
University	51.3 (60)	61.5 (362)		42.3 (94)	50.1 (552)		51.9 (4234)
Missing	4.1 (5)	3.4 (21)		6.3 (15)	5.1 (59)		13.6 (1283)
Age at menarche, years, mean (SD)	13.4 (2.0)	13.0 (1.4)	0.02	12.8 (1.5)	13.3 (1.5)	< 0.001	13.2 (1.5)
Parity, % (n)			< 0.001			0.12	
0	22.1 (27)	14.0 (85)		17.9 (42)	12.6 (144)		12.1 (1129)
1	25.4 (31)	14.0 (85)		14.5 (34)	12.9 (147)		14.5 (1354)
2	36.9 (45)	51.8 (314)		42.7 (100)	46.8 (534)		47.6 (4460)
≥ 3	15.6 (19)	20.1 (122)		24.8 (58)	27.8 (317)		25.9 (2423)
Missing	0.0 (0)	0.7 (4)		1.3 (3)	1.6 (19)		0.8 (71)
Age at first birth, years, mean (SD)	27.3 (5.6)	28.5 (5.3)	0.05	24.3 (4.4)	25.8 (5.0)	< 0.001	26.6 (5.0)
Missing	5.3 (5)	5.6 (29)		6.3 (12)	5.1 (51)		
Menopausal status, % (n)			0.97			0.86	
Premenopausal	65.6 (80)	65.4 (399)		13.5 (32)	14.0 (162)		34.1 (3216)
Postmenopausal	34.4 (42)	34.6 (211)		86.5 (205)	86.0 (999)		65.9 (6221)
OC use (ever), % (n)	73.8 (90)	85.6 (519)	0.001	66.1 (154)	75.3 (853)	0.004	79.0 (6779)
Missing	0.0 (0)	0.7 (4)		1.7 (4)	2.4 (28)		9.1 (857)
HRT, % (n)			0.23			0.52	
Never	86.8 (99)	86.9 (504)		71.2 (151)	70.6 (730)		73.6 (6400)
Former	7.9 (9)	10.5 (61)		25.5 (54)	24.3 (251)		21.9 (1909)
Current	5.3 (6)	2.6 (15)		3.3 (7)	5.1 (53)		4.8 (423)
Missing	6.6 (8)	4.9 (30)		10.5 (25)	10.9 (127)		7.5 (705)
Alcohol intake, % (n)			0.02			< 0.001	
None	27.9 (34)	17.0 (104)		44.4 (103)	17.7 (200)		18.9 (1602)
1–25 g/wk	17.2 (21)	26.2 (160)		18.5 (43)	23.2 (262)		19.3 (1643)
25–50 g/wk	32.8 (40)	27.7 (169)		16.4 (38)	29.5 (333)		32.3 (2742)
> 50 g/wk	21.3 (26)	27.9 (170)		20.7 (48)	29.5 (332)		28.5 (2508)
Missing	0.8 (1)	1.1 (7)		2.1 (5)	2.9 (34)		10.0 (942)
Physical activity, % (n)			0.07			< 0.001	
< 40 MET h/d	40.2 (47)	31.6 (188)		54.1 (120)	39.9 (443)		35.4 (2913)

Table 1 Descriptive characteristics of the study population (*Continued*)

Characteristic	Matched cohort analysis insulin-treated diabetes						Insulin genetic score analysis
	Insulin-treated T1D (n = 122)	Non-diabetics (n = 610)	P value	Insulin-treated T2D (n = 237)	Nondiabetics (n = 1161)	P value	Nondiabetics (n = 9437)
40–45 MET h/d	32.5 (38)	36.8 (219)		32.0 (71)	35.4 (393)		36.0 (2969)
45–50 MET h/d	12.8 (15)	20.8 (124)		8.6 (19)	16.5 (183)		18.6 (1535)
>50 MET h/d	14.5 (17)	10.8 (64)		5.4 (12)	8.1 (90)		10.0 (822)
Missing	4.1 (5)	2.5 (15)		6.3 (15)	4.5 (52)		12.7 (1198)
Smoking status, % (n)			0.38			0.17	
Never	52.5 (64)	53.9 (327)		41.1 (97)	46.5 (536)		46.4 (3977)
Former	32.0 (39)	34.9 (212)		44.5 (105)	42.6 (491)		41.7 (3568)
Current	15.6 (19)	11.2 (68)		14.4 (34)	10.9 (125)		11.9 (1020)
Missing	0.0 (0)	0.5 (3)		0.4 (1)	0.8 (9)		9.2 (872)
Statin therapy (current), % (n)	36.1 (44)	4.3 (26)	< 0.001	61.2 (145)	11.5 (134)	< 0.001	8.9 (839)
Low-dose aspirin (current), % (n)	15.6 (19)	2.1 (13)	< 0.001	35.0 (83)	6.5 (76)	< 0.001	5.1 (483)
Charlson comorbidity index, % (n)			< 0.001			< 0.001	
0	82.0 (100)	97.0 (592)		73.8 (175)	92.2 (1070)		94.5 (8913)
1	14.8 (18)	2.6 (16)		15.2 (36)	6.5 (75)		4.8 (452)
≥ 2	3.3 (4)	0.3 (2)		11.0 (26)	1.4 (16)		0.8 (72)
Benign breast disease, % (n)			0.77			0.78	
No	78.1 (89)	76.8 (464)		75.8 (175)	74.9 (856)		76.8 (7084)
Yes	21.9 (25)	23.2 (140)		24.2 (56)	25.1 (287)		23.2 (2145)
Missing	6.6 (8)	1.0 (6)		2.5 (6)	1.6 (18)		2.2 (208)
Family history of breast cancer, % (n)			0.05			0.04	
No	84.0 (100)	90.2 (534)		80.9 (182)	86.1 (963)		87.0 (7944)
Yes	16.0 (19)	9.8 (58)		19.1 (43)	13.9 (155)		13.0 (1188)
Missing	2.5 (3)	3.0 (18)		5.1 (12)	3.7 (43)		3.2 (305)
Age at diagnosis, years, mean (SD)	19.9 (7.6)	–		54.8 (8.2)	–		–
Diabetes duration, years, mean (SD)	29.7 (10.2)	–		4.9 (2.5)	–		–
Insulin therapy, % (n)							
Glargine insulin	53.3 (65)	–		31.2 (74)	–		–
Nonglargine insulin	46.7 (57)	–		68.8 (163)	–		–
Comedication metformin, % (n)							
No	95.9 (117)	–		47.3 (112)	–		–
Yes	4.1 (5)	–		52.7 (125)	–		–

Abbreviations: T1D Type 1 diabetes, *T2D* Type 2 diabetes, *BMI* Body mass index, *OC* Oral contraceptive, *HRT* Hormone replacement therapy, *MET* Metabolic equivalent of activity level

Study populations: matched cohort analysis including insulin-treated diabetes and insulin genetic score analysis including women with available genotyping data and no known diabetes. All women in the study population were free of cancer at study entry (i.e., the baseline screening visit). In total, 21 T2D patients could not be matched to a maximum of 5 individuals (i.e., 20 patients were matched to 4 individuals, and 1 patient was matched to 1 individual), leaving 610 and 1161 age-matched women without diabetes for insulin-treated T1D and T2D analyses, respectively. Participant characteristics were compared using *t* tests for continuous data and chi-squared tests for categorical variables

Table 2 Geometric means and percentage differences of volumetric mammographic density comparing insulin-treated T1D and T2D patients with age-matched individuals without diabetes

Geometric mean (95% CI)

	No. of subjects	Percent dense volume (%)		Absolute dense volume (cm³)		Absolute nondense volume (cm³)	
		Age- and BMI-adjusted	Multivariable-adjusted	Age- and BMI-adjusted	Multivariable-adjusted	Age- and BMI-adjusted	Multivariable-adjusted
Insulin-treated T1D							
Nondiabetics	610	8.7 (8.5; 9.1)	8.7 (8.4; 9.0)	59.6 (57.4; 61.9)	59.7 (57.5; 62.1)	610.3 (589.5; 631.8)	615.0 (593.8; 637.0)
T1D – insulin any	122	11.3 (10.4; 12.2)	11.4 (10.5; 12.4)	65.7 (60.4; 71.5)	64.7 (58.8; 71.1)	509.8 (471.8; 550.9)	490.5 (450.0; 534.6)
P value		<0.001	<0.001	0.01	0.14	<0.001	<0.001
Nondiabetics	610	8.7 (8.5; 9.1)	8.7 (8.4; 9.0)	59.6 (57.4; 61.9)	59.8 (57.6; 62.2)	611.0 (590.2; 632.6)	615.7 (594.5; 637.7)
T1D – nonglargine insulin	57	11.0 (9.8; 12.3)	11.5 (10.2; 13.0)	60.0 (52.7; 68.2)	59.1 (51.5; 67.9)	477.1 (423.9; 536.9)	447.2 (394.3; 507.2)
T1D – glargine insulin	65	11.5 (10.4; 12.8)	11.4 (10.2; 12.7)	70.9 (63.2; 79.6)	69.2 (61.3; 78.2)	534.1 (480.3; 593.9)	525.9 (470.8; 587.4)
P value		<0.001	<0.001	0.02	0.07	<0.001	<0.001
Insulin-treated T2D							
Nondiabetics	1161	6.5 (6.4; 6.7)	6.5 (6.3; 6.6)	52.7 (51.3; 54.1)	52.6 (51.2; 54.0)	746.9 (728.3; 766.0)	753.5 (734.5; 773.0)
T2D – insulin any	237	7.4 (6.9; 8.0)	7.8 (7.2; 8.4)	57.5 (53.5; 61.9)	58.0 (53.7; 62.7)	708.9 (661.3; 760.0)	679.1 (630.9; 731.0)
P value		0.002	0	0.004	0.03	0.20	0.02
Nondiabetics	1161	6.5 (6.4; 6.7)	6.5 (6.3; 6.7)	52.8 (51.4; 54.3)	52.7 (51.3; 54.2)	746.6 (727.8; 765.8)	753.0 (733.9; 772.6)
T2D – nonglargine insulin	163	7.1 (6.5; 7.8)	7.5 (6.8; 8.2)	55.2 (50.4; 60.4)	56.0 (50.9; 61.5)	715.3 (656.1; 779.9)	687.1 (628.0; 751.7)
T2D – glargine insulin	74	7.9 (7.1; 8.7)	8.2 (7.4; 9.1)	60.7 (54.9; 67.1)	60.7 (54.8; 67.3)	700.8 (636.7; 771.4)	669.2 (606.6; 738.3)
P value		0.002	<0.001	0.04	0.04	0.41	0.05

Percentage difference (95% CI)

	Percent dense volume		Absolute dense volume		Absolute nondense volume	
	Age- and BMI-adjusted	Multivariable-adjusted	Age- and BMI-adjusted	Multivariable-adjusted	Age- and BMI-adjusted	Multivariable-adjusted
Insulin-treated T1D						
Nondiabetics	Reference	Reference	Reference	Reference	Reference	Reference
T1D – insulin any	28.8 (18.3; 40.2)	31.2 (19.5; 44.0)	10.3 (0.5; 21.0)	8.2 (−2.6; 20.3)	−16.5 (−23.3; −9.0)	−20.2 (−27.6; −12.2)
Nondiabetics	Reference	Reference	Reference	Reference	Reference	Reference
T1D – nonglargine insulin	25.6 (11.2; 41.8)	31.8 (15.7; 50.2)	0.6 (−12.1; 15.2)	−1.2 (−14.7; 14.4)	−21.9 (−31.0; −11.6)	−27.4 (−36.5; −17.0)
T1D – glargine insulin	31.3 (17.7; 46.5)	30.7 (16.5; 46.6)	19.1 (5.4; 34.5)	15.7 (1.7; 31.7)	−12.6 (−21.8; −2.3)	−14.6 (−24.1; −3.9)
Insulin-treated T2D						
Nondiabetics	Reference	Reference	Reference	Reference	Reference	Reference
T2D – insulin any	13.7 (4.7; 23.6)	20.5 (10.3; 31.6)	9.2 (0.4; 18.7)	10.3 (0.9; 20.6)	−5.1 (−12.4; 2.8)	−9.9 (−17.2; −1.9)
Nondiabetics	Reference	Reference	Reference	Reference	Reference	Reference
T2D – nonglargine insulin	8.3 (−2.1; 19.7)	15.0 (3.6; 27.7)	4.5 (−5.5; 15.6)	6.2 (−4.5; 18.1)	−4.2 (−13.0; 5.5)	−8.8 (−17.5; 1.0)
T2D – glargine insulin	20.4 (8.3; 33.8)	26.9 (13.8; 41.6)	14.9 (3.3; 27.8)	15.2 (3.1; 28.6)	−6.1 (−15.2; 3.9)	−11.1 (−20.0; −1.3)

Abbreviations: T1D Type 1 diabetes, *T2D* Type 2 diabetes, *BMI* Body mass index

Multivariable-adjusted model: model adjusted for age (years), body mass index (kg/m²), education level (compulsory, gymnasium, university), age at menarche (years), parity, and age at first birth (nulliparous, parous/age at first birth <25 years, parous/age at first birth 25–30 years, parous/age at first birth >30 years), menopausal status (premenopausal, postmenopausal), oral contraceptives (never, ever), hormone replacement therapy (never, former, current), alcohol intake (none, 1–25 g/wk, 25–50 g/wk, >50 g/wk), physical activity (<40 MET h/d, 40–45 MET h/d, 45–50 MET h/d, >50 MET h/d), smoking status (never, former, current), statins (no, yes), low-dose aspirin (no, yes), Charlson comorbidity index (0, 1, ≥2), benign breast disease (no, yes), and family history of breast cancer (no, yes). All analyses were standard adjusted for metformin therapy greater percent dense (7.8% vs. 6.5%) and absolute dense (58.0 vs. 52.6 cm^3) volumes, as well as a smaller absolute nondense volume (754 vs. 679 cm^3). As for T1D, insulin glargine use was associated with the largest difference in absolute dense volume in T2D patients.

A positive association of insulin glargine use with the absolute dense volume was also observed in case-only analyses including insulin-treated T1D and T2D patients only (Additional file 1: Table S5), despite the lower level of statistical significance due to smaller sample size. The association of insulin glargine with the absolute non-dense volume, however, was directionally inconsistent with the association observed in analyses using age-matched nondiabetics as a comparator (Additional file 1: Table S5, Additional file 3: Figure S1). In case-only analyses, glargine insulin users had a greater (T2D) or similar-sized (T1D) absolute nondense volume (and consequently similar-sized (T2D) or greater (T1D) percent dense volume) compared with nonglargine insulin users. Associations between insulin therapy and MD were not very different in analyses comparing insulin-treated T2D patients with T2D patients receiving noninsulin glucose-lowering medication; that is, insulin-treated T2D patients had a greater percent and absolute dense volume and a smaller absolute nondense volume than non-insulin-treated T2D patients, with the

absolute dense volume association being specific for insulin glargine use (Additional file 1: Table S6).

Results of analyses by insulin treatment duration are summarized in Fig. 1 and Additional file 1: Table S7. Compared with age-matched individuals without diabetes, a gradual increase in absolute dense volume was found with duration of insulin treatment in T1D patients. In T2D patients, a similar increase in absolute dense volume was observed with treatment duration. Case-only analyses in insulin-treated T1D patients supported the presence of a treatment duration effect on the absolute dense volume (P trend = 0.04), though numbers were small, and the association with long-term therapy (beyond 28 years) attenuated following multivariable adjustment (P trend = 0.23) (Additional file 1: Table S8). No consistent evidence of a treatment duration effect was found for percent dense and absolute nondense volumes, overall and in case-only analyses (Additional file 3: Figure S1, Additional file 1: Tables S7 and S8).

Associations of the insulin genetic score with MD are shown in Fig. 2, and a summary of individual SNP estimates is provided in Additional file 1: Table S9. Genetically predicted insulin levels were positively associated with both percent dense and absolute dense volume (Fig. 2) (beta [95% CI] per 1-SD increase in genetic score = 0.80 [0.00–1.59] and 0.93 [0.05–1.81], respectively), but not

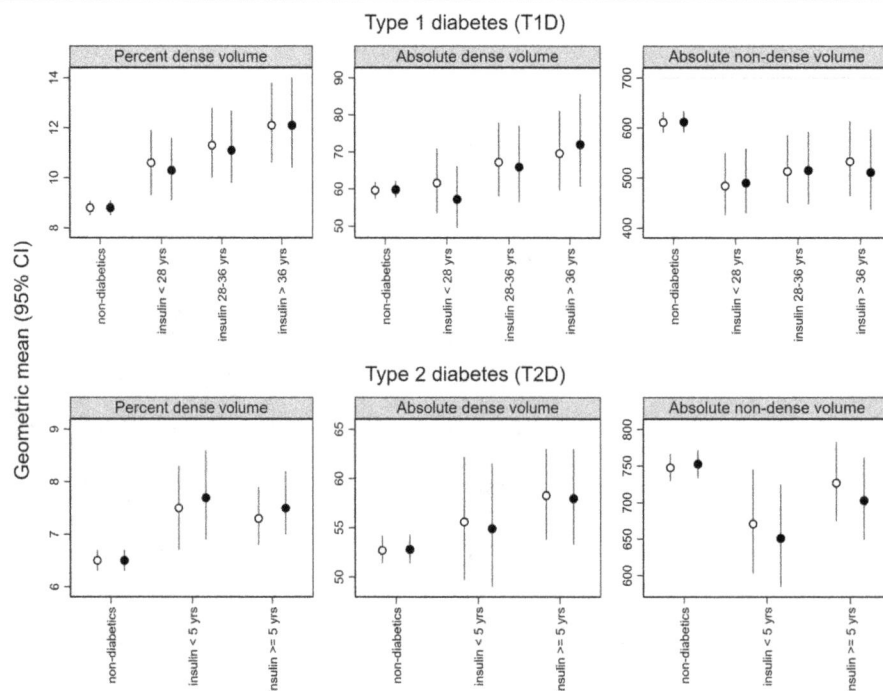

Fig. 1 Associations of duration of insulin therapy with volumetric mammographic density in type 1 diabetes (T1D) and type 2 diabetes (T2D) patients. Geometric means and 95% CIs of volumetric mammographic density by duration of insulin therapy in T1D and T2D patients. Model 1 (*open circles*): adjusted for age and body mass index. Model 2 (*closed circles*): adjusted for age, body mass index, education level, age at menarche, parity, age at first birth, menopausal status, oral contraceptives use, hormone replacement therapy, alcohol intake, physical activity, smoking status, statins, low-dose aspirin, Charlson comorbidity index, benign breast disease, family history of breast cancer, and metformin therapy

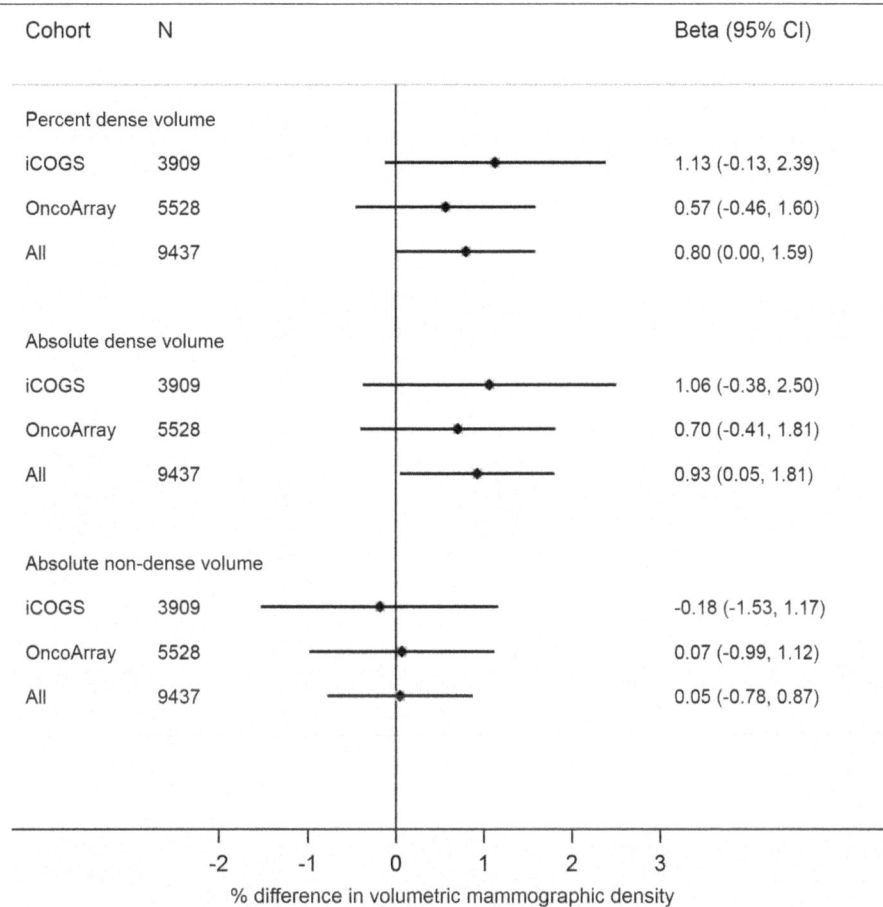

Fig. 2 Association of the insulin genetic score with volumetric mammographic density. Association of 18-single-nucleotide polymorphism insulin genetic score with volumetric mammographic density in nondiabetic women, overall and stratified by genotyping array. Associations with volumetric mammographic density were analyzed in a linear regression model, adjusted for age, body mass index, menopausal status, and six principal components. Analyses in the total study population were additionally adjusted for genotyping array. All volumetric mammographic density measures were log-transformed prior to analyses, with beta values representing percentage differences in volumetric mammographic density per 1-SD increase in insulin genetic score

with the absolute nondense volume (beta [95% CI] per 1-SD increase in genetic score = 0.05 [– 0.78; 0.87]). There was no evidence of associations being driven by potential confounders (Additional file 4: Figure S2), except for genetically elevated insulin levels being weakly associated with a lower odds of previous benign breast disease. Given the positive association between benign breast disease and MD, analyses conditioning on this variable strengthened the effect estimates (Additional file 5: Figure S3).

Discussion

In this mammography screening cohort, we found that insulin-treated T1D and T2D patients had higher MD levels as compared with age-matched individuals without diabetes and diabetes patients receiving other noninsulin glucose-lowering medication. Associations with the absolute dense volume were driven mainly by long-term insulin use and the long-acting insulin analog glargine,

whereas no associations with treatment duration or insulin type were found for the absolute nondense volume. We further observed positive associations of genetically predicted insulin levels with percent dense and absolute dense volumes, but not with absolute nondense volume. The consistency in direction of association for insulin treatment and the insulin genetic score with the absolute dense volume strengthen the evidence of a potential causal effect of long-term increased insulin exposure on mammographic dense breast tissue.

Observational studies and randomized clinical trials are limited in their ability to investigate associations of long-term insulin exposure with relatively rare outcomes such as breast cancer. As a continuous intermediate trait, MD represents an attractive endpoint for identifying potential carcinogenic effects [40]. Because MD was routinely collected in all study participants regardless of screening outcome, this outcome is also not susceptible to ascertainment bias. To date, only one study assessed associations between exogenous insulin use and MD. This study [41] reported a suggestive association of insulin therapy with a higher prevalence of mixed/dense breast density patterns, but it included only 20 diabetes patients and could not examine associations with treatment duration or insulin glargine use, nor could it distinguish associations based on fibroglandular dense and adipose nondense tissues. Though previous observational data on breast cancer risk have been somewhat conflicting, recent findings [14] of a positive association between long-term insulin glargine use and breast cancer risk cohere with the results for the absolute dense volume reported herein. Altogether, these findings suggest that the carcinogenic potential of exogenous insulins might be greatest for insulin glargine, possibly because of its unique characteristics in terms of receptor affinity and pharmacokinetic profile with prolonged duration of action.

Because our study is observational in nature, we aimed to integrate evidence from different methodological approaches to assess the likelihood of a potential causal effect of long-term insulin exposure. First, we investigated the influence of exogenous insulin use in diabetes patients. To address confounding by indication, we assessed associations with insulin-treated T1D and T2D separately. Because T1D and T2D differ in pathophysiology and underlying risk factors (with T1D being an autoimmune disease, whereas insulin resistance, driven mainly by obesity, is the hallmark of T2D), consistent results for insulin-treated T1D and T2D are suggestive of an insulin therapy effect independent of underlying disease etiology. This analysis approach using nondiabetics as a comparator, however, does not rule out confounding by the indication itself (T1D or T2D). Hence, to address possible residual confounding, we also assessed MD differences by duration of insulin treatment and insulin glargine use in case-only analyses, and we performed additional analyses using non-insulin-treated diabetes patients as an active comparator. Although none of these observational assessments may be completely free of bias, sources and directions of bias in each of these are likely to be different. Therefore, consistency of direction of association across the different approaches can be interpreted as evidence for a potential causal association. To further investigate the likelihood of a long-term insulin effect, we also explored associations with an insulin genetic score [24] as an instrument for long-term exposure to elevated circulating insulin levels. Although effect sizes for this endogenous genetic proxy are not directly comparable to those observed for exogenous insulins, because of differences in measurement scale and magnitudes of anticipated physiological effects [13], the consistency in direction of associations

observed for the absolute dense volume strengthen the evidence of a causal influence of long-term elevated insulin levels on mammographic dense tissue. On the other hand, direction of association for insulin treatment and the insulin genetic score were not consistent for the absolute nondense volume, arguing against a causal influence of insulin on adipose breast tissue.

To our knowledge, this is the first study investigating associations of long-term insulin exposure with MD combining data from observational and genetic analyses. Although absolute mammographic dense tissue is a well-known risk factor and intermediate phenotype of breast cancer, further studies investigating the effect of long-term insulin exposure on breast cancer risk are warranted, ideally with MD measurement to address the extent to which breast cancer risk associations are mediated by MD. Because long-term exogenous insulin use in diabetes patients may have a greater impact on breast tissue than genetic predisposition to long-term elevations in endogenous insulin, it will also be relevant to assess potential differential associations by exposure type. Moreover, because insulin is the mainstay of treatment for T1D and uncontrolled T2D, and because diabetes patients tend to participate less in mammography screening programs [42, 43], increasing screening awareness and participation among insulin-treated patients with diabetes may be a first step in reducing insulin-associated adverse effects from a clinical perspective.

Some limitations of the present study are noteworthy. Historical information on insulin treatment duration was not complete, because the Prescribed Drug Register has had nationwide coverage since July 2005. This limited the analysis contrasting short- vs. long-term effects of insulin use, especially in insulin-treated T2D patients, where no assumption regarding treatment initiation could be made. Also, insulin glargine and treatment duration analyses were limited by small numbers of patients, which resulted in some uncertainty in effect estimates and low statistical power when analyses were restricted to diabetes patients only. We also cannot rule out misclassification of T1D and T2D patients in instances where diagnostic age cutoffs were used. T2D incidence below the age of 30 years was low in Sweden during the study period, and most diabetes patients diagnosed before 30 years of age are likely to be true T1D cases. Finally, our study was insufficiently powered to study effects of insulin analogs other than insulin glargine. Strengths of the current study are the screening-based setting, extensive information on potential confounders, and the use of a fully automated method for MD measurement that is not prone to subjective measurement error. The unique study design further allowed us to address the likelihood of a causal association by making relevant patient comparisons and by using a genetic score robustly associated with circulating insulin levels independent of other metabolic markers and confounding factors [24].

Conclusions

Our study provides evidence of observational and genetic associations of long-term increased insulin exposure with the absolute dense volume. Apart from identifying a potential causal effect of long-term increased insulin exposure on mammographic dense breast tissue, these findings support efforts to improve screening awareness and participation among insulin-treated patients with diabetes.

Additional files

Additional file 1: Table S1. Prescriptions of insulin and insulin analogs dispensed in the year prior to study entry in T1D and T2D patients. **Table S2.** Prescriptions of glucose-lowering medication dispensed in the year prior to study entry in T2D patients not receiving insulin therapy. **Table S3.** Single-nucleotide polymorphisms included in the insulin genetic score. **Table S4.** Descriptive characteristics of insulin-treated T2D patients and non-insulin-treated T2D patients. **Table S5.** Geometric means and percentage differences of volumetric mammographic density comparing glargine insulin users to non-glargine insulin users (case only analyes). **Table S6.** Geometric means and percentage differences of volumetric mammographic density comparing insulin-treated T2D patients to non-insulin treated T2D patients. **Table S7.** Geometric means and percentage differences of volumetric mammographic density comparing insulin-treated T1D and T2D patients to age-matched individuals without diabetes by insulin treatment duration. **Table S8.** Geometric means and percentage differences of volumetric mammographic density by treatment duration in insulin-treated T1D patients (case only analyses). **Table S9.** Associations of fasting insulin single nucleotide polymorphisms with volumetric mammographic density. (DOCX 88 kb)

Additional file 2: Supplementary methods: handing of missing covariate data. (DOCX 13 kb)

Additional file 3: Figure S1. Summary of percentage differences in volumetric mammography density observed by insulin therapy across the different observational analyses. Association of insulin therapy with volumetric mammographic density in different observational analyses with age and BMI adjusted estimates (*open circles*) and multivariable adjusted estimates (*closed circles*). Betas represent % differences in percent dense, absolute dense and absolute non-dense volume for differences in insulin exposure. (PDF 476 kb)

Additional file 4: Figure S2. Association of the insulin genetic score with potential confounders. Association of 18-SNP insulin genetic score with potential confounders in Karma sub-cohort of non-diabetic women with genotyping data. Associations were tested using linear regression and (multinomial) logistic regression, adjusting for age, six principal components and genotyping array. Betas represent differences in covariate level per 1-standard deviation increment in insulin genetic score. (PDF 225 kb)

Additional file 5: Figure S3. Association of the insulin genetic score with volumetric mammographic density measures after additional adjustment for benign breast disease. Association of 18-SNP insulin genetic score with volumetric mammographic density in Karma sub-cohort of non-diabetic women with genotyping data, overall and stratified by genotyping array and with additional adjustment for benign breast disease. Associations with volumetric mammographic density were tested by linear regression, adjusting for age, body mass index, menopausal status, six principal components and benign breast disease. Analyses in total sub-cohort were additionally adjusted for genotyping array. All volumetric mammographic density measures

were log-transformed prior to analyses, with betas representing % differences in volumetric mammographic density per 1-standard deviation increment in insulin genetic score. (PDF 146 kb)

Abbreviations
ATC: Anatomical Therapeutic Chemical Classification System; BMI: Body mass index; ICD: International Classification of Diseases; iCOGS: Illumina iSelect array; IGF-1: Insulin like-growth factor 1; Karma: KARolinska MAmmography Project for Risk Prediction of Breast Cancer; MD: Mammographic density; SNP: Single-nucleotide polymorphism; T1D: Type 1 diabetes; T2D: Type 2 diabetes

Acknowledgements
The authors thank all participants of the Karma study, the study personnel for their devoted work during data collection, and Dr. Ralph Highnam and colleagues for their technical support with the Volpara software.

Funding
This work was financed by the Swedish Research Council (grant no. 2014-2271), the Swedish Cancer Society (grant no. CAN 2013/469), and the Cancer Society in Stockholm (grant no. 141092). The KARMA study is supported by the Märit and Hans Rausing Initiative Against Breast Cancer and the Cancer and Risk Prediction Center (CRisP), a Linneus Centre (grant no. 70867902) financed by the Swedish Research Council.
Genotyping of the OncoArray was principally funded from three sources: the PERSPECTIVE project, funded from the Government of Canada through Genome Canada and the Canadian Institutes of Health Research, the Ministère de l'Économie, de la Science et de l'Innovation du Québec through Genome Québec, and the Quebec Breast Cancer Foundation; the National Cancer Institute Genetic Associations and Mechanisms in Oncology (GAME-ON) initiative and Discovery, Biology and Risk of Inherited Variants in Breast Cancer (DRIVE) project (National Institutes of Health grants U19 CA148065 and X01HG007492); and Cancer Research UK (C1287/A10118 and C1287/A16563). The Breast Cancer Association Consortium (BCAC) is funded by Cancer Research UK (C1287/A16563), by the European Community's Seventh Framework Programme under grant agreement 223175 (HEALTH-F2-2009-223175) (COGS), and the European Union's Horizon 2020 Research and Innovation Programme under grant agreements 633784 (B-CAST) and 634935 (BRIDGES). Genotyping of the iCOGS array was funded by the European Union (HEALTH-F2-2009-223175), Cancer Research UK (C1287/A10710), the Canadian Institutes of Health Research for the "CIHR Team in Familial Risks of Breast Cancer" program, and the Ministry of Economic Development, Innovation and Export Trade of Quebec (grant no. PSR-SIIRI-701. The funders had no role in the design of the study; the collection, analysis, or interpretation of the data; the writing of the manuscript; or the decision to submit the manuscript for publication.

Authors' contributions
SB and JSB conceived of and designed the study with input from AHR, NBP, and MD. JSB performed the statistical analyses. SB and JSB drafted the manuscript. All authors contributed to the interpretation of the data and critically reviewed the manuscript for publication. All authors read and approved the final version submitted for publication and are accountable for the accuracy and integrity of the work.

Competing interests
MD declares being employed by Novo Nordisk (Denmark). All other authors declare that they have no competing interests. Novo Nordisk had no role in the design of the study; the collection, analysis, or interpretation of the data; the writing of the manuscript; or the decision to submit the manuscript for publication.

Author details

[1]Division of Oncology and Pathology, Clinical Sciences, Lund University, SE-221 85 Lund, Sweden. [2]Clinical Trial Unit, Skåne University Hospital, Lund, Sweden. [3]Department of Medical Epidemiology and Biostatistics, Karolinska Institute, Solna, Sweden. [4]Julius Centre University of Malaya (JCUM), Faculty of Medicine, University of Malaya, Kuala Lumpur, Malaysia. [5]Global Medical Affairs, Novo Nordisk A/S, Søborg, Denmark. [6]Institution for Clinical Sciences, Lund University, Lund, Sweden. [7]Department of Oncology, Södersjukhuset, Stockholm, Sweden. [8]Clinical Epidemiology and Biostatistics, School of Medical Sciences, Örebro University, Örebro, Sweden.

References

1. Giovannucci E, Harlan DM, Archer MC, Bergenstal RM, Gapstur SM, Habel LA, Pollak M, Regensteiner JG, Yee D. Diabetes and cancer: a consensus report. Diabetes Care. 2010;33(7):1674–85.

2. Chappell J, Leitner JW, Solomon S, Golovchenko I, Goalstone ML, Draznin B. Effect of insulin on cell cycle progression in MCF-7 breast cancer cells: direct and potentiating influence. J Biol Chem. 2001;276(41):38023–8.

3. Ish-Shalom D, Christoffersen CT, Vorwerk P, Sacerdoti-Sierra N, Shymko RM, Naor D, De Meyts P. Mitogenic properties of insulin and insulin analogues mediated by the insulin receptor. Diabetologia. 1997;40(Suppl 2):S25–31.

4. Rose DP, Vona-Davis L. The cellular and molecular mechanisms by which insulin influences breast cancer risk and progression. Endocr Relat Cancer. 2012;19(6):R225–41.

5. Wu JW, Filion KB, Azoulay L, Doll MK, Suissa S. Effect of long-acting insulin analogs on the risk of cancer: a systematic review of observational studies. Diabetes Care. 2016;39(3):486–94.

6. Bronsveld HK, ter Braak B, Karlstad O, Vestergaard P, Starup-Linde J, Bazelier MT, De Bruin ML, de Boer A, Siezen CL, van de Water B, et al. Treatment with insulin (analogues) and breast cancer risk in diabetics; a systematic review and meta-analysis of in vitro, animal and human evidence. Breast Cancer Res. 2015;17:100.

7. Formica V, Tesauro M, Cardillo C, Roselli M. Insulinemia and the risk of breast cancer and its relapse. Diabetes Obes Metab. 2012;14(12):1073–80.

8. Pisani P. Hyper-insulinaemia and cancer, meta-analyses of epidemiological studies. Arch Physiol Biochem. 2008;114(1):63–70.

9. Larsson SC, Mantzoros CS, Wolk A. Diabetes mellitus and risk of breast cancer: a meta-analysis. Int J Cancer. 2007;121(4):856–62.

10. Bordeleau L, Yakubovich N, Dagenais GR, Rosenstock J, Probstfield J, Chang Yu P, Ryden LE, Pirags V, Spinas GA, Birkeland KI, et al. The association of basal insulin glargine and/or n-3 fatty acids with incident cancers in patients with dysglycemia. Diabetes Care. 2014;37(5):1360–6.

11. Rosenstock J, Fonseca V, McGill JB, Riddle M, Halle JP, Hramiak I, Johnston P, Davis M. Similar risk of malignancy with insulin glargine and neutral protamine Hagedorn (NPH) insulin in patients with type 2 diabetes: findings from a 5 year randomised, open-label study. Diabetologia. 2009;52(9):1971–3.

12. Sturmer T, Marquis MA, Zhou H, Meigs JB, Lim S, Blonde L, Macdonald E, Wang R, Lavange LM, Pate V, et al. Cancer incidence among those initiating insulin therapy with glargine versus human NPH insulin. Diabetes Care. 2013;36(11):3517–25.

13. Suissa S, Azoulay L, Dell'Aniello S, Evans M, Vora J, Pollak M. Long-term effects of insulin glargine on the risk of breast cancer. Diabetologia. 2011;54(9):2254–62.

14. Wu JW, Azoulay L, Majdan A, Boivin JF, Pollak M, Suissa S. Long-term use of long-acting insulin analogs and breast cancer incidence in women with type 2 diabetes. J Clin Oncol. 2017;35(32):3647–53.

15. Kurtzhals P, Schaffer L, Sorensen A, Kristensen C, Jonassen I, Schmid C, Trub T. Correlations of receptor binding and metabolic and mitogenic potencies of insulin analogs designed for clinical use. Diabetes. 2000;49(6):999–1005.

16. Yehezkel E, Weinstein D, Simon M, Sarfstein R, Laron Z, Werner H. Long-acting insulin analogues elicit atypical signalling events mediated by the insulin receptor and insulin-like growth factor-I receptor. Diabetologia. 2010;53(12):2667–75.

17. Gunter MJ, Hoover DR, Yu H, Wassertheil-Smoller S, Rohan TE, Manson JE, Li J, Ho GY, Xue X, Anderson GL, et al. Insulin, insulin-like growth factor-I, and risk of breast cancer in postmenopausal women. J Natl Cancer Inst. 2009; 101(1):48–60.

18. Kabat GC, Kim M, Caan BJ, Chlebowski RT, Gunter MJ, Ho GY, Rodriguez BL, Shikany JM, Strickler HD, Vitolins MZ, et al. Repeated measures of serum glucose and insulin in relation to postmenopausal breast cancer. Int J Cancer. 2009;125(11):2704–10.

19. Lawlor DA, Smith GD, Ebrahim S. Hyperinsulinaemia and increased risk of breast cancer: findings from the British Women's Heart and Health study. Cancer Causes Control. 2004;15(3):267–75.

20. Mink PJ, Shahar E, Rosamond WD, Alberg AJ, Folsom AR. Serum insulin and glucose levels and breast cancer incidence: the atherosclerosis risk in communities study. Am J Epidemiol. 2002;156(4):349–52.

21. McCormack VA, dos Santos Silva I. Breast density and parenchymal patterns as markers of breast cancer risk: a meta-analysis. Cancer Epidemiol Biomark Prev. 2006;15(6):1159–69.

22. Wanders JO, Holland K, Veldhuis WB, Mann RM, Pijnappel RM, Peeters PH, van Gils CH, Karssemeijer N. Volumetric breast density affects performance of digital screening mammography. Breast Cancer Res Treat. 2017;162(1):95–103.

23. Boyd NF, Rommens JM, Vogt K, Lee V, Hopper JL, Yaffe MJ, Paterson AD. Mammographic breast density as an intermediate phenotype for breast cancer. Lancet Oncol. 2005;6(10):798–808.

24. Nead KT, Sharp SJ, Thompson DJ, Painter JN, Savage DB, Semple RK, Barker A, Australian National Endometrial Cancer Study Group (ANECS), Perry JR, Attia J, et al. Evidence of a causal association between insulinemia and endometrial cancer: a Mendelian randomization analysis. J Natl Cancer Inst. 2015;107(9):djv178.

25. Gabrielson M, Eriksson M, Hammarström M, Borgquist S, Leifland K, Czene K, Hall P. Cohort profile: the Karolinska Mammography Project for Risk Prediction of Breast Cancer (KARMA). Int J Epidemiol. 2017;46(6):1740–1g.

26. Ludvigsson JF, Andersson E, Ekbom A, Feychting M, Kim JL, Reuterwall C, Heurgren M, Olausson PO. External review and validation of the Swedish national inpatient register. BMC Public Health. 2011;11:450.

27. Wettermark B, Hammar N, Fored CM, Leimanis A, Otterblad Olausson P, Bergman U, Persson I, Sundstrom A, Westerholm B, Rosen M. The new Swedish prescribed drug register—opportunities for pharmacoepidemiological research and experience from the first six months. Pharmacoepidemiol Drug Saf. 2007;16(7):726–35.

28. Zendehdel K, Nyren O, Ostenson CG, Adami HO, Ekbom A, Ye W. Cancer incidence in patients with type 1 diabetes mellitus: a population-based cohort study in Sweden. J Natl Cancer Inst. 2003;95(23):1797–800.

29. Hemminki K, Liu X, Forsti A, Sundquist J, Sundquist K, Ji J. Subsequent type 2 diabetes in patients with autoimmune disease. Sci Rep. 2015;5:13871.

30. Brand JS, Czene K, Shepherd JA, Leifland K, Heddson B, Sundbom A, Eriksson M, Li J, Humphreys K, Hall P. Automated measurement of volumetric mammographic density: a tool for widespread breast cancer risk assessment. Cancer Epidemiol Biomark Prev. 2014;23(9):1764–72.

31. Highnam R, Brady M, Yaffe MJ, Karssemeijer N, Harvey J. Robust breast composition measurement - Volpara™. Lect Notes Comput Sci. 2010;6136:342–9.

32. Eng A, Gallant Z, Shepherd J, McCormack V, Li J, Dowsett M, Vinnicombe S, Allen S, dos -Santos-Silva I. Digital mammographic density and breast cancer risk: a case-control study of six alternative density assessment methods. Breast Cancer Res. 2014;16(5):439.

33. Charlson ME, Pompei P, Ales KL, MacKenzie CR. A new method of classifying prognostic comorbidity in longitudinal studies: development and validation. J Chronic Dis. 1987;40(5):373–83.

34. Michailidou K, Hall P, Gonzalez-Neira A, Ghoussaini M, Dennis J, Milne RL, Schmidt MK, Chang-Claude J, Bojesen SE, Bolla MK, et al. Large-scale genotyping identifies 41 new loci associated with breast cancer risk. Nat Genet. 2013;45(4):353–61. e2

35. Amos CI, Dennis J, Wang Z, Byun J, Schumacher FR, Gayther SA, Casey G, Hunter DJ, Sellers TA, Gruber SB, et al. The OncoArray Consortium: a network for understanding the genetic architecture of common cancers. Cancer Epidemiol Biomark Prev. 2017;26(1):126–35.

36. Scott RA, Lagou V, Welch RP, Wheeler E, Montasser ME, Luan J, Magi R, Strawbridge RJ, Rehnberg E, Gustafsson S, et al. Large-scale association analyses identify new loci influencing glycemic traits and provide insight into the underlying biological pathways. Nat Genet. 2012;44(9):991–1005.

37. Cole TJ, Altman DG. Statistics notes: percentage differences, symmetry, and natural logarithms. BMJ. 2017;358:j3683.

38. Chang CC, Chow CC, Tellier LC, Vattikuti S, Purcell SM, Lee JJ. Second-generation PLINK: rising to the challenge of larger and richer datasets. Gigascience. 2015;4:7.
39. White IR, Royston P, Wood AM. Multiple imputation using chained equations: issues and guidance for practice. Stat Med. 2011;30(4):377–99.
40. Boyd NF, Martin LJ, Yaffe MJ, Minkin S. Mammographic density and breast cancer risk: current understanding and future prospects. Breast Cancer Res. 2011;13(6):223.
41. Buschard K, Thomassen K, Lynge E, Vejborg I, Tjonneland A, von Euler-Chelpin M, Andersen ZJ. Diabetes, diabetes treatment, and mammographic density in Danish diet, Cancer, and Health cohort. Cancer Causes Control. 2017;28(1):13–21.
42. Jimenez-Garcia R, Hernandez-Barrera V, Carrasco-Garrido P, Gil A. Prevalence and predictors of breast and cervical cancer screening among Spanish women with diabetes. Diabetes Care. 2009;32(8):1470–2.
43. Lipscombe LL, Hux JE, Booth GL. Reduced screening mammography among women with diabetes. Arch Intern Med. 2005;165(18):2090–5.

16

Glucocorticoids promote transition of ductal carcinoma in situ to invasive ductal carcinoma by inducing myoepithelial cell apoptosis

Arantzazu Zubeldia-Plazaola[1,2], Leire Recalde-Percaz[1,2†], Núria Moragas[1,2†], Mireia Alcaraz[1,2], Xieng Chen[1,2], Mario Mancino[1,2], Patricia Fernández-Nogueira[1,2], Miquel Prats de Puig[2,4], Flavia Guzman[5], Aleix Noguera-Castells[1,2], Anna López-Plana[1,2], Estel Enreig[1,2], Neus Carbó[6], Vanessa Almendro[7], Pedro Gascón[1,2,3], Paloma Bragado[1,2*†] and Gemma Fuster[1,2*†] (iD)

Abstract

Background: The microenvironment and stress factors like glucocorticoids have a strong influence on breast cancer progression but their role in the first stages of breast cancer and, particularly, in myoepithelial cell regulation remains unclear. Consequently, we investigated the role of glucocorticoids in ductal carcinoma in situ (DCIS) in breast cancer, focusing specially on myoepithelial cells.

Methods: To clarify the role of glucocorticoids at breast cancer onset, we evaluated the effects of cortisol and corticosterone on epithelial and myoepithelial cells using 2D and 3D in vitro and in vivo approaches and human samples.

Results: Glucocorticoids induce a reduction in laminin levels and favour the disruption of the basement membrane by promotion of myoepithelial cell apoptosis in vitro. In an in vivo stress murine model, increased corticosterone levels fostered the transition from DCIS to invasive ductal carcinoma (IDC) via myoepithelial cell apoptosis and disappearance of the basement membrane. RU486 is able to partially block the effects of cortisol in vitro and in vivo. We found that myoepithelial cell apoptosis is more frequent in patients with DCIS+IDC than in patients with DCIS.

Conclusions: Our findings show that physiological stress, through increased glucocorticoid blood levels, promotes the transition from DCIS to IDC, particularly by inducing myoepithelial cell apoptosis. Since this would be a prerequisite for invasive features in patients with DCIS breast cancer, its clinical management could help to prevent breast cancer progression to IDC.

Keywords: Glucocorticoids, DCIS, Invasiveness, Myoepithelial cells, Apoptosis

Background

Breast cancer, the most frequent tumour among women worldwide, is a heterogeneous disease [1]. The most common non-invasive breast cancer lesion is ductal carcinoma in situ (DCIS) [2], defined as intraductal, since there is clonal proliferation of cancerous epithelial cells within the ductal lumen without spreading into the mammary stroma and with the myoepithelial cell layer and basement membrane (BM) remaining intact [2]. However, DCIS is considered a non-obligatory precursor lesion of invasive ductal carcinoma (IDC), in which the disappearance of myoepithelial cells and the BM leads to the invasion of the mammary stroma by tumour epithelial cells [3]. DCIS is a highly heterogeneous lesion and the evolution differs in each patient: some rapidly progress to IDC if untreated or undertreated, whereas others remain virtually unaltered for 5–20 years or never progress [4]. Epidemiologically,

* Correspondence: bragado@clinic.cat; gfuster@clinic.cat
†Leire Recalde-Percaz, Núria Moragas, Paloma Bragado and Gemma Fuster contributed equally to this work.
¹Institut d'Investigacions Biomèdiques August Pi i Sunyer (IDIBAPS), Barcelona, Spain
Full list of author information is available at the end of the article

DCIS accounts for 15–25% of newly diagnosed breast cancer cases in the USA and this incidence is increasing [5], while the frequency of IDC remains stable [6], indicating that some DCIS will be over treated without therapeutic benefit. Therefore, there is a need to improve the management of patients with DCIS by matching the risk to each individual, avoiding over/under treatment of patients with DCIS to prevent the transition to IDC, which is less therapeutically affordable than DCIS.

Recent efforts have focused on unravelling the role of cancerous epithelial cells in DCIS and IDC [4, 7]. However, the mechanisms regulating the transition from DCIS to invasive carcinoma remain largely unknown, hampering correct subsequent surgery and treatment. The characteristic feature in the transition from DCIS to IDC is the disappearance of the myoepithelial cell layer and its BM [8], which is closely related to the loss of function of myoepithelial cells, since the gene expression of the main component of the BM, laminin, is altered [9]. Myoepithelial cells play a crucial role as tumour suppressors of the transition to the invasiveness of DCIS [10]. However, despite recent progress in cell research [11–13], the molecular mechanisms that regulate myoepithelial cell layer disruption in the transition from DCIS to IDC remain unexamined.

Recent studies have highlighted the role of the microenvironment in the transition from DCIS to IDC [14–16]. During the transition from DCIS to IDC, epigenetic changes have been observed in stromal cells, including fibroblasts and myoepithelial cells [17], suggesting that the microenvironment plays a relevant role. The tumour microenvironment may be modulated by stress response factors such as hormones and neuronal factors [18]. In fact, the effect of stress-related neuroendocrine factors on breast cancer progression has been addressed by several research groups including ours [19–21]. However, the impact of these molecules in the transition from DCIS to IDC has not yet been studied. Thus, understanding how stress and associated neuronal factors affect the biology of DCIS and, in particular, the fate of myoepithelial cells, could be relevant to clinical management and outcomes.

Glucocorticoids are one of the most important neuronal factors involved in the stress response, and are implicated in other physiological functions, such as the inflammatory response and glucose metabolism regulation [22]. Glucocorticoids are lipophilic molecules and diffuse across the cell membrane. They act through their intracellular glucocorticoid receptors (GR) and mineralocorticoid receptors, although it is suggested they induce tumour progression activity in a GR-dependent manner [23].

Cortisol and corticosterone are the two major glucocorticoids present in humans. Blood corticosterone levels are 10–20-fold lower than cortisol, but corticosterone represents almost 40% of total active glucocorticoids in cerebrospinal fluid [24]. Corticosterone is the major glucocorticoid in rodents and has been related to cancer progression in animal models [25], although its role in the context of DCIS invasiveness is unknown.

Cortisol, the major glucocorticoid found in humans, generates a physical response to the stress signal by binding to its receptor, GR. Cortisol plays an important role in mammary gland development [26] and function and therefore increased levels caused by stress may affect the fate of the mammary tissue. In addition, cortisol has an impact on oestrogen activity in the mammary gland, inducing aromatase activity [27] and regulating breast cancer [19]. Cortisol is an immunomodulator that reduces the immune system's ability to detect and respond to tumour cells [19, 28], acts on DNA repair mechanisms, and modulates apoptosis [19, 23, 29].

GR is expressed in healthy breast tissue and in breast cancer, including DCIS and IDC [30]. GR expression diminishes with breast cancer progression and thus is higher in DCIS than in IDC [30]. Moreover, the GR antagonist, RU486 or mifepristone, has been suggested to be a normal breast epithelium protector [31], and in this context, there is an ongoing clinical trial based on the activity of RU486 in patients with breast cancer genes 1/2 (BRCA1/2) (clinical trial identifier NCT01898312). Additionally, pathological studies have found that myoepithelial cells express higher levels of GR than epithelial cells [30]. However, studies of the function of cortisol in the fate of myoepithelial cells and in the regulation of DCIS invasiveness are lacking. The purpose of this study was to investigate the effects of glucocorticoids on the transition from DCIS to IDC, paying special attention to myoepithelial cell modulation. Interestingly, our studies demonstrate that glucocorticoids foster the transition from DCIS to IDC through the induction of myoepithelial cell apoptosis and the reduction in laminin levels in in vitro and in vivo stress model experiments. Furthermore, in patients with breast cancer, myoepithelial cell apoptosis is more frequent in patients with DCIS+IDC than in patients with DCIS, implying this process may be a key factor in the evolution from DCIS to IDC.

Methods

Cell culture

MCF10DCIS (Asterand, MI, USA) and MCF10A (American Type Culture Collection (ATCC), VA, USA) human mammary cell lines were cultured at 37° in a humidified atmosphere with 5% CO_2 in Dulbecco's modified Eagle's medium nutrient mixture-F12 (DMEM-F12) (Gibco, Life Technologies, CA, USA), supplemented with 1% of L-GlutaMAX™ 200 mM (Gibco, Life Technologies CA, USA), 100 U/mL penicillin, 100 μg/mL streptomycin and 5 μg/mL Fungizone (PSF) (Gibco, Life

Technologies CA, USA), 5% of horse serum (Gibco, Life Technologies CA, USA) and, specifically, for MCF10A, 20 ng/mL epithelial growth factor (EGF) (Peprotech, NJ, USA), 0.5 µg/mL hydrocortisone (Sigma, MO, USA), 10 µg/mL insulin (Sigma, MO, USA) and 100 ng/mL cholera toxin (Sigma, MO, USA) were also added.

Primary myoepithelial cells and epithelial cells were isolated from fresh healthy mammary tissue from five women aged 20–45 years (Additional file 1: Table S1). Samples were obtained under the approval of the Institutional Review Board of the Hospital Clinic and Clinica Planas, Barcelona. To obtain mammary myoepithelial cells, epithelial cells and organoid fractions were cultured in M87A medium [32] (see Additional file 2). Cell sorting of CD10+ cells from epithelial and organoid fractions was used to isolate myoepithelial cells, as described by LaBarge and colleagues [33].

Cell viability
To analyse in vitro cell viability, 3-(4, 5-dimethylthiazol-2-yl)-2, 5-diphenyl tetrazolium bromide (MTT) assays (Promega, WI, USA) were performed. Briefly, $1.5*10^4$ cells/100 µL were seeded per well in MW96 plates. After 24 h, cells were treated for 48 h with increasing concentrations of cortisol (0.1, 0.25, 0.5, 1, 2.5, 5 and 10 µM), corticosterone (0.125, 0.25, 0.375, 0.5, 0.75, 1, 1.25 and 1.5 µM) or with the corresponding vehicle concentration (methanol). The analysis was carried out following the kit instructions (Promega, WI, USA). Absorbance was measured immediately using a microplate reader spectrophotometer (Sinergy, Bio Tek, VE, USA). Measurements were made at 492 nm (test wavelength) and at 620 nm (reference wavelength), to correct for noise.

Cell cycle
Cell cycle was analysed using bromodeoxyuridine (5-Br-2′-deoxyuridine or BrdU): $2*10^5$ cells were seeded in p60 dishes and when 70% of cell density was achieved cells were treated with 0.7 µM of cortisol or vehicle (methanol). After 48 h the cells were treated with 10 µM BrdU for 5 h. Subsequently, BrdU (10 µM) was added to each well and left to be incorporated into the newly synthesized DNA of replicating cells for 3 h. Cells were harvested with PBS and fixed with ethanol O/N. The next day, cells were permeabilized and denaturalized by HCl 2 M and 0.5% Triton X-100 for 1 h at room temperature (RT); 0.1 M $Na_2B_4O_7$ was then used to neutralize HCl for 20 min at RT. Anti-BrdU-fluorescein isothiocyanate (FITC) antibody (1:20, #F7210, Dako, Denmark) was added and the mixture kept in the dark for 1 h after PBS washing. Next, cells were suspended in 500 µL of propidium iodide (PI) buffer (PBS, 0.4 mg/mL RNase A, 0.2 µg/mL PI) and incubated in darkness for 15–20 min. The cells were analysed by flow cytometry (BD LSRFortessa)

and the results evaluated by FACSDiva software (Becton-Dickinson, NJ, USA).

Cell apoptosis
To determine cell apoptosis, an Annexin V assay (BD Annexin V: FITC Apoptosis Detection Kit I, (BD Biosciences, CA, USA) was performed in semi-confluent cell cultures: $3*10^5$ cells were seeded in p60 dishes until the plates were 70% confluent. The cells were then treated with 0.1, 0.25 and 1 µM cortisol or with 0.25, 0.6 and 1 µM of corticosterone for 48 h or vehicle (methanol). The assay was performed following the manufacturer's instructions (BD Biosciences, CA, USA) and analysed using flow cytometry (FORTESSA LSR, Becton-Dickinson, NJ, USA). The results were evaluated by FACSDiva software (Becton-Dickinson).

Three-dimensional cell culture
The functional characteristics of the cells and their ability to form proper acinar structures were evaluated by three-dimensional (3D) cultures using BD Matrigel™ Basement Membrane Matrix (BD Biosciences, CA, USA) under corticosterone and cortisol treatment. On-top 3D cell cultures were made in MW24 plates and $1*10^5$ of a mix of primary epithelial and myoepithelial cells/well were seeded in 500 µL of M87A medium supplemented with 4% of matrigel on a matrigel pre-coated MW24 well. Medium was changed three times per week and 1 mL of M87A medum with 4% of matrigel was added to each well. Cells were seeded on top of matrigel cultures and treatment was started after 5 days. Briefly, the cell medium was discarded and new M87A medium was mixed with the desired amount of the molecule of interest and 4% of matrigel on ice. Cortisol 0.7 µM, corticosterone 1 µM and RU486 0.5 µM (Sigma, MO, USA) was used as treatment. Treatment was administered three times per week until day 14 after seeding.

In vivo experiments
In vivo experiments were performed in female NUDE mice aged 3–4 weeks that were bred at the medical school's animal facility laboratory and kept under specific pathogen-free conditions at constant ambient temperature (22–24 °C) and humidity (30–50%). The mice had access to sterilized food and tap water *ad libitum*. In vivo experiments were performed according to Catalan Government Animal Experimentation Ethics Committee regulations (*Comitè Ètic d'Experimentació Animal*(CEEA)).

The MCF10DCIS cell line, which forms DCIS in mice and spontaneously evolves to invasive carcinoma, was used [18]. Mice were anaesthetized using ketamine/xylazine to inoculate the mammary fat pad with cancer cells:

10^5 cells diluted in PBS-matrigel (BD Biosciences, CA, USA) (1:1) were then injected orthotopically into each mouse mammary fat pad with a total volume of 100 µL.

In vivo time course

Tumour growth and animal weight were monitored twice a week for 29 days after MCF10DCIS inoculation. Mice were killed at days 7, 22 and 29 after inoculation. Tumours were extracted, fixed in paraformaldehyde (PFA) 4% and stored as paraffin-embedded tissue.

In vivo immobilization stress model

Mice were subjected to immobilization stress 7 days after inoculation of MCF10DCIS cells into the mammary fat pad. Briefly, mice were placed into 50-mL Falcon tubes where various holes ensured proper ventilation for 2 h, 5 days per week, for 3 weeks [34, 35]. We consider our in vivo stress model a chronic stress model because acute stress is a type of punctual and short-term stress [36]. On the other hand, chronic stress implies a more repetitive and/or long-term exposure to the stress source [37]. In parallel, blood was extracted from the mouse tail vein twice per week, starting before the inoculation of cells and continuing until sacrifice. Blood was extracted using EDTA-coated eppendorf tubes (Microvette® CB 300, Sarstedt, Germany), kept on ice and then centrifuged at 10,000 rpm for 5 min at 4 °C. Plasma was recovered and stored at − 80 °C.

Corticosterone ELISA in stress experiments in vivo

Circulating levels of corticosterone in murine plasma were measured using an ELISA kit according to the manufacturer's instructions (Abnova, China). Colour intensity was measured at 450 nm in a spectrophotometer (Sinergy, BioTek, VE, USA). Corticosterone levels were determined using a standard sigmoidal curve and comparing it with the standard curve.

In vivo chicken embryo model

The chicken chorioallantoic membrane (CAM) model has been previously described [38–40]. For the CAM xenografts we used premium specific pathogen-free (SPF), fertile, 9-day- incubated embryonated chicken eggs supplied by Gibert farmers: $2*10^6$ MCF10DCIS cells diluted in PBS and matrigel were inoculated on CAMs and tumours were grown for 6 days. The day after inoculation, the tumours were treated with cortisol 0.7 µM or/and RU486 0.5 µM for 5 days. On day 6 after inoculation the tumours were excised, weighed, measured and immediately fixed in 4% formaldehyde to perform IF analysis.

Immunofluorescence

To carry out immunofluorescence in 2D cell culture systems, cells were seeded on coverslips, incubated at 37° for 24 h and treated for 24 h with 0.7 µM cortisol and 1 µM corticosterone. Immunofluorescence of K14 (1/100, #ab9220, Abcam, UK), K19 (1/10, #Troma-III, DSHB, IA, USA) and for GR distribution studies (1/100, #PA-1-511A, Thermo Fisher Scientific, MA, USA) was carried out as previously described [41]. After washing, secondary antibodies were added and cells were counterstained with Hoechst dye 2 µg/mL (Life Technologies, CA, USA) for 15 min at RT in a dark humidified chamber. Cell coverslips were mounted using ProLong® Gold antifade reagent (Life Technologies, CA, USA).

Three-dimensional immunofluorescence was carried out in 3D cell cultures for 14 days after 8 days treatment with cortisol 0.7 µM, corticosterone 1 µM and RU486 0.5 µM as previously described [41]. K14 (1/100), K19 (1/10) and laminin (1/100, #ab11575, Abcam, UK) were used as primary antibodies. Muc1-FITC (#559774, Becton Dickinson, NJ, USA) was used as primary antibody to counterstain epithelial cells. Incubation with secondary antibodies was sequentially applied after washing. Samples were then counterstained with Hoechst dye 2 µg/mL (Life Technologies, CA, USA) for 15 min and analysed by confocal microscopy (Leica TCS-SP5 Broadband Confocal and Multiphoton Microscope). Additionally, we performed immunofluorescence of α-smooth muscle actin (α-SMA) (1/100, #M0851, Dako, Denmark) in the tumour sections. Briefly, the slides were incubated at 65 °C for 30 min and hydrated following a decreasing ethanol gradient (100–70%). Then, citrate buffer (pH = 6.0) was used for immunoreactivity enhancement. The primary and secondary antibody incubation was performed as described above for the 2D immunofluorescence.

Immunohistochemical analysis

Immunohistochemical analysis of tumour samples stored as paraffin-embedded tissue was carried as previously described [42]. Laminin (1/100) and cleaved caspase 3 (1/100, #9664S, Cell Signaling, MA, USA) antibodies were used. Depending on the technique performed and the manufacturer's specifications, different antibodies were used to detect myoepithelial cells: CD10 (1/100, #M7308, Dako, CA, USA), p63 (1/100, #sc-8431, Santa Cruz Biotechnologies, TE, USA) and αSMA (1/100) were used as primary antibodies. After washing the samples were incubated in the presence of HRP-conjugated secondary antibodies. After washing, samples were incubated with Vectastain ABC for 30 min in a humidified chamber followed by incubation in the presence of DAB substrate (FAST™ 3,3′-diaminobenzidine tablets, Sigma) for 5–10 min at RT, monitoring colour development by microscopy. Slides were washed with water and counterstained in 1:3 Gill II haematoxylin (Panreac) for 1 min. The slides were mounted with Cytoseal™ 60 (Thermo Scientific), left to dry and analysed by phase contrast microscopy.

Double immunofluorescence in paraffin-embedded tissue
The first steps for double immunofluorescence in paraffin-embedded tissue were identical to those of the immunohistochemical analysis. Deparaffinization and re-hydration were carried out followed by antigen retrieval, as previously described [42]. After cooling, samples were washed with PBS and blocked with 10% normal goat serum in PBS for 10 min at RT. The primary antibodies, p63 (1/100) and cleaved caspase 3 (1/100) or laminin (1/100) were diluted in 5% normal goat serum in PBS and the mix was incubated for 2 h at RT in a humid box. After washing, the mix was incubated with secondary antibodies for 1 h at RT in a dark humid box. Slides were counterstained with Hoechst dye 2 μg/mL (Life Technologies, CA, USA) for 15 min in a dark humid box. Finally, samples were mounted with ProLong® Gold antifade reagent (Life Technologies, CA, USA) and analysed using fluorescence microscopy.

Patient samples
Samples from patients with DCIS or DCIS+IDC were obtained from the Biobank of the Hospital Clinic of Barcelona, Institut d'Investigacions Biomèdiques August Pi i Sunyer (IDIBAPS), after Institutional Ethics Committee approval. Thirteen samples from patients with DCIS and fifteen from patients with DCIS+IDC were used (lesions specified in Additional file 3: Table S2). Myoepithelial cell layer apoptosis was evaluated using immunohistochemical analysis of CD10 (1/100) and double immunofluorescence of cleaved caspase 3 (1/300) and p63 (1/100).

Statistical analysis
The results were plotted and analysed using GraphPad Prism7 software (CA, USA). The Mann-Whitney test, Wilcoxon paired test and one-way analysis of variance (ANOVA) followed by a post-hoc test were used according to the type of analysis.

Results
Cortisol inhibits myoepithelial cell growth through induction of cell cycle arrest and apoptosis
To study the effect of glucocorticoids on myoepithelial cells, we used human myoepithelial primary cell cultures isolated from reduction mammoplasties [41]. Since primary epithelial cells are difficult to maintain in culture, we used the MCF10A cell line as representative of the epithelial population. Another epithelial cell line, MCF10DCIS, which spontaneously generates DCIS when transplanted into mice [18], was also used. First, we tested the expression of glucocorticoid receptors in epithelial, myoepithelial and MCF10DCIS cells (Additional file 4: Figure S1). We found that all cell lines express the glucocorticoid receptor (GR), and that

myoepithelial cells express higher levels than MCF10A or MCF10DCIS.

Two-dimensional myoepithelial cells and epithelial cell cultures were then treated with different concentrations of cortisol for 48 h. MTT assays showed that myoepithelial cell survival was reduced dose-dependently in the presence of cortisol, reaching a reduction of almost 50% at the highest tested dose (Fig. 1a). Epithelial MCF10A cell growth was also slightly more attenuated after treatment with cortisol (Fig. 1a), suggesting it affects the proliferation of both epithelial and myoepithelial cell growth. MCF10DCIS epithelial cells were resistant to cortisol (Fig. 1a) at the maximum doses tested.

Since cortisol inhibits myoepithelial cell growth we used a BrdU assay to analyse its effect on the cell cycle. We found that treatment with cortisol arrested myoepithelial cells in both the G1 and G2 phases, further decreasing the number of cells undergoing the S phase (Fig. 1b-c). In contrast, in MCF10A cells, only a very small percentage of cells were arrested in the G2 phase and there was no arrest in the G1 phase. Therefore, the reduction in cells in the S phase was not as prominent as in the case of myoepithelial cells (Fig. 1b-c). These results suggest that myoepithelial cells are more susceptible than epithelial cells to the effects of cortisol on their cell cycle. Thus, cortisol inhibits epithelial and, in a stronger way, myoepithelial cell growth partially through the induction of cell cycle arrest.

However, the effect of cortisol on the cell cycle did not explain the differences in survival between myoepithelial and epithelial cells after glucocorticoid treatment. Therefore, we also investigated the induction of apoptosis by glucocorticoids. We used an Annexin V binding assay to determine whether these cells were undergoing apoptosis and found that myoepithelial cell apoptosis increased in a dose-dependent manner by around 15% (Fig. 1d): however, the percentage of apoptotic cells was always below 5% for MCF10A epithelial cells and the MCF10DCIS cell line (Fig. 1d). Thus, we speculate that the induction of apoptosis might explain the reduction observed in the survival of myoepithelial cells after glucocorticoid treatment, an effect that seems to be restricted to the myoepithelial cell lineage.

Cortisol hampers the formation of 3D acinar-like structures in vitro
After observing that glucocorticoids inhibited the proliferation of myoepithelial cells by causing apoptosis and cell cycle arrest, we studied how glucocorticoids influenced the formation and structure of 3D *acini* using on-top matrigel cultures of a mix of healthy primary mammary epithelial cells and myoepithelial cells that, when grown in 3D systems, can form acinar structures [41].

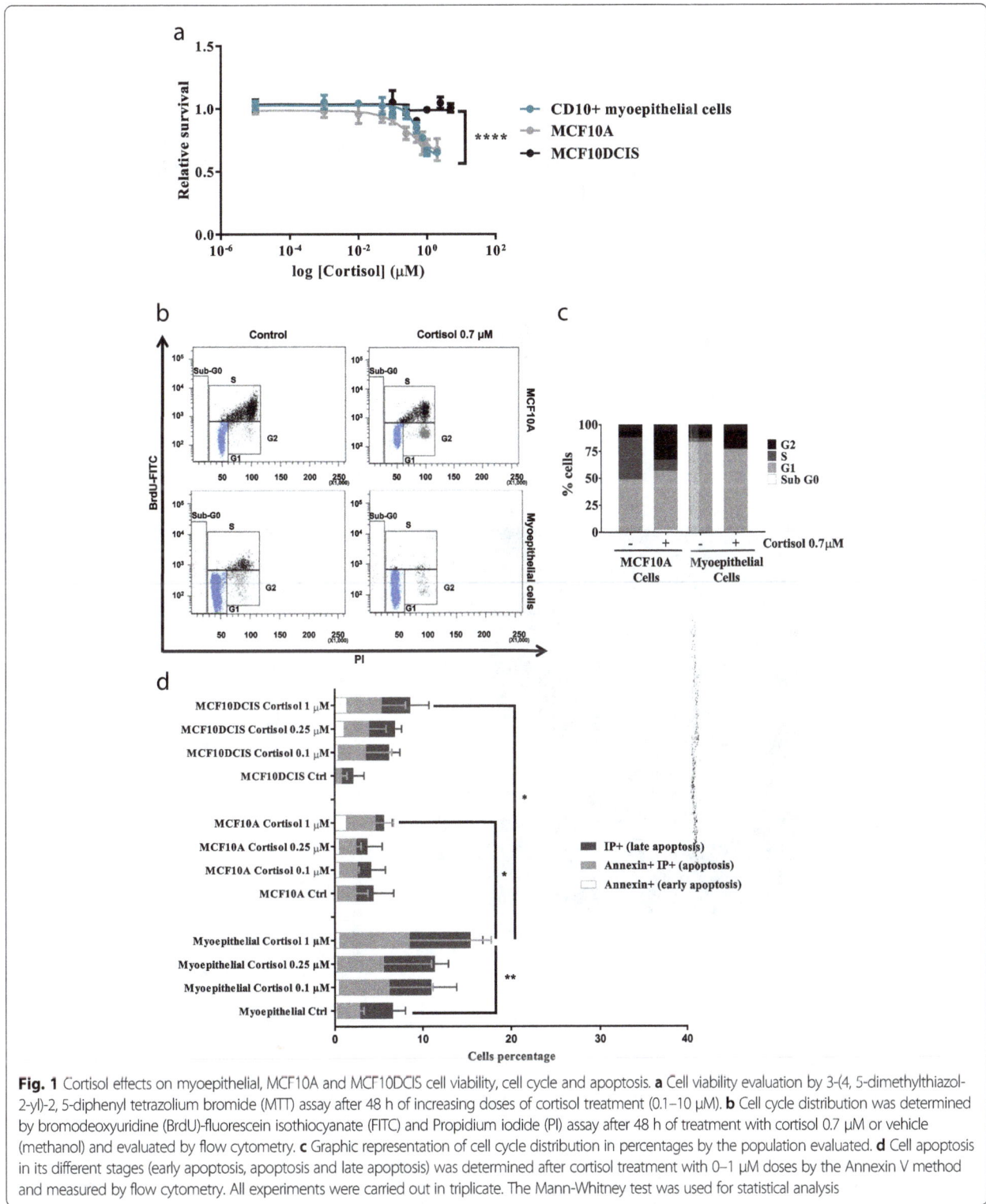

Fig. 1 Cortisol effects on myoepithelial, MCF10A and MCF10DCIS cell viability, cell cycle and apoptosis. **a** Cell viability evaluation by 3-(4, 5-dimethylthiazol-2-yl)-2, 5-diphenyl tetrazolium bromide (MTT) assay after 48 h of increasing doses of cortisol treatment (0.1–10 μM). **b** Cell cycle distribution was determined by bromodeoxyuridine (BrdU)-fluorescein isothiocyanate (FITC) and Propidium iodide (PI) assay after 48 h of treatment with cortisol 0.7 μM or vehicle (methanol) and evaluated by flow cytometry. **c** Graphic representation of cell cycle distribution in percentages by the population evaluated. **d** Cell apoptosis in its different stages (early apoptosis, apoptosis and late apoptosis) was determined after cortisol treatment with 0–1 μM doses by the Annexin V method and measured by flow cytometry. All experiments were carried out in triplicate. The Mann-Whitney test was used for statistical analysis

We seeded the cells on matrigel and let the *acini* grow for 5 days before treating them with cortisol for 9 days. Subsequently, we searched for epithelial cell (cytokeratin 19) and myoepithelial cell (cytokeratin 14) marker expression. We found that cortisol affected the capacity of

epithelial and myoepithelial mammary cells to form acinar structures because the number of *acini* was smaller than in untreated cell cultures (Fig. 2a). In addition, cortisol treatment seems to disrupt the myoepithelial cell layer, as the number of disrupted *acini* increased significantly

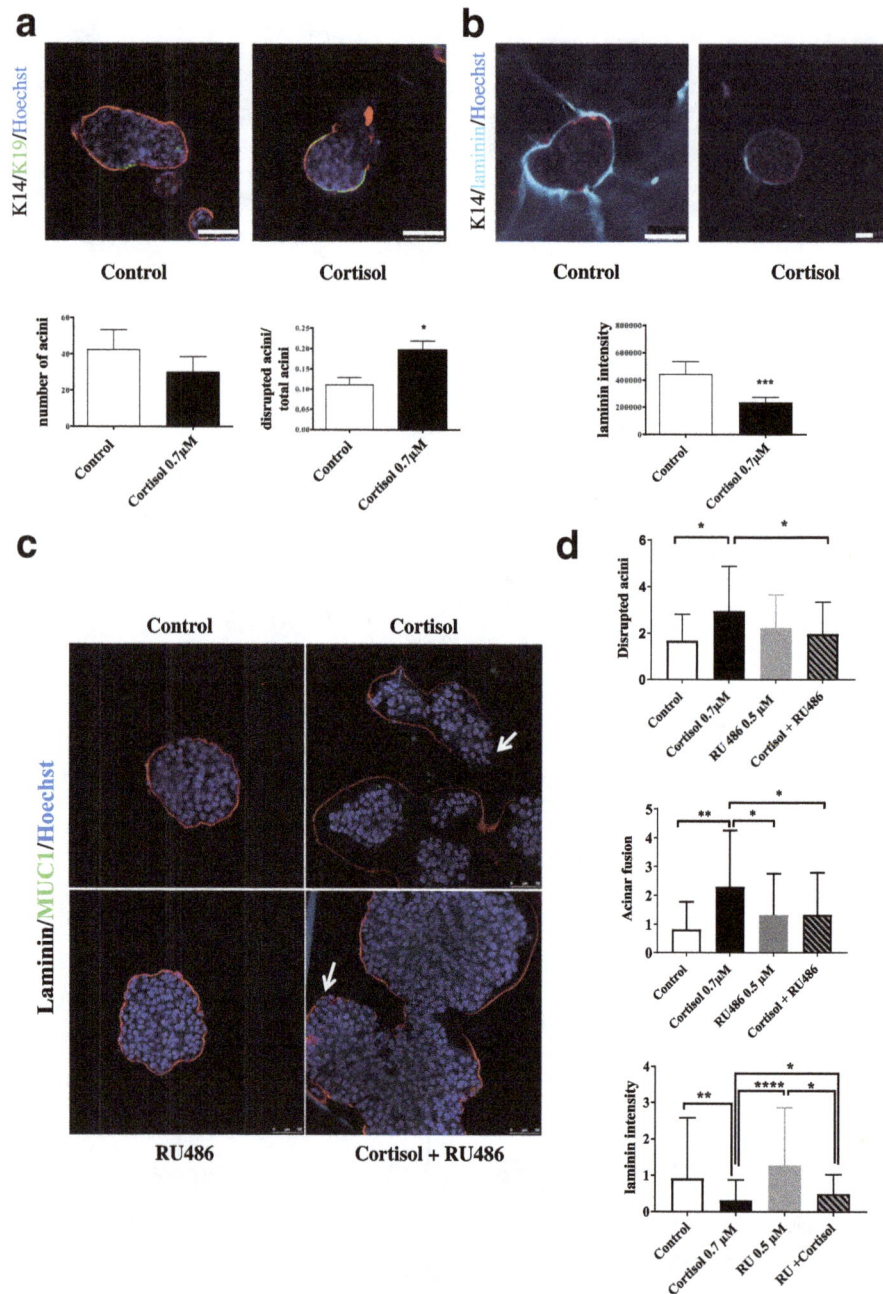

Fig. 2 Influences of cortisol treatment on 3D growth of mammary epithelial cells for 14 days identified by immunofluorescence. Cells were treated with cortisol 0.7 μM or vehicle (methanol) from day 5 after seeding until day 14. **a** Upper panels: immunodetection in primary epithelial and myoepithelial cells of K14 (myoepithelial cells), K19 (epithelial cells) and Hoechst dye was used as *nuclei* counterstaining. Scale bar = 50 μm. Bottom panels: quantification of morphometric analysis in the control group and cortisol-treated group of the number of *acini* formed and quantification of disrupted *acini* per total number of *acini*. **b** Upper panels: immunofluorescence of laminin (BM), cytokeratin14 (myoepithelial cells) and Hoechst dye to counterstain *nuclei*. Scale bar = 100 μm. Bottom panels: quantification by Image J software of laminin intensity after cortisol 0.7 μM or vehicle treatment. **c** Immunofluorescence in MCF10DCIS 3D growth of laminin (basement membrane), Muc1 (epithelial cells) and Hoechst dye to stain the *nuclei* under control (vehicle), cortisol 0.7 μM, RU486 0.5 μM and cortisol 0.7 μM + RU486 0.5 μM. Arrows indicate rupture points of the *acini*. **d** Morphometric quantification of disrupted *acini* and acinar fusion and intensity of laminin determined by the integrated density parameter of Image J software. Scale bar = 50 μm. All experiments were carried out in triplicate. Statistical analysis was performed using the Mann-Whitney test or one-way analysis of variance followed by Tukey post-hoc test

(Fig. 2a). To further study myoepithelial cell layer disruption, we also stained the 3D structures for laminin, the principal component of the BM, which is usually produced by myoepithelial cells [10]. We found that, when treated with cortisol, the amount of laminin surrounding the *acini* was significantly reduced (Fig. 2b). This suggests that when treated with cortisol, the *acini* acquire a more invasive phenotype and that apoptosis or cell cycle arrest of myoepithelial cells might in part be responsible for myoepithelial layer disruption (Fig. 2a-b). These results are in agreement with our 2D results, since apoptosis of myoepithelial cells caused by cortisol may affect their capacity to form duct-like structures and would favour invasion by disrupting the myoepithelial cell layer.

We made 3D cultures of MCF10DCIS cells and treated them with cortisol to determine whether this molecule has the same effect on MCF10DCIS cells, which were resistant to cortisol in MTT experiments (Fig. 1a, Fig. 2c-d). After treatment with cortisol, laminin intensity decreased and the proportion of acinar fusion increased (Fig. 2c-d), suggesting that treatment with cortisol also promotes the invasive capacity of DCIS acinar-like structures. Additionally, treatment with the GR antagonist, RU486, was able to block the effects of cortisol on the functional abilities of the MCF10DCIS 3D cultures (Fig. 2c-d). In fact, it prevented cortisol induction of acinar fusion and disruption (Fig. 2c-d). However, RU486 treatment only partially prevented cortisol inhibition of laminin levels (Fig. 2c-d). These results suggest that cortisol via its receptor GR is responsible for the acceleration of MCF10 DCIS acquisition of invasive features.

Glucocorticoids accelerate the progression of DCIS to IDC in vivo by inducing myoepithelial cell layer disruption

To better understand the role of myoepithelial cells in the progression of breast cancer and to study the dynamics of the formation and disruption of the myoepithelial layer under stress, we established an in vivo model using immunosuppressed mice and the MCF10DCIS cell line, which generates DCIS when inoculated into immunosuppressed mice and then evolves to IDC [18]. First, we established the dynamics of the formation and disruption of the myoepithelial cell layer in a control situation (Additional file 5: Figure S2A). We inoculated 10^5 cells in the mammary fat pad of mice that were subsequently killed at different times (Additional file 5: Figure S2A). Tumours were fixed and stored as paraffin-embedded tissue to study the tumour histology with haematoxylin and eosin staining (H&E) and by immunohistochemical analysis using antibodies against the myoepithelial cell markers alpha-smooth muscle actin (αSMA) and p63 (Additional file 5: Figure S2A).

The results showed that the first duct-like structures, surrounded by a layer of cells positive for αSMA and p63 (Additional file 5: Figure S2A), were formed at day 7

after inoculation of MCF10DCIS cells. At day 22, the myoepithelial cell layer was widely ruptured and by day 29 duct organization was virtually lost. At this point, some αSMA-positive cells were tumour-associated fibroblasts, while a subset of tumour epithelial cells was p63 positive (Additional file 5: Figure S2A). To investigate whether MCF10DCIS epithelial or myoepithelial cells could respond to glucocorticoids in vivo, we analysed the expression of GR in these tumours and found that both epithelial and myoepithelial cells expressed GRs (Additional file 5: Figure S2B).

Since corticosterone is the glucocorticoid expressed in mice, we determined whether it had the same effects as cortisol (Additional file 6: Figure S3) and found that it inhibited proliferation in myoepithelial cells and to a lesser extent in MCF10A cells while MCF10DCIS cells were also resistant to corticosterone (Additional file 6: Figure S3A). Furthermore, similar to cortisol, treatment with corticosterone induced apoptosis only in myoepithelial cells (Additional file 6: Figure S3B). Moreover, corticosterone treatment also induced the disruption of 3D culture *acini* and inhibited laminin expression in a co-culture of primary epithelial and myoepithelial cells and also in the MCF10DCIS cell line (Additional file 6: Figure S3C-F). These results suggest that corticosterone might promote invasiveness through myoepithelial cell apoptosis, as did cortisol.

To determine whether glucocorticoids promote DCIS transition to IDC, MCF10DCIS cells were inoculated into mice mammary fat pads, and 9 days later when DCIS was established immobilization stress was initiated to mimic chronic stress (Fig. 3a). Blood was extracted from mice tails every 3 days and corticosterone levels were measured using ELISA (Fig. 3a-b). We have previously found that in vitro corticosterone treatment of MCF10DCIS cells produces similar effects to cortisol on cell viability, apoptosis and functional 3D abilities (Fig. 2c-d and Additional file 6: Figure S3A-B), favouring the breakdown of the myoepithelial cell layer and the disappearance of the BM in a similar fashion to cortisol.

Mice underwent stress daily until they were killed at 24 days after inoculation, when the myoepithelial cell layer was mostly ruptured (Fig. 3c). Tumours were extracted, fixed and stored as paraffin-embedded tissue. As expected, corticosterone levels significantly increased when stress began and remained elevated throughout the experiment (Fig. 3b).

To determine how the architecture of duct-like structures changed in control and stressed mice tumours, histology was examined by H&E staining and immunohistochemical analysis was performed using antibodies against the myoepithelial cell and basement membrane markers α-SMA and laminin (Fig. 3c-d). We found that although the ducts in both control and stressed tumours were starting to rupture, there was greater disorganization of the ductal architecture

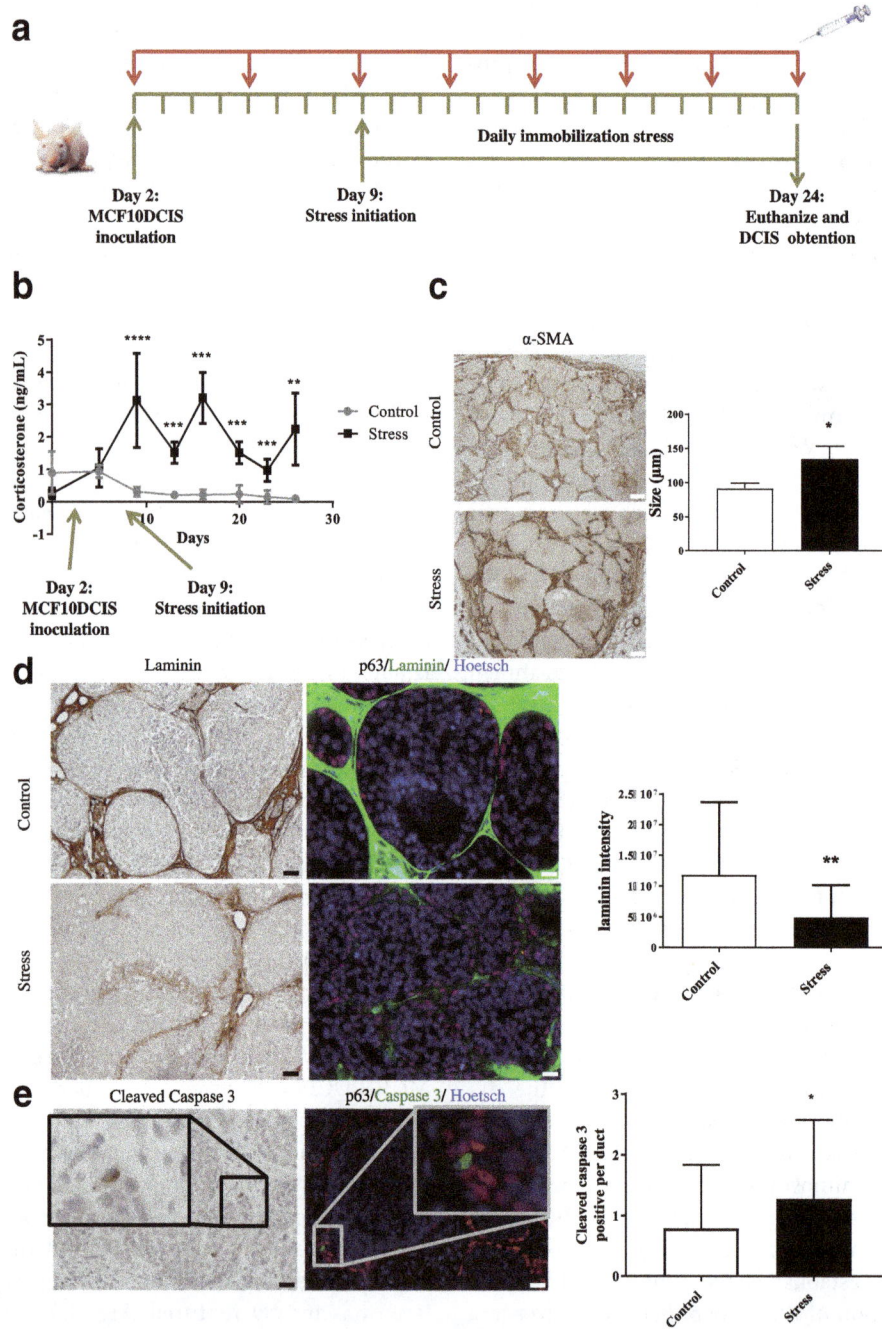

Fig. 3 In vivo stress model and the effects on evolution of the MCF10DCIS xenograft. **a** Timeline of the in vivo stress model indicating blood extraction and the immobilization method applied. **b** Corticosterone levels (ng/ml) in plasma samples obtained at different points of the in vivo stress model in mice, in the control and stressed group of MCF10DCIS xenograft. The Wilcoxon paired test was used for statistical analysis. **c** Left panel: representative image of α-smooth muscle actin (α-SMA, a myoepithelial cell marker) from immunohistochemical analysis of the control and stressed tumours in mice. Scale bar = 50 μm. **c** Right panel: duct size quantification by Image J Software. In vivo experiments were performed using five animals per group. The Mann-Whitney test was used for statistical analysis. **d** Left panel: representative laminin immunohistochemical images in control and stressed MCF10DCIS xenografts. Scale bar = 50 μm. **d** Right panel: laminin and p63 double immunofluorescence and quantification of laminin intensity images (Image J Software) of tumours derived from control and stressed mice. Hoechst dye was used to counterstain the *nuclei*. Scale bar = 20 μm. **e** Left panel: representative cleaved caspase 3 immunohistochemical image of a tumour from stressed mice. Scale bar = 20 μm. **e** Middle panel: representative cleaved caspase 3(green) and p63(red) immunofluorescence image of a tumour from stressed mice. Hoechst dye was used as the counterstain for *nuclei*. Scale bar = 20 μm. **e** Right panel: quantification of caspase 3-positive myoepithelial cells per duct in control and tumours from stressed mice; n = 5 animals/group. The Mann-Whitney test was used for statistical analysis. DCIS, ductal carcinoma in situ

when mice underwent stress (Fig. 3c-d), and the ducts were significantly larger in the tumours of stressed animals, suggesting they may have been disrupted earlier, joining together and forming larger ductal structures (Fig. 3c-d).

To determine how stress affected the invasiveness of DCIS, BM loss was also analysed by laminin staining, a key feature of invasiveness. Laminin immunohistochemical and double immunofluorescence assays, together with p63 staining, were used and the results showed stressed mice had significantly less laminin surrounding the ducts (Fig. 3d), thus showing a more invasive phenotype.

As the treatment of myoepithelial cell cultures with corticosterone in vitro caused apoptosis (Additional file 6: Figure S3B), we analysed the number of apoptotic myoepithelial cells per duct and found more apoptotic myoepithelial cells in tumours from stressed mice, who were thus exposed to higher corticosterone levels (Fig. 3e).

These results may suggest that chronic stress through sustained high blood corticosterone levels and other mechanisms promotes myoepithelial cell apoptosis, leading to disruption of the myoepithelial cell layer, favouring cell invasion and fostering progression from DCIS to IDC.

Additionally, we used the chick embryo chorioallantoic membrane (CAM) system for growing MCF10DCIS tumours (Fig. 4a). First of all, we tested whether when inoculated in CAM, MCF10DCIS form the same structures as they do in xenografts on mice (Additional file 7: Figure S4). The double p63 and laminin immunofluorescence carried out in the tumour sections showed typical organization of MCF10DCIS tumour growth and a proper laminin and p63 distribution (Additional file 7: Figure S4). Thus, we have used this model to study the effects of cortisol and the GR antagonist, RU486, on the transition of MCF10DCIS tumours to IDC in vivo (Fig. 4). Our results have shown that cortisol treatment slightly increases tumour volume, while treatment with cortisol and RU486 partially reverts this effect. In a similar way, treatment with cortisol induces acinar fusion and increases *acini* size (Fig. 4d-e). Furthermore, the myoepithelial cell layer detected by staining of αSMA positive cells was reduced after cortisol treatment (Fig. 4f). Interestingly, treatment with GC antagonist alone slightly increases αSMA staining. However, combination of cortisol and RU486, not only reverted cortisol inhibition of αSMA and disruption of the myoepithelial cell layer, but also prevented cortisol induction of acinar fusion and reduced *acini* size (Fig. 4d-f).

We also quantified myoepithelial cell apoptosis (Fig. 4g-h). In agreement with our previous in vitro results, the number of apoptotic myoepithelial cells was increased after treatment with cortisol. Interestingly, RU486 treatment partially reverted the effects of cortisol

on myoepithelial cell apoptosis (Fig. 4g-h). Thus, treatment with RU486 in vivo hampers cortisol induction of acinar fusion, degradation of the BM and myoepithelial cells apoptosis, preventing cortisol promotion of DCIS invasiveness.

Myoepithelial cell fate in patients with DCIS and DCIS+IDC

As we have found that myoepithelial cell apoptosis contributes to disruption of the myoepithelial cell layer and the BM and promotes the invasiveness of DCIS, we wondered if patients with DCIS+IDC would have more apoptotic myoepithelial cells in the ducts, indicating a more invasive DCIS phenotype. Therefore, we obtained breast tissue samples from patients with DCIS or DCIS+IDC and evaluated myoepithelial cell apoptosis. We analysed tissue samples from 13 patients with DCIS and 15 patients with DCIS+IDC (Additional file 3: Table S2) with both immunohistochemistry against CD10 (myoepithelial cells) (Fig. 5a) and double immunofluorescence against p63 (myoepithelial cells) and cleaved caspase 3 (apoptosis marker) (Fig. 5b-c and Additional file 8: Figure S5). The results showed that patients with DCIS+IDC lost most of the continuous p63 staining (Fig. 5b bottom part, 5C and Additional file 8: Figure S5) and exhibited myoepithelial cell apoptosis in some ducts, whereas patients with DCIS did not present apoptosis of myoepithelial cells in most ducts, although isolated apoptotic events were detected (Fig. 5b upper part, 5C and Additional file 8: Figure S5), suggesting myoepithelial cell apoptosis is a prerequisite for DCIS invasiveness (Fig. 6) and that the use of RU486 could partially prevent this event.

Discussion

Understanding the mechanisms that initiate and trigger DCIS invasiveness is relevant because understanding how DCIS evolves into invasive carcinoma could enable the design of interventional strategies to prevent breast cancer progression. The most widely accepted hypothesis on the mechanisms regulating the transition from DCIS to IDC suggests the microenvironment is involved, in particular fibroblasts and myoepithelial cells [14, 15, 43]. Despite recent progress in myoepithelial cell research suggesting that they may act as tumour suppressors [11], the mechanism of myoepithelial cell layer disruption remains elusive.

In this scenario, the present study investigated the role of glucocorticoids in the transition of DCIS to invasiveness. The effect of stress-related factors, studied as microenvironmental elements, in the progression of breast cancer has been investigated [18, 44]. However, the impact of glucocorticoids in the transition from DCIS to IDC has not yet been studied. To the best of our knowledge, this is the first study to suggest that glucocorticoids contribute to the transition from DCIS to IDC, particularly through the disappearance of the basal lamina and the induction of myoepithelial cell apoptosis.

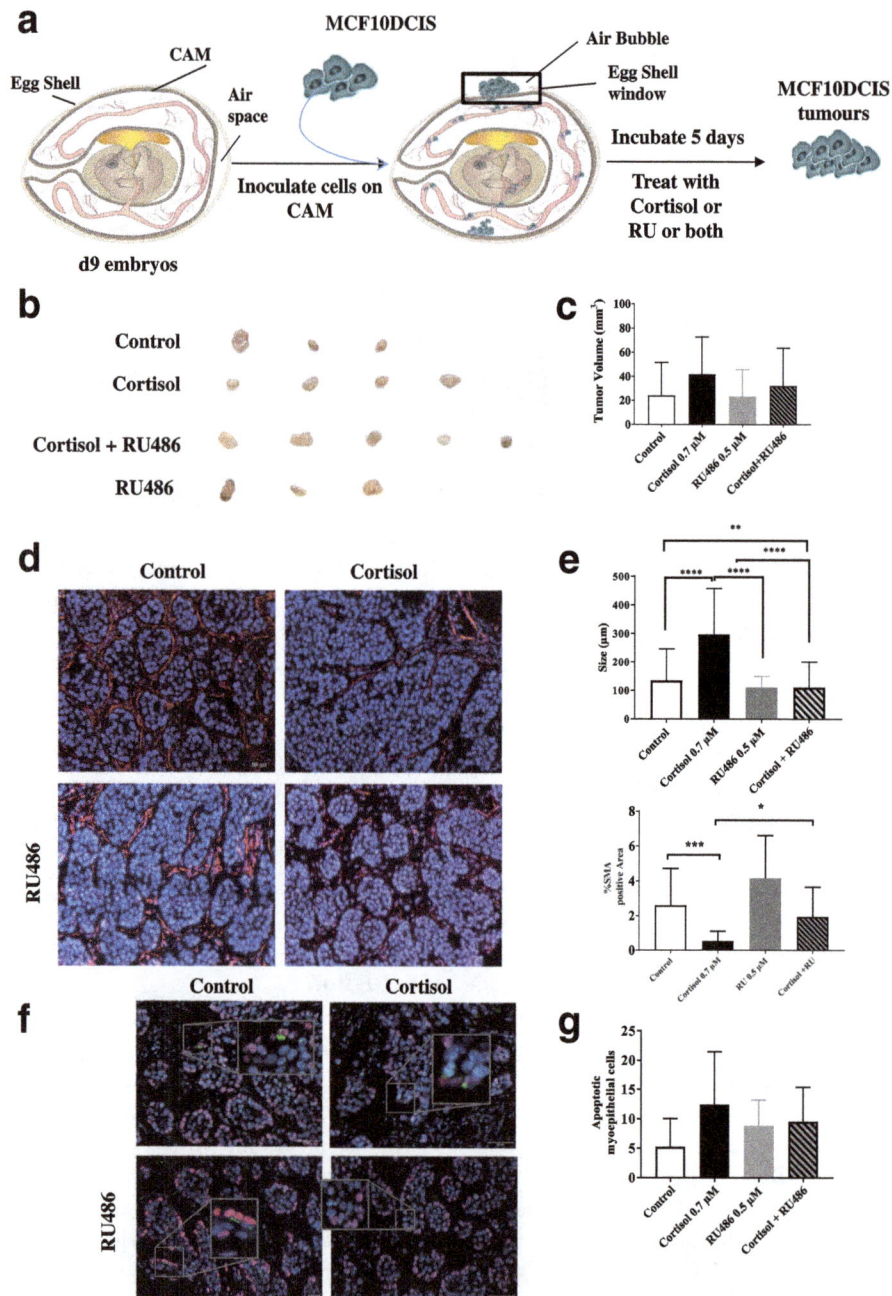

Fig. 4 In vivo chicken embryo chorioallantoic membrane (CAM) system for growing MCF10DCIS tumours. **a** Timeline of CAM model indicating how the inoculation of MCF10DCIS cells was performed and how the tumours were treated. **b** Representative tumour images after treating with control, cortisol 0.7 μM, RU486 0.5 μM and cortisol + RU486 for 5 days. **c** Graphical representation of tumour volume in mm^3. **d** α-Smooth muscle actin (α-SMA) (in red) immunofluorescence of the tumours after treatment with cortisol 0.7 μM, RU486 0.5 μM and cortisol + RU486. Hoechst dye was used to counterstain *nuclei*. Scale bar =20 μm. **e** Quantification of *acini* size (μm). Bottom panel: representation of percentage of α-SMA-positive area in tumours. Scale bar = 50 μM. **f** Images of double p63 (myoepithelial cells) and cleaved caspase 3 immunofluorescence in tumours. Scale bar = 50 μM. **g** Graphical representation of apoptotic myoepithelial cells quantification in tumours under the different treatments. One-way analysis of variance was used for statistical analysis followed by Tukey post-hoc test

In addition, myoepithelial cell apoptosis is prominent in breast cancer tumours that have progressed to IDC, suggesting apoptosis could be a preliminary, essential factor that precedes invasiveness.

Glucocorticoids have been shown in studies to mediate growth inhibition in some mammary tumour cell lines [45], and to induce G1/G0 cell cycle arrest [46], and if administration persists, to lead to cell apoptosis [47].

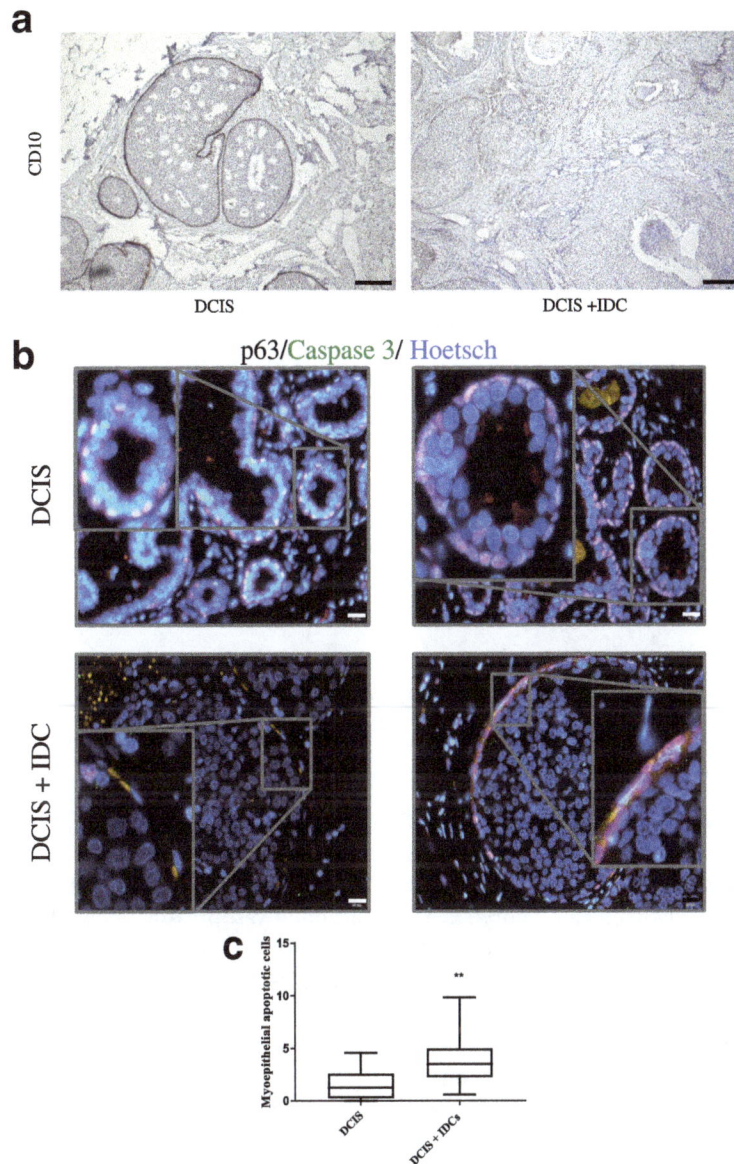

Fig. 5 Immunohistochemical and immunofluorescence images of human samples from patients with ductal carcinoma in situ (DCIS) and DCIS + invasive ductal carcinoma (IDC). **a** CD10 (myoepithelial cells) immunohistochemical analysis of samples from patients. Scale bar = 100 μm. **b** Double immunofluorescence of p63 (myoepithelial cells) and cleaved caspase 3 and Hoechst dye as a *nuclei* counterstain. Upper panel: patients with DCIS; bottom panel: patients with DCIS + IDC. White scale bar = 20 μm and red scale bar = 50 μm. **c** Quantification of apoptotic myoepithelial cells in DCIS (13 patients) and DCIS + IDC (15 patients). The Mann-Whitney test was used for statistical analysis

However, there are contrasting results on the effect of glucocorticoids on cell survival and proliferation [45, 48]. For instance, in breast invasive tumours, glucocorticoids promote cell survival through the induction of anti-apoptotic genes [29]. In contrast, glucocorticoids trigger apoptosis in hematopoietic cells and lymphocytes [28], suggesting they may act differently depending on the cell subtype. GRs are expressed in luminal epithelial cells and occasionally in stromal cells, but predominantly in myoepithelial cells [30], suggesting that GR are expressed in a cell-lineage-dependent manner in breast

tissue [30] as reported in other tissues [45, 46], and that myoepithelial cells may play a physiological role in mediating the effects of glucocorticoid hormones in the breast.

Furthermore, our results showed that glucocorticoids induce the degradation of the BM and the disruption of acinar structures through a significant loss of laminin in healthy human mammary epithelial and myoepithelial cells and in MCF10DCIS 3D cultures. Laminin is a prominent and influential component of the BM, which constitutes a physical barrier for invasive epithelial cells

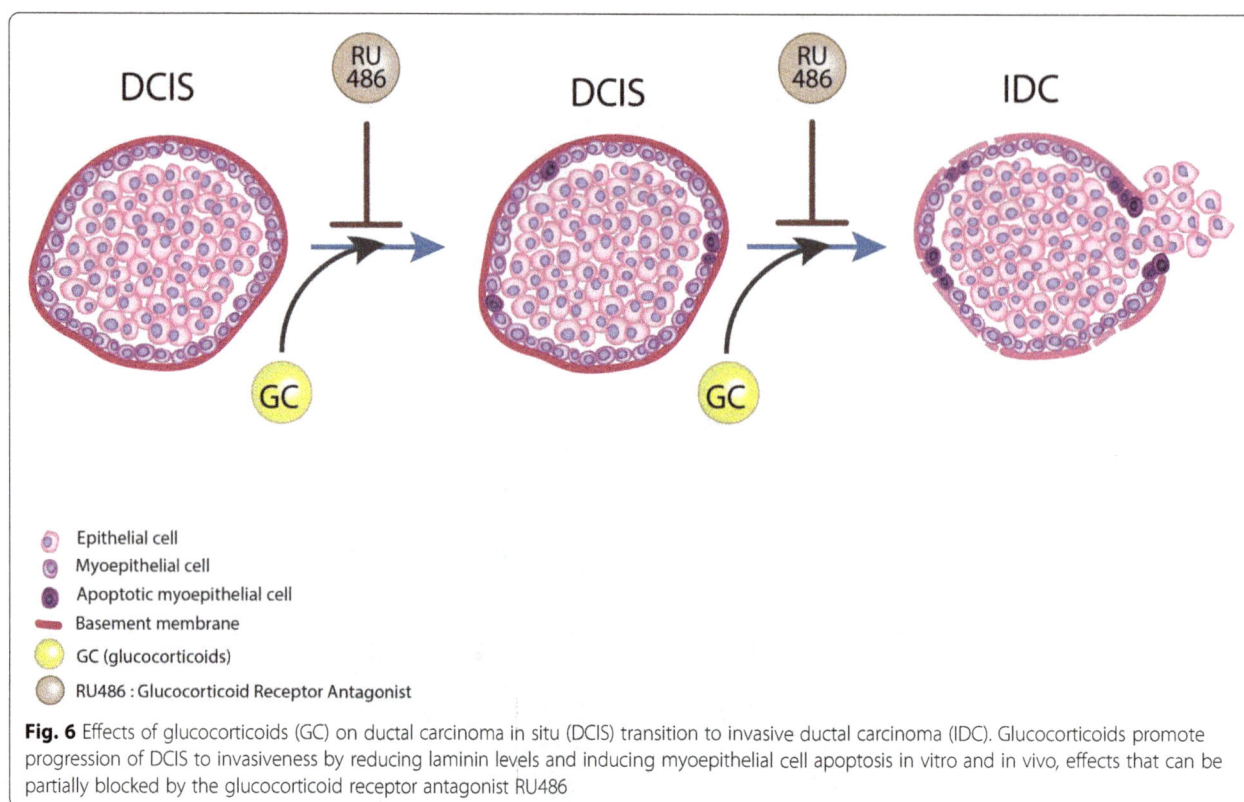

Fig. 6 Effects of glucocorticoids (GC) on ductal carcinoma in situ (DCIS) transition to invasive ductal carcinoma (IDC). Glucocorticoids promote progression of DCIS to invasiveness by reducing laminin levels and inducing myoepithelial cell apoptosis in vitro and in vivo, effects that can be partially blocked by the glucocorticoid receptor antagonist RU486

[49–51]. Laminin expression and αSMA levels are both related to tumour malignancy [52, 53]. Similarly, our in vivo stress model and our in vivo chicken embryo CAM system showed indicators of higher invasiveness after stress challenge [10], in particular increased acinar rupture and reduced laminin levels or αSMA levels. Moreover, treatment of MCF10DCIS 3D cultures with the GR antagonist, RU486, blocked the effects of cortisol on the integrity of the acinar structures and also on the BM, highlighting the influence of cortisol on the early acquisition of invasive features in breast cancer cells. We hypothesize that the loss of laminin is directly related to myoepithelial cell loss by apoptosis. However, more experiments are needed to confirm this idea.

In this context, repeated immobilization has been described as a model of chronic stress since in our case it was applied for 2 h every day for a period of 4 weeks. In addition, the repeated immobilization model is reported to increase corticosterone plasma levels among other changes [54]. In fact, chronic stress situations initiate a cascade of pathways in the central nervous system and periphery, triggering fight-or-flight stress responses in the autonomic nervous system (ANS) or defeat/withdrawal responses in the hypothalamic-pituitary-adrenal axis (HPA) [55]. ANS responses to stress are mediated by the activation of the sympathetic nervous system (SNS) and the following release of cathecolamines [56].

HPA responses to stress include hypothalamic production of corticotrophin-releasing hormone (CRH) and arginine vasopressin (AVP). These molecules activate the secretion of pituitary hormones and adrenocorticotropic hormones (ACTH), which induces the release of glucocorticoids from the adrenal cortex [55]. In this scenario, glucocorticoids are the final effectors of the HPA axis, which regulate CRH and ACTH secretion and limit the duration of the total tissue exposure of the organism to glucocorticoids [57].

In agreement with our findings connecting glucocorticoids with the invasiveness of DCIS, several studies have linked glucocorticoids to the progression and malignancy of breast cancer. In animal models, glucocorticoid regulation following exposure to social isolation was associated with an increased mammary tumour burden [28], while acute stressors were linked to abnormal glucocorticoid regulation and increased mammary tumour growth [58]. Pan et al. identified correlation between the expression of GRs in estrogen receptor (ER)⁻ breast tumours with shorter relapse-free survival [59]. In addition, women with metastatic breast cancer frequently have flatter-than-normal diurnal cortisol patterns and the degree of diurnal variation of glucocorticoids may predict earlier breast cancer mortality [60]. Glucocorticoids have also been linked to reduced immunosurveillance, which is associated with the induction of tumour progression [61, 62]. These studies and our results suggest that a possible side effect of glucocorticoid therapy would be a higher risk of evolution to invasive breast cancer in patients who might have preneoplastic lesions that have not been diagnosed.

After stress challenge or glucocorticoid treatment, apoptotic myoepithelial cells were more frequent in patients with DCIS+IDC than in patients with DCIS, in agreement with a study that described apoptosis in the myoepithelial cell layer in comedo-type DCIS [13]. The authors claimed that it was an early event associated with the central necrosis of this type of DCIS, both in MCF10DCIS xenografts and patient samples [13]. Samples from our patients with DCIS+IDC seemed to display more malignant characteristics than those from patients with DCIS. Since the apoptotic myoepithelial cells are in the intact DCIS, this suggests that myoepithelial cell apoptosis might be a prerequisite for disruption of the myoepithelium and the consequent invasion of the epithelial compartment into the stroma.

Conclusions

In conclusion, we found that chronic stress, through sustained glucocorticoid treatment, plays a role in the progression of DCIS to invasiveness, particularly by promoting myoepithelial cell apoptosis in vitro and in vivo. Myoepithelial cell apoptosis differentiates patients with DCIS from those with DCIS+IDC, and might be a prerequisite for invasive features. Thus, the use of glucocorticoid inhibitors or other therapies that might prevent myoepithelial cell apoptosis could potentially interfere with and prevent the progression of DCIS to invasiveness. In addition, the prevalence of apoptosis in myoepithelial cells in DCIS samples might be used as a prognostic factor for progression to IDC.

Additional file

Additional file 1: Table S1. Description of patient samples used for the primary mammary epithelial and myoepithelial cells. Internal codes, histological description and age of patients. (PPTX 53 kb)

Additional file 2: Tissue digestion and cell fraction separation protocol. (PDF 231 kb)

Additional file 3: Table S2. Description of patient samples used to confirm apoptosis in human myoepithelial cell samples. Internal codes, histopathological description and receptor characteristics of patient samples. ND: not detectable. NA: not applicable. A: amplified. (PPTX 90 kb)

Additional file 4: Figure S1. Immunofluorescence of glucocorticoid receptor in myoepithelial, MCF10A and MCF10DCIS cells. Hoechst was used to counterstain nuclei. Scale bar= 20 μm. (PPTX 917 kb)

Additional file 5: Figure S2. In vivo progression of MCF10DCIS xenografts. **a** Histology of tumours (H&E) and expression of α-SMA and p63 were analysed at the indicated time points after injection (n=5 animals). Scale bar= 100 μm. **b** Representative image of glucocorticoid receptor immunohistochemistry in in vivo samples. Scale bar= 20 μm.

Red arrow indicates myoepithelial positive cells for GR and black arrow shows positivity in epithelial cells. (PPTX 5642 kb)

Additional file 6: Figure S3. Corticosterone effects on mammary epithelial cells viability, apoptosis and functional abilities. **a** MCF10A epithelial, primary myoepithelial cells and MCF10DCIS cell viability evaluated by MTT assay after 48h of increasing doses of corticosterone treatment (0.125-1.5 μM). **b** MCF10A epithelial, primary myoepithelial cells and MCF10DCIS determination of cell apoptosis in its different stages (early, apoptosis, late and total) after treatment with corticosterone 0-1 μM by the Annexin V method and measured by flow cytometry. All experiments were carried out in triplicate. Statistical analysis was made using ANOVA followed by Dunn's multiple test. **c** and **d**. Influence of corticosterone treatment on 3D growth of primary epithelial and myoepithelial cells and on MCF10DCIS for 14 days by immunofluorescence. Treatment with corticosterone 1 μM or vehicle (methanol) was carried out from day 5 after seeding until day 14. **c** Upper part. Immunodetection of K14 (myoepithelial cells), K19 (epithelial cells), with hoechst used as nuclei counterstaining. Scale bar=50 μm. **c** Bottom part. Quantification of morphometric analysis in control group and corticosterone-treated group of number of acini formed and related quantification of disrupted acini per total number of acini. **d** Upper part. Immunofluorescence of laminin (basement membrane), K14 (myoepithelial cells) and hoechst to counterstain nuclei. Scale bar=100 μm. **d** Bottom part. Quantification of laminin intensity after treatment with corticosterone 1 μM or vehicle by Image J software comparison test. **e** Immunofluorescence in MCF10DCIS 3D growth of laminin (basement membrane), Muc1 (epithelial cells) and hoechst to stain the nuclei. Arrows indicated rupture points of the acini showed. F. Morphometric quantification of disrupted acini and acinar fusion and intensity of laminin determined by integrated density parameter of Image J software. Scale bar=50μm. All experiments were carried out in triplicate. Statistical analysis was made using the Mann-Whitney test. (PPTX 3174 kb)

Additional file 7: Figure S4. Representative immunofluorescence images of MCF10DCIS xenografts in chicken embryo CAM membrane.**a** Hoechst in blue, p63 in red and laminin in green. **b** Merge of p63 and laminin double immunofluorescence images and zoom in showing an acini detail. Scale bar=20 μm. (PPT 4617 kb)

Additional file 8: Figure S5. Representative immunofluorescence images of human samples of DCIS (6 patients) and DCIS + IDC (6 patients).**a** Double immunofluorescence of p63 (myoepithelial cells) and cleaved caspase 3 indicated with red arrows and hoechst as a nuclei counterstainer in DCIS sample patients and **b** in DCIS + IDC sample patients. White scale bar=20 and red scale bar=50 μm. (PPTX 13532 kb)

Abbreviations

ACTH: Adrenocorticotropic hormone; ANS: Autonomic nervous system; α-SMA: α-Smooth muscle actin; 3D: Three-dimensional; BM: Basement membrane; BrdU: Bromodeoxyuridine; CAM: Chorioallantoic membrane; CRH: Corticotrophin-releasing hormone; DCIS: Ductal carcinoma in situ; ELISA: Enzyme-linked immunosorbent assay; FITC: Fluorescein isothiocyanate; GR: Glucocorticoid receptor; HPA: Hypothalamic-pituitary-adrenal axis; HRP: Horseradish-peroxidase conjugated; IDC: Invasive ductal carcinoma; IDIBAPS: Institut d'Investigacions Biomèdiques August Pi i Sunyer; MTT: 3-(4, 5-Dimethylthiazol-2-yl)-2, 5-diphenyl tetrazolium bromide; PBS: Phosphate-buffered saline; PI: Propidium iodide; RT: Room temperature

Acknowledgements

This work was performed at Institut d'Investigacions Biomèdiques August Pi i Sunyer (IDIBAPS) (CERCA Programme/Generalitat de Catalunya) and was developed at the Centre de Recerca Biomèdica Cellex, Barcelona. We are particularly grateful to Prof. Prats Esteve for providing healthy mammary material and Darya Kulyk for image creation. We thank our colleagues from the Laboratory of Molecular and Translational Oncology in Barcelona for their valuable assistance: E. Ametller, R. Alonso, and P. Jauregui. We thank M. Sols, G. Guillardin, J. Borras, M.J. Vidal, and E. Payá for their help with the collection of mammoplasty samples in Clinica Planas; the plastic surgery staff (Dr J. Planas, Dr. G.Planas, Dr. X. Bisbal, Dr. C. Del Cacho, Dr. A. Carbonell and Dr. J. Masià) in Clinica Planas; and Dr. Llebaria, A.Viña, E. Sanfeliu and other members of the histopathology laboratory for their help with the collection of mammoplasty samples in Llebalust Serveis S.A. We thank M. Calle for her statistical assistance. We are indebted to the Biobank core facility and Citomics core facility of IDIBAPS and also to the microscopy facility of Universitat de Barcelona for the technical help.

Funding

This work was sponsored by the Instituto de Salud Carlos III (ISCIII) through the Plan Estatal de Investigación Científica y Técnica y de Innovación, project reference number PI08022 and PI15/00661. This work was co-funded by the European Regional Development Fund (ERDF); the Fundación Cellex; Rede-sTemáticas de Investigación en Cáncer (RTICC, RD12/00360055); PhD program of the Department of Education, Language policy and Culture of the Government of the Basque Country (AZ;BFI- 2011-59); the Juan de la Cierva Fellowship programme (GF; JCI-2011-10799); APIF fellowships from the University of Barcelona, School of Medicine (PFN, EE, AL-N); Ayuda del Programa de Formación de Profesorado Universitario (FPU16/02744) (LR-P); Sara Borrell Fellowship programme (MM); Fundació per a la Recerca en Oncologia i Immunologia (FROI) (NM) and Beatriu Pinós postdoctoral fellowship "AGAUR; BP-B 00160" (co-funded by the European Union) (PB). This work has been developed in a consolidated group by Secretaria d'Universitats i Recerca del Departament d'Economia i Coneixement (2014_SGR_530).

Authors' contributions

AZ-P conducted most of the experiments for this work, evaluated the data and interpreted the results. LR-P, NM, MA and XC carried out and analysed some of the experiments. AN-C, AL-P and EE provided technical support in the experiments. MP and FG contributed with the healthy patient samples and their histological analysis and diagnosis. AZ-P, VA, PG, PB and GF contributed to study design and critically evaluated the data analysis/interpretation. GF, PB and PG wrote the manuscript. AZ-N, LR-P, NM, AN-C, MM, PF-N, NC and PG critically edited the manuscript. All authors read and approved the final manuscript version.

Competing interests

The authors declare that they have no competing interests.

Author details

[1]Institut d'Investigacions Biomèdiques August Pi i Sunyer (IDIBAPS), Barcelona, Spain. [2]Department of Medicine, University of Barcelona, Barcelona, Spain. [3]Department of Medical Oncology, Hospital Clínic, Barcelona, Spain. [4]Department of Senology, Clínica Planas, Barcelona, Spain. [5]Histopathology-Citology, Anatomical Pathology Service, Centro Médico Teknon, Barcelona, Spain. [6]Department of Biochemistry and molecular Biomedicine, University of Barcelona, Barcelona, Spain. [7]Division of Medical Oncology, Department of Medicine, Harvard Medical School, Dana-Farber Cancer Institute, Brigham and Women's Hospital, Boston, MA, USA.

References

1. Torre LA, Bray F, Siegel RL, Ferlay J, Lortet-Tieulent J, Jemal A. Global cancer statistics, 2012. CA Cancer J Clin. 2015;65(2):87–108.
2. Burstein HJ, Polyak K, Wong JS, Lester SC, Kaelin CM. Ductal carcinoma in situ of the breast. N Engl J Med. 2004;350(14):1430–41.
3. Polyak K. Is breast tumor progression really linear? Clin Cancer Res. 2008; 14(2):339–41.
4. Yao J, Weremowicz S, Feng B, Gentleman RC, Marks JR, Gelman R, Brennan C, Polyak K. Combined cDNA array comparative genomic hybridization and serial analysis of gene expression analysis of breast tumor progression. Cancer Res. 2006;66(8):4065–78.
5. Siegel RL, Miller KD, Jemal A. Cancer statistics, 2017. CA Cancer J Clin. 2017; 67(1):7–30.
6. Groen EJ, Elshof LE, Visser LL, Rutgers EJ, Winter-Warnars HA, Lips EH, Wesseling J. Finding the balance between over- and under-treatment of ductal carcinoma in situ (DCIS). Breast. 2017;31:274–83.
7. Chin K, de Solorzano CO, Knowles D, Jones A, Chou W, Rodriguez EG, Kuo WL, Ljung BM, Chew K, Myambo K, et al. In situ analyses of genome instability in breast cancer. Nat Genet. 2004;36(9):984–8.
8. Claus EB, Stowe M, Carter D. Breast carcinoma in situ: risk factors and screening patterns. J Natl Cancer Inst. 2001;93(23):1811–7.
9. Morrow M, Schnitt SJ, Norton L. Current management of lesions associated with an increased risk of breast cancer. Nat Rev Clin Oncol. 2015;12(4):227–38.
10. Polyak K, Hu M. Do myoepithelial cells hold the key for breast tumor progression? J Mammary Gland Biol Neoplasia. 2005;10(3):231–47.
11. Deugnier MA, Teuliere J, Faraldo MM, Thiery JP, Glukhova MA. The importance of being a myoepithelial cell. Breast Cancer Res. 2002; 4(6):224–30.
12. Xiao G, Liu YE, Gentz R, Sang QA, Ni J, Goldberg ID, Shi YE. Suppression of breast cancer growth and metastasis by a serpin myoepithelium-derived serine proteinase inhibitor expressed in the mammary myoepithelial cells. Proc Natl Acad Sci USA. 1999;96(7):3700–5.
13. Shekhar MP, Tait L, Pauley RJ, Wu GS, Santner SJ, Nangia-Makker P, Shekhar V, Nassar H, Visscher DW, Heppner GH, et al. Comedo-ductal carcinoma in situ: a paradoxical role for programmed cell death. Cancer Biol Ther. 2008; 7(11):1774–82.
14. Jang M, Kim E, Choi Y, Lee H, Kim Y, Kim J, Kang E, Kim SW, Kim I, Park S. FGFR1 is amplified during the progression of in situ to invasive breast carcinoma. Breast Cancer Res. 2012;14(4):R115.
15. Hu M, Yao J, Cai L, Bachman KE, van den Brule F, Velculescu V, Polyak K. Distinct epigenetic changes in the stromal cells of breast cancers. Nat Genet. 2005;37(8):899–905.
16. Cowell CF, Weigelt B, Sakr RA, Ng CK, Hicks J, King TA, Reis-Filho JS. Progression from ductal carcinoma in situ to invasive breast cancer: revisited. Mol Oncol. 2013;7(5):859–69.
17. Obeid EI, Conzen SD. The role of adrenergic signaling in breast cancer biology. Cancer Biomark. 2013;13(3):161–9.
18. Hu M, Yao J, Carroll DK, Weremowicz S, Chen H, Carrasco D, Richardson A, Violette S, Nikolskaya T, Nikolsky Y, et al. Regulation of in situ to invasive breast carcinoma transition. Cancer Cell. 2008;13(5):394–406.
19. Duijts SF, Zeegers MP, Borne BV. The association between stressful life events and breast cancer risk: a meta-analysis. Int J Cancer. 2003; 107(6):1023–9.
20. Ben-Eliyahu S, Yirmiya R, Liebeskind JC, Taylor AN, Gale RP. Stress increases metastatic spread of a mammary tumor in rats: evidence for mediation by the immune system. Brain Behav Immun. 1991;5(2):193–205.
21. Sternlicht MD, Kedeshian P, Shao ZM, Safarians S, Barsky SH. The human myoepithelial cell is a natural tumor suppressor. Clin Cancer Res. 1997;3(11): 1949–58.
22. Coutinho AE, Chapman KE. The anti-inflammatory and immunosuppressive effects of glucocorticoids, recent developments and mechanistic insights. Mol Cell Endocrinol. 2011;335(1):2–13.
23. Wu W, Pew T, Zou M, Pang D, Conzen SD. Glucocorticoid receptor-induced MAPK phosphatase-1 (MPK-1) expression inhibits paclitaxel-associated MAPK activation and contributes to breast cancer cell survival. J Biol Chem. 2005; 280(6):4117–24.
24. Valles SL, Benlloch M, Rodriguez ML, Mena S, Pellicer JA, Asensi M, Obrador E, Estrela JM. Stress hormones promote growth of B16-F10 melanoma metastases: an interleukin 6- and glutathione-dependent mechanism. J Transl Med. 2013;11:72.
25. De la Roca-Chiapas JM, Barbosa-Sabanero G, Martinez-Garcia JA, Martinez-Soto J, Ramos-Frausto VM, Gonzalez-Ramirez LP, Nowack K. Impact of stress and levels of corticosterone on the development of breast cancer in rats. Psychol Res Behav Manag. 2016;9:1–6.
26. Wintermantel TM, Bock D, Fleig V, Greiner EF, Schutz G. The epithelial glucocorticoid receptor is required for the normal timing of cell proliferation during mammary lobuloalveolar development but is dispensable for milk production. Mol Endocrinol. 2005;19(2):340–9.

27. Spiegel D, Giese-Davis J. Depression and cancer: mechanisms and disease progression. Biol Psychiatry. 2003;54(3):269–82.
28. Pufall MA. Glucocorticoids and cancer. Adv Exp Med Biol. 2015;872:315–33.
29. Moran TJ, Gray S, Mikosz CA, Conzen SD. The glucocorticoid receptor mediates a survival signal in human mammary epithelial cells. Cancer Res. 2000;60(4):867–72.
30. Lien HC, Lu YS, Cheng AL, Chang WC, Jeng YM, Kuo YH, Huang CS, Chang KJ, Yao YT. Differential expression of glucocorticoid receptor in human breast tissues and related neoplasms. J Pathol. 2006;209(3):317–27.
31. Engman M, Skoog L, Soderqvist G, Gemzell-Danielsson K. The effect of mifepristone on breast cell proliferation in premenopausal women evaluated through fine needle aspiration cytology. Hum Reprod. 2008;23(9):2072–9.
32. Garbe JC, Bhattacharya S, Merchant B, Bassett E, Swisshelm K, Feiler HS, Wyrobek AJ, Stampfer MR. Molecular distinctions between stasis and telomere attrition senescence barriers shown by long-term culture of normal human mammary epithelial cells. Cancer Res. 2009;69(19):7557–68.
33. Labarge MA, Garbe JC, Stampfer MR. Processing of human reduction mammoplasty and mastectomy tissues for cell culture. J Vis Exp. 2013;71: e50011.
34. Kandere-Grzybowska K, Gheorghe D, Priller J, Esposito P, Huang M, Gerard N, Theoharides TC. Stress-induced dura vascular permeability does not develop in mast cell-deficient and neurokinin-1 receptor knockout mice. Brain Res. 2003;980(2):213–20.
35. Su F, Ouyang N, Zhu P, Jia W, Gong C, Ma X, Xu H, Song E. Psychological stress induces chemoresistance in breast cancer by upregulating mdr1. Biochem Biophys Res Commun. 2005;329(3):888–97.
36. Yamada S, Nankai M, Toru M. Acute immobilization stress reduces (+/−) DOI induced 5-HT2-mediated head shakes in rats. Jpn J Psychiatry Neurol. 1993; 47(2):414–5.
37. Dhabhar FS, McEwen BS. Acute stress enhances while chronic stress suppresses cell-mediated immunity in vivo: a potential role for leukocyte trafficking. Brain Behav Immun. 1997;11(4):286–306.
38. Fluegen G, Avivar-Valderas A, Wang Y, Padgen MR, Williams JK, Nobre AR, Calvo V, Cheung JF, Bravo-Cordero JJ, Entenberg D, et al. Phenotypic heterogeneity of disseminated tumour cells is preset by primary tumour hypoxic microenvironments. Nat Cell Biol. 2017;19(2):120–32.
39. Kain KH, Miller JW, Jones-Paris CR, Thomason RT, Lewis JD, Bader DM, Barnett JV, Zijlstra A. The chick embryo as an expanding experimental model for cancer and cardiovascular research. Dev Dyn. 2014;243(2):216–28.
40. Ossowski L, Reich E. Changes in malignant phenotype of a human carcinoma conditioned by growth environment. Cell. 1983;33(2):323–33.
41. Zubeldia-Plazaola A, Ametller E, Mancino M, Prats de Puig M, Lopez-Plana A, Guzman F, Vinyals L, Pastor-Arroyo EM, Almendro V, Fuster G, et al. Comparison of methods for the isolation of human breast epithelial and myoepithelial cells. Front Cell Dev Biol. 2015;3:32.
42. Garcia-Recio S, Fuster G, Fernandez-Nogueira P, Pastor-Arroyo EM, Park SY, Mayordomo C, Ametller E, Mancino M, Gonzalez-Farre X, Russnes HG, et al. Substance P autocrine signaling contributes to persistent HER2 activation that drives malignant progression and drug resistance in breast cancer. Cancer Res. 2013;73(21):6424–34.
43. Sprague BL, Trentham-Dietz A, Nichols HB, Hampton JM, Newcomb PA. Change in lifestyle behaviors and medication use after a diagnosis of ductal carcinoma in situ. Breast Cancer Res Treat. 2010;124(2):487–95.
44. Lutgendorf SK, Sood AK. Biobehavioral factors and cancer progression: physiological pathways and mechanisms. Psychosom Med. 2011;73(9):724–30.
45. Lippman M, Bolan G, Huff K. The effects of glucocorticoids and progesterone on hormone-responsive human breast cancer in long-term tissue culture. Cancer Res. 1976;36(12):4602–9.
46. Goya L, Maiyar AC, Ge Y, Firestone GL. Glucocorticoids induce a G1/G0 cell cycle arrest of Con8 rat mammary tumor cells that is synchronously reversed by steroid withdrawal or addition of transforming growth factor-alpha. Mol Endocrinol. 1993;7(9):1121–32.
47. Ploner C, Schmidt S, Presul E, Renner K, Schrocksnadel K, Rainer J, Riml S, Kofler R. Glucocorticoid-induced apoptosis and glucocorticoid resistance in acute lymphoblastic leukemia. J Steroid Biochem Mol Biol. 2005;93(2–5): 153–60.
48. Wu W, Chaudhuri S, Brickley DR, Pang D, Karrison T, Conzen SD. Microarray analysis reveals glucocorticoid-regulated survival genes that are associated with inhibition of apoptosis in breast epithelial cells. Cancer Res. 2004;64(5): 1757–64.
49. Hanahan D, Weinberg RA. Hallmarks of cancer: the next generation. Cell. 2011;144(5):646–74.
50. Murrell TG. The potential for oxytocin (OT) to prevent breast cancer: a hypothesis. Breast Cancer Res Treat. 1995;35(2):225–9.
51. Hench PS, Kendall EC, Slocumb CH, Polley HF. Effects of cortisone acetate and pituitary ACTH on rheumatoid arthritis, rheumatic fever and certain other conditions. Arch Intern Med (Chic). 1950;85(4):545–666.
52. Akhavan A, Griffith OL, Soroceanu L, Leonoudakis D, Luciani-Torres MG, Daemen A, Gray JW, Muschler JL. Loss of cell-surface laminin anchoring promotes tumor growth and is associated with poor clinical outcomes. Cancer Res. 2012;72(10):2578–88.
53. Verbeke S, Richard E, Monceau E, Schmidt X, Rousseau B, Velasco V, Bernard D, Bonnefoi H, MacGrogan G, Iggo RD. Humanization of the mouse mammary gland by replacement of the luminal layer with genetically engineered preneoplastic human cells. Breast Cancer Res. 2014;16(6):504.
54. Makino S, Asaba K, Nishiyama M, Hashimoto K. Decreased type 2 corticotropin-releasing hormone receptor mRNA expression in the ventromedial hypothalamus during repeated immobilization stress. Neuroendocrinology. 1999;70(3):160–7.
55. Antoni MH, Lutgendorf SK, Cole SW, Dhabhar FS, Sephton SE, McDonald PG, Stefanek M, Sood AK. The influence of bio-behavioural factors on tumour biology: pathways and mechanisms. Nat Rev Cancer. 2006;6(3):240–8.
56. Cole SW, Nagaraja AS, Lutgendorf SK, Green PA, Sood AK. Sympathetic nervous system regulation of the tumour microenvironment. Nat Rev Cancer. 2015;15(9):563–72.
57. Charmandari E, Tsigos C, Chrousos G. Endocrinology of the stress response. Annu Rev Physiol. 2005;67:259–84.
58. Patarroyo M, Tryggvason K, Virtanen I. Laminin isoforms in tumor invasion, angiogenesis and metastasis. Semin Cancer Biol. 2002;12(3):197–207.
59. Holliday DL, Brouilette KT, Markert A, Gordon LA, Jones JL. Novel multicellular organotypic models of normal and malignant breast: tools for dissecting the role of the microenvironment in breast cancer progression. Breast Cancer Res. 2009;11(1):R3.
60. Hermes GL, Delgado B, Tretiakova M, Cavigelli SA, Krausz T, Conzen SD, McClintock MK. Social isolation dysregulates endocrine and behavioral stress while increasing malignant burden of spontaneous mammary tumors. Proc Natl Acad Sci USA. 2009;106(52):22393–8.
61. Thaker PH, Han LY, Kamat AA, Arevalo JM, Takahashi R, Lu C, Jennings NB, Armaiz-Pena G, Bankson JA, Ravoori M, et al. Chronic stress promotes tumor growth and angiogenesis in a mouse model of ovarian carcinoma. Nat Med. 2006;12(8):939–44.
62. Volden PA, Conzen SD. The influence of glucocorticoid signaling on tumor progression. Brain Behav Immun. 2013;30(Suppl):S26–31.

17

Disrupted circadian clocks and altered tissue mechanics in primary human breast tumours

Eleanor Broadberry, James McConnell, Jack Williams, Nan Yang, Egor Zindy, Angela Leek, Rachel Waddington, Leena Joseph, Miles Howe, Qing-Jun Meng[*†] and Charles H Streuli[*†] (iD)

Abstract

Background: Circadian rhythms maintain tissue homeostasis during the 24-h day-night cycle. Cell-autonomous circadian clocks play fundamental roles in cell division, DNA damage responses and metabolism. Circadian disruptions have been proposed as a contributing factor for cancer initiation and progression, although definitive evidence for altered molecular circadian clocks in cancer is still lacking. In this study, we looked at circadian clocks in breast cancer.

Methods: We isolated primary tumours and normal tissues from the same individuals who had developed breast cancer with no metastases. We assessed circadian clocks within primary cells of the patients by lentiviral expression of circadian reporters, and the levels of clock genes in tissues by qPCR. We histologically examined collagen organisation within the normal and tumour tissue areas, and probed the stiffness of the stroma adjacent to normal and tumour epithelium using atomic force microscopy.

Results: Epithelial ducts were disorganised within the tumour areas. Circadian clocks were altered in cultured tumour cells. Tumour regions were surrounded by stroma with an altered collagen organisation and increased stiffness. Levels of *Bmal1* messenger RNA (mRNA) were significantly altered in the tumours in comparison to normal epithelia.

Conclusion: Circadian rhythms are suppressed in breast tumour epithelia in comparison to the normal epithelia in paired patient samples. This correlates with increased tissue stiffness around the tumour region. We suggest possible involvement of altered circadian clocks in the development and progression of breast cancer.

Keywords: Circadian clocks, Epithelial cells, Breast cancer, Mammographic density

Background

Circadian clocks maintain tissue homeostasis during the 24-h day-night cycle. They exist in most cell types and are active after birth. Peripheral clocks are entrained by a central core clock located in the hypothalamus, and are integral to normal tissue function [9, 14, 19, 31, 41]. Cell-autonomous circadian clocks are fundamental in gating cell division, regulating DNA damage responses, and temporally controlling cell metabolism [43]. Altered clocks may contribute to the onset of certain types of tumour, including breast [30, 39]. Interestingly, epidemiological studies indicate that long-term night shift workers have a higher risk of developing breast cancer [22]. Moreover, animal studies reveal an association between clock gene mutations and the initiation, growth rate, and metastasis of mammary tumours [4, 16].

The breast is a regenerative organ that undergoes frequent periods of tissue remodelling [38]. Mouse models have been used to reveal the changes found in mammary gland tissue that are associated with the oestrous cycle, pregnancy, and lactation. During each oestrous cycle, cells proliferate to form alveolar buds on the tertiary side branches and then regress in an ordered fashion [37]. Lobulo-alveolar growth and differentiation takes place in pregnancy, when the epithelial structures expand

* Correspondence: qing-jun.meng@manchester.ac.uk; cstreuli@manchester.ac.uk
†Qing-Jun Meng and Charles H Streuli contributed equally to this work.
Wellcome Centre for Cell-Matrix Research and Manchester Breast Centre, Faculty of Biology, Medicine and Health, University of Manchester, Manchester M13 9PT, UK

dramatically to fill the whole fat pad with milk-secreting alveoli [18]. Upon weaning, involution is triggered to remove the milk-secreting cells and return the gland to a non-pregnant state [2]. These developmental processes repeat with each oestrus cycle or pregnancy.

One consequence of the highly proliferative nature of mammary gland biology is that it is subject to abnormalities, which can result in cancer. Breast is the tissue that is most subject to cancer in the human female population worldwide, and causes a high degree of patient mortality [48]. Apart from a small percentage of cancers arising in women with inherited mutations, for example in the *Brca* genes, the cause of breast cancer is poorly understood. One of the biggest risk factors is stromal composition, where women with stroma that has a high mammographic density (MD) have a greater risk of developing cancer [46].

We have shown that circadian clocks are present in the mammary gland, and that they are required for maintaining the tissue stem cell population [53]. Moreover, the breast circadian clock amplitude changes during ageing. Approximately 600 genes are under circadian control in mouse mammary gland, and the oscillation amplitude of the circadian clocks is controlled by the biomechanical stiffness of the tissue stroma.

This is potentially relevant to breast cancer because high MD is linked to stiffer micro-scale stromal tissue [35]. This suggests that a stiffer tissue microenvironment could have an impact in causing cancer. However, it remains unclear whether stromal regions around early human breast tumours are indeed stiffer than those surrounding normal breast tissue, and how a stiffer stroma might promote cancer. One possible mechanism could be through alteration of circadian "time-keeping" clocks that are present in almost all the major body organs, including the breast [4].

There have been a few reports of changes in clock genes/circadian rhythm in immortalized breast tumour cell lines [10, 17, 42, 54]. However, to the best of our knowledge, it has not yet been established if the molecular circadian timing mechanism alters in primary tissue in patients with breast cancer.

The purpose of this study was to investigate whether the breast circadian clock changes during the progression of healthy to cancerous tissue in human patients. Through unique access to tissues from a Manchester patient cohort undergoing mastectomies, we were able to examine tissue structure and circadian rhythms within normal regions of breast tissue and in the early non-metastatic cancers in the same individuals.

We now reveal that circadian clocks, which are present within the normal human breast epithelium, are disrupted in the tumour cells isolated from the same individuals. Moreover, there are alterations in the cellular

composition, the organisation and the biomechanical stiffness of tumour stroma, in comparison to the stroma around the normal epithelium of the same patients. Given that the clocks within cells isolated from these individuals are down-regulated in the tumours, we suggest that the altered tumour stroma may contribute to the disrupted clocks.

Results

The cellular microenvironment of normal and breast cancer tissue

A cohort of women (aged 46–78 years) was recruited from the Nightingale Centre breast-screening centre (Table 1). These patients were diagnosed with breast cancer, but they did not have metastases. A clinical radiologist assessed the mammograms from each patient and suitable sample areas of normal tissue, at least 4 cm away from the tumour margin, and tumour tissue were identified (Additional file 1: Figure S1). After mastectomy, a clinical histopathologist took biopsies from the highlighted tissue areas in the resected breast for laboratory analysis, and confirmed the absence and presence of neoplasia in normal and tumorous regions.

To identify the ductal and stromal regions, tissue sections from the same individuals were stained with H&E (Fig. 1a; Additional file 2: Figure S2). The epithelia formed ducts with hollow lumens. Ductal structures were also present in the tumour tissue. However, the tumour cells invaded the ducts and filled the lumens, and tumour cells around the ducts formed abnormal growths. Stromal cells surrounded the ducts, and in the tumour tissue they were arranged in arrays of cells (Fig. 1b; Additional file 2: Figure S2).

To determine whether there were any changes within the breast microenvironment of early cancers in comparison to normal epithelia, serial tissue sections corresponding to the H&E-stained regions were immuno-stained for cytokeratin 8 (CK8) (Fig. 1c, Additional file 3: Figure S3). In normal tissue, the luminal layers of ducts were strongly stained for CK8, revealing hollow tubular structures with no cellular obstructions. In malignant tissue, regions of CK8 staining were present in the ducts, confirming the presence of epithelial cells. Transformed cells were also inside ducts and had broken through the ductal walls and were invading the surrounding tissue.

Stromal fibroblasts are actively involved in tumour progression [21]. Serial tissue sections were stained with the fibroblast intermediate filament marker, vimentin (Fig. 1d, Additional file 3: Figure S3). In normal breast, fibroblasts were present in the stroma that neighboured the mammary ducts, while the stroma at a distance from the ducts contained fibroblasts scattered in smaller numbers. Throughout tumour regions, there were more fibroblasts;

Table 1 Disease status of breast tissue examined in this study

Patient number	Age (years)	Ethnicity	BMI	Tumour details	Histology	Grade	Size (mm)	ER	PR	Her2	Her2 status	Overall tumour phenotype
Patient-1	46	White	33.7	Left breast - lower outer quadrant (LOQ)	IDC	2	23	6	8	1	Neg	ER/PR/Her2-Neg
Patient-2	77	White	36.9	Left breast - upper outer quadrant (UOQ) Mass 29 mm + 2 similar densities USS - 26 mm 3 o'clock - 21 mm	Sarcomastoid/spindle cell/ metaplastic carcinoma	3	22					
Patient-3	78		27.8	Right breast - upper half	IDC	3	70	0	0	1	Neg	ER/PR/Her2-Neg
Patient-4	55	white	38.6	Right breast - UOQ. MRI scan	ILC	2	62	8	7	1	Neg	ER/PR/Her2-Neg
Patient-5	69		37.2	Left breast - UOQ 3 cm	Invasive mucinous carcinoma	3	50	5	0	3	Pos	ER/Her2
Patient-6	67	White	34.3	Left Breast - UOQ - 2 o'clock. T2 N0	IDC	2	22	8	7	0	Neg	ER/PR/Her2-Neg
Patient-7	53		34.4	Right breast lobular cancer	ILC, multifocal	2	52	8	7	1	Neg	ER/PR/Her2-Neg
Patient-8	52	White	28.7	Left Breast - UOQ	Lobulated mass IDC	2/3	24	8	0	2 (non-amp)	Neg	ER/Her2-Neg

Details of the age, ethnicity, body mass index (BMI), and tumour status of breast tissue were analysed. We used breast tumour material, plus normal tissue from the same breast that was located at least 4 cm from the tumours

Abbreviations: ER oestrogen receptor, PR progesterone receptor, Her2 human epidermal growth factor receptor, IDC invasive ductal carcinoma, Neg negative, MRI magnetic resonance imaging, non-amp non amplified

they were concentrated around ductal epithelia, and their numbers increased in the tumour microenvironment.

These results show that there are differences in structural organisation between normal and malignant tissues from the same breasts, with the tumour epithelium disorganised and infiltrating the stroma. Thus, the organisation and composition of breast tissue change in early malignancy.

Breast cancer epithelia are altered in cell culture

To determine whether there are any changes in the growth potential of epithelial cells in early cancers in comparison to normal breast, the patient tissues were digested overnight with collagenase, and the epithelial cells were then isolated for cell culture. Primary mammary epithelial cells (MECs), isolated from normal and cancerous regions in the same individuals, were seeded as single cells at the same cell density, and cultured on Matrigel®. The cells isolated from the tumour formed larger clusters than those from normal breast (Fig. 2a). Thus, there are differences in the behaviour of epithelial cells from normal vs tumour regions in the same breasts, when they are cultured on 3D extracellular matrix (ECM).

Breast cancer epithelia have dampened circadian clocks

We have previously established that the mouse mammary gland and isolated mammary epithelia have autonomous circadian clocks. Robust 24-h rhythms were demonstrated in mammary tissue explants and in

primary MECs isolated from mice expressing the luciferase clock (protein fusion) reporter, PER2::Luc [53].

To determine whether there are any changes in circadian rhythms in the epithelia of early breast cancers in comparison to normal tissue, primary human MECs were transduced with a Per2::Luc clock reporter via lentiviral infection. The cycling of Per2::Luc levels, which faithfully reflects endogenous circadian clock activities, was then examined. The epithelial cells from normal human breast had a robust ~ 24 h Per2::Luc rhythm, indicating the presence of strong clock machinery (Fig. 2b). In contrast, MECs isolated from the adjacent cancerous tissue from the same individuals displayed a weakened rhythm, with much lower amplitude, and the rhythm was not sustained. This was the case for all three patients examined, confirming that breast tumours had suppressed circadian clocks (Additional file 4: Figure S4). These results indicate that the circadian clock mechanism is compromised in cancer epithelium, in comparison to that in the normal ductal epithelium of the same individual.

Collagen is more organised in the periductal stroma of tumour tissue

We have previously shown that the robustness of the breast circadian clock is determined by the stiffness of the extracellular environment [53]. In postmenopausal patients without breast cancer, stromal collagen

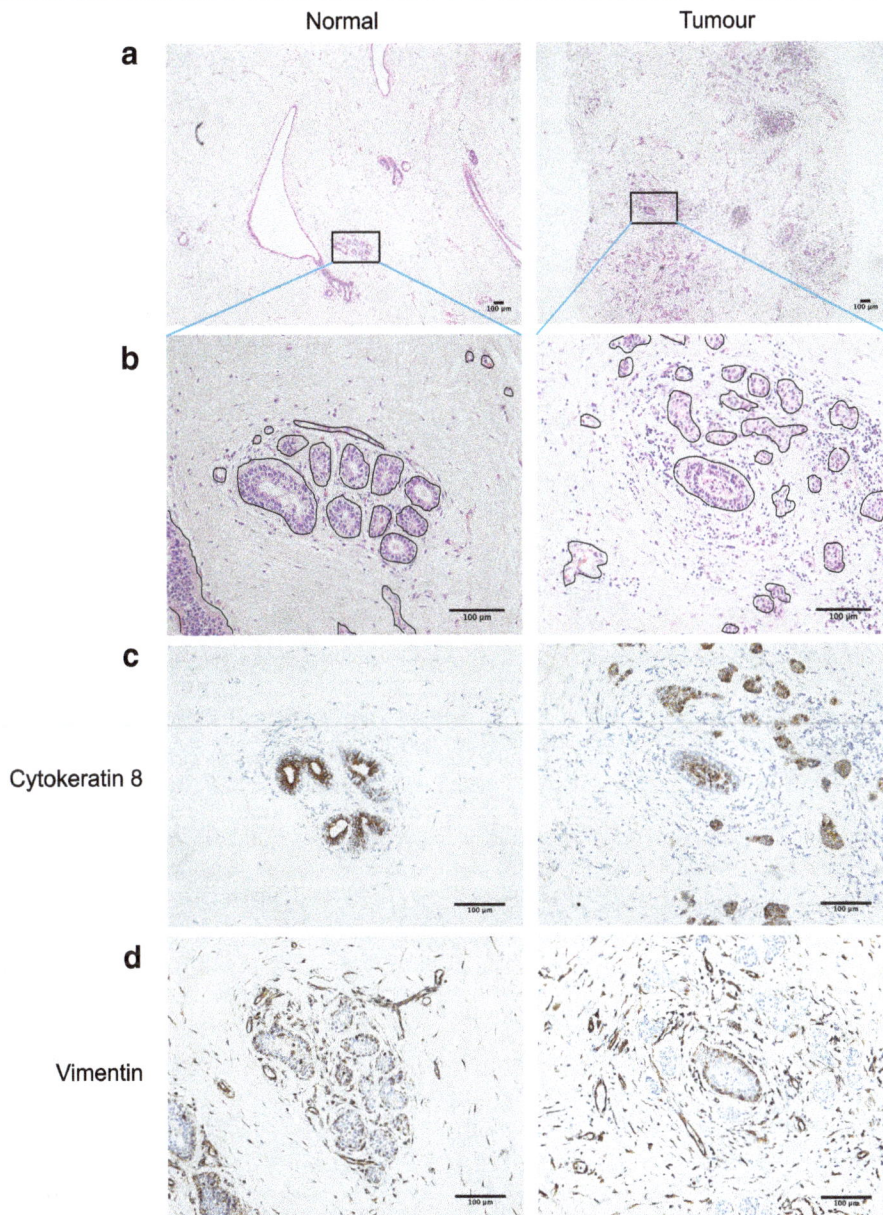

Fig. 1 Breast tissue morphology and composition. **a** Representative low power view (× 4) of H&E stained paraffin sections from normal and tumour human breast tissue (patient-6). Additional samples are shown in Additional file 2: Figure S2 and Additional file 3: Figure S3. **b** High magnification (× 20) view of the H&E stained area within the box in the image (**a**). **c** Cytokeratin 8 expression in ductal regions of breast, counterstained with haematoxylin**d** Vimentin expression in similar regions

organisation correlates with ECM stiffness [35]. We therefore hypothesised that the stromal collagen in tumour tissue may be more organised, stiffening the ECM and dampening the circadian clock in the cancerous regions of the same breasts. To investigate the organisation of stromal collagen, sections were stained with Picrosirius Red. This enables the histological abundance of collagen bundles to be detected, and when visualised under polarised light microscopy, the organisation of these collagen fibres can be quantified.

Both normal and tumour tissue contained significant levels of collagen (Fig. 3a). However, when viewed through perpendicular polarizing microscopy, most of the tumour areas showed considerably more organized collagen bundles (Fig. 3b; Additional file 5: Figure S5). A semi-quantitative estimate of the organised collagen content, determined by the percentage of collagen visible under polarised light, in relation to the total collagen present, showed more fibrillar collagen-I in the tumour regions (Fig. 3c). Thus, in

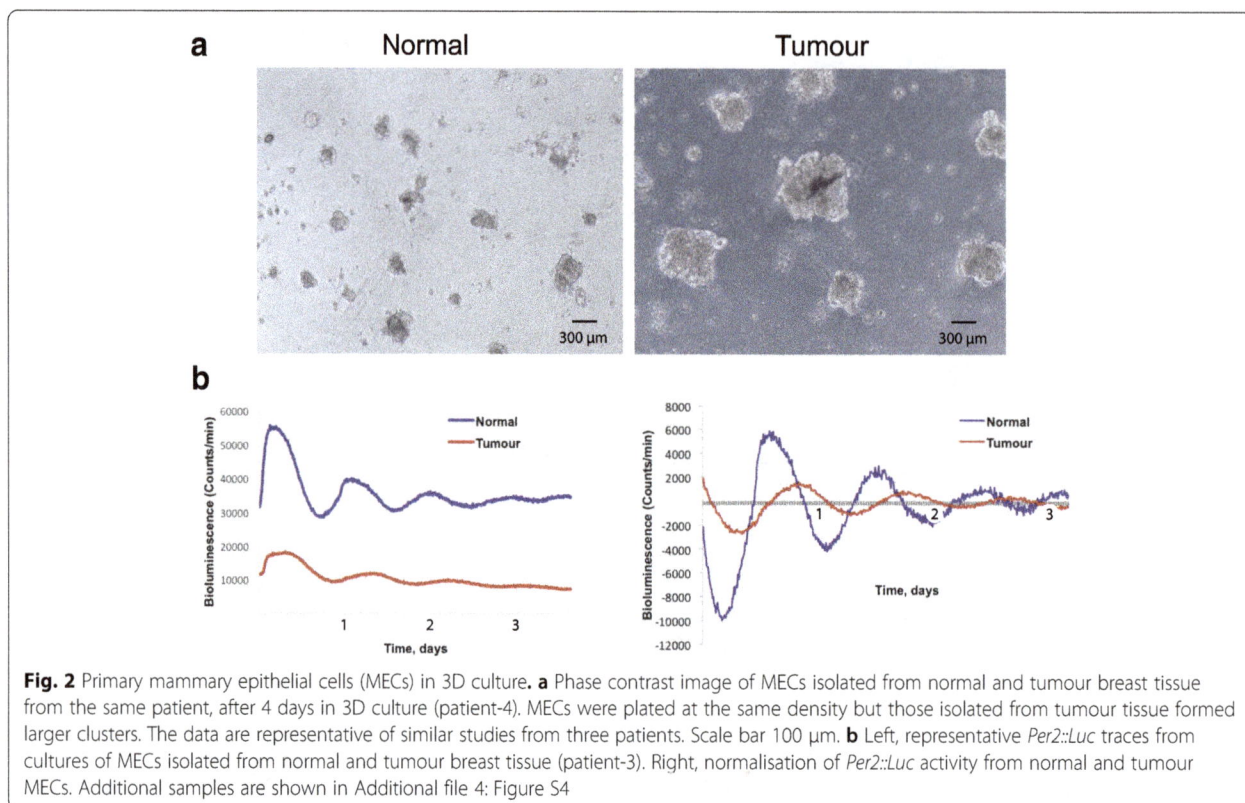

Fig. 2 Primary mammary epithelial cells (MECs) in 3D culture. **a** Phase contrast image of MECs isolated from normal and tumour breast tissue from the same patient, after 4 days in 3D culture (patient-4). MECs were plated at the same density but those isolated from tumour tissue formed larger clusters. The data are representative of similar studies from three patients. Scale bar 100 μm. **b** Left, representative *Per2::Luc* traces from cultures of MECs isolated from normal and tumour breast tissue (patient-3). Right, normalisation of *Per2::Luc* activity from normal and tumour MECs. Additional samples are shown in Additional file 4: Figure S4

most cases the collagen adjacent to epithelial ducts is more highly organised in cancerous regions than in those adjacent to normal tissue from the same patient.

Tumour stroma is stiffer than that of normal breast

We utilised atomic force microscopy (AFM) to determine whether the altered collagen organisation seen in tumours led to stiffened ECM within the stromal regions of the tissue. Indentations were made on 5 μm cryosections, in regions of stroma adjacent to mammary ducts in both the normal and tumour tissue from the same patients (Additional file 6: Figure S6). In each tissue, 2500 indentations were made, enabling analysis of data point distributions.

There was a positive (right) shift in the distribution of reduced moduli (a measure of tissue stiffness) in tumour tissue compared to the normal breast (Fig. 4a). Our data revealed that there was an average 30% increase in stromal stiffness adjacent to the tumour in comparison to the normal areas (Fig. 4b). Thus, breast tumours have a stiffer ECM adjacent to the epithelial regions than the normal tissue in the same patients.

The profile of clock genes is deregulated in breast cancer

Previous studies have identified PER1 and PER2, components of the negative arm of the molecular

clock, as tumour suppressor genes [24]. A significant decrease in PER1 and PER2 expression has been demonstrated in sporadic and familial primary breast tumours when compared to normal breast tissue [11]. However, few studies have examined the expression of positive clock factors (BMAL1 and CLOCK) in human breast cancer, largely due to the lack of reliable antibodies.

To gain an insight into how breast circadian clocks are altered in cancerous tissue in comparison to the normal breast in the same patients, quantitative PCR (qPCR) of endogenous clock genes (*Bmal1*, *Clock* and *Nr1d1*) was performed in the resected specimens.

Both the normal and cancerous regions expressed *Bmal1* messenger RNA (mRNA). In each case, the levels of *Bmal1* mRNA expression was stronger in normal tissue in comparison to tumour tissue from the same patient ($p < 0.0005$, $n = 8$) (Fig. 5a). In contrast to *Bmal1*, the expression of *Clock* (the binding partner of *Bmal1*) and *Nr1d1* (the negative transcriptional regulator of *Bmal1*) was more variable and showed no consistent changes (Fig. 5b, c).

Our findings of consistent reduction of *Bmal1* mRNA levels, together with reports from others of altered PER proteins, confirms that the intrinsic feedback machinery regulating clock expression is disrupted in early breast cancer [11]. Thus, the altered clock dynamics that we

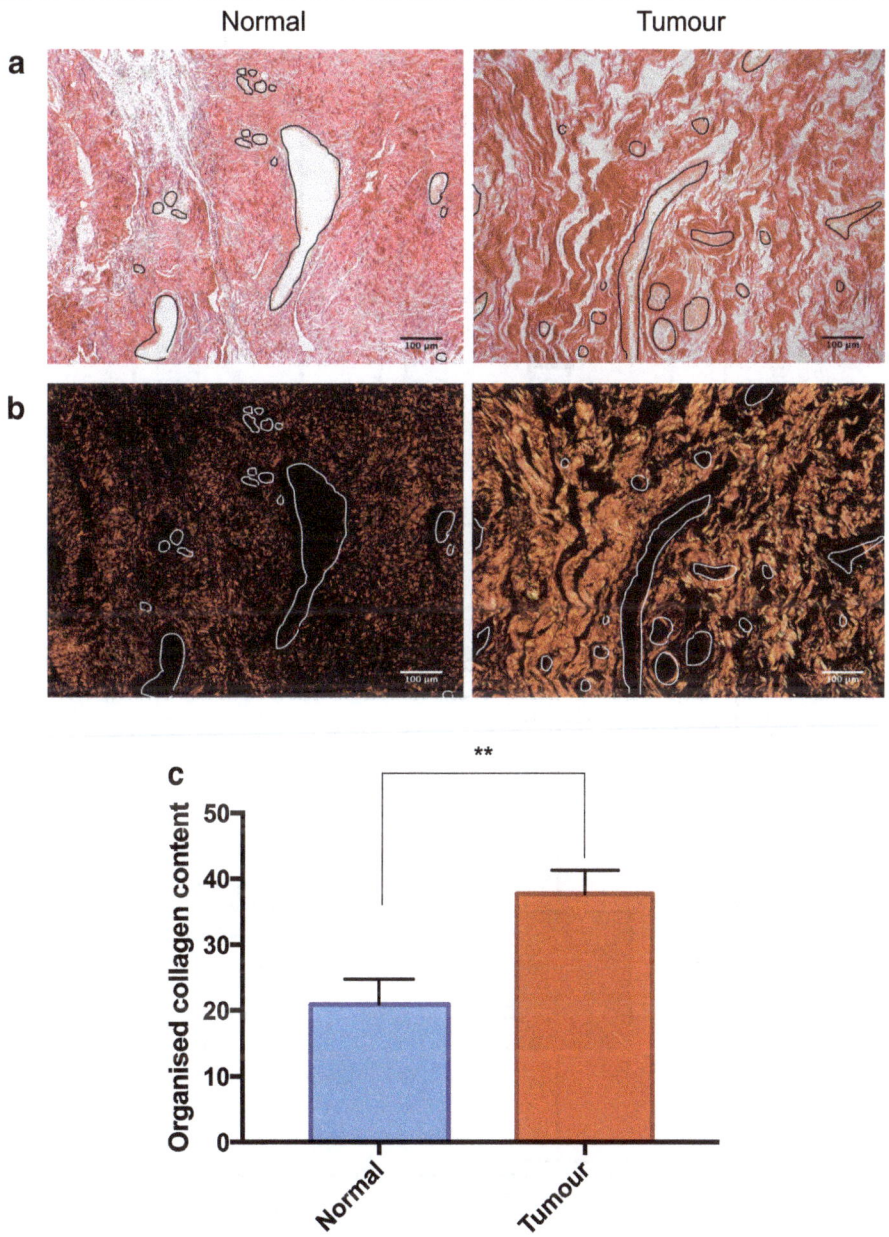

Fig. 3 Collagen organisation in periductal stroma. **a**, **b** Picrosirius-Red-stained paraffin sections (patient-6) visualised in bright-field light (**a**) and under polarised light (**b**). Ducts are outlined in black or white. Additional samples are shown in Additional file 5: Figure S5. **c** Percentage organised fibrillar collagen content after quantification, in the normal and tumour tissues: $n = 6$; mean ± SEM; unpaired t test

observed in primary cultures of normal versus cancerous tissue reflects different levels of circadian regulators in cancerous breast tissue in patients.

Discussion
Overall conclusions
Cell-autonomous circadian clocks are fundamental in cell fate and functions [43]. Disrupted circadian rhythms have been suggested as a risk factor for the development of breast cancer [39]. However definitive evidence linking clock dysregulation with tumour progression in

humans is missing [23, 50]. This is partly because there has been a lack of direct comparison of circadian clock properties between cells from tumorous and non-tumourous regions of the same patients. Our study has now compared primary tumours to regions of normal breast within the same individuals.

By monitoring rhythmic activities of a clock gene reporter (*Per2*::luciferase), we discovered that circadian clocks in cancerous epithelium have compromised clock machinery. To the best of our knowledge, this is the first demonstration of mammary clock disruption in epithelial

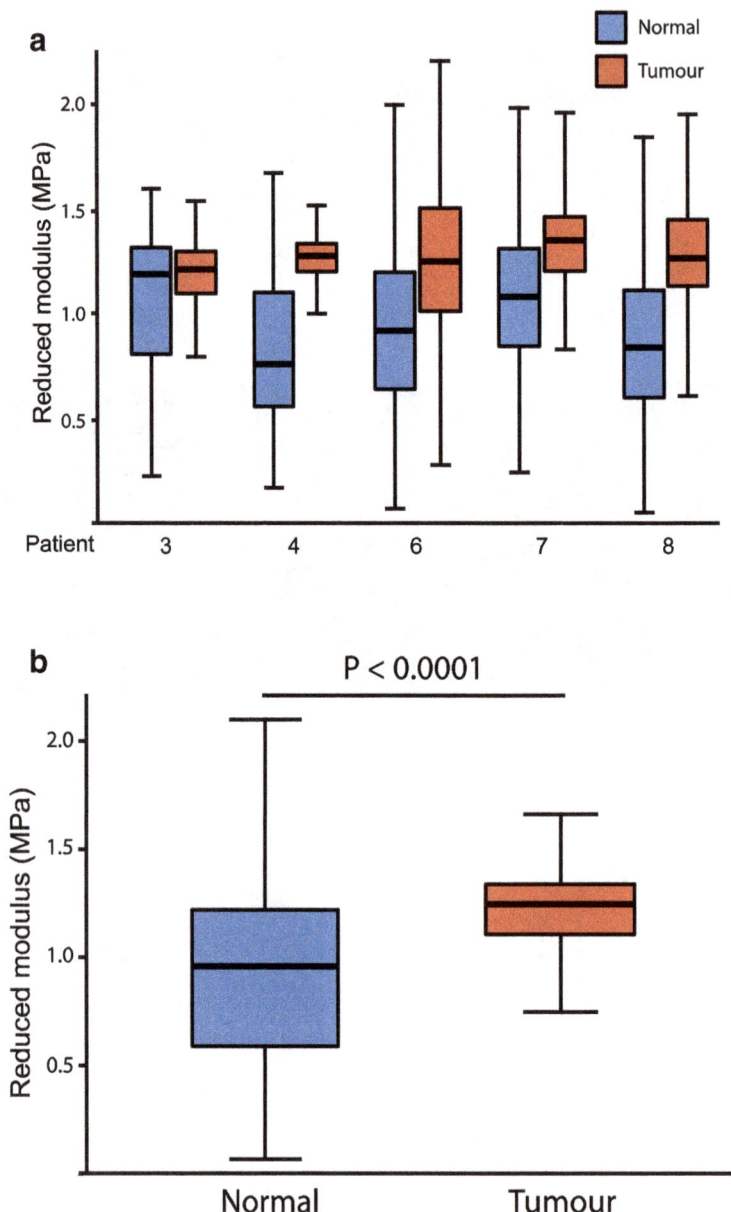

Fig. 4 Micromechanical stiffness of periductal stroma. **a** Mean reduced modulus for periductal regions of the stroma in normal (blue) versus tumour (red) tissue sections from five patients. The regions analysed are shown in Additional file 6: Figure S6. **b** Mean reduced modulus for periductal regions of the stroma in tumour tissue compared with normal breast tissue (in all five patients assessed). Tumour periductal stroma (reduced modulus = 1.21 MPa) was significantly stiffer than normal periductal stroma (reduced modulus = 0.90 MPa, $p < 0.0001$, $n = 5$)

cells freshly isolated from primary tumours of patients with breast cancer. Our data support the hypothesis that the circadian rhythm is suppressed in breast cancer.

Compositional and mechanical changes in the stroma of breast cancer

By staining breast tissue sections with H&E, cytokeratin and vimentin, we identified distinct structural and compositional changes to the breast tumour microenvironment. In cancerous breast tissue, malignant epithelial cells invade the duct and infiltrate the stroma. In addition, there is an accumulation of fibroblasts within the tumour region. Fibroblasts are key stromal cells that contribute to the interaction of MECs with their associated stroma [6]. This occurs through secretion of ECM components such as collagen and growth factors, enabling the stroma to actively participate in malignant epithelial cell transformation [28]. Our future work will examine how aberrant stromal-tumour cell interactions contribute to the maintenance of a tumour microenvironment.

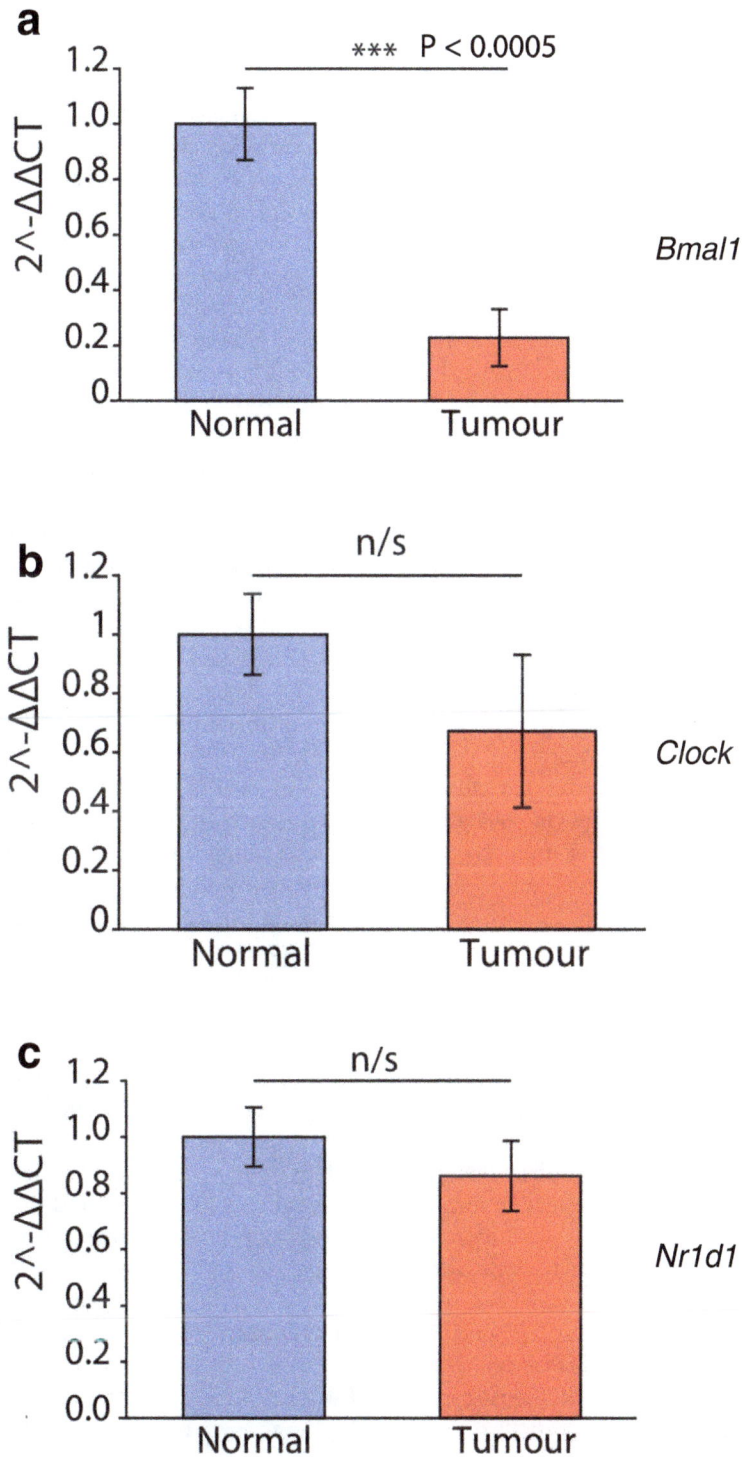

Fig. 5 Clock genes expressed in normal and tumour breast tissue. Representative quantitative PCR levels in breast tumour material, plus normal tissue from the same breast that was located at least 4 cm from the tumours. Here, samples from eight separate patients with invasive lobular and invasive ductal carcinoma were used. In each case, RNA levels were normalised to a β-actin loading control, with ΔΔ cycle threshold (CT) quantification of expression. **a** *Bmal1*; **b** *Clock*; **c** *Nr1d1*

We also found mechanical changes in the microenvironment of cancerous breast tissue, and suggest that altered stromal stiffness contributes to tumour formation. We know that mammographic density represents the second highest risk factor for breast cancer, and have shown that stiffness is related to differences in collagen organisation [35]. Very little is known about the molecular basis for how different collagen-I networks are formed in either normal or cancer-associated stroma. However, our data suggest that tumour stroma has increased fibrillar collagen organisation compared to matched non-tumour tissue. Indeed, others have shown that the stromal collagen network is reorganised in early desmoplastic tumour progression [3, 29]. Although alterations in stromal organisation and stiffness during tumour progression have been well-characterised, the pathways orchestrating these changes are less understood [1]. Breast tumour-associated fibroblasts over-express lysyl oxidase, stiffening the matrix and leading to increased tumour cell invasion [20]. Lysyl oxidase cross-links collagen fibres, and changing its levels alters collagen organisation, matrix stiffness and the metastatic potential of cell lines [12]. This may be coordinated by hypoxia inducible factors, indeed silencing these factors alters fibrillar collagen synthesis, deposition and degradation in MDA-MB-231 cells [44, 45]. We are currently elucidating the effect of these pathways on collagen deposition in the peri-tumour stroma by examining protein expression with mass spectrometry.

Altered circadian clocks in breast cancers

Breast epithelium contains circadian clocks, but their amplitude declines during ageing when the stromal areas surrounding the epithelium become stiffer [4, 53]. We now show that the stroma adjacent to human breast tumours is significantly stiffer than it is close to normal epithelium in the same individuals. Given that extracellular stiffness dampens the epithelial circadian clock, our findings begin to explain how the clock may become reduced in breast cancer. However, there are varying explanations of which clock components become altered in cancer to suppress the clock itself.

A possible role of altered BMAL1 in breast cancer

Our data at the RNA level reveals that in breast cancers some genes contributing to core clock mechanisms, such as that encoding BMAL1, become reduced. BMAL1 is a key circadian transcription factor with central roles in fine-tuning the behaviour of epithelial cells. Currently, we do not know if altered levels of clock gene expression have direct functions in breast cancer or if they are simply correlative. Our future studies will use overexpression and gene deletion approaches in both culture and mouse models to determine their downstream

transcriptional targets in breast epithelia, and their role in 3D models of cell growth and survival.

We think it likely that altered stoichiometry of clock factors contributes to altered clocks both in primary tumour cell culture and in the breast itself [8, 32]. Given that circadian dimers such as BMAL1-CLOCK are involved with chromatin opening and transcription of downstream genes, this would not be surprising [36]. Indeed, loss of coordinated Per3/Cry2 gene expression is associated with worse prognosis, particularly in patients with less oestrogen receptor (ER) and with human epidermal growth factor receptor 2 (Her2) amplification [7]. In future we aim to determine whether alterations in the levels of specific clock RNAs, and their encoded proteins, are linked to different types of breast cancers, such as the ER, progesterone receptor (PR)-positive or triple-negative cases. Moreover, further studies on the control of clock gene expression in breast cancer by methylation, is also warranted [33].

Previous work on pancreatic cancer demonstrated that BMAL1 expression was lower in malignant tissues than in tissue from non-cancerous controls [26], as we have also found in malignant breast tissue. BMAL1 was proposed to have an inhibitory effect on cell cycle progression and invasion, suggesting it is protective in this type of cancer. In contrast, over-expression of BMAL1 contributes to the aggressiveness of malignant pleural mesothelioma, with knockdown of BMAL1 suppressing cell proliferation [15]. Consistent with this study, agonists of REV-ERB, which is the main suppressor of Bmal1 transcription, are lethal to cancer cells and oncogene-induced senescent cells [49].

Altered BMAL1 also influences the development of squamous tumours [25]. In the U2OS osteosarcoma line, BMAL1 over-expression induces apoptosis, while in CA46 lymphoma cells it increases apoptosis and reduces proliferation, leading to smaller tumours when the cells are injected into mice [5]. Stromal cells are the origin of osteosarcoma cells, and we have examined clocks in stromal cells [52]. We found that stromal clocks are regulated oppositely to those in epithelial cells in normal tissues, so it will be interesting to determine possible alterations of clock gene expression in the normal and tumour-associated stromal regions of breast tissue.

Conclusion

We examined tumour and adjacent normal regions of breast tissue in patients with cancer, and discovered that circadian clocks are suppressed in the tumour epithelium. We also found that there are alterations in the cellular composition, the organisation and the biomechanical stiffness of tumour stroma. The implication is that there is a novel link between ECM stiffening and the control of circadian rhythms in early human breast cancers. This is the first step towards understanding how microenvironmental remodelling alters the circadian clock in breast cancer. At this stage, we still do not know whether the reduction of circadian rhythm is just a consequence of tumorigenesis, or an early event in the establishment of breast cancer. Further investigation into the relationship between cell-matrix interactions and circadian clock gene expression will provide a new understanding about how breast cancer initiates and progresses.

Methods
Reagents
We used foetal bovine serum (Labtech), DMEM (Lonza), Matrigel (Corning), insulin, hydrocortisone, epidermal growth factor (EGF), cholera toxin, trypsin-EDTA, bovine pituitary extract (BPE), antibiotic antimycotic solution, collagenase D and hyaluronidase (Sigma).

Cohort and breast tissue samples used in this study
A radiologist assessed digital mammograms, and putative areas of tumour and normal tissue were identified and then verified by a histopathologist. These areas were excised following mastectomy and transported on ice to the laboratory. Tissue samples were bisected, one part being used for primary culture of epithelial cells and the other for histological analysis, stromal composition and assessment of stiffness and the levels of circadian clocks.

Human mammary tissue dissection and epithelial isolation
Biopsies were kept in chilled RPMI medium until ready for digestion, then MECs were isolated [47]. The tissue was chopped manually with a scalpel for 10 min and placed into a conical flask containing collagenase mix (3 mg/ml collagenase, 0.7 mg/ml hyaluronidase and 0.2 mg antibiotics), then digested overnight at 37 °C with constant agitation. The following morning, the digest mix was transferred into a Falcon tube and left for 5 min to allow separation, the layer of fat was removed and the sample centrifuged at 1500 rpm for 5′. The resulting pellet was kept on ice whilst the supernatant was transferred into a new Falcon tube and centrifuged for a further 5′, washed twice and resuspended in 10 ml DMEM and 10% FBS and was left for up to 3 h on a 10 cm dish to deplete fibroblasts. The medium containing unbound cells was aspirated, centrifuged at 1000 rpm for 5′, the pellet was resuspended in human growth medium and cultured in complete medium (mammary epithelial cell growth medium (MEBM) supplemented with 52 μg/ml BPE, 5 μg/ml insulin, 500 ng/ml hydrocortisone, 10 ng/ml human EGF and 10% fetal calf serum (Biowittaker). All cells were cultured at 37 °C with 5% CO2.

Tissue architecture
A portion of tissue sample was fixed in 4% paraformaldehyde in PBS before processing overnight using an automated tissue processor (Shandon Citadel 2000). Samples were embedded in molten paraffin wax using a Leica EG1150H embedding station, sectioned at 3 μm, and mounted onto positively charged slides using a Leica RM 2155 microtome. Sections were dewaxed, rehydrated through a descending alcohol gradient into distilled water, then stained with H&E using a Thermo Fisher Scientific Shandon Varistain 24-4 autostainer, then mounted in DPX mounting medium (Sigma, MO, USA) and left to dry overnight before imaging using an Olympus Slide Scanner.

Immunohistochemical analysis
Tissue sections were dewaxed and rehydrated through a descending alcohol gradient, then immersed in boiled 10 mM sodium citrate, 0.005% Tween 20, pH 6.0 for 20 min to expose antigen sites. Endogenous peroxidase activity was quenched with H2O2 before staining with primary antibody (diluted in PBS with 0.1% Triton-X 100 and 3% goat serum) overnight at 4 °C in a humidified chamber, then biotinylated secondary antibody was applied (Vector Laboratories, CA, USA) for 2 h at room temperature (RT), and streptavidin-conjugated-Horseradish Peroxidase (Sigma, MO, USA) was added for 1 h. Chromogenic detection was with 3,3-diaminobenzidine (DAB) in the presence of H2O2 for 5 min, slides were counterstained for 2 min in Methyl Green (Sigma, MO, USA), washed in H_2O or water dehydrated and mounted in DPX mounting medium. The images were viewed using an Olympus Slide Scanner.

RNA expression
Breast tissue from normal and tumour areas was selected from a subset of patients in the study previously described. Tissue pieces were homogenized using a TissueRuptor II (QIAGEN), and mRNA extracted using an RNeasy Micro Kit (QIAGEN) according to the manufacturer's protocol. For qPCR, RNA concentrations were determined using a NanoDrop Lite (Thermo Fisher), and equal amounts of RNA were converted to complementary DNA (cDNA) using the High-Capacity cDNA Reverse Transcription Kit (Thermo Fisher). TaqMan-based qPCR was performed using a StepOnePlus Real-Time PCR System (Thermo Fisher) with FAST Blue qPCR MasterMix (Eurogentec). TaqMan primers and probes were purchased from Applied Biosystems (Thermo Fisher). The following probe IDs were used: Actb Hs99999903_m1, Bmal1/Arntl Hs00154147_m1, Clock Hs00231857_m1, Nr1d1 Hs00253876_m1.

Real-time recording of clock activities

Cells were synchronised an hour before recording with 100 nM dexamethasone (Sigma, MO, USA). Cells were then washed and cultured in warmed HEPES-buffered and sodium bicarbonate-buffered recording medium containing luciferin and sealed with UV-irradiated vacuum grease and 40 mm glass coverslips (Thermo Fisher Scientific, MA, USA). Dishes were placed into photomultiplier tubes (PMTs) or into LumiCyclr apparatus (Actimetrics, IL, USA). Bioluminescence was measured with LumiCycle software and curves were normalised using a 24 h moving average baseline correction.

Lentiviral packaging

HEK293FT cells were co-transfected with the transfer vector pLV-*Per2-luc* and the packaging plasmids pMD2-VSV-G, pMDLg/pRRE and pRSV-REV [34] using the calcium phosphate method on day 1 [27]. Medium was changed on day 2, collected and changed on day 3, collected on day 4 and then the supernatants were combined and centrifuged at 200 g for 5 min. The resulting supernatant was then centrifuged at 2000 g for 40 min using Vivaspin 20 Centrifugation Columns (Sartorius AG, Göttingen, Germany). The fraction remaining in the column was stored at – 80 °C or used immediately.

Transducing primary human MECs with a *Per2::Luc* clock reporter

For lentiviral transduction, human MECs were grown to 80% confluence in 35 mm dishes. Cells were transduced with 50 μl lentiviral particles, and the medium was changed to fresh medium after 16 h. For cells transduced with the *mPer2::luc* reporter, this was changed to recording medium and recorded for bioluminescent activity in PMTs.

Real-time recording of clock activities

Cells cultured in 35 mm dishes were synchronised with 100 nM dexamethasone. Prior to placing in the Lumicycle, normal culture medium was removed and rapidly replaced with pre-warmed HEPES-buffered and sodium bicarbonate-buffered recording medium. The bioluminescence values for all cell types were recorded in this medium. Culture dishes were sealed with coverslips and vacuum grease and placed into the LumiCycle or photomultiplier devices. Baseline subtraction was performed using a 24 h moving average algorithm.

Collagen organisation

Tissue sections were rehydrated through a descending alcohol gradient into distilled water before staining with Picrosirius Red (Sigma, MO, USA) for 1 h. Sections were washed twice in 5% HAc solution and gently blotted with filter paper to remove any excess stain. Slides were dehydrated, cleared through an ascending alcohol gradient into xylene, before mounting in DPX mounting medium, dried overnight and then imaged on an Olympus Slide Scanner under normal and polarised light. Collagen organisation was assessed from the Picrosirius red staining [40, 51]).

Atomic force microscopy

Breast tissue was embedded in optimal cutting temperature cryo-sectioning medium in a 2.5 cm mould at – 20 °C, sectioned at 5 μm using an HM560 automated cryostat and stored at – 80 °C. Cryosections were air-dried overnight at RT then examined by AFM. Micro-indentation was carried out using 5 μm cryo-sections and a Nanowizard 4 AFM (JPK, Cambridge, UK) mounted onto an Axiovert T1 inverted optical microscope (Zeiss, Cambridge, UK) fitted with a spherically tipped cantilever (nominal radius and spring constant of 1 μm and 3 Nm^{-1}, respectively: Windsor Scientific Ltd., Slough, UK,) running SPM software v 8.15 (JPK, Cambridge, UK). The local reduced modulus was determined for each of 2500 points in a 50 × 50 μm region, indented at a frequency of 1 Hz. The extend curve was used in conjunction with a contact-point-based model to calculate the reduced modulus for each indentation [13]. Post hoc analyses of force curves were performed using SPM analysis software v 1.40 (JPK, Cambridge, UK), whereby a baseline correction was applied to each curve before a force fit was applied using the Herzian (spherical) model and a maximum force fit of 70%. Once all force curves had been generated, quality control was applied, whereby any force values falling more than two standard deviations away from the mean value were discarded to account for failed indents (fewer than 10% of force curves).

Statistical analysis

Statistical analysis was done using Microsoft Excel or GraphPad PRISM Data Analysis software. Statistical significance was determined by Student's t test for paired samples when comparing two groups. One-way analysis of variance (ANOVA) was used when comparing more than two groups. Differences between samples were significantly different when $p = < 0.05$. For all graphs shown, error bars represent +/– standard error of the mean. The means have 1–4 asterisks centred over the error bar to indicate the relative level of the p value: *$p < 0.05$, **$p < 0.01$, ***$p < 0.001$ and ****$p < 0.0001$.

Additional files

Additional file 1: Figure S1. Breast tissues used in this study. Mammograms of patients examined in this study. The regions used for analysis were visually alike in most of the patients, and are outlined - red is tumour tissue, while green is normal. (PDF 698 kb)

Additional file 2: Figure S2. Histology of tissues used in this study. Histology of normal and tumour regions obtained for this study. In each case the normal regions were 4 cm or more away from the primary tumours in the same breasts. (PDF 41755 kb)

Additional file 3: Figure S3. Cytokeratin and vimentin staining of the tissues used in this study. Cytokeratin 8 and vimentin staining of normal and tumour regions used in this study. (PDF 144000 kb)

Additional file 4: Figure S4. Circadian clocks in breast tissue. Left - representative Per2::Luc traces from cultures of MECs isolated from the normal and tumour regions of patients with breast cancer. Right - normalisation of Per2::Luc activity from normal and tumour MECs. (PDF 287 kb)

Additional file 5: Figure S5. Collagen organisation in normal and tumour stroma. Picrosirius-Red-stained paraffin sections visualised in bright-field or polarised light. Samples of normal (left) and tumour (right) tissue from the same individuals are shown in each case. Ducts are outlined in black and white. (PDF 82243 kb)

Additional file 6: Figure S6. Stromal regions analysed by AFM. H&E staining of the normal and tumour regions of breasts from each individual that were examined by AFM (see Fig. 4a). The black squares represent the exact regions that were analysed. (PDF 36538 kb)

Abbreviations
AFM: Atomic force microscopy; BPE: Bovine pituitary extract; DAB: 3,3-Diaminobenzidine; DMEM: Dulbecco's modified Eagle's medium; ECM: Extracellular matrix; EGF: Epidermal growth factor; ER: Oestrogen receptor; FBS: Foetal bovine serum; H&E: Haematoxylin and eosin; Her2: Human epidermal growth factor receptor 2; MD: Mammographic density; MEC: Mammary epithelial cell; mRNA: Messenger RNA; PBS: Phosphate-buffered saline; PMT: Photomultiplier tube; PR: Progesterone receptor; qPCR: Quantitative PCR

Acknowledgements
Thanks for support from the Medical Research Council (MRC) for Q-JM, Prevent Breast Cancer for JM, the Biotechnology and Biological Sciences Research Council for JW, and the Wellcome Trust for supporting The Wellcome Centre for Cell-Matrix Research.

Funding
This work was supported by an MRC Centenary Award, a Prevent Breast Cancer grant, a Biotechnology and Biomedical Sciences Research Council (BBSRC) studentship and Wellcome Trust core funding.

Authors' contributions
EB, JM, JW and NY conducted the experimental work. EZ constructed imaging software. AL, RW, LJ and MH collected the patient material. CHS and QJM were involved in experimental planning and study design. CHS, QJM and EB wrote the manuscript. All authors read and agreed to the manuscript in its submitted form.

Competing interests
The authors declare that they have no competing interests.

References
1. Acerbi I, Cassereau L, Dean I, Shi Q, Au A, Park C, Chen YY, Liphardt J, Hwang ES, Weaver VM. Human breast cancer invasion and aggression correlates with ECM stiffening and immune cell infiltration. Integr. Biol. Quant. Biosci. Nano Macro. 2015;7:1120–34.
2. Akhtar N, Li W, Mironov A, Streuli CH. Rac1 controls both the secretory function of the mammary gland and its remodeling for successive gestations. Dev Cell. 2016;38:522–35.
3. Barcus CE, O'Leary KA, Brockman JL, Rugowski DE, Liu Y, Garcia N, Yu M, Keely PJ, Eliceiri KW, Schuler LA. Elevated collagen-I augments tumor progressive signals, intravasation and metastasis of prolactin-induced estrogen receptor alpha positive mammary tumor cells. Breast Cancer Res BCR. 2017;19:9.
4. Blakeman V, Williams JL, Meng Q-J, Streuli CH. Circadian clocks and breast cancer. Breast Cancer Res. 2016;18:89.
5. Bu Y, Yoshida A, Chitnis N, Altman BJ, Tameire F, Oran A, Gennaro V, Armeson KE, McMahon SB, Wertheim GB, et al. A PERK-miR-211 axis suppresses circadian regulators and protein synthesis to promote cancer cell survival. Nat Cell Biol. 2018;20:104–15.
6. Buchsbaum RJ, Oh SY. breast cancer-associated fibroblasts: where we are and where we need to go. Cancers. 2016;8(2):19.
7. Cadenas C, van de Sandt L, Edlund K, Lohr M, Hellwig B, Marchan R, Schmidt M, Rahnenführer J, Oster H, Hengstler JG. Loss of circadian clock gene expression is associated with tumor progression in breast cancer. Cell Cycle Georget Tex. 2014;13:3282–91.
8. Casey TM, Crodian J, Erickson E, Kuropatwinski KK, Gleiberman AS, Antoch MP. Tissue-specific changes in molecular clocks during the transition from pregnancy to lactation in mice. Biol Reprod. 2014;90:127.
9. Cermakian N, Sassone-Corsi P. Multilevel regulation of the circadian clock. Nat Rev Mol Cell Biol. 2000;1:59–67.
10. Chacolla-Huaringa R, Moreno-Cuevas J, Trevino V, Scott SP. Entrainment of Breast Cell Lines Results in Rhythmic Fluctuations of MicroRNAs. Int. J. Mol. Sci. 2017;18.18(7):1499.
11. Chen S-T, Choo K-B, Hou M-F, Yeh K-T, Kuo S-J, Chang J-G. Deregulated expression of the PER1, PER2 and PER3 genes in breast cancers. Carcinogenesis. 2005;26:1241–6.
12. Cox TR, Bird D, Baker A-M, Barker HE, Ho MW-Y, Lang G, Erler JT. LOX-mediated collagen crosslinking is responsible for fibrosis-enhanced metastasis. Cancer Res. 2013;73:1721–32.
13. Crick SL, Yin FC-P. Assessing micromechanical properties of cells with atomic force microscopy: importance of the contact point. Biomech Model Mechanobiol. 2007;6:199–210.
14. Dudek M, Meng Q-J. Running on time: the role of circadian clocks in the musculoskeletal system. Biochem J. 2014;463:1–8.
15. Elshazley M, Sato M, Hase T, Yamashita R, Yoshida K, Toyokuni S, Ishiguro F, Osada H, Sekido Y, Yokoi K, et al. The circadian clock gene BMAL1 is a novel therapeutic target for malignant pleural mesothelioma. Int J Cancer. 2012; 131:2820–31.
16. Fu L, Pelicano H, Liu J, Huang P, Lee C. The circadian gene Period2 plays an important role in tumor suppression and DNA damage response in vivo. Cell. 2002;111:41–50.
17. Gery S, Virk RK, Chumakov K, Yu A, Koeffler HP. The clock gene Per2 links the circadian system to the estrogen receptor. Oncogene. 2007;26:7916–20.
18. Glukhova MA, Streuli CH. How integrins control breast biology. Curr Opin Cell Biol. 2013;25:633–41.
19. Gossan N, Zeef L, Hensman J, Hughes A, Bateman JF, Rowley L, Little CB, Piggins HD, Rattray M, Boot Handford RP, et al. The circadian clock in murine chondrocytes regulates genes controlling key aspects of cartilage homeostasis. Arthritis Rheum. 2013;65:2334–45.
20. Hanley CJ, Noble F, Ward M, Bullock M, Drifka C, Mellone M, Manousopoulou A, Johnston HE, Hayden A, Thirdborough S, et al. A subset of myofibroblastic cancer-associated fibroblasts regulate collagen fiber elongation, which is prognostic in multiple cancers. Oncotarget. 2016;7: 6159–74.
21. Hasebe T. Tumor-stromal interactions in breast tumor progression-significance of histological heterogeneity of tumor-stromal fibroblasts. Expert Opin Ther Targets. 2013;17:449–60.
22. Haus EL, Smolensky MH. Shift work and cancer risk: potential mechanistic roles of circadian disruption, light at night, and sleep deprivation. Sleep Med Rev. 2013;17:273–84.

23. Hu M-L, Yeh K-T, Lin P-M, Hsu C-M, Hsiao H-H, Liu Y-C, Lin HY-H, Lin S-F, Yang M-Y. Deregulated expression of circadian clock genes in gastric cancer. BMC Gastroenterol. 2014;14:67.

24. Hwang-Verslues WW, Chang P-H, Jeng Y-M, Kuo W-H, Chiang P-H, Chang Y-C, Hsieh T-H, Su F-Y, Lin L-C, Abbondante S, et al. Loss of corepressor PER2 under hypoxia up-regulates OCT1-mediated EMT gene expression and enhances tumor malignancy. Proc Natl Acad Sci U S A. 2013;110:12331–6.

25. Janich P, Pascual G, Merlos-Suárez A, Batlle E, Ripperger J, Albrecht U, Cheng H-YM, Obrietan K, Di Croce L, Benitah SA. The circadian molecular clock creates epidermal stem cell heterogeneity. Nature. 2011;480:209–14.

26. Jiang W, Zhao S, Jiang X, Zhang E, Hu G, Hu B, Zheng P, Xiao J, Lu Z, Lu Y, et al. The circadian clock gene Bmal1 acts as a potential anti-oncogene in pancreatic cancer by activating the p53 tumor suppressor pathway. Cancer Lett. 2016;371:314–25.

27. Jones VC, McKeown L, Verkhratsky A, Jones OT. LV-pIN-KDEL: a novel lentiviral vector demonstrates the morphology, dynamics and continuity of the endoplasmic reticulum in live neurones. BMC Neurosci. 2008;9:10.

28. Kaukonen R, Mai A, Georgiadou M, Saari M, De Franceschi N, Betz T, Sihto H, Ventelä S, Elo L, Jokitalo E, et al. Normal stroma suppresses cancer cell proliferation via mechanosensitive regulation of JMJD1a-mediated transcription. Nat Commun. 2016;7:12237.

29. Kaushik S, Pickup MW, Weaver VM. From transformation to metastasis: deconstructing the extracellular matrix in breast cancer. Cancer Metastasis Rev. 2016;35:655–67.

30. Kelleher FC, Rao A, Maguire A. Circadian molecular clocks and cancer. Cancer Lett. 2014;342:9–18.

31. Ko, C.H., and Takahashi, J.S. (2006). Molecular components of the mammalian circadian clock. Hum Mol Genet 15 Spec No 2, R271

32. Kondratov RV, Kondratova AA, Gorbacheva VY, Vykhovanets OV, Antoch MP. Early aging and age-related pathologies in mice deficient in BMAL1, the core componentof the circadian clock. Genes Dev. 2006;20:1868–73.

33. Kuo S-J, Chen S-T, Yeh K-T, Hou M-F, Chang Y-S, Hsu NC, Chang J-G. Disturbance of circadian gene expression in breast cancer. Virchows Arch Int J Pathol. 2009;454:467–74.

34. Lu W, Meng Q-J, Tyler NJC, Stokkan K-A, Loudon ASI. A circadian clock is not required in an arctic mammal. Curr Biol CB. 2010;20:533–7.

35. McConnell JC, O'Connell OV, Brennan K, Weiping L, Howe M, Joseph L, Knight D, O'Cualain R, Lim Y, Leek A, et al. Increased peri-ductal collagen micro-organization may contribute to raised mammographic density. Breast Cancer Res. 2016;18:5.

36. Menet JS, Pescatore S, Rosbash M. CLOCK:BMAL1 is a pioneer-like transcription factor. Genes Dev. 2014;28:8–13.

37. Metcalfe AD, Gilmore A, Klinowska T, Oliver J, Valentijn AJ, Brown R, Ross A, MacGregor G, Hickman JA, Streuli CH. Developmental regulation of Bcl-2 family protein expression in the involuting mammary gland. J Cell Sci. 1999; 112(Pt 11):1771–83.

38. Muschler J, Streuli CH. Cell-matrix interactions in mammary gland development and breast cancer. Cold Spring Harb Perspect Biol. 2010;2:a003202.

39. Reszka E, Przybek M, Muurlink O, Pepłonska B. Circadian gene variants and breast cancer. Cancer Lett. 2017;390:137–45.

40. Rich L, Whittaker P. Collagen and picrosirius red staining: a polarized light assessment of fibrillar hue and spatial distribution. Braz J Morphol Sci. 2005;22: 97–104.

41. Roenneberg T, Merrow M. Circadian clocks - the fall and rise of physiology. Nat. Rev Mol Cell Biol. 2005;6:965–71.

42. Rossetti S, Esposito J, Corlazzoli F, Gregorski A, Sacchi N. Entrainment of breast (cancer) epithelial cells detects distinct circadian oscillation patterns for clock and hormone receptor genes. Cell Cycle. 2012;11:350–60.

43. Sahar S, Sassone-Corsi P. Metabolism and cancer: the circadian clock connection. Nat Rev Cancer. 2009;9:886–96.

44. Schito L, Semenza GL. Hypoxia-inducible factors: master regulators of cancer progression. Trends Cancer. 2016;2:758–70.

45. Semenza GL. The hypoxic tumor microenvironment: a driving force for breast cancer progression. Biochim Biophys Acta. 2016;1863:382–91.

46. Sherratt MJ, McConnell JC, Streuli CH. Raised mammographic density: causative mechanisms and biological consequences. Breast Cancer Res. 2016;18:45.

47. Sokol ES, Miller DH, Breggia A, Spencer KC, Arendt LM, Gupta PB. Growth of human breast tissues from patient cells in 3D hydrogel scaffolds. Breast Cancer Res. 2016;18:19.

48. Streuli CH. Integrins as architects of cell behavior. Mol Biol Cell. 2016;27: 2885–8.

49. Sulli G, Rommel A, Wang X, Kolar MJ, Puca F, Saghatelian A, Plikus MV, Verma IM, Panda S. Pharmacological activation of REV-ERBs is lethal in cancer and oncogene-induced senescence. Nature. 2018;553:351–5.

50. Wang Y, Hua L, Lu C, Chen Z. Expression of circadian clock gene human Period2 (hPer2) in human colorectal carcinoma. World J Surg Oncol. 2011;9:166.

51. Whittaker P, Kloner RA, Boughner DR, Pickering JG. Quantitative assessment of myocardial collagen with picrosirius red staining and circularly polarized light. Basic Res Cardiol. 1994;89:397–410.

52. Williams J, Yang N, Wood A, Zindy E, Meng QJ, Streuli CH. Epithelial and stromal circadian clocks are inversely regulated by their mechano-matrix environment. J. Cell Sci. 2018;131(5):e0505.

53. Yang N, Williams J, Pekovic-Vaughan V, Wang P, Olabi S, McConnell J, Gossan N, Hughes A, Cheung J, Streuli CH, et al. Cellular mechano-environment regulates the mammary circadian clock. Nat Commun. 2017;8:14287.

54. Yang X, Wood PA, Oh E-Y, Du-Quiton J, Ansell CM, Hrushesky WJM. Down regulation of circadian clock gene Period 2 accelerates breast cancer growth by altering its daily growth rhythm. Breast Cancer Res Treat. 2009; 117:423–31.

18

HER4 expression in estrogen receptor-positive breast cancer is associated with decreased sensitivity to tamoxifen treatment and reduced overall survival of postmenopausal women

Anja Kathrin Wege[1†], Dominik Chittka[1,2†], Stefan Buchholz[1], Monika Klinkhammer-Schalke[3], Simone Diermeier-Daucher[1], Florian Zeman[4], Olaf Ortmann[1] and Gero Brockhoff[1*] [iD]

Abstract

Background: The sensitivity of estrogen receptor-positive breast cancers to tamoxifen treatment varies considerably, and the molecular mechanisms affecting the response rates are manifold. The human epidermal growth factor receptor-related receptor HER2 is known to trigger intracellular signaling cascades that modulate the activity of coregulators of the estrogen receptor which, in turn, reduces the cell sensitivity to tamoxifen treatment. However, the impact of HER2-related receptor tyrosine kinases HER1, HER3, and, in particular, HER4 on endocrine treatment is largely unknown.

Methods: Here, we retrospectively evaluated the importance of HER4 expression on the outcome of tamoxifen- and aromatase inhibitor-treated estrogen receptor-positive breast cancer patients ($n = 258$). In addition, we experimentally analyzed the efficiency of tamoxifen treatment as a function of HER4 co-expression in vitro.

Results: We found a significantly improved survival in tamoxifen-treated postmenopausal breast cancer patients in the absence of HER4 compared with those with pronounced HER4 expression. In accordance with this finding, the sensitivity to tamoxifen treatment of estrogen and HER4 receptor-positive ZR-75-1 breast cancer cells can be significantly enhanced by HER4 knockdown.

Conclusion: We suggest an HER4/estrogen receptor interaction that impedes tamoxifen binding to the estrogen receptor and reduces treatment efficiency. Whether the sensitivity to tamoxifen treatment can be enhanced by anti-HER4 targeting needs to be prospectively evaluated.

Keywords: HER4 receptor, Estrogen receptor positive breast cancer, Tamoxifen treatment

Background

Tamoxifen (TAM) treatment of hormone receptor-positive breast cancer (BC) has proved to be a pioneering target-specific therapy regimen [1] that was introduced more than four decades ago [2]. The main indication for an ad-juvant treatment of breast cancer with anti-estrogens is the immunohistochemical identification of estrogen receptor (ER)-positive tumor cells that was suggested in 1987 [3] and has since evolved into a standardized diagnostic procedure. TAM is being frequently applied in the adjuvant (i.e., postsurgery) setting and in terms of remission maintenance and according to the treatment guidelines released by the American Society of Clinical Oncology (ASCO) and the German Gynecologic-Oncology Working Group (AGO) the application of the

* Correspondence: gero.brockhoff@ukr.de
†Anja Kathrin Wege and Dominik Chittka contributed equally to this work.
[1]Clinic of Gynecology and Obstetrics, University Medical Center Regensburg, Regensburg, Germany
Full list of author information is available at the end of the article

antiestrogen is conceived as a long-term (up to 10 years) therapy [4, 5].

From a molecular point of view TAM has been developed to competitively bind ERs located in the cell nucleus and thereby to competitively hamper the binding of estradiol. As a result, estradiol-specific (e.g., pro-proliferative) effects are inhibited and tumor growth becomes retarded or ideally even blocked [6, 7]. However, clinically short- and long-term remissions achieved by endocrine (TAM-based) treatment are often followed by the acquisition of resistance and, ultimately, disease relapse [8]. Treatment guidelines released by internationally recognized expert organizations such as the *Arbeitsgemeinschaft der Wissenschaftlichen Medizinischen Fachgesellschaften* e.V. (Berlin, Germany), the National Comprehensive Cancer Network NCCN™ (PA, USA), and the European Society for Medical Oncology (ESMO; Viganello-Lugano, Switzerland) all strongly recommend including an aromatase inhibitor (AI) into the treatment regimens for postmenopausal women (level of evidence 1b). AIs are designed to inhibit the endogenous synthesis of the estrogen receptor ligand estradiol and it has been demonstrated that a sequential targeting of the endocrine receptor ligand system prolongs the period of remission by circumventing molecular mechanism that cause treatment resistance [9, 10].

Both the ER and the human epidermal growth factor-related receptor 2 (HER2) represent dominant drivers for the genesis and progression of BC [11]. The sensitivity to target (i.e., ER and HER2 receptor) specific treatments is affected by an extensive crosstalk of receptor-triggered pathways [12]. Mechanistically, the HER2 receptor tyrosine kinase triggers a variety of downstream signaling pathways, such as the RAF/RAS/MAPK cascade that results in phosphorylation of the ER and co-regulatory molecules such as AIB1/Src-3 [12–17]. As a final consequence, TAM binding to the ER is ineffective since it does not weaken the transcriptional and pro-proliferative activity of the malignant cells. Nevertheless, HER2-induced TAM resistance is clinically manageable by switching from the anti-estrogen to an AI or by extending the treatment by an anti-HER2 targeting [18–20]. Indeed, a number of options to target alternate intracellular pathways are available to overcome HER2-induced TAM resistance [20]. However, HER2 does not work as a stand-alone receptor but forms a functional unit with its relatives HER1, HER3, and HER4. All HER receptors have prognostic impact on BC disease [21–23]; however, the extent to which HER1, HER3, and HER4 affect the sensitivity of ER-positive BC cancers to TAM treatment is hardly known. Amongst the four cognate receptor tyrosine kinases the HER4 receptor might play an exceptional role in BC biology because it has been associated either with a disadvantageous [24] or with a favorable [21, 22] impact on the course and

outcome of disease. For instance, we previously reported a positive impact of a gain of the HER4 gene locus on the outcome of HER2-positive and trastuzumab-treated BC patients [21, 23]. This finding has been later confirmed by others [25]. By way of contrast, the presence of HER4 has been associated with acquired resistance to HER2 inhibitors such as lapatinib [26].

Here, we retrospectively analyzed the impact of HER4 expression on the course and outcome of ER-positive breast cancer patients. To this end, we determined the HER4 mRNA level of 258 ER-positive BC samples by quantitative polymerase chain reaction (qPCR). Subcohorts of pre- and postmenopausal patients were analyzed independently and as a function of treatment with TAM and AIs. These analyses were complemented by in vitro TAM treatment of the strongly ER-positive ZR-75-1 BC cell line. The impact of HER4 on the TAM treatment efficiency was evaluated by siRNA-based HER4 receptor knockdown.

Compared with the cohort of BC patients without or with only low HER4 expression we found poor overall survival of ER-positive and TAM-treated breast cancer patients when the HER4 expression was high. This phenomenon was pronounced and highly significant in postmenopausal women. In contrast to the TAM-treated patients, within the cohort of AI-treated women no impact of HER4 expression on the course and outcome of disease could be observed. In accordance with the analysis on primary tumor samples, the sensitivity of ER- and HER4-positive ZR-75-1 cells to TAM treatment could be significantly enhanced by siRNA-based HER4 knockdown. Taken together, the HER4 expression seems to impair the efficiency of TAM but not AI treatment, even though the predictive value of HER4 in ER-positive BC patients needs to be prospectively evaluated.

Material and methods
ER-positive BC database
The pathological diagnostics were performed at the Institute of Pathology at the University of Regensburg (Regensburg, Germany). BC tissues were (immuno)histochemically analyzed based on the estrogen/progesterone receptor, Ki67, and Her2 receptor status and grading and, if applicable, by fluorescence in situ hybridization. Clinicopathological parameters were documented by the Institute of Pathology and the Breast Cancer Center of the University Cancer Center Regensburg. Clinical follow-up was correlated with data from the Tumor Center Regensburg, a population-based regional cancer registry covering a population of more than 2.2 million people including Upper Palatinate and Lower Bavaria. The documentation comprises individual patient data, information on primary diagnosis, treatment regimens, course of disease, and the complete

follow-up. Table 1 lists the demographic and clinicopathological data of the patient collective $n = 258$ subjected to this study.

Tissue embedding, processing, and immunohistochemistry
All specimens were acquired from the tissue archive of the Institute of Pathology, University of Regensburg,

Table 1 Demographic data of 258 evaluated hormone receptor-positive patients

Clinicopathological parameter	Premenopausal ($n = 67$)		Postmenopausal ($n = 191$)	
	n	%	n	%
Tumor stage				
I	32	48	111	58
II	28	42	67	35
III	4	6	8	4
IV	0	0	0	0
Unknown	3	4	5	3
Subtype				
Invasive ductal	56	84	151	79
Invasive lobular	7	10	24	13
Others	4	6	16	8
Grading				
1	5	7	25	13
2	44	66	110	58
3	17	25	52	27
Unknown	1	1	4	2
Lymph node status				
0	30	45	116	61
1	19	28	52	27
2	10	15	13	7
3	6	9	6	3
Unknown	2	3	4	2
Endocrine treatment				
Tamoxifen	43	64	66	35
Aromatase inhibitor	24	36	125	65
Surgery				
Mastectomy	27	40	51	27
Breast-conserving therapy	40	60	140	73
Radiation				
Yes	50	75	151	79
No	7	10	23	12
Unknown	10	15	17	9
Cytotoxicity treatment				
Yes	56	84	85	44
No	1	1	3	2
Unknown	10	15	103	54

Germany. The embedding procedure was performed as described elsewhere [27]. Immediately after surgery, the breast tissues were transferred into the formalin fixative (4% formaldehyde, 1% sodium phosphate; SG Planung, Holzkirchen, Germany). The total fixation time was between 12 h (minimum) and 36 h (maximum). The specimens were then subjected to automated dehydration and paraffin immersion. Tissue dehydration was performed by subjecting the tissues to a series of ascending ethanol concentrations (70% for 30 min, 70% for 60 min, 96% for 60 min, 96% for 50 min, 100% for 50 min, and 100% for 90 min), and was completed by incubation in 100% xylene (2×50 min). Finally, the tissues were embedded in paraffin with a Shandon Hypercenter XP (2×30 min; 2×60 min) and 1.5-μm paraffin sections were prepared from the embedded tissue blocks. Specimens were deparaffinized and pretreated by microwave heating for 30 min at 320 W in 0.1 M citrate buffer adjusted to pH 7.3. The immunostaining was automatically performed on a Ventana Nexes autostainer (Ventana, Tucson, USA) by using the streptavidin–biotin peroxidase complex method and 3,3'-diaminobenzidine (DAB) as a chromogen. The autostainer was programmed based on the instructions given by the OptiView DAB detection kit (Ventana). The mouse monoclonal anti-ER antibody clone 6F11 (Leica Microsystems GmbH, Novocastra, Wetzlar, Germany) was used at a dilution of 1:35. The specimens were analyzed by conventional bright field microscopy. ER positivity was rated based on the recommendations given by Remmele and Stegner [3].

RNA isolation, cDNA synthesis, and HER4-specific real-time qPCR
Four different HER4 isoforms, namely JM-a/CYT1, JM-a/CYT2, JM-b/CYT1, and JM-b/CYT2, resulting from differential splicing have been described while the juxtamembrane (JM)-a variant represents the cleavable form [28]. It has been shown that in BC only the cleavable JM-a isoforms are expressed [23, 29]. Accordingly, we used only HER4/JM-a isoform-specific primers in this study. Base sequences of primers and probes were as follows: forward 5' CCA CCC ATC CCA TCC AAA-3', reverse 5' CCA ATT ACT CCA GCT GCA ATC A-3', Probe 5' Fam-ATG GAC GGG CAA TTC CAC TTT ACC A-Dabcyl-3'. We have previously described the qPCR procedure in detail [23]. Briefly, the miRNeasy RNA Isolation Kit (Qiagen, Hilden, Germany) was used to extract RNA from formalin-fixed and paraffin-embedded tissue samples. For synthesis of cDNA, a template of 0.5 μg total RNA was used. According to the manufacturer's instructions (Transcriptor First Strand cDNA Synthesis Kit; Roche Diagnostics, Mannheim, Germany), the reaction contains random hexamers (Promega, Mannheim, Germany), reverse transcriptase

(Promega), dNTP-mixture, and RNAse inhibitor. All reactions were performed in duplicate in the presence and absence of reverse transcriptase. Real-time PCR was performed using fluorescent oligonucleotide LC480 hybridization probes (Metabion, Martinsried, Germany). A calibration standard as well as probes and primers annealing to mRNA of β-actin were used as internal reference and for comparison of successive experiments. PCR was carried out in a final volume of 10 µl containing 2.5 µl cDNA template (1:5 attenuation), 5 µl LC480 Probes Master (Roche), 1 µl probe, and 1.5 µl primers (0.75 µl primer β-actin, 0.75 µl primer target). Probes were labeled with fluorescent reporter dyes FAM (Her4 isoform probes) or LC Red (β-actin probes). Thermal cycling started with the pre-incubation at 95 °C for 10 min. Then amplification was carried out by running 45 cycles, initiated with 30 s at 60 °C followed by 15 s at 95 °C on a LC480 device.

ZR-75-1 cell line incubation, TAM treatment, and siRNA-based HER4 knockdown

The ZR-75-1 BC cell line was purchased from the American Type Culture Collection (ATCC number CRL-1500, Manassas, VA, USA). For this study, the cell line was authenticated by the Leibniz-Institute "German Collection of Microorganisms and Cell Culture" GmbH (DSMZ, Braunschweig, Germany).

ZR-75-1 cells were cultured in Roswell Park Memorial Institute 1640 medium (RPMI-1640) supplemented with 5% fetal calf serum (FCS) (both from PAN Biotech, Aidenbach, Germany). Cells were commonly seeded at densities of 2×10^5 cells per T75 tissue flask (Greiner Bio-One, Frickenhausen, Germany) and were incubated in a humidified atmosphere containing 5% CO_2 at 37 °C. Culture medium was refreshed every 2 days. For harvesting, cells were washed with phosphate-buffered saline (PBS; pH 7.4, Biochrom, Berlin, Germany) and were detached from culture flasks by incubating for 3 min at 37 °C in a PBS solution supplemented with 0.05% trypsin and 0.02% ethylenediaminetetraacetic acid.

For the siRNA-mediated HER4 downregulation, 5×10^5 ZR-75-1 cells were seeded in a T25 tissue flask in RPMI-1640 medium supplemented with 5% FCS on day 0. The next day, the medium was removed and 2.5, 2.3, and 2.1 ml (untreated sample/DharmaFECT-treated sample/ siRNA sample) fresh RPMI/1% FCS was added, respectively. The transfection mix was prepared by incorporation of 10 µl DharmaFECT (Dharmacon, Lafayette, CO, USA) with 190 µl Opti-MEM (Invitrogen, Karlsruhe, Germany) in tube 1 and 12.5 µl of 10 µM anti-HER4 siRNA (L-003128-00-0005 ON-TARGETplus SMARTpool Human ERBB4 2066, Dharmacon) and 187.5 µl Opti-MEM in tube 2. For control purposes we exposed the cells to non-targeting siRNA (D-001810-10-05 ON-TARGETplus

Non-targeting Pool; Horizon Discovery Ltd., CA, USA) which is expected to cause no effect on receptor expression and cell proliferation. After 5 min incubation at room temperature the contents of tube 1 and tube 2 were pooled and subsequently thoroughly mixed. After a further incubation step of 20 min at room temperature the 400-µl transfection mix was added per flask to give a final siRNA concentration of 50 nM. From day 2 on, the cells were treated with 5 µM TAM for 96 h (Sigma-Aldrich Chemie GmbH, Deisenhofen, Germany).

Western blotting

Treated and untreated ZR-75-1 cells were lysed for total protein analysis in cell-lysis buffer (Cell Signaling, Danvers, MA, USA) supplemented with Halt™ Protease and Phosphatase Inhibitor Cocktail (Thermo Fisher Scientific, Bremen, Germany). After calculating the protein concentration with the Pierce BCA protein assay kit (ThermoFisher), 25 µg total protein per lane were separated in 7.5% SDS-PAGE under reducing conditions (mercaptoethanol) and blotted onto polyvinylidene difluoride (PVDF) membranes. Membranes were blocked with Tris-buffered saline supplemented with 5% low-fat milk and 2% Tween for 2 h and then incubated overnight at 4 °C using the following primary antibodies: rabbit anti-human HER1 (D38B1; 1:1000), rabbit anti-human HER2 (29D8; 1:4000), rabbit anti-human HER3 (D22C5; 1:200), rabbit anti-human HER4/ErbB4 (111B2; 1:1000) (all from Cell Signaling Technology), rabbit anti-human β-actin (A2066; 1:5000, Sigma-Aldrich Chemie GmbH), and mouse anti-estrogen receptor (NCL-L-ER-6F11; 1:500, Leica Microsystems). The next day, after washing the membrane, incubation with secondary antibodies (goat anti-rabbit 7074 HRP-conjugated and horse anti-mouse (7076) HRP-conjugated; both 1:2000, and both from Cell Signaling Technology) was performed for 1 h at room temperature. The blots were visualized using the chemiluminescent Western blotting detection system (GE Healthcare, Amersham, UK) and analyzed by ImageQuant LAS 4000 mini-imager (GE Healthcare).

Proliferation assessment by flow cytometry

BrdU/Hoechst quenching measurements (i.e., the assessment of G0-phase fraction) were performed as described previously [30]. This approach is based on continuous labeling of cells in vitro with BrdU which is incorporated into the DNA instead of thymidine during the cell cycle S phase. BrdU incorporation results in quenching of Hoechst 33258 but not of propidium iodide upon DNA double staining. Thus, actively proliferating cells and quiescent (i.e., G0 phase) cells can be differentiated and separately quantified. For flow cytometric cell analyses, 5×10^5 cells were seeded on day 0 into T25 culture flasks and were incubated for 7 days. At day 4, 120 µM

BrdU was added to the culture flasks and cells were incubated in the presence of BrdU for an additional 72 h. To minimize potential disturbance in the nucleotide pathway due to BrdU treatment, the medium was also supplemented with half-equimolar 2'deoxycytidine. After detachment the cells were stored at −20 °C at a concentration of 10^6 cells/ml in freezing medium (RPMI-1640 medium + 10% FCS + 10% dimethyl sulfoxide (DMSO)) until flow cytometric analysis. For cell staining, thawed cells were washed twice with 2 ml ice-cold DNA-staining buffer (100 mM Tris-HCl, pH 7.4, 154 mM NaCl, 1 mM $CaCl_2$, 0.5 mM $MgCl_2$, 0.1% IGEP AL CA-630 (Nonylphenylpolyethylenglycol), 0.2% bovine serum albumin (BSA)); 5×10^5 cells were resuspended in 1 ml buffer supplemented with 40 g/ml (2–4 units/ml) RNase and 1.2 µg/ml Hoechst 33258 (Sigma-Aldrich) and incubated for 15 min at 37 °C. Cellular DNA content was stained with propidium iodide (1.5 µg/ml) for 15 min on ice. Samples were passed through a 70-µm nylon mesh to remove cell aggregates prior to flow cytometric analysis. Flow cytometric measurements were performed on a FACSCanto II flow cytometer (BD Biosciences, San Jose, CA) equipped with a blue (488 nm), red (633 nm), and violet (405 nm) laser and a standard optical configuration. Sample measurements and data analysis were performed with FACSDiva Software v7.0 (BD Biosciences), and 50,000 events/sample were collected. As described previously in detail, the G0 cell fraction was calculated by taking into account the fraction of cells that had divided once, twice, or three times within the period of observation [31].

Statistical analyses

Overall survival (OS) was calculated from the date of diagnosis to the date of death of any cause. Patients who survived were classified as censored cases at the latest date they were confirmed to be alive. Disease-free survival (DFS) was calculated as the period of time after (successful) primary treatment without any evidence of cancer-related signs, symptoms, or death. Patients without any cancerous disease and being alive were classified as censored cases at the latest date they were confirmed to be disease free and alive. Maximum follow-up time was set to 10 years. Patients with a longer follow-up were classified as censored cases after 10 years. The

impact of HER4 expression on DFS and OS was calculated for all patients and subcohorts (i.e., pre- versus postmenopausal, TAM- versus AI-treated patients). Survival curves were estimated using the Kaplan–Meier method and hazard ratios (HRs) and corresponding 95% confidence intervals (Cis) were calculated by Cox proportional hazards regression models for the univariate as well as for the multivariable models. An optimal cut-off for HER4 values for predicting OS and DFS was estimated based on log-rank statistics. All reported p values were two-sided. A p value lower than 0.05 was considered to indicate a significant difference. All statistical analyses were performed using R version 3.3.3 (The R Foundation for Statistical Computing) or GraphPad Prism (Ver. 6, GraphPad Software, La Jolla, CA, USA).

Results

Considering the entire collective HER4 expression has no significant impact on the outcome of disease

No correlation of HER4 expression (continuously or dichotomized) with the DFS or the OS could be found when all patients (i.e., without regard to the treatment regimen and age) were included into the analysis (Table 2).

HER4 expression has a significant impact on the outcome of TAM-treated but not on the outcome of AI-treated patients

When considering TAM-treated patients, a significant impact of HER4 expression on the OS was found (HR = 1.28 HER4 continuous; HR 3.22, HER4 ≥ 1, respectively; Table 3). Further analyses identified a better cut-off for the HER4 expression of the TAM-treated group, with HER4 < 1 (HER4-negative) versus HER4 ≥ 1 (HER4-positive). In contrast to the TAM-treated cohort, in the AI-treated subpopulation no correlation of HER4 expression to the OS (HR = 0.86 and 0.68, respectively) or DFS (HR = 0.85 and 0.72, respectively) was seen (Table 3).

Further stratification of the TAM-treated group based on the pre- and postmenopausal status (< 46 years vs. ≥ 46 years) revealed that HER4 expression had a significant impact on the OS (HR =1.43, HER4 continuous; HR −4.98, HER4 ≥ 1) and DFS (HR = 1.81, HER4 continuous) only in postmenopausal but not in premenopausal women (Table 4).

Table 2 Impact of HER4 expression on the overall survival (OS) and disease-free survival (DFS) in all patients (independent of menopausal status and treatment)

Predictor	OS				DFS			
	HR	95% CI		p value	HR	95% CI		p value
HER4 continuous	1.08	0.87	1.35	0.474	1.00	0.80	1.25	0.993
HER4-positive (ref. no HER4 expression)	0.90	0.49	1.66	0.736	0.91	0.54	1.55	0.733

CI confidence interval, *HR* hazard ratio

Table 3 Impact of HER4 expression on the overall survival (OS) and disease-free survival (DFS) in patient subcohorts stratified by treatment (TAM or AI)

Subgroup	Predictor	OS				DFS			
		HR	95% CI		p value	HR	95% CI		p value
TAM treated	HER4 continuous	**1.28**	**1.01**	**1.62**	**0.040**	1.16	0.89	1.52	0.270
	HER4 expression (ref. no HER4 expression)	1.63	0.52	5.06	0.399	1.23	0.54	2.84	0.622
	HER4 ≥ 1 (ref. HER4 < 1)	**3.22**	**1.17**	**8.86**	**0.024**	1.36	0.63	2.97	0.436
AI treated	HER4 continuous	0.86	0.60	1.22	0.393	0.85	0.61	1.18	0.338
	HER4 expression (ref. no HER4 expression)	0.68	0.31	1.50	0.339	0.72	0.36	1.44	0.352

Significant values are shows in bold typeface
AI aromatase inhibitor, *CI* confidence interval, *HR* hazard ratio, *TAM* tamoxifen

Kaplan–Meier survival curves confirmed that the OS of TAM-treated patients was significantly (p = 0.0167) improved in HER4-negative BC patients, which was independent of their menopausal status (Fig. 1, left column). No significant difference (p = 0.433) was detectable with respect to the DFS (Fig. 1, right column). Classification by age revealed no significant differences for DFS (p = 0.37) or OS (p = 0.652) in TAM-treated premenopausal (< 46 years of age) patients (Fig. 1, middle row). However, the OS (p = 0.0087) was significantly impaired in postmenopausal HER4-positive patients (≥ 46 years of age; Fig. 1, bottom row). The DFS of postmenopausal and TAM-treated women tends to be significantly better in case of HER4-negative BC compared with HER4-positive BC (p = 0.0477; Fig. 1, bottom row).

Patients treated with AIs did not display any significant HER4 dependency with respect to OS and DFS, neither in pre- nor in postmenopausal patients (all p values greater than 0.05, Fig. 2). However, a trend towards an improved (rather than to an impaired) course and outcome of disease in HER4-positive patients compared with women with HER4-negative tumors became apparent.

To assess if HER4 is an independent predictor for OS and DFS within the TAM-treated postmenopausal women, a multivariable Cox regression model was applied (Table 5). Due to the limited number of events only two further covariables were added to the model. Based on clinical relevance and statistical significance, patient age and tumor staging (pT) were selected. In the adjusted models, HER4

as a continuous variable remains a significant predictor for both OS (p = 0.035, HER4 continuous) and DFS (p = 0.003, HER4 continuous).

HER4 downregulation enhanced efficiency of TAM treatment in vitro

HER4 knockdown in ER-positive ZR-75-1 breast cancer cells resulted in about 90% reduced HER4 protein levels (Fig. 3a). Off-target effects on the other members of the HER receptor family (i.e., HER1, HER2, and HER3) could be excluded (Fig. 3b–d). The unaffected ER expression in ZR-75-1 cells is exemplarily shown in Fig. 4a. BrdU/Hoechst quenching assay was applied to quantify the different TAM efficiencies in wild-type (WT) and HER4 knockdown cells. This technique allows the quantitative assessment of proliferating and resting cells. Cells which stop proliferation are considered to become quiescent and to enter the G0/G1 resting phase. Repeated measurements revealed a significantly increased fraction of G0-phase cells in the presence of TAM treatment compared with untreated cells (Fig. 4b). This observation applies to both WT (p < 0.001) cells and cells treated with non-targeting siRNA (p < 0.001). However, TAM treatment efficiency is significantly enhanced in ZR-75-1 cells upon HER4 receptor knockdown compared with ZR-75-1 cells with regular HER4 expression (on average 19% versus 47.0%, p < 0.0001). Flow cytometric example measurements are shown in Fig. 4c. An increased fraction of G0/G1 resting cells upon TAM

Table 4 Impact of HER4 expression on the overall survival (OS) and disease-free survival (DFS) in tamoxifen-treated patients stratified by menopausal status

Strata	Predictor	OS				DFS			
		HR	95% CI		p value	HR	95% CI		p value
Premenopausal (< 46 years)	HER4 continuous	1.06	0.59	1.89	0.845	0.77	0.43	1.38	0.380
	HER4 ≥ 1 (ref. HER4 < 1)	1.51	0.25	9.01	0.655	0.56	0.15	2.03	0.377
Postmenopausal (≥ 46 years	HER4 continuous	**1.43**	**1.09**	**1.86**	**0.009**	**1.81**	**1.25**	**2.63**	**0.002**
	HER4 ≥ 1 (ref. HER4 < 1)	**4.98**	**1.32**	**18.80**	**0.018**	2.94	0.96	9.00	0.059

Significant values are shows in bold typeface
CI confidence interval, *HR* hazard ratio

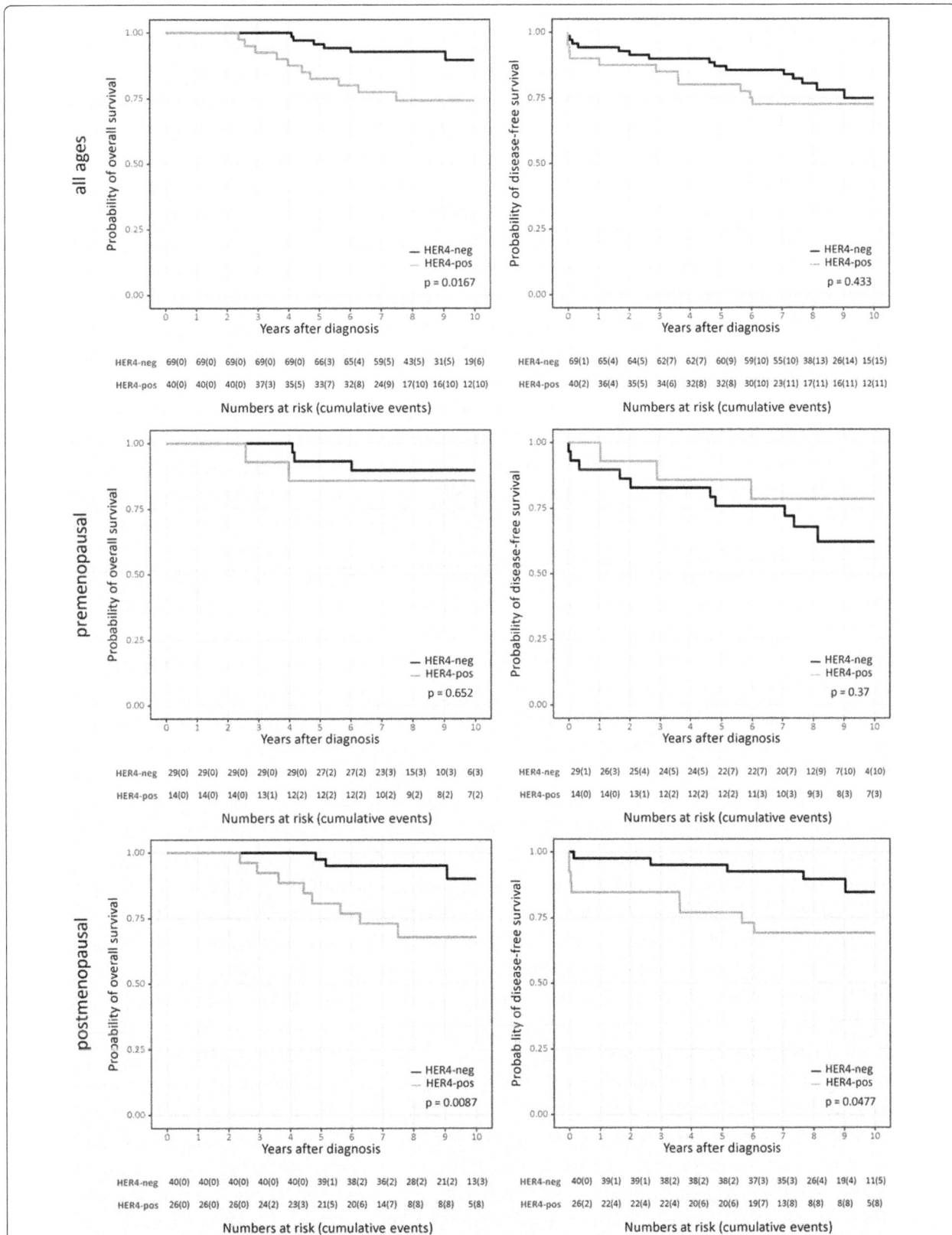

Fig. 1 Disease outcome of TAM-treated ER-positive breast cancer patients. OS and DFS are displayed for all patients (top row), only premenopausal (< 46 years; middle row), and only postmenopausal (≥ 46 years, bottom row) breast cancer patients treated with TAM. The p values were calculated using the log-rank test (Mantel–Cox) and are indicated in each graph

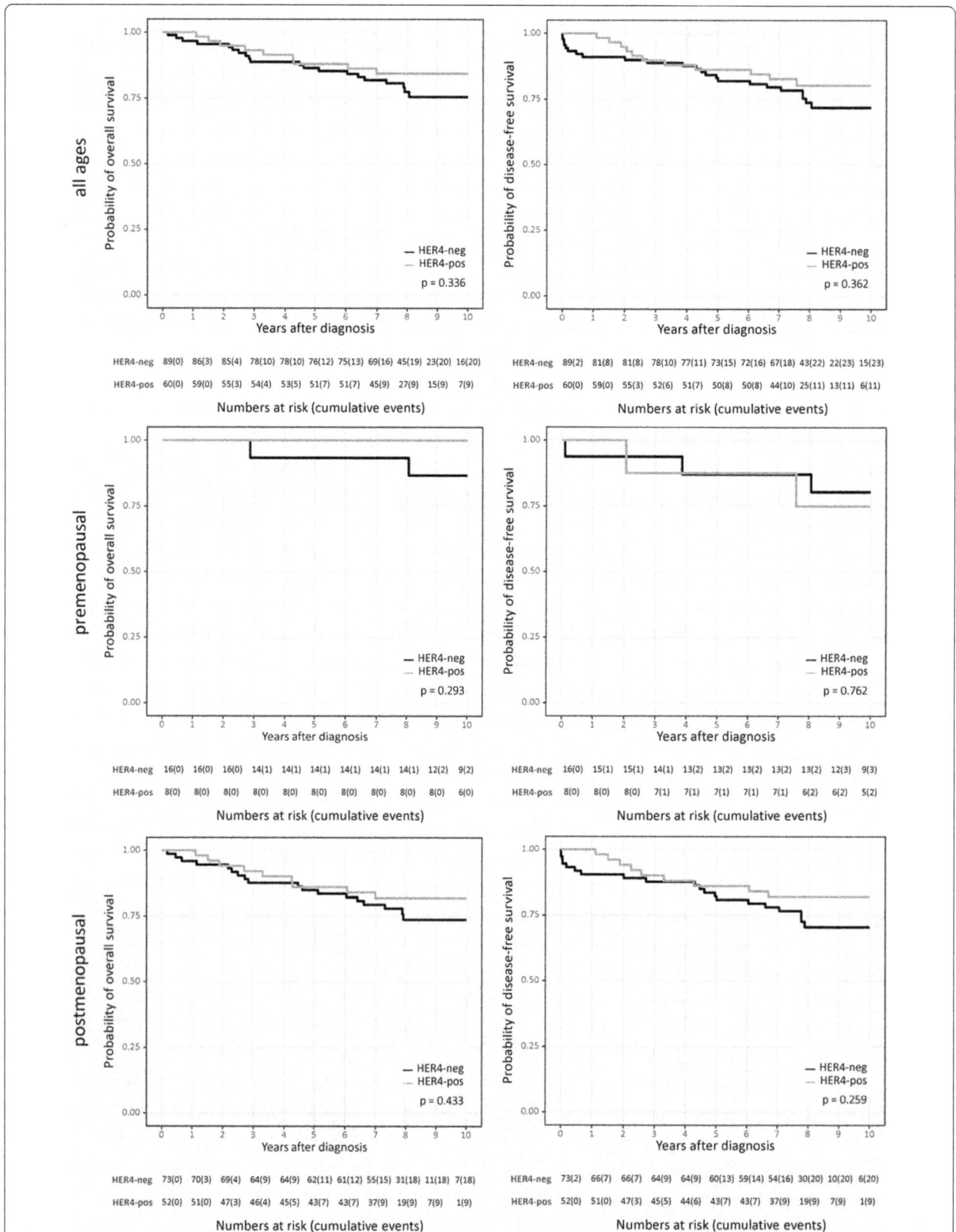

Fig. 2 Disease outcome of AI-treated ER-positive breast cancer patients. OS and DFS are displayed for all patients (top row), premenopausal (< 46 years; middle row), and postmenopausal (≥ 46 years, bottom row) breast cancer patients treated with AI. The *p* values were calculated using the log-rank test (Mantel–Cox) and are indicated in each graph

Table 5 Multivariable Cox regression analysis of tamoxifen-treated postmenopausal women on the overall survival (OS) and disease-free survival (DFS) including HER4, patient age, and tumor stage

	OS ($n = 64$, events $= 12$)				DFS ($n = 64$, events $= 12$)			
	HR	95% CI		p value	HR	95% CI		p value
Model 1								
HER4 continuous	**1.41**	**1.02**	**1.95**	**0.035**	**2.34**	**1.34**	**4.06**	**0.003**
Age	1.14	1.07	1.21	< 0.001	1.11	1.05	1.18	< 0.001
pT stage (ref. pT1)	4.98	1.11	22.37	0.036	4.01	1.10	14.64	0.035
Model 2								
HER4 ≥ 1 (ref. HER4 < 1)	**3.89**	**0.92**	**16.37**	**0.064**	2.38	0.71	8.00	0.161
Age	1.12	1.05	1.18	< 0.001	1.09	1.04	1.15	0.001
pT2 or higher (ref. pT1)	6.68	1.60	27.93	0.009	3.80	1.13	12.80	0.031

Significant values that refer to HER4 are shown in bold typeface
CI confidence interval, HR hazard ratio, pT tumor stage

treatment was measured in ZR-75-1 wild-type cells (6% in untreated vs. 19% in treated cells). This effect was significantly enhanced upon HER4 knockdown (9.2% in untreated vs. 47% in treated cells; p = 0.0001). The quiescent cells were not able to proceed with cycling within the period of treatment/observation and are blocked in G0/G1 of the first cycle.

Discussion

For about four decades, TAM (which binds to and antagonizes the ER) has been the mainstay of endocrine therapy in both early and advanced breast cancer patients. Although the hormone treatment has brought significant benefit to hormone receptor-positive BC patients, up to 50% of patients with advanced disease do not respond to first-line treatment but show de novo resistance. Another significant cohort of advanced BC patients in the adjuvant setting acquire resistance while treated with TAM and later on develop tumor relapse [20]. Mechanisms that contribute to or directly cause resistance to the TAM treatment are manifold [19], although receptor tyrosine kinases (e.g., HER2) are frequently involved. In order to evade TAM resistance, AIs that inhibit the endogenous synthesis of the native ER activating ligand estrogen can be administered sequentially with TAM [20] or as first-line treatment, especially for postmenopausal women. Here, we retrospectively analyzed the impact of HER4 on the course and outcome of TAM- or AI-treated patients with ER-positive BC. In addition, we evaluated the TAM treatment efficiency of ER-positive ZR-75-1 BC cells in vitro as a function of HER4 receptor expression.

We found a significant unfavorable effect of HER4 in patients treated with TAM but not in women treated with AIs. A detailed analysis of sample subcohorts further disclosed a strong and significant impact in postmenopausal but not in premenopausal patients. In vitro analyses revealed that the proliferation of markedly ER-positive ZR-75-1 cells was inhibited when exposed to

TAM. However, the treatment efficiency was significantly enhanced upon siRNA-based HER4 knockdown.

Apparently, HER4 impedes the efficiency of TAM but not AI treatments. The unfavorable impact of HER4 on the outcome of TAM- but not AI-treated patients suggests a direct interaction of HER4 with the ER. A possible explanation is the ER-stimulating activity of the intracellular HER4 domain when translocated into the tumor cell nucleus [32, 33] (Fig. 5). A nuclear localization can be explained by a two-step intramembrane proteolysis of the HER4 receptor [34]. First, a metalloproteinase called tumor necrosis factor α converting enzyme (TACE) can cleave and release the HER4 ectodomain. Second, this proteolysis can be followed by an intracellular cleavage performed by γ-secretase that releases an intracellular domain (4ICD) into inner cell compartments. Depending upon specific molecular interactions [35], the 4ICD either translocates to the nucleus or remains in the cytosol where mitochondrial accumulation has been observed. As a protein with pronounced BCL-2 homology-3, the 4ICD can interact with pro-apoptotic molecules located in the mitochondrial membrane and initiate apoptotic cell death by cytochrome-c release [33, 36]. In contrast, when transferred into the nucleus, 4ICD can work as a co-activator of the estrogen receptor and - in the presence of exogenous estrogen - contribute to enhanced (tumor) cell growth [32] and thereby possibly account for an unfavorable disease course [37, 38]. The subcellular localization might also be determined by a differential expression of intracellular isoform domains [33, 34, 38–40]. Even if only the juxtamembranous cleavable isoform JM-a (but never JM-b) is expressed in BC [28, 29, 39, 40], two different cytoplasmatic domains (i.e., CYT1 and CYT2) potentially occur also in the sample cohort of this study. Notably, CYT1 and CYT2 domains have been shown to interact with different intracellular molecules that are involved in cell compartment (cytoplasm vs. nucleus)-specific 4ICD routing [41]. In this study, we did not differentiate the two

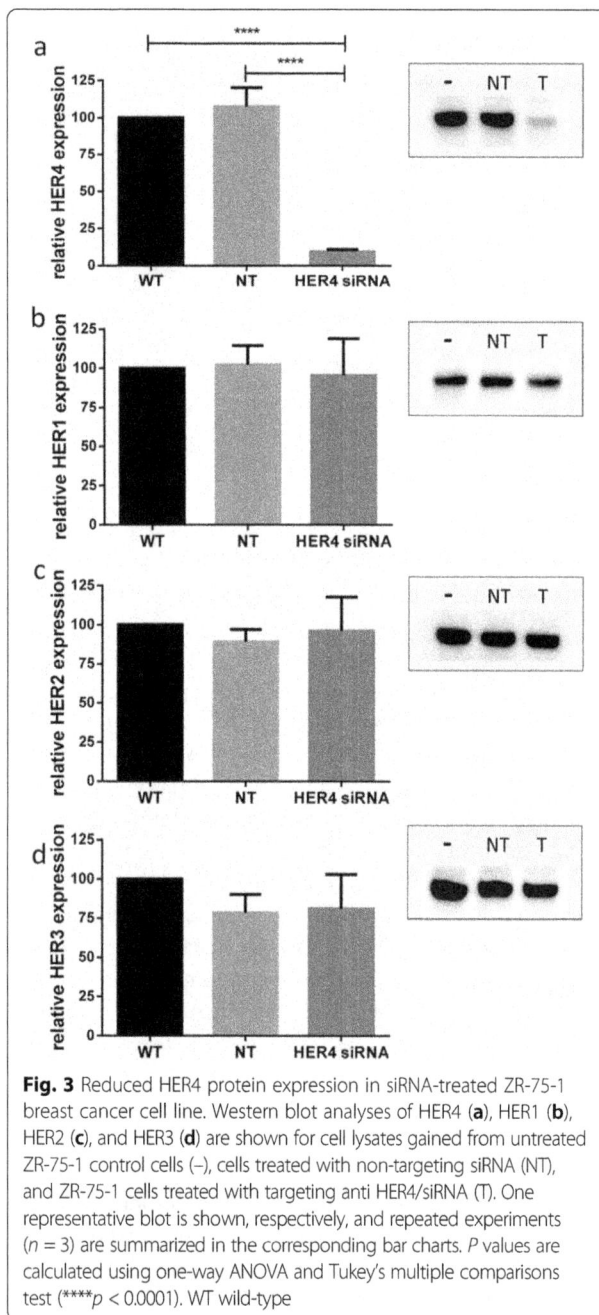

Fig. 3 Reduced HER4 protein expression in siRNA-treated ZR-75-1 breast cancer cell line. Western blot analyses of HER4 (**a**), HER1 (**b**), HER2 (**c**), and HER3 (**d**) are shown for cell lysates gained from untreated ZR-75-1 control cells (–), cells treated with non-targeting siRNA (NT), and ZR-75-1 cells treated with targeting anti HER4/siRNA (T). One representative blot is shown, respectively, and repeated experiments ($n = 3$) are summarized in the corresponding bar charts. P values are calculated using one-way ANOVA and Tukey's multiple comparisons test (****$p < 0.0001$). WT wild-type

HER4-specific intracellular domains; however, a preferred routing to the cell nucleus might have contributed to the unfavorable impact of HER4 expression on ER-positive/TAM-treated patients. The assumed mechanisms of ER action in the presence and absence of HER4/4ICD are illustrated in Fig. 5. The two-step proteolytic activation of HER4 by TACE and γ-secretase [29] causes the release of 4ICD into inner cell compartments. If translocated into the nucleus, 4ICD, as an ER co-activator, enhances the pro-proliferative effect of estrogen. Within an autoloop, 4ICD also enhances the transcription of HER4 itself. In contrast, HER4 receptor knockdown eliminates the

co-stimulatory activity of 4ICD. As a consequence, appropriately dosed TAM can competitively replace the estrogen and binds to the ER. As a result, pro-proliferative activity of the ER is inhibited.

We previously associated the presence of HER4 with an improved outcome in BC patients [21, 22]. In contrast to former studies, however, we herein explicitly explored hormone receptor (i.e., ER)-positive BCs, and HER4 might mediate different effects in different BC subtypes. Indeed, it has been experimentally shown that TAM disrupts an estrogen-driven interaction between ER and 4ICD while promoting mitochondrial accumulation of the 4ICD/BH3-only protein [36]. Accordingly, it seems plausible that a 4ICD/ER interaction impairs TAM binding and reduces treatment efficiency both in vivo and in vitro. The increased sensitivity of ZR-75-1 cells to TAM treatment on HER4 knockdown supports the assumption that the HER4/4ICD directly interferes with the TAM-ER binding. Nevertheless, other mechanisms that underlie HER4/4ICD-mediated reduced TAM efficiency cannot be excluded.

An ER/4ICD interaction would explain the reduced efficiency of TAM treatment in the presence of HER4/4ICD and the improved outcome of patients with ER$^+$/HER4^{low} tumors compared with patients who suffer from ER$^+$/HER4^{high} tumors. Moreover, it would also be compatible with the lack of impact of HER4 in AI-treated patients. Since AIs do not affect the ER function but inhibit the synthesis of the ER ligand, a direct ER/4ICD interaction would neither be affected by an administration of AIs, nor would the AI treatment efficiency be affected by the presence of HER4 (i.e., the 4ICD/ER crosstalk).

In AI-treated patients we found a trend towards an improved (rather than to an impaired) course and outcome of disease in HER4-positive patients. Notably, this trend is in reverse to the negative significant effect of HER4 in TAM-treated patients and might be explained by the absence (or reduced systemic level) of estrogen in AI-treated women. A reduced presence of ER might entail a pronounced accumulation of 4ICD in the cytoplasm where it induces a rather tumor-suppressive effect by a pro-apoptotic (i.e., favorable) activity [33, 42, 43].

Notably, stratified analyses revealed a significant impact of HER4 in ER-positive and TAM-treated BC patients for postmenopausal but not for premenopausal women. This finding might to some extent be explained by different age-related estrogen synthesis. In premenopausal women estrogens are mainly synthesized in the ovaries, whereas in postmenopausal women the final synthesis occurs in peripheral tissues such as mesenchymal cells from adipose tissue (including the breast), bones, muscle, or brain. Important for the final synthesis is aromatase which can be detected in non-malignant

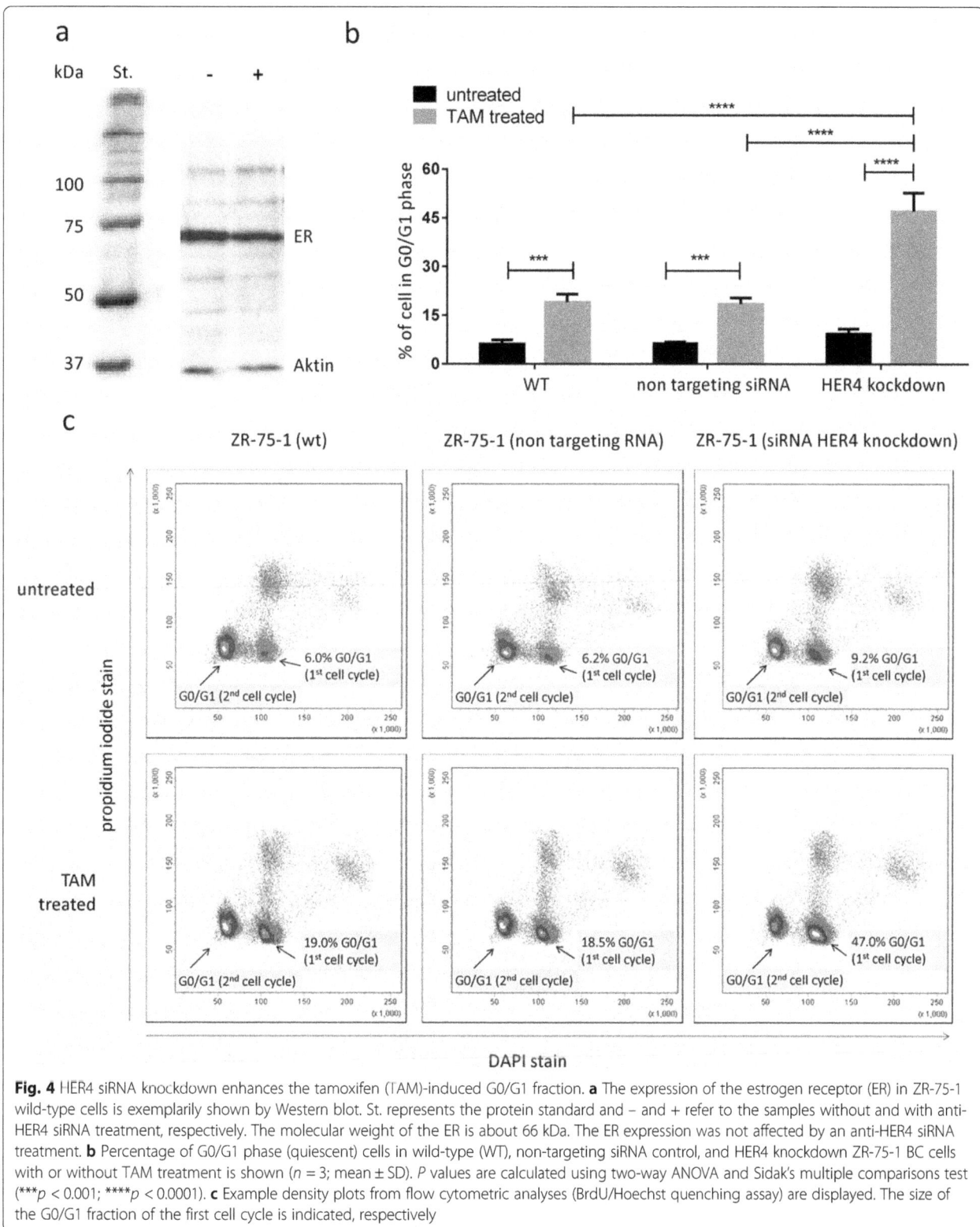

Fig. 4 HER4 siRNA knockdown enhances the tamoxifen (TAM)-induced G0/G1 fraction. **a** The expression of the estrogen receptor (ER) in ZR-75-1 wild-type cells is exemplarily shown by Western blot. St. represents the protein standard and – and + refer to the samples without and with anti-HER4 siRNA treatment, respectively. The molecular weight of the ER is about 66 kDa. The ER expression was not affected by an anti-HER4 siRNA treatment. **b** Percentage of G0/G1 phase (quiescent) cells in wild-type (WT), non-targeting siRNA control, and HER4 knockdown ZR-75-1 BC cells with or without TAM treatment is shown ($n = 3$; mean ± SD). P values are calculated using two-way ANOVA and Sidak's multiple comparisons test (***$p < 0.001$; ****$p < 0.0001$). **c** Example density plots from flow cytometric analyses (BrdU/Hoechst quenching assay) are displayed. The size of the G0/G1 fraction of the first cell cycle is indicated, respectively

adipose tissue but also in breast tumors [43]. Indeed, the estrogen level in the peripheral blood in premenopausal women is higher compared with postmenopausal women [44]. However, the tissue concentration of estrogen sulfate, sulfatase, and aromatase activities was significantly higher in postmenopausal women [45]. In addition, significantly higher estrogen concentrations could be even found in malignant versus normal tissues

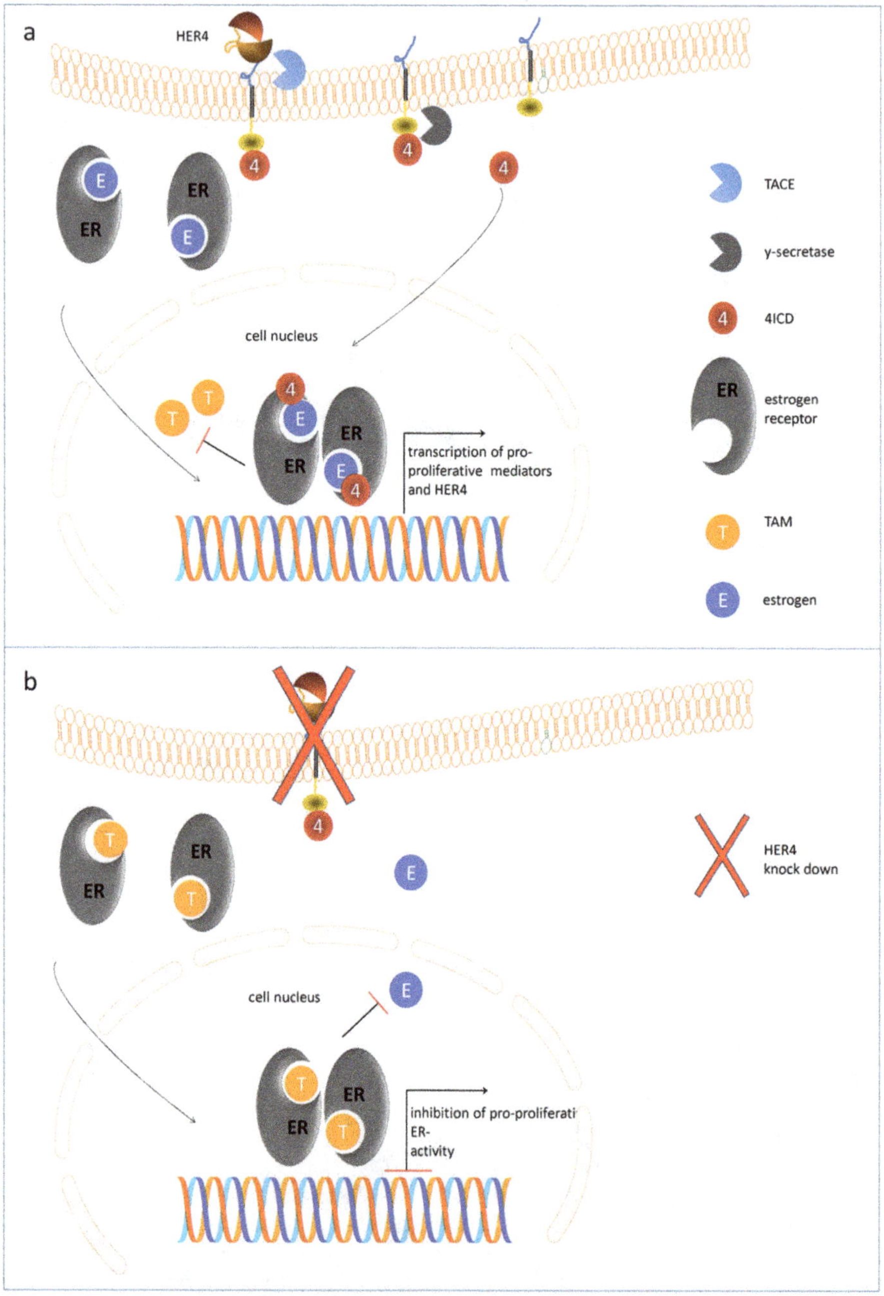

Fig. 5 Suggested mechanism of estrogen receptor (ER) action in the presence and absence of HER4. **a** HER4 can be processed by a two-step proteolytic activation. First tumor necrosis factor α converting enzyme (TACE) cleaves the extracellular domain, and subsequently y-secretase cleaves the intracellular domain of HER4 (4ICD) which is released into inner cell compartments. If translocated into the nucleus, 4ICD as an ER co-activator enhances the pro-proliferative effects of estrogen. Within an autoloop, 4ICD also enhances the transcription of HER4 itself. **b** HER4 receptor knockdown eliminates the co-stimulatory activity of 4ICD. As a consequence, appropriately dosed tamoxifen (TAM) can competitively replace the estrogen and binds to the ER. As a result, pro-proliferative activity of the ER is inhibited

[46, 47]. Moreover, the ER level affects the estradiol levels found in tissues and can cause a significant (up to 8-fold) increased estradiol level in ER-positive tumor tissue [48]. Hence, the local estrogen synthesis is increased especially in ER-positive tumors. Provided that the anti-estrogen TAM is mainly effective in the (local) presence of estradiol it appears plausible that an ER-TAM-HER4/4ICD interaction is relevant in particular in postmenopausal women. Thus, a reduced efficiency of TAM treatment in elderly BC patients becomes mainly apparent in the presence of HER4. This finding might to some extent also be due to the larger sample cohort of

HER4 expression in estrogen receptor-positive breast cancer is associated with decreased...

239

postmenopausal women compared with the number premenopausal patients.

The finding of impaired TAM treatment efficiency in the presence of HER4 might have clinical implications and might promote alternate therapeutic strategies, particularly in postmenopausal women. Analogously to ER and HER2 testing, the BC diagnostics could be extended by the evaluation of HER4 expression. If the TAM treatment efficiency is low in an ER/HER4 double-positive tumor one might preferably switch to an AI treatment. Alternatively, combined ER/HER4 receptor targeting might restore TAM sensitivity or even enhance the endocrine treatment efficiency. Anti-HER4 targeting can be performed based on different strategies. On the one hand, an HER4 JM-a type-specific anti-HER4 monoclonal antibody, called Ab1479, has been reported to block HER4 cleavage in BC cells and to suppress BC cell growth in vivo and in vitro [34, 49]. A systematic clinical trial on ER/HER4 double-positive BC could potentially result in clinical approval of Ab1479 for the treatment of this BC entity. Alternatively, pan-HER-receptor inhibitors, e.g., afatinib or neratinib, could be administered in combination with an anti-estrogen [50, 51]. By using the latter strategy not only HER4 but also the potentially expressed HER2 receptor, which is frequently involved in TAM resistance, would be targeted at the same time. After all, in addition to immunohistochemistry and in-situ hybridization, a number of quantitative and multiplexed HER1–4 analytics became available to quantify HER1–4 receptors and categorize the patients for individualized treatments [21, 52, 53]. However, all the suggested strategies require prospective clinical testing and approval in advance.

Conclusion

Here we provide evidence for the HER4 receptor as a new predictive marker for the sensitivity of ER-positive BC to TAM treatment, especially in postmenopausal patients. Dual ER/HER4 targeting might improve the treatment efficiency of hormone receptor-positive BC but needs to be prospectively evaluated in an appropriate preclinical and clinical setting.

Abbreviations

4ICD: Intracellular domain of HER4; AI: Aromatase inhibitor; BC: Breast cancer; CI: Confidence interval; CYT: Cytoplasmatic domain; DFS: Disease-free survival; ER: Estrogen receptor; HER: Human epidermal growth factor-related receptor; HR: Hazard ratio; JM: Juxtamembrane; OS: Overall survival; TACE: Tumor necrosis factor a converting enzyme; TAM: Tamoxifen; WT: Wild-type

Acknowledgements

We thank Dr. Florian Weber (Institute of Pathology, University of Regensburg, Germany) for the careful and professional inspection of the histological BC specimens. We would like to thank Prof. Christoph Klein (Dept. of Experimental Medicine and Therapy Research, University of Regensburg) for providing access to the LC480 technology. The authors are also grateful to Gerhard Piendl and Veruschka Albert (both Department of Gynecology, University of Regensburg) who supported the project with their perfect technical assistance.

Funding

This work has been funded by the German research foundation (Deutsche Forschungsgemeinschaft), project number BR1873/9–1.

Authors' contributions

AKW provided analysis of the ex-vivo and in vitro data, and was a co-author of the manuscript. DC performed the in vitro experiments. SB co-authored the manuscript. FZ provided statistical analyses. MKS provided documentation and processing of clinicopathological data. SDD assisted vitally in the in vitro experiments. OO co-authored the manuscript. GB provided study design and supervision, wrote the manuscript, and was principle investigator. All authors read and approved the final manuscript.

Competing interests

The authors declare that they have no competing interests.

Author details

[1]Clinic of Gynecology and Obstetrics, University Medical Center Regensburg, Regensburg, Germany. [2]Department of Nephrology, University Hospital Regensburg, Regensburg, Germany. [3]Tumor Center Regensburg, University of Regensburg, Regensburg, Germany. [4]Center for Clinical Studies, University Hospital Regensburg, Regensburg, Germany.

References

1. Jordan VC. Tamoxifen as the first targeted long-term adjuvant therapy for breast cancer. Endocr Relat Cancer. 2014;21:R235–46.
2. Lippman ME, Bolan G. Oestrogen-responsive human breast cancer in long term tissue culture. Nature. 1975;256:592–3.
3. Remmele W, Stegner HE. Vorschlag zur einheitlichen Definition eines Immunreaktiven Score (IRS) für den immunhistochemischen Ostrogenrezeptor-Nachweis (ER-ICA) im Mammakarzinomgewebe. Pathologe. 1987;8:138–40.
4. Burstein HJ, Temin S, Anderson H, Buchholz TA, Davidson NE, Gelmon KE, Giordano SH, Hudis CA, Rowden D, Solky AJ, Stearns V, Winer EP, Griggs JJ. Adjuvant endocrine therapy for women with hormone receptor-positive breast cancer: American Society of Clinical Oncology clinical practice guideline focused update. J Clin Oncol. 2014;32:2255–69.
5. Thomssen C, Augustin D, Ettl J, Haidinger R, Lück H-J, Lüftner D, Marmé F, Marschner N, Müller L, Overkamp F, Ruckhäberle E, Thill M, Untch M, Wuerstlein R, Harbeck N. ABC3 Consensus: assessment by a German group of experts. Breast Care (Basel, Switzerland). 2016;11:61–70.
6. Allred DC, Anderson SJ, Paik S, Wickerham DL, Nagtegaal ID, Swain SM, Mamounas EP, Julian TB, Geyer CE, Costantino JP, Land SR, Wolmark N. Adjuvant tamoxifen reduces subsequent breast cancer in women with estrogen receptor-positive ductal carcinoma in situ: a study based on NSABP protocol B-24. J Clin Oncol. 2012;30:1268–73.
7. Bartlett JMS, Brookes CL, Robson T, van de Velde CJH, Billingham LJ, Campbell FM, Grant M, Hasenburg A, Hille ETM, Kay C, Kieback DG, Putter H, Markopoulos C, Kranenbarg EM-K, Mallon EA, Dirix L, Seynaeve C, Rea D. Estrogen receptor and progesterone receptor as predictive biomarkers of response to endocrine therapy: a prospectively powered pathology study in the Tamoxifen and Exemestane Adjuvant Multinational trial. J Clin Oncol. 2011;29:1531–8.

8.   Viedma-Rodríguez R, Baiza-Gutman L, Salamanca-Gómez F, Diaz-Zaragoza M, Martínez-Hernández G, Ruiz Esparza-Garrido R, Velázquez-Flores MA, Arenas-Aranda D. Mechanisms associated with resistance to tamoxifen in estrogen receptor-positive breast cancer (review). Oncol Rep. 2014;32:3–15.

9.   Peddi PF. Hormone receptor positive breast cancer: state of the art. Curr Opin Obstet Gynecol. 2018;30:51–4.

10. Tremont A, Lu J, Cole JT. Endocrine therapy for early breast cancer: updated review. Ochsner J. 2017;17:405–11.

11. Alqaisi A, Chen L, Romond E, Chambers M, Stevens M, Pasley G, Awasthi M, Massarweh S. Impact of estrogen receptor (ER) and human epidermal growth factor receptor-2 (HER2) co-expression on breast cancer disease characteristics: implications for tumor biology and research. Breast Cancer Res Treat. 2014;148:437–44.

12. Giuliano M, Trivedi MV, Schiff R. Bidirectional crosstalk between the estrogen receptor and human epidermal growth factor receptor 2 signaling pathways in breast cancer: molecular basis and clinical implications. Breast Care (Basel, Switzerland). 2013;8:256–62.

13. Osborne CK, Schiff R. Growth factor receptor cross-talk with estrogen receptor as a mechanism for tamoxifen resistance in breast cancer. Breast (Edinburgh, Scotland). 2003;12:362–7.

14. Schiff R, Massarweh SA, Shou J, Bharwani L, Mohsin SK, Osborne CK. Cross-talk between estrogen receptor and growth factor pathways as a molecular target for overcoming endocrine resistance. Clin Cancer Res. 2004;10:331S–6S.

15. Shou J, Massarweh S, Osborne CK, Wakeling AE, Ali S, Weiss H, Schiff R. Mechanisms of tamoxifen resistance: increased estrogen receptor-HER2/neu cross-talk in ER/HER2-positive breast cancer. JNCI J Natl Cancer Inst. 2004;96:926–35.

16. Arpino G, Wiechmann L, Osborne CK, Schiff R. Crosstalk between the estrogen receptor and the HER tyrosine kinase receptor family: molecular mechanism and clinical implications for endocrine therapy resistance. Endocr Rev. 2008;29:217–33.

17. Osborne CK, Schiff R. Mechanisms of endocrine resistance in breast cancer. Annu Rev Med. 2011;62:233–47.

18. Mehta A, Tripathy D. Co-targeting estrogen receptor and HER2 pathways in breast cancer. Breast (Edinburgh, Scotland). 2014;23:2–9.

19. Clarke R, Tyson JJ, Dixon JM. Endocrine resistance in breast cancer—an overview and update. Mol Cell Endocrinol. 2015;418(Pt 3):220–34.

20. Brufsky AM. Long-term management of patients with hormone receptor-positive metastatic breast cancer: concepts for sequential and combination endocrine-based therapies. Cancer Treat Rev. 2017;59:22–32.

21. Sassen A, Rochon J, Wild P, Hartmann A, Hofstaedter F, Schwarz S, Brockhoff G. Cytogenetic analysis of HER1/EGFR, HER2, HER3 and HER4 in 278 breast cancer patients. Breast Cancer Res. 2008;10:R2.

22. Sassen A, Diermeier-Daucher S, Sieben M, Ortmann O, Hofstaedter F, Schwarz S, Brockhoff G. Presence of HER4 associates with increased sensitivity to herceptin in patients with metastatic breast cancer. Breast Cancer Res. 2009;11:R50.

23. Machleidt A, Buchholz S, Diermeier-Daucher S, Zeman F, Ortmann O, Brockhoff G. The prognostic value of Her4 receptor isoform expression in triple-negative and Her2 positive breast cancer patients. BMC Cancer. 2013;13:437.

24. Lodge AJ, Anderson JJ, Gullick WJ, Haugk B, Leonard RCF, Angus B. Type 1 growth factor receptor expression in node positive breast cancer: adverse prognostic significance of c-erbB-4. J Clin Pathol. 2003;56:300–4.

25. Portier BP, Minca EC, Wang Z, Lanigan C, Gruver AM, Downs-Kelly E, Budd GT, Tubbs RR. HER4 expression status correlates with improved outcome in both neoadjuvant and adjuvant trastuzumab treated invasive breast carcinoma. Oncotarget. 2013;4:1662–72.

26. Canfield K, Li J, Wilkins OM, Morrison MM, Ung M, Wells W, Williams CR, Liby KT, Vullhorst D, Buonanno A, Hu H, Schiff R, Cook RS, Kurokawa M. Receptor tyrosine kinase ERBB4 mediates acquired resistance to ERBB2 inhibitors in breast cancer cells. Cell Cycle (Georgetown, Tex). 2015;14:648–55.

27. Brockhoff G, Seitz S, Weber F, Zeman F, Klinkhammer-Schalke M, Ortmann O, Wege AK. The presence of PD-1 positive tumor infiltrating lymphocytes in triple negative breast cancers is associated with a favorable outcome of disease. Oncotarget. 2018;9:6201–12.

28. Junttila TT, Sundvall M, Määttä JA, Elenius K. Erbb4 and its isoforms: selective regulation of growth factor responses by naturally occurring receptor variants. Trends Cardiovasc Med. 2000;10:304–10.

29. Junttila TT, Sundvall M, Lundin M, Lundin J, Tanner M, Härkönen P, Joensuu H, Isola J, Elenius K. Cleavable ErbB4 isoform in estrogen receptor-regulated growth of breast cancer cells. Cancer Res. 2005;65:1384–93.

30. Brockhoff G, Heckel B, Schmidt-Bruecken E, Plander M, Hofstaedter F, Vollmann A, Diermeier S. Differential impact of cetuximab, pertuzumab and trastuzumab on BT474 and SK-BR-3 breast cancer cell proliferation. Cell Prolif. 2007;40:488–507.

31. Diermeier-Daucher S, Breindl S, Buchholz S, Ortmann O, Brockhoff G. Modular anti-EGFR and anti-Her2 targeting of SK-BR-3 and BT474 breast cancer cell lines in the presence of ErbB receptor-specific growth factors. Cytometry A. 2011;79:684–93.

32. Rokicki J, Das PM, Giltnane JM, Wansbury O, Rimm DL, Howard BA, Jones FE. The ERalpha coactivator, HER4/4ICD, regulates progesterone receptor expression in normal and malignant breast epithelium. Mol Cancer. 2010;9:150.

33. Jones FE. HER4 intracellular domain (4ICD) activity in the developing mammary gland and breast cancer. J Mammary Gland Biol Neoplasia. 2008;13:247–58.

34. Hollmén M, Liu P, Kurppa K, Wildiers H, Reinvall I, Vandorpe T, Smeets A, Deraedt K, Vahlberg T, Joensuu H, Leahy DJ, Schöffski P, Elenius K. Proteolytic processing of ErbB4 in breast cancer. PLoS One. 2012;7:e39413.

35. Komuro A, Nagai M, Navin NE, Sudol M. WW domain-containing protein YAP associates with ErbB-4 and acts as a co-transcriptional activator for the carboxyl-terminal fragment of ErbB-4 that translocates to the nucleus. J Biol Chem. 2003;278:33334–41.

36. Naresh A, Thor AD, Edgerton SM, Torkko KC, Kumar R, Jones FE. The HER4/4ICD estrogen receptor coactivator and BH3-only protein is an effector of tamoxifen-induced apoptosis. Cancer Res. 2008;68:6387–95.

37. Mohd Nafi SN, Generali D, Kramer-Marek G, Gijsen M, Strina C, Cappelletti M, Andreis D, Haider S, Li J-L, Bridges E, Capala J, Ioannis R, Harris AL, Kong A. Nuclear HER4 mediates acquired resistance to trastuzumab and is associated with poor outcome in HER2 positive breast cancer. Oncotarget. 2014;5:5934–49.

38. Thor AD, Edgerton SM, Jones FE. Subcellular localization of the HER4 intracellular domain, 4ICD, identifies distinct prognostic outcomes for breast cancer patients. Am J Pathol. 2009;175:1802–9.

39. Muraoka Cook RS, Sandahl MA, Strunk KE, Miraglia LC, Husted C, Hunter DM, Elenius K, Chodosh LA, Earp HS. ErbB4 splice variants Cyt1 and Cyt2 differ by 16 amino acids and exert opposing effects on the mammary epithelium in vivo. Mol Cell Biol. 2009;29:4935–48.

40. Elenius K, Corfas G, Paul S, Choi CJ, Rio C, Plowman GD, Klagsbrun M. A novel juxtamembrane domain isoform of HER4/ErbB4. Isoform-specific tissue distribution and differential processing in response to phorbol ester. J Biol Chem. 1997;272:26761–8.

41. Veikkolainen V, Vaparanta K, Halkilahti K, Iljin K, Sundvall M, Elenius K. Function of ERBB4 is determined by alternative splicing. Cell Cycle (Georgetown, Tex.). 2011;10:2647–57.

42. Guler G, Iliopoulos D, Guler N, Himmetoglu C, Hayran M, Huebner K. Wwox and Ap2gamma expression levels predict tamoxifen response. Clin Cancer Res. 2007;13:6115–21.

43. Miller WR. Aromatase and the breast: regulation and clinical aspects. Maturitas. 2006;54:335–41.

44. Shimizu H, Ross RK, Bernstein L, Pike MC, Henderson BE. Serum oestrogen levels in postmenopausal women: comparison of American whites and Japanese in Japan. Br J Cancer. 1990;62:451–3.

45. Pasqualini JR, Chetrite G, Blacker C, Feinstein MC, Delalonde L, Talbi M, Maloche C. Concentrations of estrone, estradiol, and estrone sulfate and evaluation of sulfatase and aromatase activities in pre- and postmenopausal breast cancer patients. J Clin Endocrinol Metab. 1996;81:1460–4.

46. van Landeghem AA, Poortman J, Nabuurs M, Thijssen JH. Endogenous concentration and subcellular distribution of estrogens in normal and malignant human breast tissue. Cancer Res. 1985;45:2900–6.

47. Blankenstein MA, Maitimu-Smeele I, Donker GH, Daroszewski J, Milewicz A, Thijssen JH. On the significance of in situ production of oestrogens in human breast cancer tissue. J Steroid Biochem Mol Biol. 1992;41:891–6.

48. Lønning PE, Helle H, Duong NK, Ekse D, Aas T, Geisler J. Tissue estradiol is selectively elevated in receptor positive breast cancers while tumour estrone is reduced independent of receptor status. J Steroid Biochem Mol Biol. 2009;117:31–41.

49. Hollmén M, Määttä JA, Bald L, Sliwkowski MX, Elenius K. Suppression of breast cancer cell growth by a monoclonal antibody targeting cleavable ErbB4 isoforms. Oncogene. 2009;28:1309–19.

50. Yoshioka T, Shien K, Namba K, Torigoe H, Sato H, Tomida S, Yamamoto H, Asano H, Soh J, Tsukuda K, Nagasaka T, Fujiwara T, Toyooka S. Antitumor activity of pan-HER inhibitors in HER2-positive gastric cancer. Cancer Sci. 2018. https://doi.org/10.1111/cas.13546 .

51. Zhang X, Munster PN. New protein kinase inhibitors in breast cancer:
     afatinib and neratinib. Expert Opin Pharmacother. 2014;15:1277–88.
52. Vollmann-Zwerenz A, Diermeier-Daucher S, Wege AK, Sassen A, Schmidt-
     Brücken E, Hofstaedter F, Ortmann O, Nauwelaers F, Brockhoff G.
     Multichromatic phenotyping of HER receptor coexpression in breast tumor
     tissue samples using flow cytometry—possibilities and limitations.
     Cytometry A. 2010;77:387–98.
53. Nuciforo P, Radosevic-Robin N, Ng T, Scaltriti M. Quantification of HER family
     receptors in breast cancer. Breast Cancer Res. 2015;17:53.

19

Age-specific breast cancer risk by body mass index and familial risk: prospective family study cohort (ProF-SC)

John L. Hopper[1]*[iD], Gillian S. Dite[1], Robert J. MacInnis[1,2], Yuyan Liao[3], Nur Zeinomar[3], Julia A. Knight[4,5], Melissa C. Southey[6,21], Roger L. Milne[1,2], Wendy K. Chung[7,8], Graham G. Giles[1,2], Jeanine M. Genkinger[3], Sue-Anne McLachlan[9,10], Michael L. Friedlander[11,12], Antonis C. Antoniou[13], Prue C. Weideman[1], Gord Glendon[4], Stephanie Nesci[14], kConFab Investigators[15,16], Irene L. Andrulis[4,17], Saundra S. Buys[18], Mary B. Daly[19], Esther M. John[20], Kelly Anne Phillips[1,14,15] and Mary Beth Terry[3,7*]

Abstract

Background: The association between body mass index (BMI) and risk of breast cancer depends on time of life, but it is unknown whether this association depends on a woman's familial risk.

Methods: We conducted a prospective study of a cohort enriched for familial risk consisting of 16,035 women from 6701 families in the Breast Cancer Family Registry and the Kathleen Cunningham Foundation Consortium for Research into Familial Breast Cancer followed for up to 20 years (mean 10.5 years). There were 896 incident breast cancers (mean age at diagnosis 55.7 years). We used Cox regression to model BMI risk associations as a function of menopausal status, age, and underlying familial risk based on pedigree data using the Breast and Ovarian Analysis of Disease Incidence and Carrier Estimation Algorithm (BOADICEA), all measured at baseline.

Results: The strength and direction of the BMI risk association depended on baseline menopausal status ($P < 0.001$); after adjusting for menopausal status, the association did not depend on age at baseline ($P = 0.6$). In terms of absolute risk, the negative association with BMI for premenopausal women has a much smaller influence than the positive association with BMI for postmenopausal women. Women at higher familial risk have a much larger difference in absolute risk depending on their BMI than women at lower familial risk.

Conclusions: The greater a woman's familial risk, the greater the influence of BMI on her absolute postmenopausal breast cancer risk. Given that age-adjusted BMI is correlated across adulthood, maintaining a healthy weight throughout adult life is particularly important for women with a family history of breast cancer.

Keywords: Breast cancer, Body mass index, Familial risk, Breast and Ovarian Analysis of Disease Incidence and Carrier Estimation Algorithm, Gene–environment interaction

---

* Correspondence: j.hopper@unimelb.edu.au; mt146@cumc.columbia.edu
[1]Centre for Epidemiology and Biostatistics, The University of Melbourne, Parkville, VIC, Australia
[3]Department of Epidemiology, Mailman School of Public Health, Columbia University, 722 W 168th St, 7th Floor, New York, NY, USA
Full list of author information is available at the end of the article

Background

Body mass index (BMI) is an intriguing risk factor for breast cancer because its association with the disease depends on time of life. Greater BMI has been found to be associated with an increased risk for postmenopausal women [1–9], while for premenopausal women, young women, and even adolescent girls [2, 4, 6, 8, 10–14], greater BMI has been found to be associated with a decreased risk. These findings have been consistent across different racial and ethnic subgroups [2, 14, 15] and across both case–control and cohort designs globally [1–4, 6–13], suggesting they are not a consequence of systematic biases [9].

BMI is an important risk factor because it is potentially modifiable. The fact that greater BMI appears to be protective at young ages, yet has the opposite association in later life, presents a potential problem for simple cancer control messaging; therefore, its consequences need to be quantified. A prospective study and a case-control study have found that the increased risk associated with higher BMI increases with time after menopause but is not evident until 10 years post menopause [16, 17].

A better understanding of how the BMI-associated risk varies with age and menopausal status is needed. It is interesting that, from genome-wide association studies, genetic risk scores based on single-nucleotide polymorphisms (SNPs) that predict higher BMI in childhood or adulthood are associated with lower risk of both premenopausal and postmenopausal breast cancer [18, 19]. Under the assumptions of Mendelian randomization, the authors concluded that these relationships were causal (even though those SNPs explained only a small proportion of the variation in BMI), thus lending additional support to the evidence that the effect of BMI varies by time of life.

Family history is another important risk factor for breast cancer that could not exist without there being a very strong gradient in underlying familial risk. To explain an overall average estimate of a 2-fold increased risk associated with having an affected first-degree relative, there must be at least a 20-fold inter-quartile risk ratio across the underlying familial causes [20]. This gives reason to consider family history not solely as a binary construct but rather as an underlying continuous measure that reflects this large gradient. Underlying familial risk can be predicted from family history using risk models that use pedigree information including age of onset of affected relatives. It is becoming increasingly possible to better differentiate women according to underlying genetic risk using SNP-based scores [21, 22]. Familial risk prediction is likely to improve with larger genome-wide association studies and the use of more informative statistical methods to create better SNP-based and family-history-based risk scores.

With the advent of gene panel testing for high-risk mutations in known breast cancer susceptibility genes [23–25], family cancer clinics will screen increasing numbers of women with a family history of breast cancer. The vast majority of these women will, however, not be found to carry a mutation that can currently be classified as deleterious. Therefore, a key clinical issue is risk management advice for women at familial risk who are found not to carry high-risk mutations. To resolve this issue, it is essential to know if their breast cancer risk factors are the same, and if the risk associations are of the same magnitude, as they are for women in the general population.

This issue of multiplicative and additive interaction with familial risk must be considered for each risk factor. If there is no difference in strength of associations by familial risk and the study is well-powered, advice on that risk factor's relevance can be confidently given to women across the full spectrum of familial risk. In theory, if there are no interactions between risk factors on the multiplicative scale then there will be additive interactions [26, 27]. Knowledge of the extent of disease association by familial risk will enable prevention and screening measures to be appropriately offered to women.

To address the issues of whether breast cancer risk associated with BMI depends on the age of a woman, her menopausal status, and her underlying familial risk, we conducted a prospective study of women across broad ranges of age and familial risk at baseline.

Methods

The Breast Cancer Prospective Family Study Cohort (ProF-SC) comprises baseline and follow-up data from the Breast Cancer Family Registry (BCFR) and the Kathleen Cuningham Foundation Consortium for Research into Familial Breast Cancer (kConFab) (for full details see [28]). These prospective family cohorts are enriched for familial risk of breast cancer and have accumulated up to 20 years of follow up. The BCFR is a collaboration of six breast cancer family studies from the USA, Canada and Australia, and the protocols and data collection have previously been reported for the baseline studies [29] and the follow-up studies [28]. kConFab is an Australian and New Zealand breast cancer family study, and details of the core resource [30] and follow-up study [28, 31] have been previously reported. Ethics approval for the six sites of the BCFR and for kConFab was granted by the applicable human research ethics committees at the participating institutions. All participants in the BCFR and kConFab provided written informed consent before participation.

Recruitment and follow up

Probands and their family members were recruited to the BCFR and kConFab according to site-specific protocols

[28–30, 32]. At a minimum, first-degree female relatives of the probands were recruited, and at some sites second-degree and more distant female relatives of the probands were also recruited. In the BCFR, most of the families were recruited from 1996 to 2000, with some sites recruiting new families after that time; all sites continued to recruit additional participants within these families on an ongoing basis as relatives decided to join or attained the minimum eligibility age of 18 years. Australian families recruited to an earlier study from 1992 to 1995 [33, 34] were also included, while the North American sites extended the recruitment of specific subgroups from 2001 to 2011 (minorities in Philadelphia, New York, Ontario, and Northern California; *BRCA1* and *BRCA2* mutation carriers in Utah; Ashkenazim in Ontario). For kConFab, participants were recruited continuously from 1997 onwards.

For the BCFR, systematic follow ups were conducted 10 years and 15 years after the first round of recruitment to the BCFR, while the kConFab participants have been followed up every 3 years. At follow-up, the risk factor and cancer family history questionnaires were updated and participants were asked to provide the date of death of any deceased relatives.

Baseline questionnaires

The BCFR and kConFab used the same risk factor questionnaire [28]. At baseline, questionnaires were interviewer administered, either in person or by telephone, or administered by mail. The risk factor questionnaire asked about each participant's demographic characteristics, height, weight, history of benign breast disease, breast and ovarian surgeries, reproductive history, and lifestyle factors. The cancer family history questionnaire asked about breast and other cancers (excluding non-melanoma skin cancer) in the participants and their first-degree and second-degree relatives. Each participant's cancer information was obtained from one or more sources and was usually self-reported or reported by a first-degree relative. Where possible, verification of cancer diagnosis was sought through pathologist review of tissue samples, pathology reports, cancer registries, medical records, or death certificates [28–30].

Statistical methods

We studied women who were initially unaffected by invasive breast cancer or ductal carcinoma in situ of the breast up until 3 months following completion of their baseline questionnaires. To be eligible, women also had to be aged 18 to 79 years at baseline, have at least 2 months of follow up (either by completing a questionnaire before 30 June 2011 or having a family member update their cancer and vital status), and not have had a bilateral risk-reducing mastectomy at baseline. For these analyses, we excluded 331 women for whom we did not

have complete data for BMI, 1220 women for whom we were unable to determine menopausal status, and 42 women for whom we did not have complete data for both BMI and menopausal status. From the original cohort of 17,628 women, this left 16,035 (91.0%) available for analysis.

Baseline BMI was calculated as current weight (kg) divided by squared height (m) using information captured by the baseline risk factor questionnaire. We used log-transformed BMI in analyses. Baseline menopausal status was determined from questions asking about time since last menstrual period and reason for cessation of menstruation. For each participant, the 1-year risk of invasive breast cancer and the lifetime risk (risk to age 80 years from birth) were calculated using the Breast and Ovarian Analysis of Disease Incidence and Carrier Estimation Algorithm (BOADICEA) version 3 using pedigree information at baseline. This algorithm uses information on breast, ovarian, and male breast cancer and age at diagnosis for first, second, and third-degree relatives, along with date of birth, vital status, age at interview or death, and country-specific age-specific incidences [35, 36] to calculate risk. Where available, information on *BRCA1* and *BRCA2* mutation testing was also used to calculate risk. Mutations were protein-truncating or missense mutations classified as deleterious by the Breast Cancer Information Core [37]. Details of testing are given elsewhere [38]. Sensitivity of the mutation detection technique was assumed to equal 70% and 80% for *BRCA1* and *BRCA2*, respectively.

Time in the study began 2 months after the age of completion of the baseline questionnaire and ended at whichever came first of the following: age last known to be alive, diagnosis of invasive or in situ breast cancer, bilateral risk-reducing mastectomy, age 80 years, or age at death. We conducted sensitivity analyses by including only invasive breast cancers and by excluding the 652 *BRCA1* and 519 *BRCA2* mutation carriers. We also conducted sensitivity analyses by including women with missing menopausal status and including a parameter for this group.

To investigate whether the hazard ratios (HRs) for the associations between risk of breast cancer and BMI differed by the underlying familial risk, we used Cox proportional hazard models with age as the time axis and stratified by study site and birth cohort in 10-year groups. Familial risk was defined as the log 1-year incidence of breast cancer predicted by BOADICEA adjusted for age and birth cohort. We fitted interaction terms between risk factors and familial risk.

Statistical inference was made under maximum likelihood theory, including consideration of the changes in log likelihood between nested models compared with appropriate chi-squared (χ^2) distributions (likelihood ratio criterion). We considered many reproductive and other factors (e.g. ever use of hormonal contraceptives, number of live births, ever use of hormone replacement therapy, benign breast disease, ever smoked, ever consumed alcohol, race/ethnicity, and highest education level) as potential confounders and retained only those that were nominally statistically significant. Analyses were therefore adjusted for history of benign breast disease, race/ethnicity

and education. Because the cohort included families with multiple members, robust estimates of confidence intervals (CI) were calculated accounting for clustering by family. Tests of the proportional hazards assumption were based on Schoenfeld residuals. From the test for proportional hazards, we found evidence for non-proportionality

Table 1 Baseline characteristics of study cohort and unadjusted hazard ratios (HRs) and 95% confidence intervals (CIs) from Cox proportional hazards analysis

	Unaffected		Affected		HR	95% CI	P
	Number	Percentage	Number	Percentage			
Age at baseline, years							
18–29	2407	15.9	49	5.5	1.00	(referent)	
30–39	3087	20.4	182	20.3	1.34	0.81, 2.20	0.3
40–49	3189	21.1	231	25.8	1.18	0.65, 2.14	0.6
50–59	2869	19.0	232	25.9	1.20	0.60, 2.40	0.6
60–69	2179	14.4	166	18.5	0.98	0.46, 2.11	1.0
70–79	1408	9.3	36	4.0	0.53	0.20, 1.38	0.2
1-year BOADICEA, %							
Q1: 0–0.13	4010	26.5	84	9.4	1.00	(referent)	
Q2: 0.14–0.34	3167	23.9	188	21.0	2.14	1.51, 3.04	< 0.001
Q3: 0.35–0.53	3672	24.3	241	26.9	3.41	2.38, 4.89	< 0.001
Q4: 0.54–7.94	3840	25.4	383	42.8	5.20	3.65, 7.42	< 0.001
Body mass index, kg/m^2							
Q1: 14.69–21.86	3811	25.2	194	21.7	1.00	(referent)	
Q2: 21.87–24.60	3766	24.9	227	25.3	1.07	0.89, 1.30	0.5
Q3: 24.61–28.56	3771	24.9	252	28.1	1.17	0.96, 1.41	0.1
Q4: 28.57–58.86	3791	25.0	223	24.9	1.05	0.87, 1.28	0.6
History of benign breast disease							
No	10,953	72.4	551	61.5	1.00	(referent)	
Yes	3878	25.6	323	36.1	1.33	1.15, 1.54	< 0.001
Menopausal status							
Premenopausal	8669	57.3	467	52.1	1.00	(referent)	
Postmenopausal	6470	42.7	429	47.9	1.02	0.81, 1.29	0.8
Race/ethnicity							
Non-Hispanic white	11,969	79.1	750	83.7	1.00	(referent)	
Black	726	4.8	29	3.2	0.60	0.40, 0.89	0.01
Hispanic	1310	8.7	52	5.8	0.74	0.53, 1.04	0.08
Asian	574	3.8	39	4.4	0.87	0.60, 1.26	0.5
Other	417	2.8	17	1.9	0.72	0.45, 1.15	0.2
Missing	143	0.9	9	1.0			
Education, highest completed							
High school or general education development	5031	33.2	260	29.0	1.00	(referent)	
Vocational, technical, or some college or university	5709	37.7	319	35.6	1.15	0.97, 1.37	0.1
Bachelor or graduate degree	4341	28.7	313	34.9	1.42	1.18, 1.70	< 0.001
Missing	58	0.4	4	0.5			

HRs are unadjusted but stratified by birth cohort (10-year groups) and study site; to account for clustering by family, robust 95% CIs are reported
Q1–Q4 quartiles 1–4

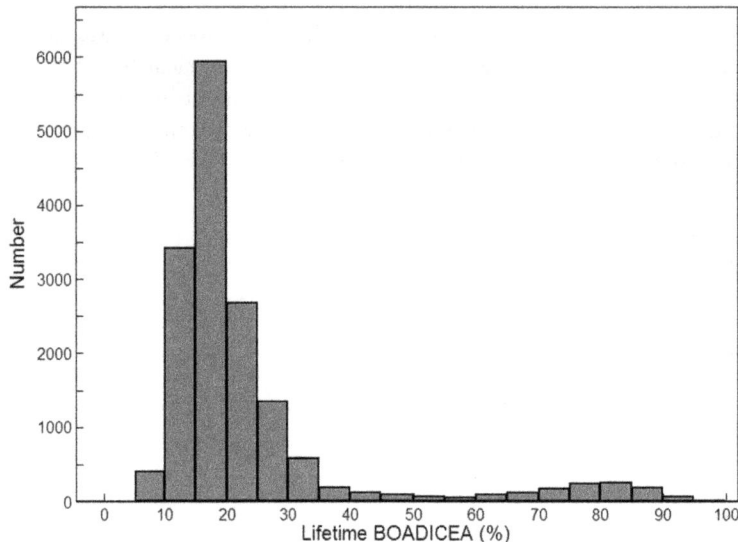

Fig. 1 Distribution of lifetime risk from birth to age 80 years (as a percent) predicted from baseline pedigree data using the Breast and Ovarian Analysis of Disease Incidence and Carrier Estimation Algorithm (BOADICEA) for the cohort

only for study site. We therefore stratified all analyses by study site and there was no longer any evidence of non-proportionality. Stata version 14 [39] was used for all statistical analyses.

We plotted the predicted age-specific absolute cumulative risk for women with different BMIs and different familial risks based on BOADICEA and underlying age-specific incidences from the Surveillance, Epidemiology, and End Results Program [40–43]. We chose three scenarios of familial risk: 12% (population average), 20% and 30%, and four scenarios of BMI (20, 25,

30 and 35 kg/m²). All statistical tests were two sided, and P values < 0.05 were considered nominally statistically significant.

Results

For the 16,035 women from 6701 families (mean 2.4 participants per family; standard deviation (SD) = 2.4; median = 2; range = 1–75), the mean age at enrollment was 47.3 years (SD = 15.4; median = 46.6; range = 18.0–79.8) and the mean duration of follow up was 10.5 years (SD = 4.7). There were 896 reported incident breast cancers

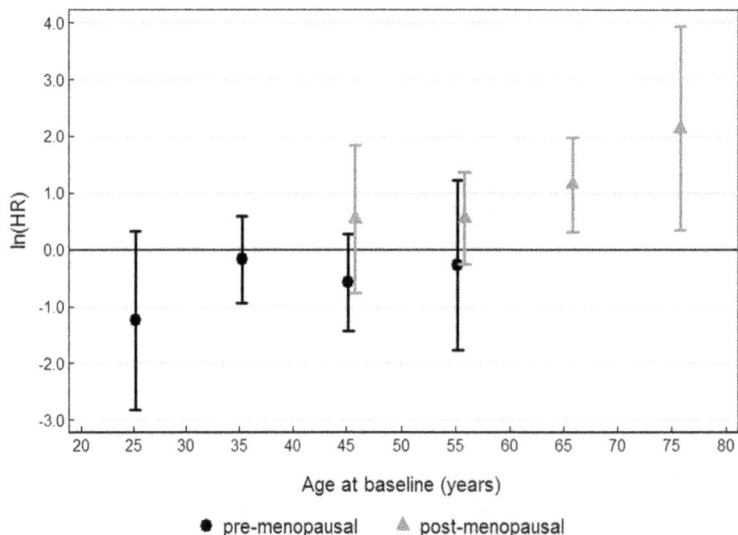

Fig. 2 Estimated log hazard ratio, ln(HR), for log body mass index (per 5 kg/m²) for premenopausal and postmenopausal women as a function of age at baseline (in 10-year groups)

(mean age at diagnosis 55.7 years, SD = 12.6). Details of the participants from the seven study sites are given in Table 1.

Figure 1 shows the distribution of predicted lifetime breast cancer risk based on BOADICEA. The second peak starting at 60% lifetime risk is almost entirely due to identified *BRCA1* and *BRCA2* mutation carriers.

Figure 2 shows that the HR estimates for the association between greater BMI and breast cancer risk change from all being negative to all being positive when moving from age at baseline < 40 years to age > 60 years. The same changes in risk occur in moving from pre- to postmenopausal status.

The results from multivariable Cox models are shown in Tables 2 and 3. In Table 2, we show that the strength and direction of the BMI risk association depended on age at baseline (model II, HR = 1.05, $P = 0.002$) and on menopausal status (model III, HR = 3.68, $P < 0.001$) at baseline. When we modeled both together, the most important factor was baseline menopausal status because once this had been taken into account (HR = 2.91, $P = 0.07$), the BMI risk association with age at baseline (HR = 1.01, $P = 0.6$) was no longer significant. Comparison of log likelihoods from model IV versus model III shows that there was no evidence for an interaction between age at baseline and menopausal status ($\chi_1^2 = 0.01$). A subsequent analysis found that there was also no evidence for an association with age at baseline for postmenopausal women (HR = 1.00, $P = 1.0$). Therefore, the best-fitting model for the BMI association included an interaction term between BMI and menopausal status only (model III).

Table 3 shows the model fits after taking familial risk into account. The most parsimonious best fitting model was model V, which shows that after the BMI association was fitted as a function of menopausal status (HR = 3.36, $P < 0.001$), there was evidence of an association with familial risk (as represented by the log 1-year BOADICEA estimate in model V; HR = 2.05, $P < 0.001$). The other models show that there was no evidence for an interaction of 1-year BOADICEA score with menopausal status (model VI, HR = 1.00, $P = 1.0$), with BMI (model VII, HR = 1.13, $P = 0.5$), or with the interaction of BMI and menopausal status (model VIII, HR = 0.73, $P = 0.4$). That is, there was no evidence that the multiplicative interaction between BMI and menopausal status differed by familial risk irrespective of how we modeled the BMI association We also re-analyzed the data by including women with missing menopausal status and putting them in a category of their own. This made no difference to our general findings of no evidence for gene–environment interactions on the multiplicative scale.

Figure 3 shows the overall implications of the study estimates on the predicted age-specific cumulative risk for women with different baseline BMI and familial risk and

Table 2 Adjusted hazard ratios (HRs) and 95% confidence intervals (CIs) from Cox proportional hazards modeling of body mass index, menopausal status and age at baseline

Model		HR[b]	95% CI	P	ΔLL[c]
I	Log body mass index[a] (per 5 kg/m²)	1.28	0.91, 1.81	0.2	2.38
	Age at baseline, years	0.98	0.96, 1.00	0.1	
	Menopause, no/yes	1.12	0.88, 1.43	0.4	
II	Log body mass index[a] (per 5 kg/m²)	0.13	0.03, 0.56	0.006	7.36
	Age at baseline, years	0.98	0.96, 1.00	0.1	
	Menopause, no/yes	1.12	0.88, 1.44	0.4	
	Log body mass index (per 5 kg/m²) × Age at baseline, years	1.05	1.02, 1.08	0.002	
III	Log body mass index[a] (per 5 kg/m²)	0.68	0.41, 1.01	0.1	9.14
	Age at baseline, years	0.98	0.96, 1.00	0.1	
	Menopause, no/yes	1.12	0.87, 1.44	0.4	
	Log body mass index (per 5 kg/m²) × Menopause, no/yes	3.68	1.86, 7.28	< 0.001	
IV	Log body mass index[a] (per 5 kg/m²)	0.40	0.06, 2.89	0.4	9.32
	Age at baseline, years	0.98	0.96, 1.00	0.1	
	Menopause, no/yes	1.12	0.88, 1.44	0.4	
	Log body mass index (per 5 kg/m²) × Age at baseline, years	1.01	0.97, 1.06	0.6	
	Log body mass index (per 5 kg/m²) × Menopause, no/yes	2.91	0.91, 9.31	0.07	

To account for clustering by family, robust 95% CIs are reported

LL log likelihood

[a]Adjusted for log baseline age as a quadratic

[b]Adjusted for history of benign breast disease, race/ethnicity, and education; stratified by year of birth (10-year groups) and study site

[c]Change in LL from the base model that includes benign breast disease, race/ethnicity, and education

age 50 years at menopause. In terms of absolute risk, the risk difference for premenopausal women is small when comparing those in the lowest BMI category with those in the highest BMI category. In contrast, the corresponding risk difference for postmenopausal women is much larger and in the opposite direction. The latter difference in absolute risk is even more so for women with a greater familial risk (e.g. for cumulative risk to age 80 years, 8% for women with high familial risk versus 4% for population risk).

Discussion

Using a large international prospective cohort enriched for women with a family history of breast cancer [28] we have found that the *absolute* breast cancer risk gradient with

Table 3 Adjusted hazard ratios (HRs) and 95% confidence intervals (CIs) from Cox proportional hazards modelling of body mass index, menopausal status, age, and BOADICEA 1-year risk of breast cancer at baseline

Model		HR[b]	95% CI	P	ΔLL[c]
V	Log body mass index[a] (per 5 kg/m^2)	0.75	0.46, 1.22	0.2	158.03
	Log 1-year BOADICEA[a] (%)	2.05	1.89, 2.23	< 0.001	
	Age at baseline, years	0.98	0.96, 1.00	0.1	
	Menopause, no/yes	1.04	0.81, 1.32	0.8	
	Log body mass index (per 5 kg/m^2) × Menopause, no/yes	3.36	1.71, 6.62	< 0.001	
VI	Log body mass index[a] (per 5 kg/m^2)	0.75	0.46, 1.22	0.2	158.03
	Log 1-year BOADICEA[a] (%)	2.05	1.86, 2.26	< 0.001	
	Age at baseline, years	0.98	0.96, 1.00	0.1	
	Menopause, no/yes	1.03	0.80, 1.34	0.8	
	Log body mass index (per 5 kg/m^2) × Menopause, no/yes	3.36	1.71, 6.63	< 0.001	
	Menopause, no/yes × Log 1-year BOADICEA[a] (%)	1.00	0.85, 1.19	1.0	
VII	Log body mass index[a] (per 5 kg/m^2)	0.70	0.41, 1.18	0.2	158.24
	Log 1-year BOADICEA[a] (%)	2.06	0.89, 2.24	< 0.001	
	Age at baseline, years	0.98	0.96, 1.00	0.1	
	Menopause, no/yes	1.04	0.81, 1.32	0.8	
	Log body mass index (per 5 kg/m^2) × Menopause, no/yes	3.46	1.75, 6.84	< 0.001	
	Log body mass index[a] (per 5 kg/m^2) × log 1-year BOADICEA[a] (%)	1.13	0.79, 1.62	0.5	
VIII	Log body mass index[a] (per 5 kg/m^2)	0.66	0.38, 1.14	0.1	158.54
	Log 1-year BOADICEA[a] (%)	2.07	1.90, 2.25	< 0.001	
	Age at baseline, years	0.98	0.96, 1.00	0.1	
	Menopause, no/yes	1.04	0.82, 1.32	0.8	
	Log body mass index (per 5 kg/m^2) × Menopause, no/yes	3.92	1.86, 8.28	< 0.001	
	Log body mass index[a] (per 5 kg/m^2) × Log 1-year BOADICEA[a] (%)	1.27	0.81, 2.00	0.3	
	Menopause, no/yes × Log body mass index[a] (per 5 kg/m^2) × Log 1-year BOADICEA[a] (%)	0.73	0.34, 1.57	0.4	

To account for clustering by family, robust 95% CIs are reported
LL log likelihood, *BOADICEA* Breast and Ovarian Analysis of Disease Incidence and Carrier Estimation Algorithm
[a]Adjusted for log baseline age as a quadratic
[b]Adjusted for history of benign breast disease, race/ethnicity, and education; stratified by year of birth (10-year groups) and study site
[c]Change in LL from the base model that includes history of benign breast disease, race/ethnicity, and education

BMI increases with age after menopause, and with underlying familial risk. There are three key findings of clinical and biological significance and they are illustrated in Fig. 3.

First, we found that greater BMI at a young adult age is associated with a decreased risk of breast cancer, as have others [44]. We have shown that this negative association with BMI does not translate into a substantial influence on absolute risk of breast cancer.

Second, our modeling confirms that BMI is associated with an increase in risk once a woman becomes postmenopausal. In terms of differences in absolute risk, it is not until a woman is in her mid to late 50s that the risk manifests; the influence on absolute risk then increases with age.

Third, our modeling predicts that the greater a woman's familial risk, the greater the influence of BMI on her absolute postmenopausal breast cancer risk. We base this on

our finding that, in terms of multiplicative risk, the association of breast cancer with BMI did not differ for women at different underlying familial risk (Table 3). Unlike most other cohorts, our enriched cohort has adequate statistical power to examine interactions with underlying familial risk [28, 45, 46]. We also created a continuous measure of familial risk using multi-generational pedigree information and the BOADICEA model to estimate 1-year and lifetime (from birth) risk of breast cancer [35, 36, 43].

As illustrated in Fig. 1, about one third of our cohort has a lifetime risk above the clinically relevant cutoff of 20% [47, 48]. Figure 3 shows that our observed lack of multiplicative interaction means that the difference in absolute risk between women at higher compared with lower BMI is greater for those women who are at higher underlying familial risk. Our finding of a lack of

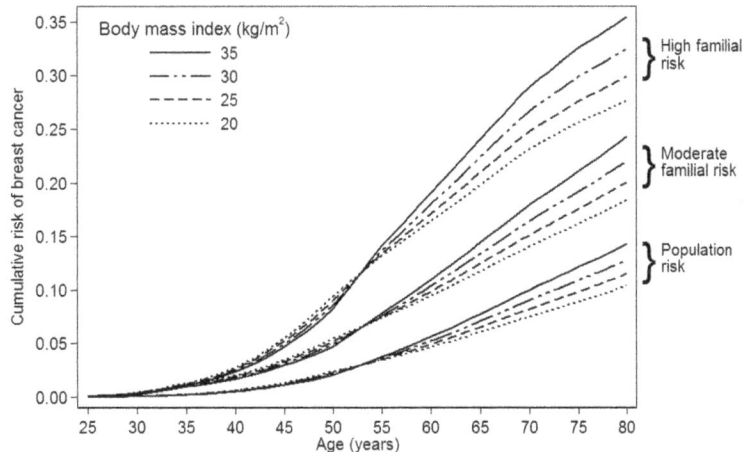

Fig. 3 Predicted age-specific cumulative risk (from birth) of breast cancer, based on model V (see Table 3), by body mass index and familial risk at baseline, where moderate familial risk is equivalent to having one affected first-degree relative and high familial risk is equivalent to having two affected first-degree relatives

multiplicative interaction between BMI and 1-year BOA-DICEA score is consistent with the lack of multiplicative interactions with BMI and more than 100 genetic variants found by a large pooled case–control analysis of almost 60,000 women [49].

One potential limitation is that a change in the BMI association with baseline menopausal status could be due to unmeasured confounders. For this to happen, such confounders would have to have a similar menopausal-dependent risk association. As most risk factors related to BMI (e.g., physical activity) do not have clear differences in association by menopausal status, unmeasured confounding is not likely. Other limitations include limited power to address issues specific to mutation carriers and hormone receptor status of tumors. The evidence of whether the protective association of BMI in early life applies solely to estrogen receptor negative disease is less consistent, with contradictory findings from two meta-analyses [50, 51] and a recent study based on a pooled study [52].

Although the negative breast cancer risk association with childhood and adolescent BMI is small in terms of absolute risk, understanding this in the light of the genome-wide association studies results [18, 19], which also support a negative association of BMI with breast cancer risk at a young age, could aid in understanding the role of breast development in breast cancer susceptibility. While increased glucose and other nutrients might alter the ability of BRCA1 to function as a tumor suppressor [53], pre-pubertal estrogen exposure could increase the ability of major breast cancer susceptibility genes to prevent breast cancer through cellular differentiation [54].

An explanation of the negative association with childhood and adolescent BMI might be found in the growth of mammographically dense tissue and changes to the

architecture surrounding the mammographically dense tissue, which develops and grows rapidly in adolescence [55]. Importantly, as we show here, although higher BMI is associated with reduced breast cancer risk before menopause, the direction of the association is reversed post-menopause and is of far more consequence in terms of absolute risk.

Laboratory studies have given insights into the mechanisms that might explain why weight gain and metabolically rich environments increase postmenopausal breast cancer risk, with implications for prevention [56]. These mechanisms include conversion of androgens to estrogens in adipose tissue [57], but could also include inflammation and metabolic processes related to cancer risk [58, 59] and changes to epigenetically regulated genes such as BRCA1 [53].

Conclusions

In summary, the negative association with BMI in premenopausal women has a much smaller influence on absolute risk than the positive association with BMI in postmenopausal women. Women at higher familial risk have a much larger difference in absolute risk depending on their BMI than women at lower familial risk.

Our modeling predicted that, for young and premenopausal women, the decrease in breast cancer risk associated with increasing BMI does not have a substantial influence on absolute risk in those periods of life. Our modeling also predicted that the *absolute* breast cancer risk gradient with BMI increases with age post menopause, and with underlying familial risk. We argue, therefore, that there is no discrepancy between the conclusions of the Mendelian randomization studies [18, 19] and the epidemiological literature (see "Background"). The genetically driven protective role of BMI on breast cancer risk in early adulthood appears to be of little consequence in terms of absolute risk and is overtaken by an environmentally driven deleterious role of greater adult BMI in later life that is even more important for women at increased genetic risk. Given that age-adjusted BMI is correlated between early and mid-adulthood [60], maintaining a healthy weight throughout adult life is of clinical significance for all women, and especially those with a family history of breast cancer.

Abbreviations
BCFR: Breast Cancer Family Registry; BMI: Body mass index; BOADICEA: Breast and Ovarian Analysis of Disease Incidence and Carrier Estimation Algorithm; kConFab: Kathleen Cuningham Foundation Consortium for Research into Familial Breast Cancer; Prof-SC: Breast Cancer Prospective Family Study Cohort; SNP: Single-nucleotide polymorphism

Acknowledgements
We thank Heather Thorne, Eveline Niedermayr, Lucy Stanhope, Yasmin Rady, Sandra Picken, all the BCFR and kConFab research nurses and staff, the heads and staff of the Family Cancer Clinics, and the many families who contribute to the BCFR and kConFab for their contributions to this resource.

Funding
This work was supported by the National Institute of Health USA. (grant number 1RO1CA159868). The ABCFR was supported in Australia by the National Health and Medical Research Council, the New South Wales Cancer Council, the Victorian Health Promotion Foundation, the Victorian Breast Cancer Research Consortium, Cancer Australia, and the National Breast Cancer Foundation. The six sites of the Breast Cancer Family Registry (BCFR) were supported by grant UM1 CA164920 from the USA National Cancer Institute. The content of this manuscript does not necessarily reflect the views or policies of the National Cancer Institute or any of the collaborating centers in the BCFR, nor does mention of trade names, commercial products, or organizations imply endorsement by the USA Government or the BCFR. This work was supported by grants to kConFab and the kConFab follow-up study from Cancer Australia (grant number 809195), the Australian National Breast Cancer Foundation (grant number IF 17 kConFab), the National Health and Medical Research Council (grant numbers 454508, 288704, 145684), the National Institute of Health USA (grant number 1RO1CA159868), the Queensland Cancer Fund, the Cancer Councils of New South Wales, Victoria, Tasmania and South Australia, and the Cancer Foundation of Western Australia (grant numbers not applicable). KAP is a National Breast Cancer Foundation (Australia) Practitioner Fellow (grant number PRAC-17-004). ACA is supported by Cancer Research (UK grant C12292/A20861).

Authors' contributions
JLH and MBT conceived the study, obtained funding, collected data, analyzed data, interpreted the findings, and co-led the writing of the manuscript. ILA, SSB, MBD, EMJ, and KAP conceived the study, obtained funding, collected data, interpreted the findings, and contributed to writing the manuscript. GSD collected data, analyzed data, interpreted the findings, and was a major contributor to writing the manuscript. RJM programmed the BOADICEA model, analyzed data, interpreted the findings, and was a major contributor to writing the manuscript. YL and NZ analyzed data, interpreted the findings, and contributed to writing the manuscript. JAK, MCS, RLM, WKC, GGG, JMG, SAM, and MLF helped conceive the study, helped obtain funding, collected data, interpreted the findings and contributed to writing the manuscript. ACA developed the BOADICEA model, trained RJM in its use, and oversaw its application. PCW, GG, SN, and the kConFab Investigators co-ordinated the data collection, interpreted the findings, and contributed to writing the manuscript. All authors read approved the final manuscript.

- Northern California – Cancer Prevention Institute of California, Institutional Review Board (2001–033)
- New York – Columbia University Medical Center, Institutional Review Board (AAA7794)
- Philadelphia – Fox Chase Cancer Center, Institutional Review Board (95–009)
- Utah – Huntsman Cancer Institute, University of Utah, Institutional Review Board (00004965)
- Ontario – Mount Sinai Hospital Research Ethics Board (#02–0076-U) and University Health Network Research Ethics Board (#96-U107-CE)
- Australia – University of Melbourne, Human Ethics Sub-Committee (1441420.1)
- kConFab – Peter MacCallum Cancer Centre, the Peter Mac Ethics Committee (97/27)

Competing interests
The authors declare that they have no competing interests.

Author details
[1]Centre for Epidemiology and Biostatistics, The University of Melbourne, Parkville, VIC, Australia. [2]Cancer Epidemiology and Intelligence Division, Cancer Council Victoria, Melbourne, VIC, Australia. [3]Department of Epidemiology, Mailman School of Public Health, Columbia University, 722 W 168th St, 7th Floor, New York, NY, USA. [4]Lunenfeld-Tanenbaum Research Institute, Sinai Health System, Toronto, ON, Canada. [5]Dalla Lana School of Public Health, University of Toronto, Toronto, ON, Canada. [6]Department of Pathology, Genetic Epidemiology Laboratory, The University of Melbourne, Parkville, VIC, Australia. [7]Herbert Irving Comprehensive Cancer Center, Columbia University Medical Center, New York, NY, USA. [8]Departments of Pediatrics and Medicine, Columbia University, New York, NY, USA. [9]Department of Medicine, St Vincent's Hospital, The University of Melbourne, Parkville, VIC, Australia. [10]Department of Medical Oncology, St Vincent's Hospital, Fitzroy, VIC, Australia. [11]Prince of Wales Clinical School, University of New South Wales, Sydney, NSW, Australia. [12]Department of Medical Oncology, Prince of Wales Hospital, Randwick, NSW, Australia. [13]Department of Public Health and Primary Care, Centre for Cancer Genetic Epidemiology, University of Cambridge, Cambridge, UK. [14]Division of Cancer Medicine, Peter MacCallum Cancer Centre, Melbourne, VIC, Australia. [15]Sir Peter MacCallum Department of Oncology, The University of Melbourne, Melbourne, VIC, Australia. [16]The Research Department, The Peter MacCallum Cancer Centre, Melbourne, VIC, Australia. [17]Departments of Molecular Genetics and Laboratory Medicine and Pathobiology, University of Toronto, Toronto, ON, Canada. [18]Department of Medicine and Huntsman Cancer Institute, University of Utah Health Sciences Center, Salt Lake City, UT, USA. [19]Department of Clinical Genetics, Fox Chase Cancer Center, Philadelphia, PA, USA. [20]Department of Medicine and Stanford Cancer Institute, Stanford University School of Medicine, Stanford, CA, USA. [21]Precision Medicine, School of Clinical Sciences at Monash Health, Monash University, Clayton, CA VIC 3168, USA.

References
1. Baer HJ, Tworoger SS, Hankinson SE, Willett WC. Body fatness at young ages and risk of breast cancer throughout life. Am J Epidemiol. 2010; 171(11):1183–94.

2. Bandera EV, Chandran U, Zirpoli G, Ciupak G, Bovbjerg DH, Jandorf L, et al. Body size in early life and breast cancer risk in African American and European American women. Cancer Causes Control. 2013;24(12):2231–43.

3. Bardia A, Vachon CM, Olson JE, Vierkant RA, Wang AH, Hartmann LC, et al. Relative weight at age 12 and risk of postmenopausal breast cancer. Cancer Epidemiol Biomark Prev. 2008;17(2):374–8.

4. Berkey CS, Frazier AL, Gardner JD, Colditz GA. Adolescence and breast carcinoma risk. Cancer. 1999;85(11):2400–9.

5. Bodicoat DH, Schoemaker MJ, Jones ME, McFadden E, Griffin J, Ashworth A, et al. Timing of pubertal stages and breast cancer risk: the Breakthrough Generations Study. Breast Cancer Res. 2014;16(1):R18.

6. Robinson WR, Tse CK, Olshan AF, Troester MA. Body size across the life course and risk of premenopausal and postmenopausal breast cancer in Black women, the Carolina Breast Cancer Study, 1993-2001. Cancer Causes Control. 2014;25(9):1101–17.

7. Rosner B, Eliassen AH, Toriola AT, Chen WY, Hankinson SE, Willett WC, et al. Weight and weight changes in early adulthood and later breast cancer risk. Int J Cancer. 2017;140(9):2003–14.

8. Shawon SR, Eriksson M, Li J. Body size in early life and risk of breast cancer. Breast Cancer Res. 2017;19(1):84.

9. Terry MB. Consistency, now what? Breast Cancer Res. 2017;19(1):85.

10. Baer HJ, Colditz GA, Rosner B, Michels KB, Rich-Edwards JW, Hunter DJ, et al. Body fatness during childhood and adolescence and incidence of breast cancer in premenopausal women: a prospective cohort study. Breast Cancer Res. 2005;7(3):R314–25.

11. Coates RJ, Uhler RJ, Hall HI, Potischman N, Brinton LA, Ballard-Barbash R, et al. Risk of breast cancer in young women in relation to body size and weight gain in adolescence and early adulthood. Br J Cancer. 1999;81(1):167–74.

12. Michels KB, Terry KL, Willett WC. Longitudinal study on the role of body size in premenopausal breast cancer. Arch Intern Med. 2006;166(21):2395–402.

13. Weiderpass E, Braaten T, Magnusson C, Kumle M, Vainio H, Lund E, et al. A prospective study of body size in different periods of life and risk of premenopausal breast cancer. Cancer Epidemiol Biomark Prev. 2004;13(7):1121–7.

14. John EM, Sangaramoorthy M, Hines LM, Stern MC, Baumgartner KB, Giuliano AR, et al. Body size throughout adult life influences postmenopausal breast cancer risk among hispanic women: the breast cancer health disparities study. Cancer Epidemiol Biomark Prev. 2015;24(1):128–37.

15. Bandera EV, Maskarinec G, Romieu I, John EM. Racial and ethnic disparities in the impact of obesity on breast cancer risk and survival: a global perspective. Adv Nutr. 2015;6(6):803–19.

16. MacInnis RJ, English DR, Gertig DM, Hopper JL, Giles GG. Body size and composition and risk of postmenopausal breast cancer. Cancer Epidemiol Biomark Prev. 2004;13(12):2117–25.

17. John EM, Phipps AI, Sangaramoorthy M. Body size, modifying factors, and postmenopausal breast cancer risk in a multiethnic population: the San Francisco Bay Area Breast Cancer Study. Springerplus. 2013;24(1):239.

18. Gao C, Patel CJ, Michailidou K, Peters U, Gong J, Schildkraut J, et al. Mendelian randomization study of adiposity-related traits and risk of breast, ovarian, prostate, lung and colorectal cancer. Int J Epidemiol. 2016;45(3):896–908.

19. Guo Y, Warren Andersen S, Shu XO, Michailidou K, Bolla MK, Wang Q, et al. Genetically predicted body mass index and breast cancer risk: Mendelian randomization analyses of data from 145,000 women of European descent. PLoS Med. 2016;13(8):e1002105.

20. Hopper JL, Carlin JB. Familial aggregation of a disease consequent upon correlation between relatives in a risk factor measured on a continuous scale. Am J Epidemiol. 1992;136(9):1138–47.

21. Mavaddat N, Pharoah PD, Michailidou K, Tyrer J, Brook MN, Bolla MK, et al. Prediction of breast cancer risk based on profiling with common genetic variants. J Natl Cancer Inst. 2015;107(5):djv036.

22. Dite GS, Macinnis RJ, Bickerstaffe A, Dowty JG, Allman R, Apicella C, et al. Breast cancer risk prediction using clinical models and 77 independent risk-associated SNPs for women aged under 50 years: Australian Breast Cancer Family Registry. Cancer Epidemiol Biomark Prev. 2016;25(2):359–65.

23. Easton DF, Pharoah PD, Antoniou AC, Tischkowitz M, Tavtigian SV, Nathanson KL, et al. Gene-panel sequencing and the prediction of breast-cancer risk. N Engl J Med. 2015;372(23):2243–57.

24. Nguyen-Dumont T, Teo ZL, Pope BJ, Hammet F, Mahmoodi M, Tsimiklis H, et al. Hi-Plex for high-throughput mutation screening: application to the breast cancer susceptibility gene PALB2. BMC Med Genet. 2013;6:48.

25. Nguyen-Dumont T, Mahmoodi M, Hammet F, Tran T, Tsimiklis H, Kathleen Cuningham Foundation Consortium for Research into Familial Breast Cancer, et al. Hi-Plex targeted sequencing is effective using DNA derived from archival dried blood spots. Anal Biochem. 2015;470:48–51.

26. Hopper JL. Genetics for population and public health. Int J Epidemiol. 2017;46(1):8–11.

27. Rothman KJ, Greenland S, Lash TL. Modern epidemiology. 3rd ed. Philadelphia: Lippincott Williams & Winkins; 2013.

28. Terry MB, Phillips KA, Daly MB, John EM, Andrulis IL, Buys SS, et al. Cohort profile: The Breast Cancer Prospective Family Study Cohort (ProF-SC). Int J Epidemiol. 2016;45(3):683–92.

29. John EM, Hopper JL, Beck JC, Knight JA, Neuhausen SL, Senie RT, et al. The Breast Cancer Family Registry: an infrastructure for cooperative multinational, interdisciplinary and translational studies of the genetic epidemiology of breast cancer. Breast Cancer Res. 2004;6(4):R375–89.

30. Mann GJ, Thorne H, Balleine RL, Butow PN, Clarke CL, Edkins E, et al. Analysis of cancer risk and BRCA1 and BRCA2 mutation prevalence in the kConFab familial breast cancer resource. Breast Cancer Res. 2006;8(1):R12.

31. Phillips KA, Butow PN, Stewart AE, Chang JH, Weideman PC, Price MA, et al. Predictors of participation in clinical and psychosocial follow-up of the kConFab breast cancer family cohort. Familial Cancer. 2005;4(2):105–13.

32. Neuhausen SL, Ozcelik H, Southey MC, John EM, Godwin AK, Chung W, et al. BRCA1 and BRCA2 mutation carriers in the Breast Cancer Family Registry: an open resource for collaborative research. Breast Cancer Res Treat. 2009;116(2):379–86.

33. McCredie MR, Dite GS, Giles GG, Hopper JL. Breast cancer in Australian women under the age of 40. Cancer Causes Control. 1998;9(2):189–98.

34. Hopper JL, Giles GG, McCredie MRE, Boyle P. Background, rationale and protocol for a case-control-family study of breast cancer. Breast. 1994;3(2):79–86.

35. Antoniou AC, Cunningham AP, Peto J, Evans DG, Lalloo F, Narod SA, et al. The BOADICEA model of genetic susceptibility to breast and ovarian cancers: updates and extensions. Br J Cancer. 2008;98(8):1457–66.

36. Antoniou AC, Pharoah PP, Smith P, Easton DF. The BOADICEA model of genetic susceptibility to breast and ovarian cancer. Br J Cancer. 2004;91(8):1580–90.

37. Breast cancer information core. National Human Genome Research Institute. 2017 https://research.nhgri.nih.gov/bic/. Accessed 20 May 2018.

38. Dite GS, Whittemore AS, Knight JA, John EM, Milne RL, Andrulis IL, et al. Increased cancer risks for relatives of very early-onset breast cancer cases with and without BRCA1 and BRCA2 mutations. Br J Cancer. 2010;103(7):1103–8.

39. StataCorp. Stata Statistical Software, Release 14. College Station: StataCorp LP; 2015.

40. Surveillance Epidemiology and End Results (SEER) Program. SEER*stat database: incidence - SEER 13 regs research data, Nov 2011 Sub (1992–2009) <Katrina/Rita Population Adjustment> – Linked To County Attributes - Total U.S.; 2011.

41. Surveillance Epidemiology and End Results (SEER) Program. SEER*stat database: incidence - SEER 18 regs research data, Nov 2011 Sub (2000–2009) <Katrina/Rita Population Adjustment> – Linked To County Attributes - Total U.S.; 2011.

42. Surveillance Epidemiology and End Results (SEER) Program. SEER*stat database: incidence - SEER 9 regs research data, Nov 2011 Sub (1973–2009) <Katrina/Rita Population Adjustment> – Linked To County Attributes - Total U.S.; 2011.

43. Lee AJ, Cunningham AP, Kuchenbaecker KB, Mavaddat N, Easton DF, Antoniou AC, et al. BOADICEA breast cancer risk prediction model: updates to cancer incidences, tumour pathology and web interface. Br J Cancer. 2014;110(2):535–45.

44. Amadou A, Ferrari P, Muwonge R, Moskal A, Biessy C, Romieu I, et al. Overweight, obesity and risk of premenopausal breast cancer according to ethnicity: a systematic review and dose-response meta-analysis. Obes Rev. 2013;14(8):665–78.

45. Dite GS, MacInnis RJ, Bickerstaffe A, Dowty JG, Milne RL, Antoniou AC, et al. Testing for gene-environment interactions using a prospective family cohort design: body mass index in early and later adulthood and risk of breast cancer. Am J Epidemiol. 2017;185(6):487–500.

46. Shen J, Liao Y, Hopper JL, Goldberg M, Santella RM, Terry MB. Dependence of cancer risk from environmental exposures on underlying genetic susceptibility: an illustration with polycyclic aromatic hydrocarbons and breast cancer. Br J Cancer. 2017;116(9):1229–33.

47. Quante AS, Herz J, Whittemore AS, Fischer C, Strauch K, Terry MB. Assessing absolute changes in breast cancer risk due to modifiable risk factors. Breast Cancer Res Treat. 2015;152(1):193–7.

48. Quante AS, Whittemore AS, Shriver T, Hopper JL, Strauch K, Terry MB. Practical problems with clinical guidelines for breast cancer prevention based on remaining lifetime risk. J Natl Cancer Inst. 2015;107(7):djv124.

49. Milne RL, Gaudet MM, Spurdle AB, Fasching PA, Couch FJ, Benitez J, et al. Assessing interactions between the associations of common genetic susceptibility variants, reproductive history and body mass index with breast cancer risk in the breast cancer association consortium: a combined case-control study. Breast Cancer Res. 2010;12(6):R110.

50. Renehan AG, Tyson M, Egger M, Heller RF, Zwahlen M. Body-mass index and incidence of cancer: a systematic review and meta-analysis of prospective observational studies. Lancet. 2008;371(9612):569–78.

51. Munsell MF, Sprague BL, Berry DA, Chisholm G, Trentham-Dietz A. Body mass index and breast cancer risk according to postmenopausal estrogen-progestin use and hormone receptor status. Epidemiol Rev. 2014;36:114–36.

52. Ma H, Ursin G, Xu X, Lee E, Togawa K, Malone KE, et al. Body mass index at age 18 years and recent body mass index in relation to risk of breast cancer overall and ER/PR/HER2-defined subtypes in white women and African-American women: a pooled analysis. Breast Cancer Res. 2018;20(1):5.

53. Di LJ, Byun JS, Wong MM, Wakano C, Taylor T, Bilke S, et al. Genome-wide profiles of CtBP link metabolism with genome stability and epithelial reprogramming in breast cancer. Nat Commun. 2013;4:1449.

54. Cabanes A, Wang M, Olivo S, DeAssis S, Gustafsson JA, Khan G, et al. Prepubertal estradiol and genistein exposures up-regulate BRCA1 mRNA and reduce mammary tumorigenesis. Carcinogenesis. 2004;25(5):741–8.

55. Sherratt MJ, McConnell JC, Streuli CH. Raised mammographic density: causative mechanisms and biological consequences. Breast Cancer Res. 2016;18(1):45.

56. Picon-Ruiz M, Morata-Tarifa C, Valle-Goffin JJ, Friedman ER, Slingerland JM. Obesity and adverse breast cancer risk and outcome: mechanistic insights and strategies for intervention. CA Cancer J Clin. 2017;67(5):378–97.

57. Siiteri PK. Adipose tissue as a source of hormones. Am J Clin Nutr. 1987;45(1 Suppl):277–82.

58. Hudis C, Dannenberg A. Obesity and breast cancer: narrowing the focus. JAMA Oncol. 2015;1(5):622–3.

59. Iyengar NM, Gucalp A, Dannenberg AJ, Hudis CA. Obesity and cancer mechanisms: tumor microenvironment and inflammation. J Clin Oncol. 2016;34(35):4270–6.

60. Ester WA, Houghton LC, Lumey LH, Michels KB, Hoek HW, Wei Y, et al. Maternal and early childhood determinants of women's body size in midlife: overall cohort and sibling analyses. Am J Epidemiol. 2017;185(5):1–10.

20

Sulfatide decreases the resistance to stress-induced apoptosis and increases P-selectin-mediated adhesion: a two-edged sword in breast cancer progression

Jaroslaw Suchanski[1], Jedrzej Grzegrzolka[2], Tomasz Owczarek[1,7], Pawel Pasikowski[3], Aleksandra Piotrowska[2], Bartlomiej Kocbach[4], Aleksandra Nowak[2], Piotr Dziegiel[2,5], Andrzej Wojnar[6] and Maciej Ugorski[1,4*]

Abstract

Background: We have previously shown that galactosylceramide (GalCer) affects the tumourigenic and metastatic properties of breast cancer cells by acting as an anti-apoptotic molecule. Since GalCer is a precursor molecule in the synthesis of sulfatides, the present study was aimed to define the role of sulfatides in apoptosis and breast cancer progression.

Methods: Expression of GAL3ST1 in breast cancer cell lines and breast cancer tissue specimens was analysed using real-time PCR, western blotting and immunohistochemistry analysis. The amount of sulfatide, GalCer and ceramide was analysed by thin-layer chromatography binding assay and by the modified hydrophilic interaction liquid chromatography coupled with electrospray mass spectrometry methodology. The tumourigenicity of cancer cells was analysed by an in-vivo tumour growth assay. Apoptotic cells were detected based on caspase-3 activation and the TUNEL assay. The interaction of breast cancer cells with P-selectin or E-selectin was analysed using the flow adhesion assay. The ability of sulfatide-expressing cells to activate and aggregate platelets was studied using the flow-cytometry-based aggregation assay.

Results: Using two models of breast cancer, T47D cells with blocked synthesis of sulfatide and MDA-MB-231 cells with neosynthesis of this glycosphingolipid, we showed that high sulfatide levels resulted in increased sensitivity of cancer cells to apoptosis induced by hypoxia and doxorubicin in vitro, and decreased their tumourigenicity after transplantation into athymic nu/nu mice. Accordingly, a clinical study on GAL3ST1 expression in invasive ductal carcinoma revealed that its elevated level is associated with better prognosis. Using MDA-MB-231 cells with neosynthesis of sulfatide we also showed that sulfatide is responsible for adhesion of breast cancer cells to P-selectin-expressing cells, including platelets. Sulfatide also acted as an activating molecule, increasing the expression of P-selectin.

Conclusions: This study demonstrates that increased synthesis of sulfatide sensitises cancer cells to microenvironmental stress factors such as hypoxia and anticancer drugs such as doxorubicin. However, sulfatide is probably not directly involved in apoptotic cascades, because its increased synthesis by GAL3ST1 decreased the amounts of its precursor, GalCer, a known anti-apoptotic molecule. On the other hand, our data support the view that sulfatides are malignancy-related adhesive molecules involved in activating and binding P-selectin-expressing platelets to breast cancer cells.

Keywords: Breast cancer, Sulfatide, Galactosyloceramide, Apoptosis, Platelets, P-selectin, Adhesion

* Correspondence: maciej.ugorski@upwr.edu.pl
[1]Department of Biochemistry and Molecular Biology, Faculty of Veterinary Medicine, Wroclaw University of Environmental and Life Sciences, C.K. Norwida 31, 50-375 Wroclaw, Poland
[4]Laboratory of Glycobiology, Hirszfeld Institute of Immunology and Experimental Therapy, Polish Academy of Sciences, Wroclaw, Poland
Full list of author information is available at the end of the article

Background

Sulfatides (SM4) are sulfated galactosylceramides (GalCer) present in the external leaflet of the plasma membrane in a variety of mammalian cells. Increased amounts of sulfatides have been found in colon, ovarian and gastric cancers [1–4], as well as renal cell and hepatocellular carcinomas [5, 6]. Differential expression of sulfatides was observed in lung carcinoma, with higher levels in adenocarcinomas than in squamous cell carcinoma and undifferentiated small cell carcinoma [7]. In colorectal and ovarian carcinoma, an increase in sulfatides correlated with poor prognosis [8, 9]. However, little is known about the biological role of sulfatides in cancer progression. It has been proposed, but not experimentally proven, that sulfatides present on the surface of cancer cells are ligands for P-selectin expressed by activated endothelial cells, and such interactions facilitate the formation of aggregates, which in turn increase their metastatic potential [10]. More recently, sulfated galactocerebroside was described as a P-selectin ligand on MC-38 murine colon carcinoma cells [11]. These studies revealed that in-vitro adhesion of activated platelets expressing P-selectin to MC-38 cells is mediated solely through sulfatides present on the latter. Such interactions were also observed in vivo. When mice were transplanted intravenously with MC-38 cells, their aggregates with platelets were observed in the lungs after 30 min.

It has been shown that SM4 is produced by several breast cancer cell lines [12]. In mammalian cells, sulfatides are synthesised by highly specific, late Golgi apparatus-localised 3′-phosphoadenosine-5′-phosphosulfate galactosylceramide sulfotransferase (GAL3ST1) (cerebroside sulfotransferase (CST); EC 2.8.2.11), which is responsible for 3-O-sulfation of galactose residue in GalCer molecules [13]. We recently showed that GalCer affects the tumourigenic and metastatic properties of breast cancer cells and acts as an anti-apoptotic molecule [14]. Since it was proposed that the balance between specific sphingolipid species is a critical rheostat for regulation of cellular apoptosis [15], the present study was undertaken to define the role of sulfatides in apoptosis and breast cancer progression. We show for the first time that sulfatides act not only as adhesive molecules, but are also involved in programmed cell death together with GalCer [14]. This highlights the importance of the glycolipids as regulators of cancer progression.

Methods

Breast cancer tissue specimens

The study was carried out on archival paraffin blocks of 232 randomly selected breast cancer patients (mean age 58.25 years) diagnosed between 2004 and 2009 at the Lower Silesian Oncology Centre in Wroclaw, Poland. All patients were treated by mastectomy, quadrantectomy and/or axillary lymph node resection. Of the patients,

94.4% (219 patients) and 85.34% (198 patients) were treated by adjuvant chemotherapy and hormonotherapy, respectively. All HER2-positive patients (14.66%, 34 patients) were additionally subjected to immunotherapy. The patients' clinical and pathological data (presented in Table 1) were obtained from the hospital archives. Tumour histological type and malignancy grade (G) were determined according to World Health Organization (WHO) criteria [16]. The patients were followed for 121.41 months (range 1–161 months) and the median follow-up was 141.9 months.

Cell lines

The breast cancer cell lines MCF7, SKBR3 and BT-474 were obtained from the Cell Line Collection of the Hirszfeld Institute of Immunology and Experimental Therapy (Wroclaw, Poland). T47D and MDA-MB-231 breast cancer cell lines as well as CHO-Pro5 cells were obtained from the American Type Culture Collection (Manassas, VA, USA). CHO-Pro5 cells that expressed human E-selectin have been described elsewhere [17]. All human cell lines were authenticated by the ATCC Cell Line Authentication Service using Short Tandem Repeat analysis. The cells were cultured in α-minimum essential medium (αMEM) supplemented with 10% fetal calf serum (FCS; Cytogen, Lodz, Poland), 2 mM L-glutamine and antibiotics.

In-vivo tumour growth assay

The animal study was approved by the Second Local Ethic Committee for Animal Experimentation (Wroclaw, Poland). Six-week-old athymic nude Crl:NU(Ncr)-Foxn1nu female mice were purchased from Charles River Laboratories (Sulzfeld, Germany) and kept under specific pathogen-free conditions at room temperature (RT). Human breast cancer cells were harvested by trypsinisation, washed with PBS and resuspended in the same buffer. Cell suspensions (2×10^6 cells/100 μl PBS) were mixed with the same volume of ice-cold BD Matrigel Matrix High Concentration (Becton Dickinson, San Jose, CA, USA) and the entire mixture was inoculated subcutaneously (s.c.). Tumour growth was monitored once a week by measuring the tumour diameter with a caliper. Tumour volume (TV) was calculated as TV $(mm^3) = (d^2 \times D) / 2$, where d is the shortest diameter and D is the longest diameter. Mice were sacrificed after 10 weeks of experiment by cervical dislocation following light anaesthesia by isoflurane inhalation. Samples were collected in 10% buffered formalin and were subjected to histological studies.

Vector construction, virus production, transfections and transductions

The cDNA for P-selectin, amplified using the pCMV6-Entry vector containing P-selectin cDNA (2490 bp; OriGene, Rockville, MD, USA) as a template and primers

Table 1 Clinical and pathological characteristics of breast cancer cases

Parameter	Patients		GAL3ST1		
	IHC (N = 232)	%	IHC negative	IHC positive	p value (chi-square[a] or Fisher exact test[b])
Age					
≤ 50 years	56	24.14	25	31	0.0904[b]
> 50 years	176	75.86	102	74	
Tumour grade					
G1	67	28.88	30	38	**0.0215[b]**
G2	96	41.38	53	42	
G3	55	23.71	38	17	
No data	14	6.03			
Tumour size					
pT1	119	51.29	66	53	0.8706[b]
pT2	75	32.33	45	31	
pT3	4	1.72	2	2	
pT4	22	9.48	11	11	
	14	6.03			
Lymph nodes					
pN0	87	37.50	53	34	0.4386[b]
pN1–pN3	67	28.88	46	30	
pNx		0.00			
No data	12	5.17			
Stage					
I	53	22.84	33	20	0.6406[a]
II	60	25.86	35	25	
III	41	17.67	24	17	
IV	1	0.43	0	1	
No data	78	33.62			
Oestrogen receptor					
Negative	52	22.41	36	16	**0.0203[b]**
Positive	167	71.98	85	82	
No data	13	5.60			
Progesterone receptor					
Negative	69	29.74	40	28	0.4503[b]
Positive	150	64.66	80	70	
No data	13	5.60			
HER2					
Negative	188	81.03	97	90	0.0894[b]
Positive	34	14.66	23	11	
No data	10	4.31			
Molecular tumour types					
Triple negative	18	7.6	11	7	0.5492[b]
Other types	199	85.78	107	92	

Table 1 Clinical and pathological characteristics of breast cancer cases *(Continued)*

Parameter	Patients		GAL3ST1		
	IHC (N = 232)	%	IHC negative	IHC positive	p value (chi-square[a] or Fisher exact test[b])
No data	10	4.31			
Chemotherapy					
Negative	13	5.60	8	5	0.7764[b]
Positive	219	94.4	119	100	
Hormonal therapy					
Negative	32	13.79	20	12	0.3398[b]
Positive	198	85.34	103	95	
No data	2	0.8			

Bold values (p < 0.05) are statistically significant
HER2 human epidermal growth factor receptor 2, *IHC* immunohistochemistry, *Gal3ST1* galactosylceramide sulfotransferase

(Additional file 1: Table S1), was cloned into the pSG5 plasmid (Agilent Technologies, Palo Alto, CA, USA). The resulting pSG5/SELP vector was used together with the pSV2neo vector (Invitrogen, Carlsbad, CA, USA) to co-transfect CHO-Pro5 cells using polyethylenimine (Sigma-Aldrich, Buchs, Switzerland). G418-resistant colonies were screened for the presence of P-selectin by flow cytometry.

For generation of the GAL3ST1-expressing vector, the human GAL3ST1 cDNA was amplified by PCR from the MCF7 cDNA library using the primers presented in Additional file 1: Table S1. The resulting insert was cloned into a pRRL-CMV-IRES-PURO vector as described previously [18] and named here as pRRL-CMV-GAL3ST1-IRES-PURO. For lentivirus production, packaging LentiX 293 T cells were co-transfected at 50–60% confluence with 20 μg of expression or control vector, 10 μg pMDL-g/p-RRE, 5 μg pRSV-REV and 5 μg pMk-VSVG (kindly provided by Dr D. Trono, École Polytechnique Fédérale de Lausanne, Switzerland) using polyethylenimine (Sigma-Aldrich). The production of virus particles and transduction of cells have been described previously [14].

For silencing *GAL3ST1*, a GAL3ST1 CRISPR/Cas9 knockout plasmid encoding the Cas9 nuclease and GAL3ST1-specific 20 nucleotide guide RNA (gRNA-AGTGATCCGGGCCAACGGCT) was purchased from Applied Biological Materials Inc. (Richmond, BC, Canada). For lentivirus production the same procedure as already described was used [14]. *GAL3ST1* knockout cells were selected with puromycin (1 μg/ml). Antibiotic-resistant cells were detached by trypsinisation and subcloned using a limiting dilution technique.

Real-time PCR

Purification of RNA from tissues and cells was performed using the RNeasy Mini Kit (Qiagen, Hilden,

Germany) according to the manufacturer's instructions. The SuperScript RT (Thermo Fisher Scientific) was used to synthesise cDNA. The relative amounts of GAL3ST1 were determined by real-time PCR assay (qPCR) with iQ™ SYBR Green Supermix (Bio-Rad, Hercules, CA, USA) according to the manufacturer's protocol, using iQ5 Optical System (Bio-Rad). β-actin was used as a reference gene. The primers used for the real-time PCR assay are presented in Additional file 1: Table S1. Gene expression was calculated using the $\Delta\Delta$Ct method [19].

Western blotting analysis

Western blotting analysis was performed as described previously [18]. The antibodies used are presented in Additional file 2: Table S2.

Flow cytometry

Flow cytometry with specific antibodies was performed as described previously [20]. The antibodies used are presented in Additional file 2: Table S2. For analysis of tumour cell–platelet aggregates, tumour cells and platelets were stained, respectively, with lipophilic fluorescence dyes DiD (red fluorescence) and DiO (green fluorescence) (Thermo Fisher Scientific) for 1 h at 37 °C. After washing, tumour cells and platelets were mixed and incubated for another 1 h at 37 °C. Cells stained with antibodies or tumour cell–platelet aggregates were resuspended in PBS and analysed using the BD FACS Canto II instrument (Becton-Dickinson). Data were processed and analysed using Flowing Software version 2.

Purification of gangliosides and neutral glycolipid, thin-layer chromatography and thin-layer chromatogram binding assay (TLC binding assay)

Gangliosides and neutral glycolipids were purified as described previously [21]. Glycolipids were extracted from 10^8–10^9 cells using the chloroform–methanol extraction method. HP-TLC was performed on Silica Gel 60 high-performance TLC (HPTLC) plates (Merck Millipore). For ganglioside/sulfatide separation, a chloroform:methanol:0.2% $CaCl_2$ solvent system (60:40:9, v/v/v) was used, while neutral glycolipids were separated in a 2-isopropanol:methyl acetate:15 M ammonium hydroxide:water solvent system (75:10:5:15, v/v/v/v). The glycolipids were visualised by spraying the plate with primuline reagent (0.05% primuline in acetone/water, 4:1 by volume) and heated for 1 min at 120 °C.

Sulfatide and GalCer were detected by TLC binding assay primarily as described previously [14]. The antibodies used are presented in Additional file 2: Table S2.

Hydrophilic interaction liquid chromatography coupled with electrospray mass spectrometry (HILIC-ESI-MS/MS)

Hydrophilic interaction liquid chromatography (HILIC) separations were carried out on the Dionex Ultimate 3000 RSCL chromatographic system (Thermo Scientific) equipped with an Atlantis HILIC column (Waters, Saint-Quentin, France). The system used 10 mM ammonium acetate with the addition of 0.1% formic acid (solution A) and acetonitrile with 0.1% formic acid (solution B) as mobile phases. The column was operated at 30 °C at a flow rate of 0.3 ml/min. The gradient started at 95% solution B for the first 0.5 min and went down to 50% solution B at 6.5 min and back up to 95% solution B at 7.5 min. The column was then stabilised for another 5 min. The chromatographic system was coupled to the maXis impact q-TOF mass spectrometer (Bruker Daltonics, Billerica, MA, USA) with the electrospray ion source operated in positive ion mode. The spectrometer parameters were set as follows: mass range 50–1300 m/z, spectra rate 4 Hz, nebulising gas pressure 1.5 bar, drying gas flow 8 L/min, capillary voltage 4500 eV, source energy 5 eV and collision energy 10 eV. To obtain the fragmentation spectra of the standards, the auto-MS/MS function was set for the three most abundant peaks. For the SIM experiment, the broadband collision-induced dissociation (bbCID) fragmentation was set at an energy of 35 eV. Three biological replicates of ceramide extracts were run for each examined cell line.

Cell proliferation assay (SRB assay)

Cells (5×10^3 cells) were grown in individual wells of 96-well plates (Greiner, Germany) in complete αMEM. After 24, 48, 72 and 96 h, the cells growing in successive wells were fixed in 10% trichloroacetic acid for 30 min at 4 °C, washed with water and dried. Fixed cells were incubated with 0.4% sulforhodamine B (SRB; Sigma-Aldrich) in 1% acetic acid for 20 min at RT. After washing with 1% acetic acid, the protein-bound dye was extracted with 10 mM Tris. Absorbance at 492 nm was measured on an EnSpire 2300 Multilabel Reader (Perkin-Elmer, Waltham, MA, USA). Data are presented as mean ± SD from two independent assays.

Apoptotic assays

Caspase-3 activation was determined using the CaspGLOW fluorescein active caspase-3 staining kit (BioVision, Milpitas, CA, USA) according to the manufacturer's instructions. The cells were seeded in six-well plates (Greiner) at a density of 5×10^5 cells/ml. The following day, the cells were treated with three different concentrations (0.1, 0.5 and 1 μM) of doxorubicin hydrochloride (Pfizer, New York, NY, USA) for 48 h. The cells previously harvested by trypsinisation and centrifuged at 300 × g for 5 min were incubated with 1 μl of FITC-DEVD-FMK peptide for 45 min at 37 °C in an incubator with 5% CO_2. The cells were then washed twice before being subjected to FACS analysis. Fluorescence was measured in FL-1 on the BD FACSCalibur (Becton-Dickinson). Data were processed and analysed using Flowing Software version 2.

Apoptosis was also measured by FITC-Annexin V and propidium iodide (PI) staining using the FITC Annexin V Apoptosis Detection Kit (Becton-Dickinson) according to the manufacturer's instructions. Cells were subjected to fluorescence analysis using the BD FACSCalibur (Becton-Dickinson) and Flowing Software version 2. The percentage of Annexin V-positive cells corresponded to cells in early apoptosis, while Annexin V and PI-positive cells corresponded to cells in late apoptosis.

Flow adhesion assay

Adhesion under laminar flow conditions of human breast cancer MDA-MB-231 cells to P-selectin-expressing or E-selectin-expressing CHO cells was quantified using a parallel plate flow chamber [22]. P-selectin-expressing CHO-Pro5 cells, E-selectin-expressing CHO cells and control CHO cells were grown to confluence in the presence of complete αMEM on Permanox™ eight-well chamber slides (Nunc, Roskilde, Denmark). On the day of the experiment, the slides containing a monolayer of cells were assembled in the flow chamber (250 μm gap thickness; Immunetics, Boston, MA, USA), and placed on the stage of an inverted microscope (NiconN 2000TS, Tokyo, Japan) equipped with 200× objective lenses.

In the first stage, P-selectin-expressing or E-selectin-expressing CHO cells and control CHO cells were subjected to a fluid shear flow of 1 dyn/cm^2 formed by an infusion PHD 2000 pump (Harvard Apparatus, Holliston, MA, USA) for 5 min, with complete αMEM medium at room temperature. In the second stage (adhesion assay), human breast cancer cells were suspended in αMEM medium and stained with CellTracker dye (Molecular Probes, Eugene, OR, USA) at a concentration of 0.5 mg/ml for 1 h at 37 °C. After washing, cancer cells (10^6/ml cells) were re-suspended in complete αMEM, injected into the flow chamber and allowed to roll on CHO cell monolayers. Interacting cells were defined as those that rolled in the field of view. Those cells were quantified in a single 200× field of view of 0.2 mm^2, during a 5-s perfusion. Fluid shear flow was changed every 5 min in increasing order of 0.15, 0.3, 0.6, 1.0, 1.5, and 3 dyn/cm^2. Data were processed using Iris software (MEDI.COM, Wroclaw, Poland).

Platelet isolation and activation

Human platelets were isolated from whole blood according to the Springer Lab Protocol (Springer Lab separation of platelets from whole blood by Azucena Salas, Springer Lab, The CBR Institute for Biomedical Research, Inc., Boston, MA, USA). Briefly, peripheral blood from healthy volunteer donors was collected into citrate solution (BD Biosciences). Tubes were centrifuged and the upper phase, platelet-rich plasma (PRP), was transferred to a new tube containing ACD buffer (6.25 g sodium citrate·2 H_2O, 3.1 g citric acid anhydrous, and 3.4 g D-glucose in 250 ml H_2O) at a ratio of 9:1. The sample was centrifuged again at 900 × g for 5 min at RT and the platelet pellet was resuspended in 1 ml of Hepes-Tyrode buffer. Freshly isolated platelets were used within 2 h.

Platelets (10^6 platelets/ml), resuspended in Hepes-Tyrode buffer, were activated by incubation for 5 min at 37 °C with 1 μM or 5 μM ADP (Sigma-Aldrich) in ultrapure DEPC water. P-selectin expression on the platelet surfaces, analysed by flow cytometry, was used as an indicator of activation. Platelets that were not activated served as negative controls. Only single platelet suspensions, distinguished from platelet aggregates by their light-scattering properties, were subjected to flow cytometry analysis.

Platelet aggregation assay

Platelet aggregation was monitored on a U-5100 UV-Vis Ratio-Beam Spectrophotometer (Hitachi, Ibraki Prefecture, Japan) via the modified turbidimetric method described originally by Born [23]. Platelets (10^6 platelets/ml) suspended in Hepes-Tyrode buffer were activated with 1 μM or 5 μM of ADP and the formation of aggregates was analysed at 37 °C for 1 min with constant stirring (100 × g) for 500 s. The spectrophotometer was calibrated with an unstimulated suspension of platelets (10^6 platelets/ml) in Hepes-Tyrode buffer representing 0% aggregation, with the suspension of activated platelets (10^6/ml) in Hepes-Tyrode buffer (platelet-rich plasma, PRP) representing 100% aggregation [24].

The effect of sulfatide on the aggregation of platelets was studied by incubating sulfatide-expressing breast cancer cells (10^6 cells/ml) and platelets (10^6 platelets/ml) in a ratio of 1:1, at 37 °C for 1 min with constant stirring (100 × g) in the presence of ADP (1 μM and 5 μM) for 500 s.

Evaluation of immunohistochemistry reactions

The immunohistochemistry (IHC) reactions were evaluated by two independent pathologists using a BX-41 light microscope (Olympus, Tokyo, Japan). Expression of GAL3ST1 in tumour cells was evaluated using the semi-quantitative immunoreactive score (IRS) according to Remmele and Stegner [25]. The scoring system comprised the percentage of positively stained cells (0, no reaction; 1, < 10%; 2, 11–50%; 3, 51–80%; and 4, > 81% cells), as well as the intensity of staining (graded as 0 = no reaction, 1 = weak, 2 = moderate and 3 = strong staining). The lack of IHC GAL3ST1 expression (0 points using the IRS scale) was considered negative, and 1–12 points using the

IRS scale was considered positive expression. The median of IRS GAL3ST1 expression was established as the cut-off point for the aforementioned analysis. The same cut-off points (0 vs 1–12) was considered in the analysis of survival.

Terminal transferase dUTP nick end labelling assay

The apoptotic terminal transferase dUTP nick end labelling (TUNEL) assay was performed using the ApopTag® Peroxidase In Situ Apoptosis Detection Kit (Merck Millipore). Paraffin sections were de-waxed in xylene, rehydrated in alcohol, rinsed in distillate water and washed with PBS (pH 7.4). The sections were then incubated with Proteinase K (Dako) for 5 min at RT and rinsed in PBS. Endogenous peroxidase was blocked by incubation in 3% H_2O_2/PBS for 5 min. Next, the sections were incubated, first with Equilibration Buffer for 10 min at RT and then with TdT enzyme and reaction buffer at 37 °C for 1 h. The reaction was stopped using a stop buffer, and anti-digoxigenin peroxidase-conjugated antibodies were applied for 30 min at RT. To visualise the TUNEL-positive cell nuclei, the sections were incubated for 10 min with di-aminobenzidine (Dako). Finally, the sections were counterstained with Mayer's haematoxylin and after dehydration in alcohols mounted in SUB-X Mounting Medium (both Dako). TUNEL-positive cell nuclei expression in tumour cells was evaluated using a BX-41 light microscope equipped with the computer-assisted image analysis program Cell^D (Olympus). Three fields with the highest number of tumour cells yielding positive reaction (hot spots) were selected for every stained section and then analysed. The general result for every section was the average of the three hot-spot percentages of cells showing a brown reaction product.

Statistical analysis

All statistical analyses were performed using Prism 5.0 (GraphPad, La Jolla, CA, USA) and Statistica 10 (Stat-Soft Inc. Tulsa, OK, USA). The Shapiro–Wilk test was used to evaluate the normality assumption of examined groups. The paired t test was used for statistical analysis of in-vivo tumour growth experiments. The Mann–Whitney test was used to compare the groups of data that did not meet the assumptions of the parametric test. Additionally, the Spearman correlation test was used to analyse the existing correlations. The Kaplan–Meyer method was used to construct survival curves. To evaluate the survival analysis, the Mantel–Cox test was performed. A Cox proportional hazards model with forward stepwise selection was used to calculate univariate and multivariate hazard ratio for the studied parameters. In all analyses, the results were considered statistically significant when $p < 0.05$.

To statistically evaluate the significance of differences between Cer and HexCer levels obtained by MS analysis,

a one-way analysis of variance (ANOVA) test was performed. The p-value significance threshold was set at 0.01 due to a relatively low number of measured replicates.

Results

Accumulation of sulfatides in breast cancer cells correlates with increased sensitivity to doxorubicin-induced and hypoxia-induced apoptosis

We have previously shown that galactosylceramide (GalCer) increases the resistance of breast cancer MDA-MB-231 cells to doxorubicin-induced apoptosis [14]. Since GalCer is a precursor molecule in the synthesis of sulfatide, we wondered how the conversion of GalCer to sulfatide would affect the apoptotic properties of breast cancer cells. First, we examined the expression of GAL3ST1 and sulfatides in breast cancer MCF7, T47D, SKBR3, BT-474 and MDA-MB-231 cell lines. Neither galactosylceramide sulfotransferase nor sulfatides were detected in the metastatic MDA-MB-231 cells (Fig. 1a–c). Based on these results, MDA-MB-231 cells were used to create a model with overexpression of sulfatide, representing a gain-of-function phenotype. On the other hand, T47D cells with high expression of GAL3ST1 were chosen to obtain cells with inhibited synthesis of sulfatide, representing a loss-of-function phenotype. Transduction of MDA-MB-231 cells with the pRRL-CMV-GAL3ST1-IRES-PURO expression vector containing cDNA for GAL3ST1 resulted in a cell population that overexpressed sulfotransferase and sulfatide (Fig. 1d, e and Additional file 3: Figure S1A). These cells that had the same morphology and growth rate as appropriate control cells were called MDA.SUL cells (Additional file 3: Figure S1B).

In order to stably and irreversibly inhibit the expression of GAL3ST1 and therefore block the synthesis of sulfatides, we created a CRISPR-edited knockout of *GAL3ST1* in T47D cells. After transfection and selection with puromycin, 20 resistant clones were isolated, propagated and screened for the absence of GAL3ST1. Western blotting analysis demonstrated that three of these clones lacked GAL3ST1 expression on the protein level. Since they had the same morphology and proliferation rate, one of the clones was randomly chosen, named T47D.Δ.GAL3ST1.1, and used in further studies (Fig. 1f and Additional file 3: Figure S1C, D). Immunostaining of gangliosides purified from T47D.Δ.GAL3ST1.1 cells with anti-sulfatide antibody revealed the absence of sulfatide in these cells (Fig. 1g). A clone of T47D cells transduced with the control CRISPR/Cas9 plasmid encoding the Cas9 nuclease and non-specific 20 nt guide RNA (gRNA), called T47D.GAL3ST1.C, was obtained using the same approach.

To assess whether the accumulation of sulfatides can affect the sensitivity of breast cancer cells to drug-induced apoptosis, MDA.SUL and control MDA.C cells were incubated with doxorubicin for 48 h. We found that after doxorubicin treatment, the percentage of apoptotic cells was 4.2-fold higher in MDA.SUL cells than in MDA.C cells ($p < 0.05$) (Fig. 2a). We also analysed the sensitivity of modified cells to apoptosis under hypoxic conditions and observed that the percentage of apoptotic MDA.SUL cells was 3.5-fold higher than for MDA.C cells ($p < 0.01$) (Fig. 2a). We confirmed these results through the analysis of the loss-of-function phenotype. When T47D.Δ.GAL3ST1.1 cells and control T47D cells were treated with doxorubicin or subjected to hypoxic conditions, control T47D.GAL3ST1.C cells were more sensitive to apoptosis than T47D.Δ.GAL3ST1.1 cells by 2.2-fold ($p < 0.05$) and 3.8-fold ($p < 0.05$), respectively (Fig. 2b). The results obtained using the CaspGLOW fluorescein active caspase-3 staining kit were further confirmed through staining the apoptotic cells with FITC-Annexin V and PI. In the gain-of-function cellular model, the percentage of all (early and late) apoptotic cells was higher in MDA.SUL cells than in MDA.C cells by 3.4-fold after doxorubicin treatment and by 2.3-fold in hypoxic conditions (Fig. 2c). However, in doxorubicin-treated and hypoxia-treated T47D.Δ.GAL3ST1.1 cells, representing the loss-of-function cellular model, the percentage of all (early and late) apoptotic cells decreased compared to control T47D cells by 1.5-fold and 2.7-fold, respectively (Fig. 2d). Based on these results we questioned whether the pro-apoptotic effects of sulfatide accumulation could be linked to decreased amounts of anti-apoptotic GalCer [14] since the latter is the substrate for sulfotransferase. Immunostaining of neutral glycosphingolipids purified from MDA.SUL cells revealed highly decreased binding of anti-GalCer antibodies to HP-TLC plates compared to neutral glycosphingolipids from MDA.C and parental MDA-MB-231 cells (Fig. 2e). These results obtained using MDA.SUL cells were further supported by our second cellular model represented by T47D cells with knockout of the GAL3ST1. In such cells, an increased level of GalCer compared to control T47D.GAL3ST1.C and wild-type T47D was observed as a consequence of blocked sulfatide synthesis (Fig. 2f). These data raised the possibility that the reduced level of GalCer is a result of decreased expression of UGT8 or of increased conversion of GalCer to sulfatide caused by overexpression of GAL3ST1. Therefore, we analysed the expression of the UGT8. We did not find any differences between analysed cells at the mRNA or protein level (Fig. 2g, h), which strongly suggests that changes in GalCer levels are associated with enhanced synthesis of sulfatide.

Sulfatide inhibits tumour growth

To determine whether the increased synthesis of sulfatides can affect the malignant phenotype of breast

cancer cells, MDA.SUL and MDA.C cells were subcutaneously injected into nude mice. Statistically significant reductions in tumour volumes were observed in MDA.SUL tumours compared to tumours formed by MDA.C cells (Fig. 3a). In week 11, the mean volume of tumours developed by MDA.SUL cells was 28.95 mm^3, and the mean volume of tumours formed by MDA.C cells was 63.26 mm^3. Since the expression of sulfatide in breast cancer cells affects their sensitivity to apoptosis (see earlier), the apoptotic properties of MDA.SUL and MDA.C cells were analysed in vivo by TUNEL assay (Fig. 3b). Increased numbers of apoptotic cells were found in MDA.SUL tumours (Fig. 3b, I) compared to MDA.C tumours (Fig. 3b, II) ($p = 0.0494$, Mann–Whitney U test).

The anti-apoptotic effects of GalCer are not associated with changes in ceramide levels

We hypothesised previously that the anti-apoptotic effects of GalCer in breast cancer cells with high expression of UGT8 are associated with decreased levels of pro-apoptotic ceramide acting as a cellular regulator controlling cell fate by promoting cell survival [14, 15]. To quantify the amounts of ceramide in breast cancer cells with high and low expression of UGT8, we modified and applied a previously described HILIC-MS/MS methodology [26] involving monitoring of the characteristic ion at 264 m/z, a product of fragmentation of both Cer and HexCer (hexosyl-ceramide) but not oligosaccharide substituted ceramides. This method allowed us to relatively quantify Cer and HexCer in the following cell lines: control MDA/LUC cells with high expression of UGT8 and MDA/LUC-shUGT8 cells with suppressed expression of UGT8 [14], control T47D/PURO cells with no expression of UGT8 and T47D/PURO-UGT8 cells with overexpression of UGT8 (Additional file 3: Figure S1E, F). We found that HexCer levels are affected by the presence or absence of UGT8 as expected, while Cer levels do not differ significantly (Fig. 4). It must be noted that the concentration of free ceramide is almost two orders of magnitude greater than the concentration of HexCer. This may explain why a major alteration of HexCer levels does not significantly influence the Cer pool. Moreover, an almost complete absence of signals corresponding to hexosyl-ceramide in the T47D/PURO cell line, naturally not expressing UGT8, and highly decreased levels of hexosyl-ceramide-derived signals in MDA/LUC-shUGT8 cells with inhibited synthesis of GalCer strongly suggest that the HexCer pool consists mainly of galactosylceramide.

Sulfatide is responsible for binding breast cancer cells to P-selectin-expressing CHO cells and activated human platelets

It was proposed that sulfatides present on the surface of breast cancer cells are P-selectin ligands [12]. However,

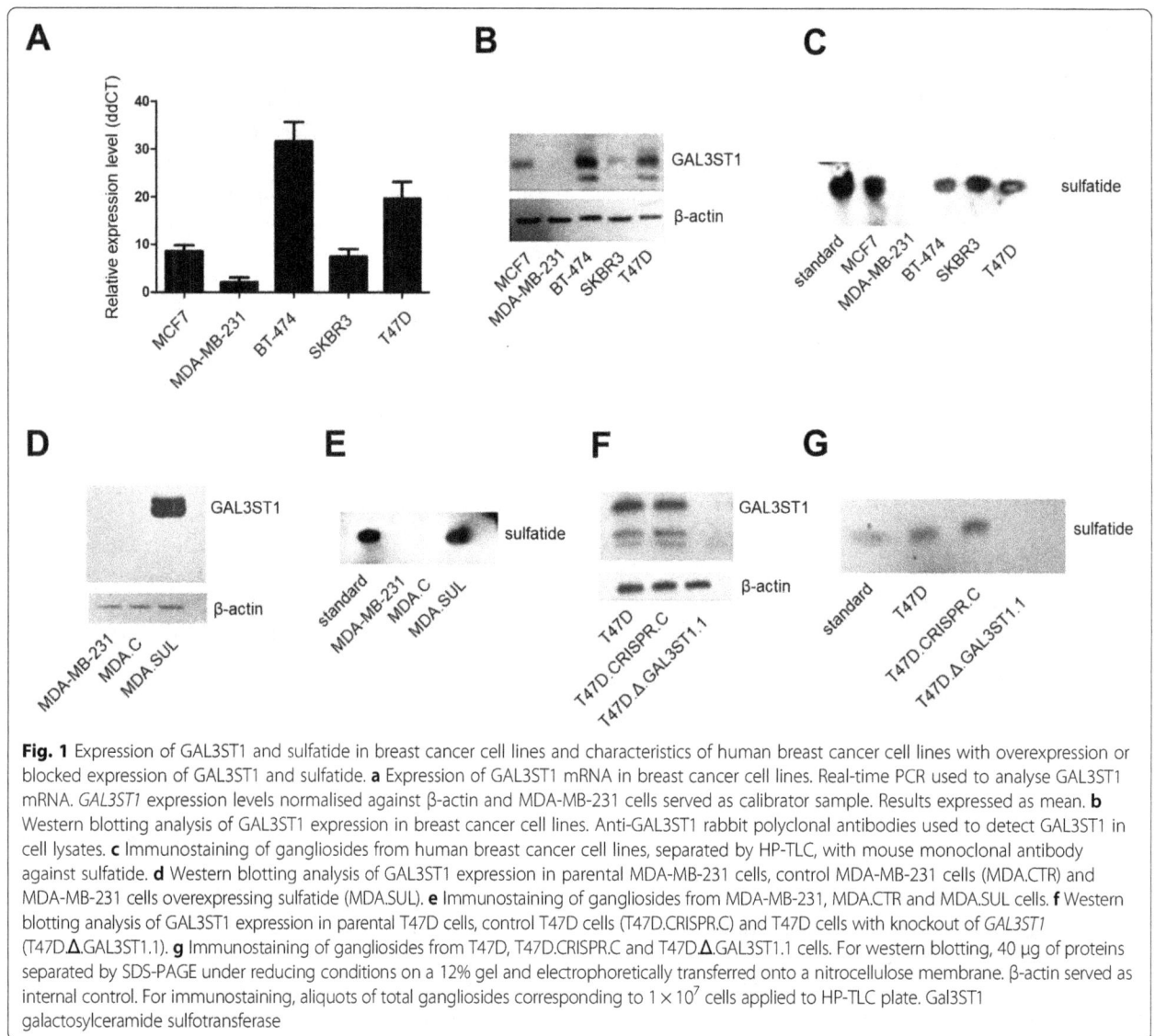

Fig. 1 Expression of GAL3ST1 and sulfatide in breast cancer cell lines and characteristics of human breast cancer cell lines with overexpression or blocked expression of GAL3ST1 and sulfatide. **a** Expression of GAL3ST1 mRNA in breast cancer cell lines. Real-time PCR used to analyse GAL3ST1 mRNA. *GAL3ST1* expression levels normalised against β-actin and MDA-MB-231 cells served as calibrator sample. Results expressed as mean. **b** Western blotting analysis of GAL3ST1 expression in breast cancer cell lines. Anti-GAL3ST1 rabbit polyclonal antibodies used to detect GAL3ST1 in cell lysates. **c** Immunostaining of gangliosides from human breast cancer cell lines, separated by HP-TLC, with mouse monoclonal antibody against sulfatide. **d** Western blotting analysis of GAL3ST1 expression in parental MDA-MB-231 cells, control MDA-MB-231 cells (MDA.CTR) and MDA-MB-231 cells overexpressing sulfatide (MDA.SUL). **e** Immunostaining of gangliosides from MDA-MB-231, MDA.CTR and MDA.SUL cells. **f** Western blotting analysis of GAL3ST1 expression in parental T47D cells, control T47D cells (T47D.CRISPR.C) and T47D cells with knockout of *GAL3ST1* (T47DΔGAL3ST1.1). **g** Immunostaining of gangliosides from T47D, T47D.CRISPR.C and T47DΔGAL3ST1.1 cells. For western blotting, 40 μg of proteins separated by SDS-PAGE under reducing conditions on a 12% gel and electrophoretically transferred onto a nitrocellulose membrane. β-actin served as internal control. For immunostaining, aliquots of total gangliosides corresponding to 1×10^7 cells applied to HP-TLC plate. Gal3ST1 galactosylceramide sulfotransferase

there is a lack of direct experimental evidence supporting this hypothesis. Therefore, the binding of breast cancer cells with neoexpression of sulfatide to P-selectin-expressing cells was studied under physiologic flow conditions. Since selectin-expressing CHO cells are a good experimental model to study ligands for selectins [17, 27], their interaction with sulfatide-expressing MDA.SUL cells and control MDA.C cells was analysed. At applied fluid shear stresses of 0.6 and 1.0 dyn/cm², which are similar to conditions found in microcirculation and postcapillary venules [28], MDA.SUL cells rolled in considerable numbers (30 and 36, respectively) on a monolayer of P-selectin-expressing CHO cells (Fig. 5a, Additional file 4: Figure S2A, Additional file 5: Video S1). In contrast, MDA.C cells did not interact with P-selectin-expressing CHO cells at any of the flow rates (Fig. 5b). Additional evidence for a specific interaction of breast cancer cells

with P-selectin came from control experiments in which parental or E-selectin-expressing CHO cells were used (Additional file 4: Figure S2B, Additional file 6: Video S2). None of the analysed breast cancer cell lines interacted with such cells.

The interaction between sulfatides and platelet P-selectin is critical for the formation of stable cancer cell–platelet aggregates, which in turn facilitates metastases [11, 29]. Here, we showed that breast cancer cells expressing sulfatide can aggregate activated human platelets in vitro, in a process called tumour cell-induced platelet aggregation (TCIPA). For this purpose, aggregation of ADP-activated platelets in the presence of MDA.SUL, MDA.C and parental MDA-MB-231 cells was examined. A significant effect of MDA.SUL cells on the aggregation of platelets after activation with 1 μM and 5 μM of ADP was observed compared to aggregation curves obtained

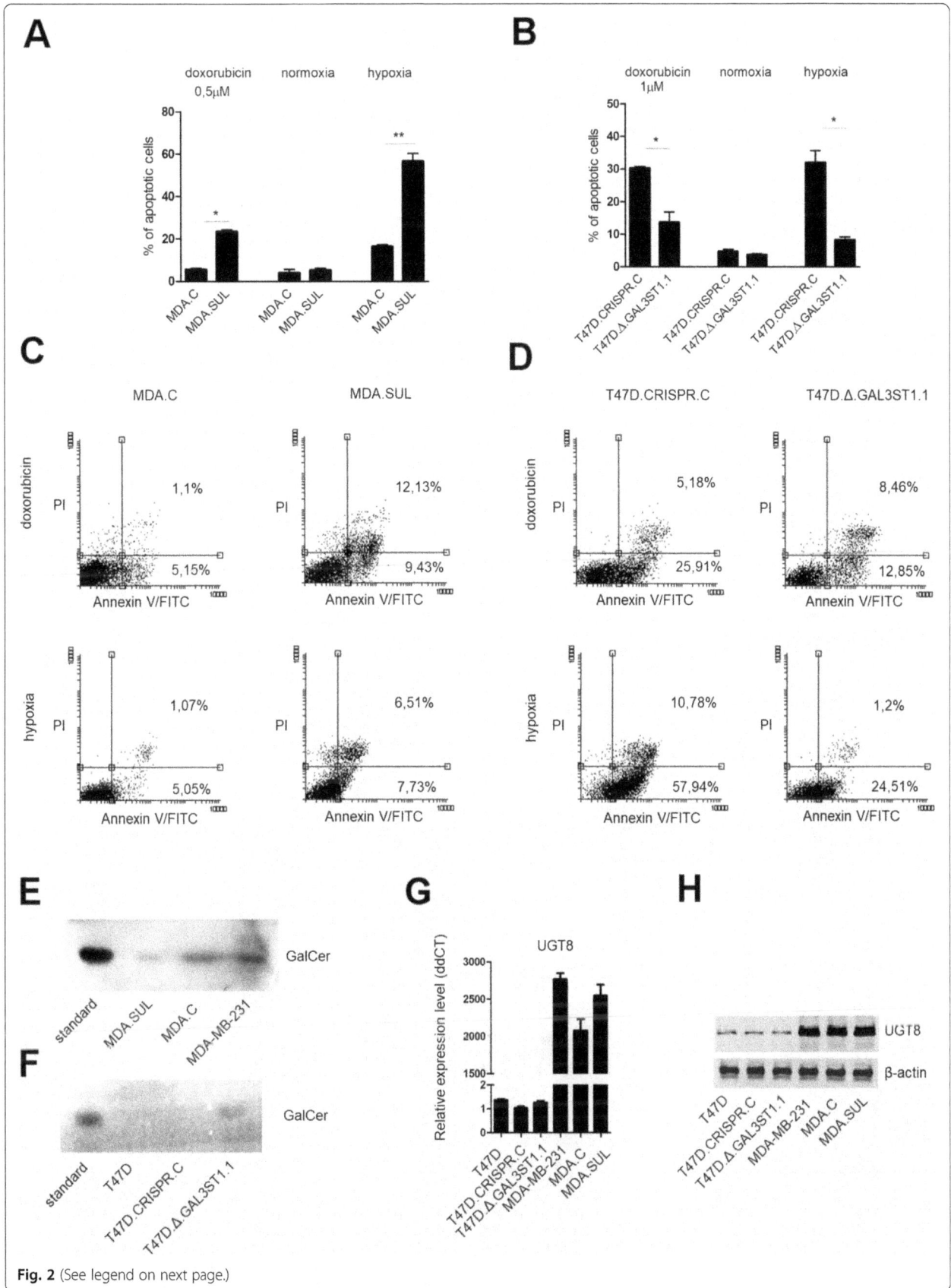

Fig. 2 (See legend on next page.)

(See figure on previous page.)

Fig. 2 Sensitivity of breast cancer MDA-MB-231 and T47D cells with varying expression of GAL3ST1 to apoptosis induced by doxorubicin and hypoxia. Cells grown in presence of doxorubicin at concentration of 0.5 μM (MDA-MB-231 cells) or 1 μM (T47D) and in hypoxic conditions (1% O_2) for 48 h. Cellular response measured by presence of active form of caspase-3 (**a, b**) or staining with Annexin V and propidium iodide (**c, d**). Statistically significant differences (**$p < 0.01$, *$p < 0.05$). Flow cytometry dot plots show percentage of early apoptotic cells (Annexin V$^+$/PI$^-$, lower right) and late apoptotic cells (Annexin V$^+$/PI$^+$, upper right). Levels of galactosyloceramide (GalCer) and UGT8 in MDA-MB-231 and T47D cells with varying expression of GAL3ST1. Immunostaining of neutral glycolipids from MDA-MB-231, MDA.C and MDA.SUL cells (**e**) and from T47D, T47D.CRISPR.C and T47D.Δ.GAL3ST1.1 cells (**f**) separated by HP-TLC. For immunostaining, aliquots of neutral glycosphingolipids corresponding to 1×10^7 cells applied to HP-TLC plate and stained with anti-GalCer rabbit polyclonal antibodies. **g** Real-time PCR used to analyse expression of UGT8 mRNA in MDA-MB-231 and T47D cell lines with varying expression levels of sulfatide. UGT8 levels normalised against β-actin and T47D.CRISPR.C cells assigned as calibrator sample. Results expressed as mean. **h** Western blotting analysis of UGT8 expression in breast cancer cell lines with different expression levels of sulfatide. Anti-UGT8 rabbit polyclonal antibodies used to detect UGT8 in cell lysates. FITC fluorescein isothiocyanate, GalCer galactosyloceramide, PI propidium iodide

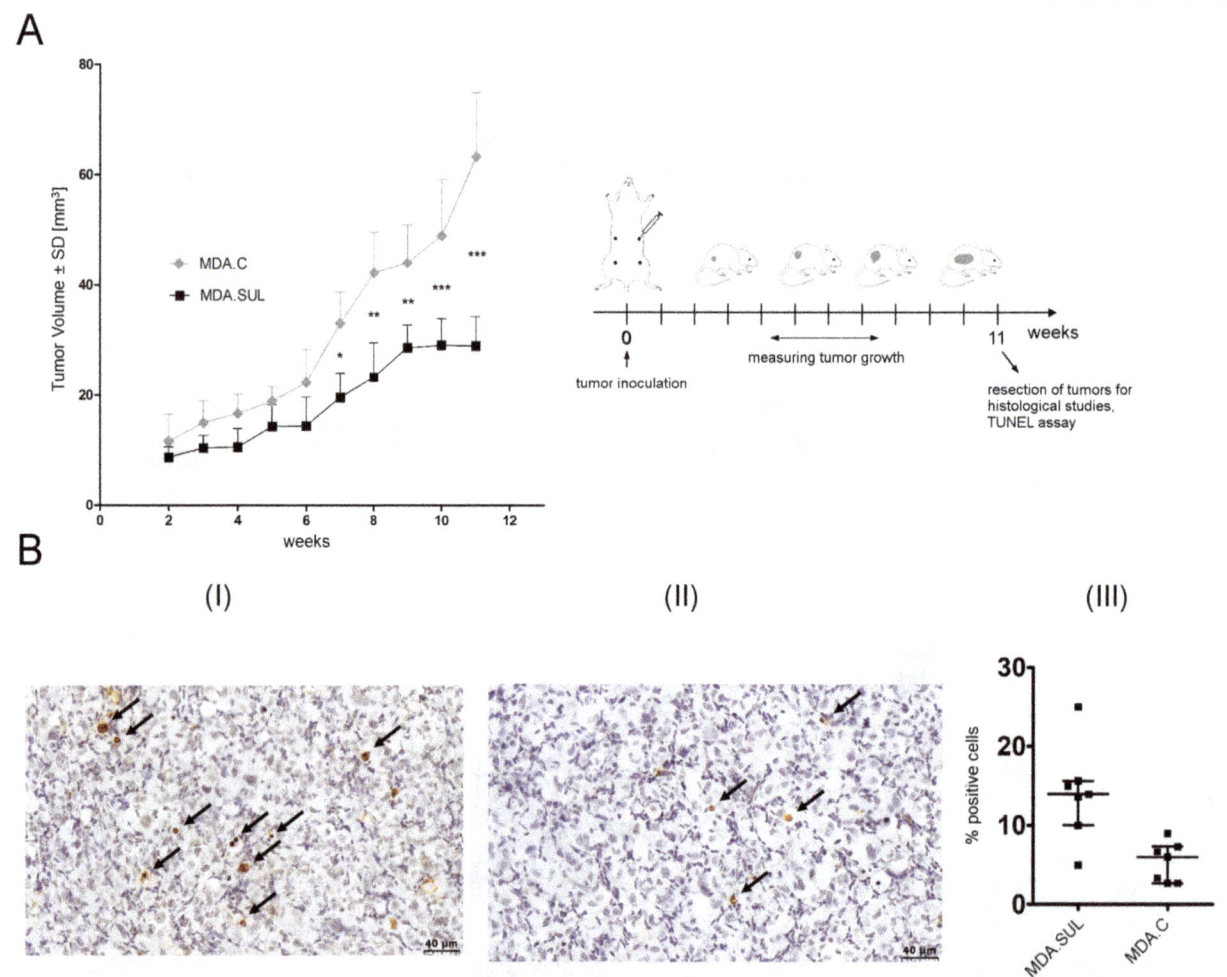

Fig. 3 Xenograft tumour growth of MDA.SUL cells with overexpression of GAL3ST1 and control MDA.C cells. **a** Tumour growth recorded once a week by measuring diameter with a calliper. Data shown as mean tumour volume for group of mice ($n = 8$ for MDA.SUL cells and $n = 9$ for MDA.C cells) ± SE at each indicated time point. Data analysed using Bonferroni multiple comparison test. *$p < 0.05$, **$p < 0.01$, ***$p < 0.001$. **b** TUNEL assay after subcutaneous implantation of MDA.SUL (I) and MDA.C (II) cells. Arrows indicate the apoptotic cells. Numbers of apoptotic cells in MDA.SUL and MDA.C tumours compared (III) by Mann–Whitney U test ($p = 0.0494$). TUNEL terminal transferase dUTP nick end labelling

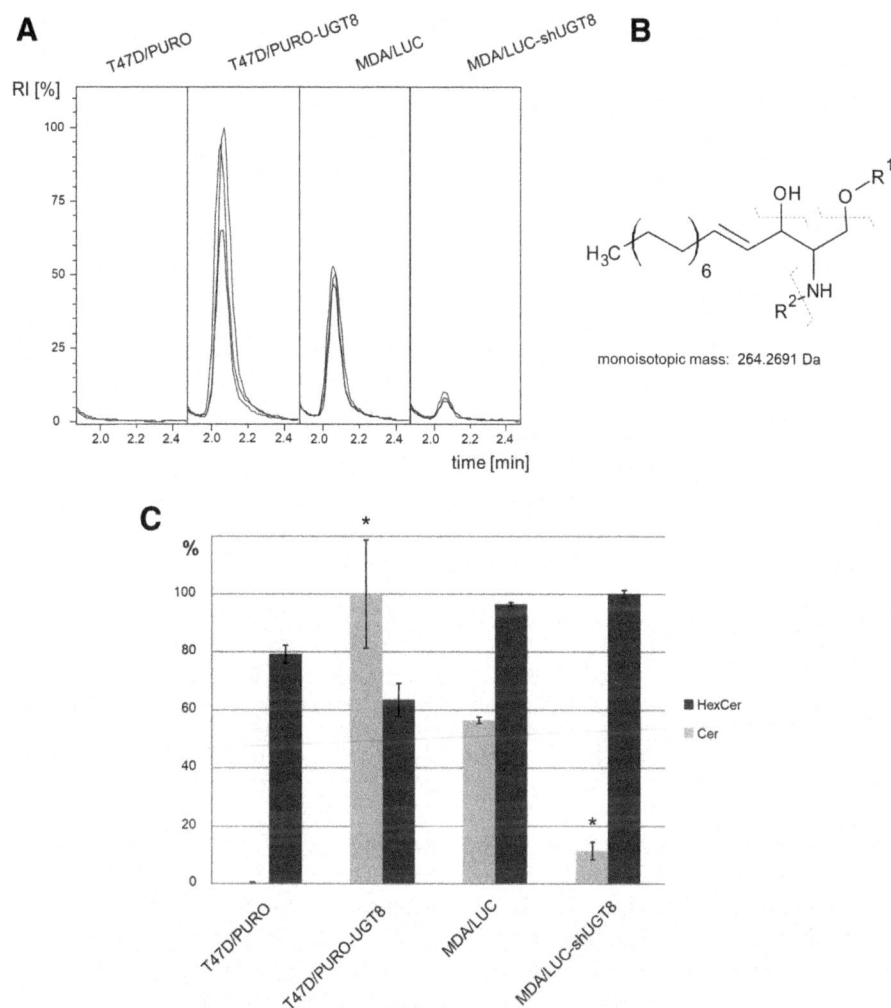

Fig. 4 Relative quantification of ceramides in selected cell lines. **a** Extracted ion chromatograms for 264.269 ± 001 m/z in cell line samples with peak at RT = 2.1 min corresponding to HexCer. RI stands for Relative Intensity. **b** Structure of reporter ion selected for relative quantification. **c** Relative quantities of Cer (dark grey) and HexCer (light grey) in breast cancer cell lines. 100% value corresponds to highest concentration of particular analyte. Error bars represent standard deviations of three biological replicates. Statistically significant differences (*$p < 0.01$) in analyte levels

for activated platelets incubated with MDA.C cells (Figs. 5c–e). These data suggest that increased aggregation of activated platelets is caused by the formation of heterotypic aggregates between platelets and tumour cells expressing sulfatide on their surface. The presence of such mixed aggregates was confirmed by flow cytometry. When breast cancer cells and platelets were labelled with fluorescence dyes DiD and DiO, respectively, considerable amounts of heterotypic tumour cell–platelet aggregates were found only in MDA.SUL cells (Figs. 6a, b).

Sulfatides present on breast cancer cells increase the expression of P-selectin in activated platelets

Merten et al. [10] showed that sulfatide is not only a ligand for P-selectin, but its presence on the surface of

platelets affects the activation of neighbouring platelets by increasing P-selectin expression. Therefore, we assessed the presence of P-selectin on the surface of activated platelets treated with ADP and found that treated platelets expressed high amounts of P-selectin (Additional file 7: Figure S3). Importantly, when activated platelets treated with 1 μM ADP were incubated with MDA.SUL cells, a subpopulation of cells with highly increased P-selectin expression was observed (Fig. 6d). Such a cell subpopulation was not observed when activated platelets were incubated with parental MDA-MB-231 and MDA.C cells. It should be stressed that the activated effect of sulfatide present on the surface of breast cancer cells was observed only in partially activated platelets since incubation of MDA.SUL cells

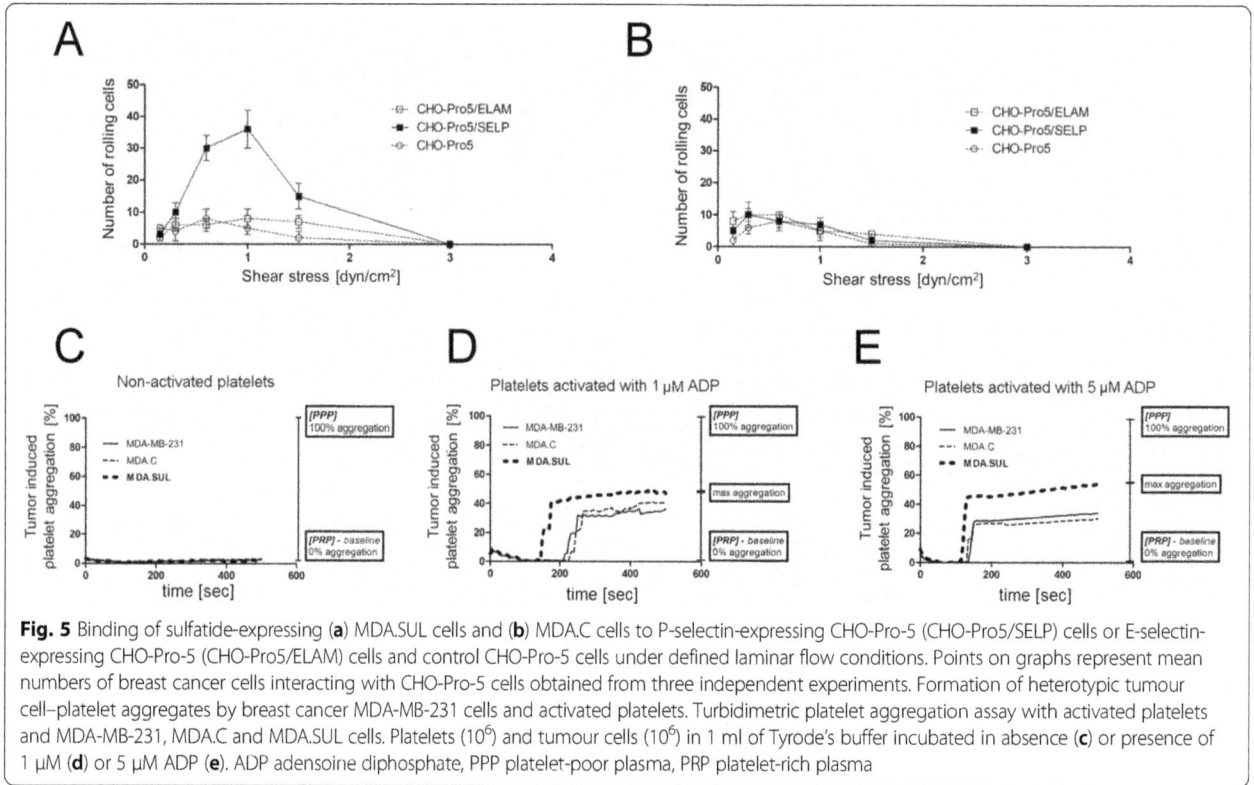

Fig. 5 Binding of sulfatide-expressing (**a**) MDA.SUL cells and (**b**) MDA.C cells to P-selectin-expressing CHO-Pro-5 (CHO-Pro5/SELP) cells or E-selectin-expressing CHO-Pro-5 (CHO-Pro5/ELAM) cells and control CHO-Pro-5 cells under defined laminar flow conditions. Points on graphs represent mean numbers of breast cancer cells interacting with CHO-Pro-5 cells obtained from three independent experiments. Formation of heterotypic tumour cell–platelet aggregates by breast cancer MDA-MB-231 cells and activated platelets. Turbidimetric platelet aggregation assay with activated platelets and MDA-MB-231, MDA.C and MDA.SUL cells. Platelets (10^6) and tumour cells (10^6) in 1 ml of Tyrode's buffer incubated in absence (**c**) or presence of 1 μM (**d**) or 5 μM ADP (**e**). ADP adensoine diphosphate, PPP platelet-poor plasma, PRP platelet-rich plasma

with resting platelets has no effect on the surface expression of P-selectin. Incubation of ADP (5 μM) activated platelets demonstrating very high P-selectin expression levels with MDA.SUL cells did not increase P-selectin expression (Fig. 6e). Our data indicate that sulfatide expressed by cancer cells is not only a ligand for P-selectin, but also plays a role as a regulatory factor affecting P-selectin expression in activated platelets.

Expression of GAL3ST1 in invasive ductal carcinoma and its correlation with patients' clinical and pathological data

The expression of GAL3ST1 in paraffin sections of invasive ductal carcinoma (IDC) specimens was studied using IHC (Fig. 7a, b). Positive cytoplasmic expression of GAL3ST1 was observed in tumour cells in 127 (54.74%) of the 232 examined cases. Higher expression of GAL3ST1 was observed in less aggressive G1 tumours than in highly aggressive G3 tumours (Mann Whitney test, $p < 0.01$; Fig. 7c). However, there were no significant associations with the expression of GAL3ST1 and other clinicopathological data (pTNM, stage, ER, PR and HER2 statuses, molecular subtypes or age at diagnosis).

To validate the predictive ability of GAL3ST1 positivity in primary breast tumours, the expression of GAL3ST1 was analysed in our cohort of breast cancer patients by IHC. Analysis of the survival rate revealed that GAL3ST1 expression in IDC cells is associated with longer overall survival (OS) (Fig. 7d, Table 2). Using cellular models, we

have shown that high expression of GAL3ST1 is associated with increased sensitivity to doxorubicin-induced apoptosis. Accordingly, a similar type of analysis was performed only for breast cancer patients who received chemotherapy. We observed a correlation between GAL3ST1 immunoreactivity in cancer cells in these chemotherapy-treated breast cancer patients. However, this was not statistically significant with the overall survival rate (Fig. 7e, Table 2).

Discussion

It is firmly established that neoplastic transformation and tumour progression are almost invariably associated with changes in the expression of surface glycosphingolipids representing ganglio-series, globo-series, lacto-series and neolacto-series [30, 31]. However, there is limited information on the role played by galactosphingolipids, including sulfatides, in human cancer progression [11, 14, 29]. Therefore, the present study was undertaken to evaluate the role of sulfatides in the malignancy-related properties of breast cancer cells. In this respect, our recent findings on the role of GalCer in breast cancer progression are of special interest [14]. We showed that GalCer affects the tumourigenic and metastatic properties of breast cancer cells as an anti-apoptotic molecule. Based on these data, we hypothesised that GalCer facilitates tumour cells to survive in the hostile tumour microenvironment [14, 32]. Since GalCer is a substrate for GAL3ST1 and a precursor

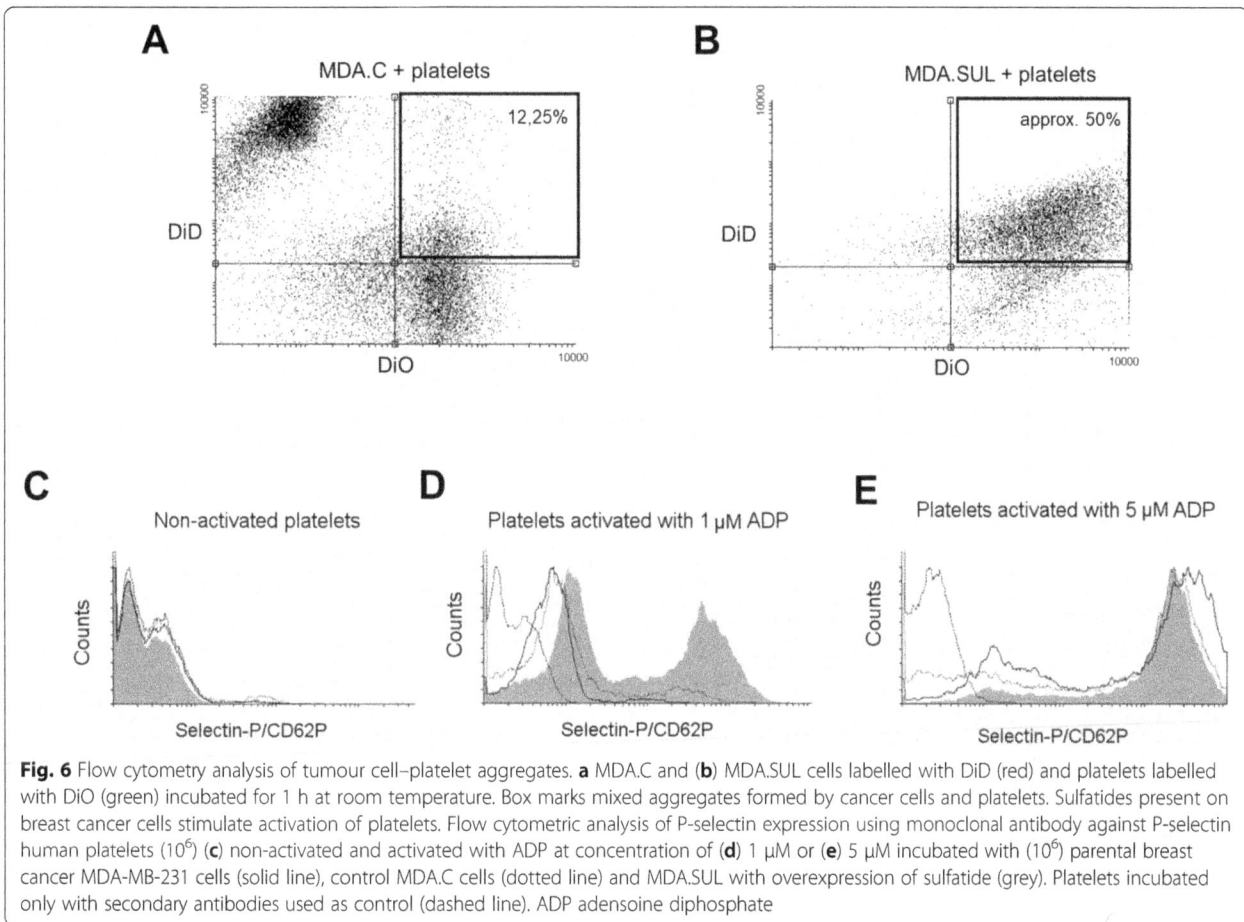

Fig. 6 Flow cytometry analysis of tumour cell–platelet aggregates. **a** MDA.C and (**b**) MDA.SUL cells labelled with DiD (red) and platelets labelled with DiO (green) incubated for 1 h at room temperature. Box marks mixed aggregates formed by cancer cells and platelets. Sulfatides present on breast cancer cells stimulate activation of platelets. Flow cytometric analysis of P-selectin expression using monoclonal antibody against P-selectin human platelets (10^6) (**c**) non-activated and activated with ADP at concentration of (**d**) 1 μM or (**e**) 5 μM incubated with (10^6) parental breast cancer MDA-MB-231 cells (solid line), control MDA.C cells (dotted line) and MDA.SUL with overexpression of sulfatide (grey). Platelets incubated only with secondary antibodies used as control (dashed line). ADP adensoine diphosphate

molecule for sulfatide, in the present study we analysed the resistance of breast cancer MDA-MB-231 cells with overexpression of sulfatide (MDA.SUL) cells and sulfatide-negative control MDA-MB-231 (MDA.C) cells to doxorubicin-induced and hypoxia-induced apoptosis. We found that MDA.SUL cells were more sensitive to apoptosis than MDA.C cells. Therefore, we quantified the amounts of GalCer in both cell types, and observed that overexpression of GAL3ST1 substantially decreased GalCer levels in breast cancer cells by increased synthesis of sulfatides, which strongly reinforces the importance of GalCer as an anti-apoptotic molecule. This hypothesis was further supported by our "loss-of-function" cellular model. T47D cells with knockout of the *GAL3ST1* demonstrated increased levels of GalCer and increased resistance to doxorubicin-induced and hypoxia-induced apoptosis. Our results suggested that sulfatide may act as a "pro-apoptotic molecule", therefore an in-vivo study was undertaken to evaluate the role of sulfatide in breast cancer progression. When MDA.SUL and MDA.C cells were subcutaneously injected into athymic nu/nu mice, control MDA-MB-231 cells formed tumours more efficiently than MDA.SUL cells. Furthermore, immunohistochemical staining of tumour specimens revealed that accumulation

of sulfatide is associated with significantly higher numbers of apoptotic cells. This correlates with data obtained using MDA-MB-231 cells with high expression of GalCer, which were significantly more tumourigenic than MDA/LUC-shUGT8 cells with decreased expression of UGT8 [14].

In our earlier study [14], we hypothesised that the anti-apoptotic effects of GalCer are associated with increased conversion of ceramide to GalCer, resulting in a decreased intracellular pool of ceramide as one of the key pro-apoptotic molecules [15]. However, the quantification of ceramide in breast cancer cells with high (MDA/LUC cells) and low (MDA/LUC-shUGT8 cells) production of GalCer revealed that both cell types contain essentially the same amounts of ceramide. Therefore, our data suggest that in breast cancer cells, glycosylation of ceramide is not a major mechanism ensuring resistance of cancer cells to drug-induced apoptosis [33]. Instead, it is likely that the key anti-apoptotic molecule in breast cancer cells is GalCer by itself since its conversion to sulfatide is directly associated with highly increased sensitivity to pro-apoptotic agents. Taken together, we propose that an increased level of sulfatide in breast cancer cells is a limiting factor in breast cancer progression. This contradicts other studies

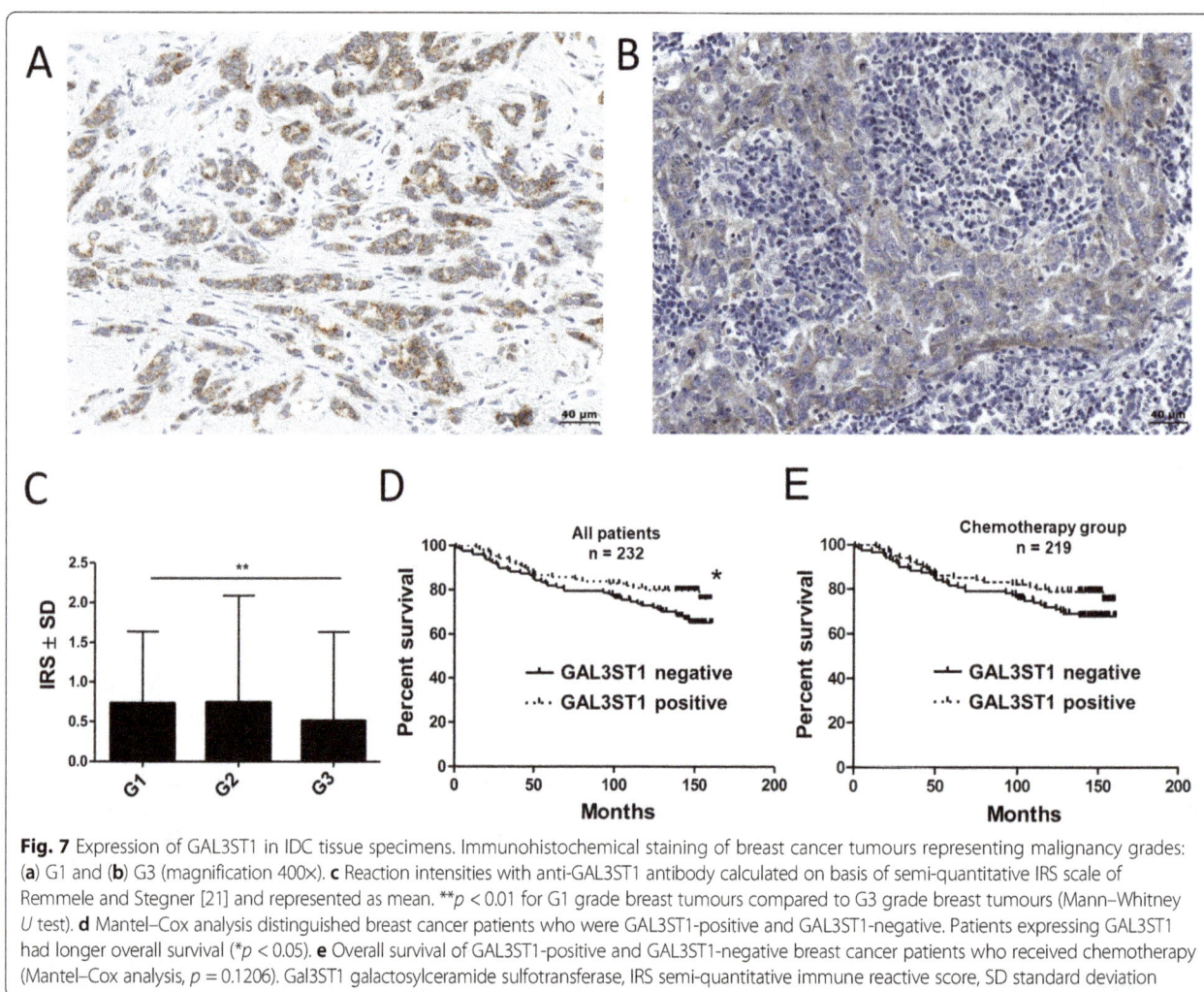

Fig. 7 Expression of GAL3ST1 in IDC tissue specimens. Immunohistochemical staining of breast cancer tumours representing malignancy grades: (**a**) G1 and (**b**) G3 (magnification 400×). **c** Reaction intensities with anti-GAL3ST1 antibody calculated on basis of semi-quantitative IRS scale of Remmele and Stegner [21] and represented as mean. **$p < 0.01$ for G1 grade breast tumours compared to G3 grade breast tumours (Mann–Whitney U test). **d** Mantel–Cox analysis distinguished breast cancer patients who were GAL3ST1-positive and GAL3ST1-negative. Patients expressing GAL3ST1 had longer overall survival (*$p < 0.05$). **e** Overall survival of GAL3ST1-positive and GAL3ST1-negative breast cancer patients who received chemotherapy (Mantel–Cox analysis, $p = 0.1206$). Gal3ST1 galactosylceramide sulfotransferase, IRS semi-quantitative immune reactive score, SD standard deviation

showing that sulfatides contribute to the malignant phenotype of cancer cells as ligands for P-selectin supporting their binding to platelets and endothelial cells [10, 12]. Therefore, to address this discrepancy, we evaluated the sulfatides expressed by breast cancer cells as adhesion molecules for endothelial and platelet P-selectin. Shear flow experiments showed for the first time that sulfatides expressed on the surface of tumour cells mediate their rolling on P-selectin-expressing cells, and do not interact with E-selectin-expressing cells. The role of sulfatides in P-selectin-mediated platelet aggregation was studied intensively [10, 34]. In murine colon cancer cells, it was shown that their removal from the cell surface decreases the formation of cancer cell–platelet aggregates, which leads to attenuation of blood-borne experimental metastases [11]. To assess the role of sulfatide in the formation of heterotypic aggregates, MDA.-SUL and MDA.C cells were incubated with activated human platelets. Only MDA.SUL cells formed aggregates with P-selectin-expressing platelets. Importantly, when partially ADP-activated platelets were mixed with

MDA.SUL cells, elevated expression of P-selectin was observed in comparison to ADP-activated platelets alone. These data are in agreement with studies showing that the treatment of platelets with exogenous sulfatides led to additional platelet aggregation and further P-selectin expression [10]. However, we have shown for the first time that sulfatide-rich tumour cells can mediate the same activating effect. Based on these results we speculate that additional activation of platelets will enhance platelet–tumour cell aggregation contributing to cancer metastasis [35–38].

Since earlier studies showed that sulfatides are malignancy-related adhesive molecules [11] and the present findings suggest that sulfatides act as pro-apoptotic molecules, we propose the following hypothesis (Fig. 8). In a primary tumour, cancer cells rich in sulfatides are more prone to apoptosis induced by microenvironmental stressors such as hypoxia, since increased synthesis of this glycolipid decreases the amounts of precursor GalCer, which acts as an anti-apoptotic molecule. However, when such cancer

Table 2 Univariate and multivariate Cox analysis of survival

Parameter	Overall survival					
	Univariate Cox analysis			Multivariate Cox analysis		
	HR	95% CI	p value	HR	95% CI	p value
Age						
≤ 50 years	**4.172**	**1.673–10.402**	**0.002**	**3.767**	**1.500–9.461**	**0.005**
> 50 years						
Tumour grade						
G1	1.235	0.887–1.719	0.212			
G2						
G3						
Tumour size						
pT1	**1.028**	**1.010–1.045**	**0.002**	**2.012**	**1.469–2.754**	**< 0.0001**
pT2						
pT3						
pT4						
Lymph nodes						
pN0	**1.921**	**1.010–1.045**	**0.038**	**2.294**	**1.295–4.065**	**0.004**
pN1–pN3						
pNx						
pM						
M0	**11.48**	**1.399–90.427**	**0.023**	7.378	0.936–58.136	0.058
M1						
Stage						
I	**1.025**	**1.006–1.045**	**0.010**	**0.512**	**0.374–0.701**	**< 0.0001**
II						
III						
IV						
Oestrogen receptor						
Negative	1.009	0.999–1.019	0.078			
Positive						
Progesterone receptor						
Negative	0.991	0.972–1.010	0.355			
Positive						
HER2						
Negative	1.002	0.983–1.021	0.847			
Positive						
Molecular tumour types						
Triple negative	1.400	0.612–3.200	0.425			
Other types						
GAL3ST1						
Negative (0)	**0.595**	**0.354–0.999**	**0.046**	0.604	0.351–1.038	0.068
Positive (1–12)						
GAL3ST1 chemotherapy subgroup						
Negative (0)	0.659	0.388–1118	0.112			
Positive (1–12)						

Bold values (p < 0.05) are statistically significant
CI confidence interval, Gal3ST1 galactosylceramide sulfotransferase, HR hazard ratio, HER2 human epidermal growth factor receptor 2

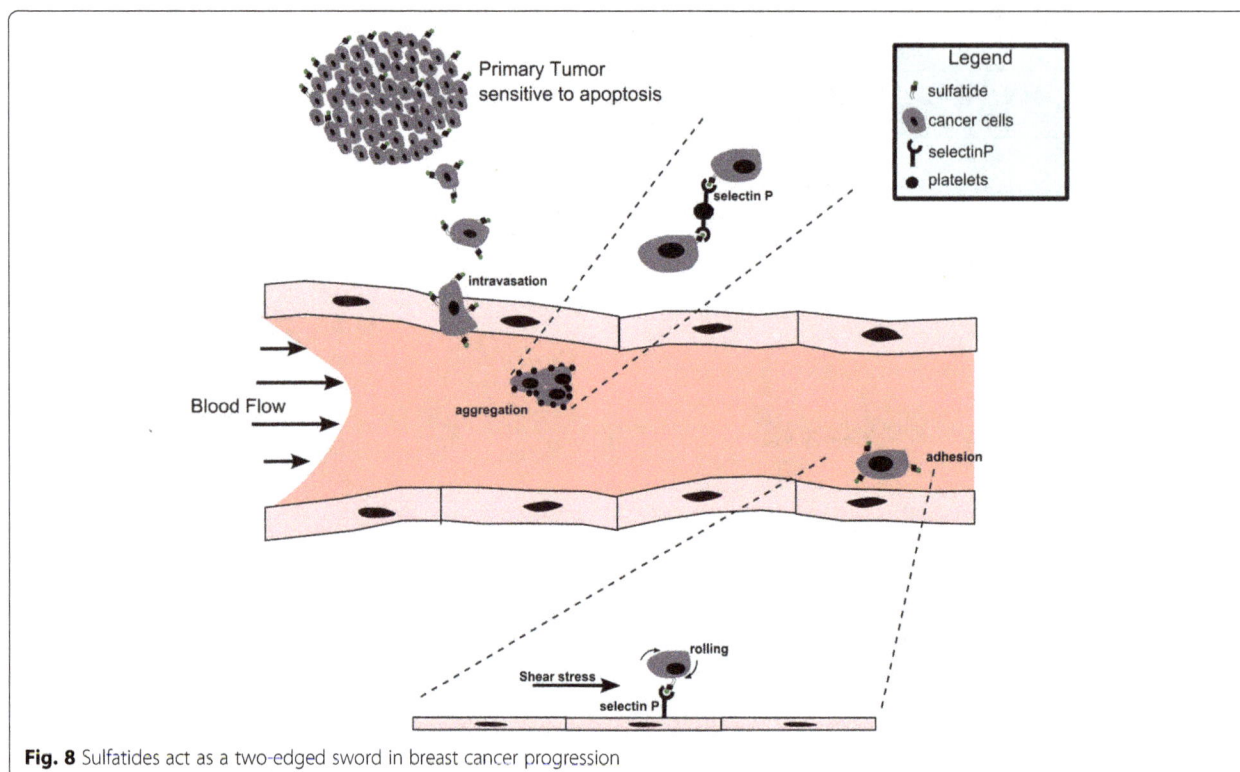

Fig. 8 Sulfatides act as a two-edged sword in breast cancer progression

cells escape from the primary tumour and invade lymphatic or blood vessels, sulfatides present on their surface act as adhesive molecules, facilitating cancer cell interactions with platelets and endothelial cells, which in turn increases their metastatic potential. Our proposal based on experimental data is supported by a clinical study with IDC patients. Using IHC, we showed that the expression of GAL3ST1 decreased with tumour malignancy grade with significant differences in GAL3ST1 expression in G1 vs G3 tumours, and that high expression of GAL3ST1 in IDC cells is associated with longer OS of patients. These results suggest that elevated GAL3ST1 levels may be associated with better prognosis.

Conclusions

We have shown for the first time that sulfatides are not only involved in adhesion of cancer cells, acting as ligands for P-selectin expressed by endothelial cells and platelets, but they also contribute to programmed cell death, acting as "pro-apoptotic molecules", making cancer cells more prone to environmental stressors such as hypoxia and anticancer drugs such as doxorubicin. Our data strongly suggest that sulfatides are not directly involved in apoptotic processes but changes in their metabolism affect the amounts of GalCer precursor; for example, increased synthesis of sulfatides decreases the amounts of GalCer,

which acts directly as an anti-apoptotic molecule [14]. Therefore our findings, which are in full agreement with the hypothesis that the balance between specific sphingolipid species is a critical rheostat for regulation of cellular apoptosis [15], highlight the importance of the sulfatide–galactosylceramide rheostat in cancer progression. Our data also suggest that both molecules can be new targets for breast cancer treatment based on the reversal of tumour cell resistance to microenvironmental-induced and drug-induced apoptosis.

Additional files

Additional file 1: Table S1. Primers used in this study (DOCX 40 kb)

Additional file 2: Table S2. Antibodies used in this study (DOCX 31 kb)

Additional file 3: Figure S1. (A) Expression of GAL3ST1 mRNA in MDA-MB-231, MDA.CTR and MDA.SUL cells. Real-time PCR used to analyse GAL3ST1 mRNA. GAL3ST1 levels normalised against β-actin and MDA-MB-231 cells served as calibrator sample. Results expressed as mean. **(B)** Proliferation of MDA.C and MDA.SUL cells determined using SRB assay. Values shown as mean of six independent replicates. **(C)** Scheme and sequencing results for PCR products of GAL3ST1 guide RNA (gRNA-bolded) targeting exon 2 in human GAL3ST1. Protospacer-adjacent motif (PAM) sequence underlined. Arrows indicate locations of PCR primers (F1: CAGCGTCCTGCTCTCCA, R1: TCACCACCGCAGGAAATC). **(D)** Proliferation of T47D.CRISPR.C and T47DΔGAL3ST1.1 cells determined using SRB assay. Values shown as mean of six independent replicates. **(E)** Western blotting analysis of UGT8 expression in parental T47D cells, control T47D/PURO transduced with pRRL-CMV-IRES-PURO vector alone and T47D/PURO-UGT8 cells transduced with pRRL-CMV-UGT8-IRES-PURO vector containing UGT8 cDNA. **(F)** Immunostaining of neutral glycolipids from T47D, T47D/PURO and T47D/PURO-UGT8 cells separated by HP-TLC with anti-GalCer rabbit polyclonal antibodies (PDF 529 kb)

Additional file 4: Figure S2. Binding of sulfatide-expressing MDA.SUL cells to (**A**) P-selectin-expressing CHO-Pro-5 (CHO-Pro/SELP) cells or (**B**) E-selectin-expressing CHO-Pro-5 (CHO-Pro/SELE) cells under flow conditions. CHO cells (dark background) and MDA.SUL cells subjected to fluid shear flow of 1 dyn/cm^2 and rolling cells shown by numbered arrows. Each image captured every 0.5 s during 5-s perfusion. Corresponding movies added as Additional files 6 and 7 (PDF 506 kb)

Additional file 5: Video S1. Binding of sulfatide-expressing MDA.SUL cells to P-selectin-expressing CHO-Pro-5 cells (MP4 290 kb)

Additional file 6: Video S2. Binding of sulfatide-expressing MDA.SUL cells to E-selectin-expressing CHO-Pro-5 cells (MP4 383 kb)

Additional file 7: Figure S3. Expression of P-selectin on surface of human platelets (10^6 platelets) activated with ADP at concentration 1 μM (grey) or 5 μM (black). Degree of platelet activation monitored by analysis of P-selectin expression using flow cytometry and monoclonal antibody against P-selectin. Expression level of selectin P in activated platelets determined relative to non-activated platelets (solid line) (PDF 50 kb)

Abbreviations
Gal3ST1: Galactosylceramide sulfotransferase; GalCer: Galactosyloceramide; HILIC: Hydrophilic interaction liquid chromatography; IDC: Invasive ductal carcinoma; IHC: Immunohistochemistry; IRS: Semi-quantitative immune reactive score; SM4: Sulfatide; SRB: Sulforhodamine B; TLC: Thin-layer chromatography; TUNEL: Terminal transferase dUTP nick end labelling

Funding
Publication was supported by Wrocław Centre of Biotechnology, Leading National Research Centre (KNOW) for 2014–2018.

Authors' contributions
JS designed and implemented experiments, analysed data and wrote the paper. JG designed and implemented data analysis. TO performed data analyses and wrote the paper. PP performed the experiments. AP performed the experiments, and designed and implemented data analysis. BK performed the experiments. AN performed the experiments. PD designed experiments, analysed data and supervised work. AW provided resources. MU designed experiments, analysed data, supervised work and wrote the paper. All authors read and approved the final manuscript.

Competing interests
The authors declare that they have no competing interests.

Author details
[1]Department of Biochemistry and Molecular Biology, Faculty of Veterinary Medicine, Wroclaw University of Environmental and Life Sciences, C.K. Norwida 31, 50-375 Wroclaw, Poland. [2]Department of Histology and Embryology, Wroclaw Medical University, Wroclaw, Poland. [3]EIT+ Wroclaw Research Center, Wroclaw, Poland. [4]Laboratory of Glycobiology, Hirszfeld Institute of Immunology and Experimental Therapy, Polish Academy of Sciences, Wroclaw, Poland. [5]Department of Physiotherapy, Wroclaw University School of Physical Education, Wroclaw, Poland. [6]Lower Silesian Oncology Center, Wroclaw, Poland. [7]Present address: Department of Medicine, Herbert Irving Comprehensive Cancer Center, Columbia University Medical Center, New York, NY, USA.

References
1. Siddiqui B, Whitehead JS, Kim YS. Glycosphingolipids in human colonic adenocarcinoma. J Biol Chem. 1978;253(7):2168–75.
2. Kiguchi K, Takamatsu K, Tanaka J, Nozawa S, Iwamori M, Nagai Y. Glycosphingolipids of various human ovarian tumors: a significantly high expression of I3SO3GalCer and Lewis antigen in mucinous cystadenocarcinoma. Cancer Res. 1992;52(2):416–21.
3. Liu Y, Chen Y, Momin A, Shaner R, Wang E, Bowen NJ, Matyunina LV, Walker LD, McDonald JF, Sullards MC, et al. Elevation of sulfatides in ovarian cancer: an integrated transcriptomic and lipidomic analysis including tissue-imaging mass spectrometry. Mol Cancer. 2010;9:186.
4. Hattori H, Uemura K, Taketomi T. The presence of blood group A-active glycolipids in cancer tissues from blood group O patients. Biochim Biophys Acta. 1981;666(3):361–9.
5. Sakakibara N, Gasa S, Kamio K, Makita A, Koyanagi T. Association of elevated sulfatides and sulfotransferase activities with human renal cell carcinoma. Cancer Res. 1989;49(2):335–9.
6. Hiraiwa N, Fukuda Y, Imura H, Tadano-Aritomi K, Nagai K, Ishizuka I, Kannagi R. Accumulation of highly acidic sulfated glycosphingolipids in human hepatocellular carcinoma defined by a series of monoclonal antibodies. Cancer Res. 1990;50(10):2917–28.
7. Yoda Y, Gasa S, Makita A, Fujioka Y, Kikuchi Y, Hashimoto M. Glycolipids in human lung carcinoma of histologically different types. J Natl Cancer Inst. 1979;63(5):1153–60.
8. Morichika H, Hamanaka Y, Tai T, Ishizuka I. Sulfatides as a predictive factor of lymph node metastasis in patients with colorectal adenocarcinoma. Cancer. 1996;78(1):43–7.
9. Makhlouf AM, Fathalla MM, Zakhary MA, Makarem MH. Sulfatides in ovarian tumors: clinicopathological correlates. Int J Gynecol Cancer. 2004;14(1):89–93.
10. Merten M, Beythien C, Gutensohn K, Kuhnl P, Meinertz T, Thiagarajan P. Sulfatides activate platelets through P-selectin and enhance platelet and platelet-leukocyte aggregation. Arterioscler Thromb Vasc Biol. 2005;25(1):258–63.
11. Garcia J, Callewaert N, Borsig L. P-selectin mediates metastatic progression through binding to sulfatides on tumor cells. Glycobiology. 2007;17(2):185–96.
12. Aruffo A, Kolanus W, Walz G, Fredman P, Seed B. CD62/P-selectin recognition of myeloid and tumor cell sulfatides. Cell. 1991;67(1):35–44.
13. Takahashi T, Suzuki T. Role of sulfatide in normal and pathological cells and tissues. J Lipid Res. 2012;53(8):1437–50.
14. Owczarek TB, Suchanski J, Pula B, Kmiecik AM, Chadalski M, Jethon A, Dziegiel P, Ugorski M. Galactosylceramide affects tumorigenic and metastatic properties of breast cancer cells as an anti-apoptotic molecule. PLoS One. 2013;8(12):e84191.
15. Bieberich E. Integration of glycosphingolipid metabolism and cell-fate decisions in cancer and stem cells: review and hypothesis. Glycoconj J. 2004;21(6):315–27.
16. Lakhani SR, Ellis IO, Schnitt SJ, Tan PH, van de Vijver MJ. WHO Classification of Tumours of the Breast. 4th ed. IARC Press, 2012.
17. Klopocki AG, Laskowska A, Antoniewicz-Papis J, Duk M, Lisowska E, Ugorski M. Role of sialosyl Lewis(a) in adhesion of colon cancer cells—the antisense RNA approach. Eur J Biochem. 1998;253(1):309–18.
18. Suchanski J, Tejchman A, Zacharski M, Piotrowska A, Grzegrzolka J, Chodaczek G, Nowinska K, Rys J, Dziegiel P, Kieda C, et al. Podoplanin increases the migration of human fibroblasts and affects the endothelial cell network formation: a possible role for cancer-associated fibroblasts in breast cancer progression. PLoS One. 2017;12(9):e0184970.
19. Livak KJ, Schmittgen TD. Analysis of relative gene expression data using real-time quantitative PCR and the 2(−Delta Delta C(T)) method. Methods. 2001;25(4):402–8.
20. Solatycka A, Owczarek T, Piller F, Piller V, Pula B, Wojciech L, Podhorska-Okolow M, Dziegiel P, Ugorski M. MUC1 in human and murine mammary carcinoma cells decreases the expression of core 2 beta1,6-N-acetylglucosaminyltransferase and beta-galactoside alpha2,3-sialyltransferase. Glycobiology. 2012;22(8):1042–54.
21. Ugorski M, Pahlsson P, Dus D, Nilsson B, Radzikowski C. Glycosphingolipids of human urothelial cell lines with different grades of transformation. Glycoconj J. 1989;6(3):303–18.
22. Lawrence MB, McIntire LV, Eskin SG. Effect of flow on polymorphonuclear leukocyte/endothelial cell adhesion. Blood. 1987;70(5):1284–90.

23. Born GVR. Quantitative investigations into the aggregation of blood platelets. J Physiol. 1962;162:67–68.

24. Phillips D. Biochemistry of Platelets. 1st ed. Academic Press, 1986.

25. Remmele W, Stegner HE. Recommendation for uniform definition of an immunoreactive score (IRS) for immunohistochemical estrogen receptor detection (ER-ICA) in breast cancer tissue. Pathologe. 1987;8(3):138–40.

26. Scherer M, Leuthauser-Jaschinski K, Ecker J, Schmitz G, Liebisch G. A rapid and quantitative LC-MS/MS method to profile sphingolipids. J Lipid Res. 2010;51(7):2001–11.

27. Sawada R, Lowe JB, Fukuda M. E-selectin-dependent adhesion efficiency of colonic carcinoma cells is increased by genetic manipulation of their cell surface lysosomal membrane glycoprotein-1 expression levels. J Biol Chem. 1993;268(17):12675–81.

28. Konstantopoulos K, Kukreti S, McIntire LV. Biomechanics of cell interactions in shear fields. Adv Drug Deliv Rev. 1998;33(1–2):141–64.

29. Borsig L, Wong R, Hynes RO, Varki NM, Varki A. Synergistic effects of L- and P-selectin in facilitating tumor metastasis can involve non-mucin ligands and implicate leukocytes as enhancers of metastasis. Proc Natl Acad Sci U S A. 2002;99(4):2193–8.

30. Hauselmann I, Borsig L. Altered tumor-cell glycosylation promotes metastasis. Front Oncol. 2014;4:28.

31. Pinho SS, Reis CA. Glycosylation in cancer: mechanisms and clinical implications. Nat Rev Cancer. 2015;15(9):540–55.

32. Dziegiel P, Owczarek T, Plazuk E, Gomulkiewicz A, Majchrzak M, Podhorska-Okolow M, Driouch K, Lidereau R, Ugorski M. Ceramide galactosyltransferase (UGT8) is a molecular marker of breast cancer malignancy and lung metastases. Br J Cancer. 2010;103(4):524–31.

33. Ogretmen B. Sphingolipid metabolism in cancer signalling and therapy. Nat Rev Cancer. 2018;18(1):33–50.

34. Merten M, Thiagarajan P. Role for sulfatides in platelet aggregation. Circulation. 2001;104(24):2955–60.

35. Erpenbeck L, Schon MP. Deadly allies: the fatal interplay between platelets and metastasizing cancer cells. Blood. 2010;115(17):3427–36.

36. Stegner D, Dutting S, Nieswandt B. Mechanistic explanation for platelet contribution to cancer metastasis. Thromb Res. 2014;133(Suppl 2):S149–57.

37. Coupland LA, Parish CR. Platelets, selectins, and the control of tumor metastasis. Semin Oncol. 2014;41(3):422–34.

38. Hyslop SR, Josefsson EC. Undercover agents: targeting tumours with modified platelets. Trends Cancer. 2017;3(3):235–46.

21

Inflammation markers and cognitive performance in breast cancer survivors 20 years after completion of chemotherapy: a cohort study

Kimberly D. van der Willik[1,2], Vincent Koppelmans[1,2,3], Michael Hauptmann[1], Annette Compter[4], M. Arfan Ikram[2] and Sanne B. Schagen[1,5*]

Abstract

Background: Inflammation is an important candidate mechanism underlying cancer and cancer treatment-related cognitive impairment. We investigated levels of blood cell–based inflammatory markers in breast cancer survivors on average 20 years after chemotherapy and explored the relation between these markers and global cognitive performance.

Methods: One hundred sixty-six breast cancer survivors who received post-surgical radiotherapy and six cycles of adjuvant cyclophosphamide, methotrexate, and fluorouracil (CMF) chemotherapy on average 20 years before enrollment were compared with 1344 cancer-free women from a population-based sample (50–80 years old). Breast cancer survivors were excluded if they used adjuvant hormonal therapy or if they developed relapse, metastasis, or second primary malignancies. Systemic inflammation status was assessed by the granulocyte-to-lymphocyte ratio (GLR), platelet-to-lymphocyte ratio (PLR), and systemic immune-inflammation index (SII). Cognitive performance was assessed using an extensive neuropsychological test battery from which the general cognitive factor was derived to evaluate global cognitive performance. We examined the association between cancer, the general cognitive factor, and inflammatory markers using linear regression models.

Results: Breast cancer survivors had a lower general cognitive factor than non-exposed participants from the comparator group (mean difference = −0.21; 95% confidence interval (CI) −0.35 to −0.06). Inflammatory markers were higher in cancer survivors compared with non-exposed participants (mean difference for log(GLR) = 0.31; 95% CI 0.24 to 0.37, log(PLR) = 0.14; 95% CI 0.09 to 0.19, log(SII) = 0.31; 95% CI 0.24 to 0.39). The association between higher levels of inflammatory markers and lower general cognitive factor was statistically significant in cancer survivors but not among non-exposed participants. We found a group-by-inflammatory marker interaction; cancer survivors showed additional lower general cognitive factor per standard deviation increase in inflammatory markers (*P* for interaction for GLR = 0.038, PLR = 0.003, and SII = 0.033).

Conclusions: This is the first study to show that (1) cancer survivors have increased levels of inflammation on average 20 years after treatment and (2) these inflammatory levels are associated with lower cognitive performance. Although this association needs verification by a prospective study to determine causality, our findings can stimulate research on the role of inflammation in long-term cognitive problems and possibilities to diminish such problems.

Keywords: Breast cancer, Inflammation, Cognitive performance, Cancer/cancer treatment-related side effects

* Correspondence: s.schagen@nki.nl
[1]Department of Psychosocial Research and Epidemiology, Netherlands Cancer Institute, Plesmanlaan 121, 1066 CX Amsterdam, the Netherlands
[5]Brain and Cognition, Department of Psychology, University of Amsterdam, Nieuwe Achtergracht 129-B, 1018 WS Amsterdam, the Netherlands
Full list of author information is available at the end of the article

Background

Patients with cancer frequently report cognitive problems that can affect their quality of life and daily functioning substantially. Studies have shown that patients with non-central nervous system (non-CNS) cancer can experience cognitive problems during and after completion of treatment including chemotherapy, and a subgroup of patients had cognitive problems up to 20 years after treatment [1, 2].

The cancer survivor population is aging and growing because of increased life expectancy and more specifically because of advances in cancer treatment and improved screening. In turn, this results in an increasing number of cancer survivors coping with cognitive problems. The driving forces underlying these cognitive problems have not been sufficiently clarified, impeding the approach and process of developing effective interventions. Cognitive problems in patients with cancer could be induced by cancer itself, cancer-related treatment, or shared risk factors for the development of both cancer and cognitive problems [3, 4]. Disentangling the effects and mechanisms of these causes of disruption of normal cognitive performance is challenging. Different mechanisms, including genetic susceptibility, telomere shortening, changes in hormone levels, and inflammation, have been proposed and revealed [3].

In recent years, inflammation in particular has been suggested as an important and potentially intervenable mechanism in the pathogenesis of cognitive problems in patients with cancer. Higher levels of inflammatory factors such as cytokines are observed in patients with cancer prior to start of any treatment [5], during chemotherapy [6–10], and after chemotherapy [11, 12] up to 5 years after treatment initiation [13]. Several studies found an association between cytokines and cognitive impairment in patients with cancer across different cognitive domains, such as psychomotor speed [8], executive functioning [14], and memory [5, 10, 11, 13]. However, these studies did not agree on the involved cytokines or on the affected cognitive domain. Moreover, because the longest follow-up in these studies was 5 years, it remains unknown whether inflammation also has a role in longer-term or late cognitive problems. Filling this knowledge gap is important as insight into underlying causes of (long-term) cognitive impairment helps to identify those cancer patients at increased risk of developing cognitive problems and opens venues for preventive and therapeutic interventions.

Most studies examined the inflammation status by investigating cytokines using different cytokine panels [5, 6, 8–19]. In contemporary studies, systemic inflammatory response markers measured in blood, including the neutrophil-to-lymphocyte ratio (NLR), platelet-to-lymphocyte ratio (PLR), and systemic immune-inflammation index (SII), are increasingly used. These markers have reliable prognostic and predictive value in patients with cancer and can easily be calculated from readily available standard full blood examination, making them more convenient to use in a clinical setting [20–24]. If related to cognitive problems, these markers could potentially be used as biomarkers for cancer-related cognitive impairment.

In this study, we investigated global cognitive performance, levels of blood cell–based inflammatory markers, and their relation in breast cancer survivors who had received post-surgical radiotherapy and six cycles of adjuvant cyclophosphamide, methotrexate, and fluorouracil (CMF) chemotherapy on average more than 20 years previously. We furthermore examined whether inflammation and cognitive performance were differentially associated between breast cancer survivors and cancer-free women from a population-based sample.

Methods

Study population

In this study, we selected women who had survived breast cancer and had received adjuvant CMF chemotherapy. We compared them with women from the general population, who were cancer-free and had never received chemotherapy.

Breast cancer survivors

Women with a history of unilateral, invasive breast cancer were identified on the basis of registries of the Netherlands Cancer Institute in Amsterdam and the Daniel den Hoed Cancer Clinic of the Erasmus Medical Center in Rotterdam as described previously [2]. Briefly, women were selected if they had received post-surgical radiotherapy and six cycles of adjuvant CMF chemotherapy between 1976 and 1995.

Breast cancer survivors were eligible if they were 50–80 years old at the time of inclusion in 2008, if invasive breast cancer was their first and only malignancy, if they had not developed relapse or distant metastasis, if they had sufficient command of the Dutch language, and if they did not have any contraindications for magnetic resonance imaging (MRI). In addition, ever use of hormonal therapy was applied as an exclusion criterion. Because adjuvant hormonal therapy was not part of the standard treatment for patients with breast cancer in the Netherlands until the mid-1990s, only a few women received this treatment. To enhance homogeneity within the group of breast cancer survivors, we included hormone treatment-naïve cancer survivors only.

Three hundred fifty-nine breast cancer survivors were assessed for eligibility and 292 were selected. Of these 292 women, 196 agreed to participate and provided informed consent. We previously reported on cognitive performance of these survivors in comparison with cancer-free women identified within the Rotterdam Study [2]. For the present study, the following additional inclusion criteria were defined: availability of blood measurements and completeness of neuropsychological test data to calculate the general cognitive factor. Thirty of the 196 (15.3%) breast cancer survivors were excluded because of missing data on blood measurements ($n = 5$) and incomplete data of neuropsychological tests ($n = 25$, Fig. 1a). Because breast cancer survivors did not receive an extensive dementia screening, history of dementia was not applied as an exclusion criterion. However, based on the interviews with a trained psychologist, subjective memory complaints, cognitive tests, and brain MRI, it is unlikely that the included breast cancer survivors had dementia at the time of examinations.

Population-based non-exposed participants

Cancer-free women were selected from the Rotterdam Study, an ongoing population-based prospective cohort that started in 1990 in Rotterdam, the Netherlands. The main objective of the Rotterdam Study is to investigate risk factors of diseases in the elderly. By the end of 2008, the Rotterdam Study consisted of three subcohorts, comprising 14,926 individuals. The design of the Rotterdam Study was described in detail previously [25].

The third subcohort (RS-III) started in 2006 and was the first cohort in which an extensive set of neuropsychological tests was implemented at baseline. For this reason, RS-III was chosen as the reference subcohort, which was composed of 3392 participants (65% out of invitees). From these participants, women 50–80 years old without a history of cancer or dementia were eligible as non-exposed participants ($n = 1574$). This sample comprised the non-exposed participants used in our previous cognitive study [2]. Two hundred thirty persons were additionally excluded because of lack of blood measurements ($n = 39$) and incomplete data of

neuropsychological tests ($n = 191$), resulting in 1344 non-exposed participants (Fig. 1b).

Assessment of inflammatory markers

All participants had fasting blood samples taken during the research center visit. Full blood count measurements were performed by using a COULTER® Ac·T diff2™ Hematology Analyzer (Beckman Coulter, San Diego, CA, USA) directly after the blood sample was drawn. Hematologic measurements included absolute granulocyte, lymphocyte, and platelet counts in 10^9 per liter.

We used the granulocyte count as proxy for the neutrophil count because we did not have this measurement available in our sample. Because most of the granulocytes are represented by neutrophils, we believe this did not affect our results [26, 27]. For accuracy purposes, we will refer to the granulocyte-to-lymphocyte ratio (GLR) instead of using the term NLR.

The GLR and PLR were calculated as the ratio of granulocyte count to lymphocyte count and as the ratio of platelet count to lymphocyte count, respectively [28]. The SII was defined as platelet count times the GLR [22]. Because they are either ratios or indices, the derived inflammatory markers did not have a unit.

Assessment of cognitive performance

Cognitive performance was evaluated between November 2009 and June 2010 for breast cancer survivors and between February 2006 and December 2008 for non-exposed participants on the same day the blood sample was drawn. Cognitive performance was assessed by a neuropsychological battery in the research center of the Rotterdam Study. Six tests were administered: the Mini–Mental State Examination, Letter-Digit Substitution Test (LDST), Word Fluency Test (WFT), Stroop Test (reading, naming, and interference), Purdue Pegboard Test (PPB) (right, left, and both hands), and 15-Word Learning Test (15-WLT) (immediate recall, delayed recall, and recognition). Global cognitive

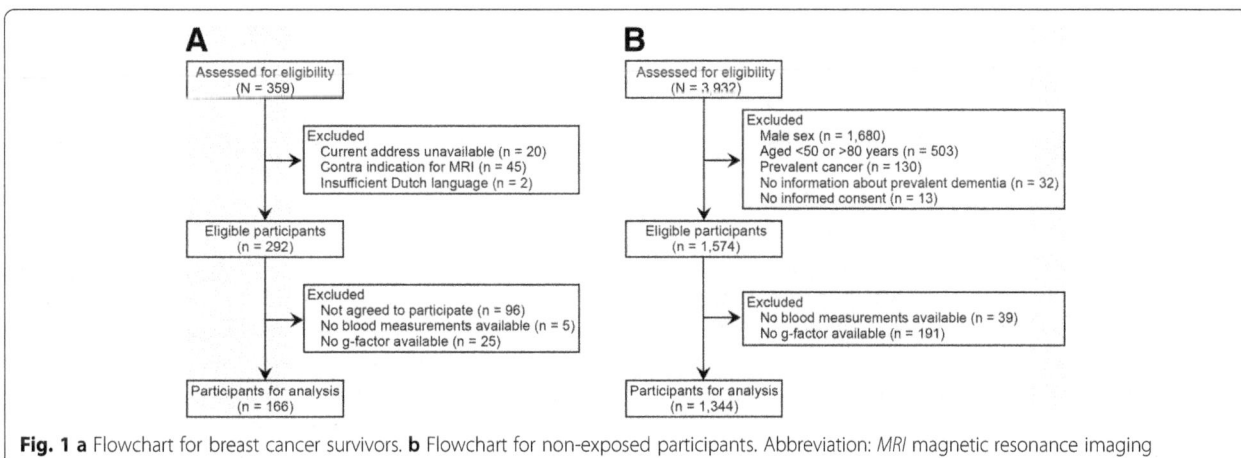

Fig. 1 a Flowchart for breast cancer survivors. **b** Flowchart for non-exposed participants. Abbreviation: *MRI* magnetic resonance imaging

performance was assessed via the general cognitive factor, which was generated by using principal component analysis of the following tests: LDST (total completion time), WFT (number of words), Stroop interference (time in seconds, adjusted for errors), PPB test (total number of pins across three subtasks), and 15-WLT (number of words during delayed recall) [29].

Other assessments

We assessed education level (primary: primary education; lower: lower general education, intermediate general education, or lower vocational education; intermediate: intermediate vocational education or higher general education; higher: higher vocational education or university) and smoking status (current, former, or never) by interview. Body mass index (BMI) (in kilograms per square meter) was computed from measurements of height and weight. Diabetes mellitus was defined as use of antidiabetic medication, a fasting serum glucose level of at least 7.1 mmol/L, or a random serum glucose level of at least 11.1 mmol/L [30]. History of stroke or myocardial infarction was assessed by interview [31, 32]. Symptoms of depression were evaluated with the Center for Epidemiologic Studies Depression scale (CES-D), which was converted to a sum-score [33]. We had no information about anxiety and fatigue and therefore could not control for these symptoms.

Statistical analyses

Linear regression models were used to investigate mean differences in the general cognitive factor and inflammatory markers between breast cancer survivors and non-exposed participants. Inflammatory markers were log-transformed because of their skewed distribution. We constructed two nested models: model I was adjusted for age (continuous) and education (four categories), and model II was additionally adjusted for smoking status (three categories), BMI (continuous), diabetes mellitus (yes/no), history of stroke (yes/no), history of myocardial infarction (yes/no), and CES-D sum-score (continuous). To investigate whether levels of the general cognitive factor were explained by different inflammatory markers, we adjusted additionally for each inflammatory marker separately.

The association between the general cognitive factor and inflammatory markers was investigated for breast cancer survivors and non-exposed participants using linear regression models. To study whether this association was stronger in breast cancer survivors than in non-exposed participants, we computed interaction terms between history of cancer/cancer treatment and each inflammatory marker. We explored effect modification by stratifying for mean BMI.

Since mean age was higher in the breast cancer survivors compared with the non-exposed participants (Table 1), we repeated all analyses using age-matched non-exposed participants to minimize residual confounding. These analyses provided estimates comparable to the analyses using all non-exposed participants and therefore are not reported separately.

Multiple imputation was used for missing data on covariates (generally between 0.07% and 0.3% with a maximum of 1.8% for the CES-D sum-score) with five imputed datasets, based on history of cancer/cancer treatment, inflammatory markers, general cognitive factor, and other covariates (that is, age, sex, education, BMI, smoking status, presence of diabetes mellitus, history of stroke, history of myocardial infarction, and CES-D sum-score). Rubin's method was used for pooled regression coefficients (β) and 95% confidence intervals (CIs) [34]. All analyses were performed by using IBM SPSS Statistics Version 24.0 and RStudio Version 3.3.2. All statistical tests were two-sided, and a P value of less than 0.05 was considered statistically significant.

Results

Characteristics of breast cancer survivors and non-exposed participants are presented in Table 1. Breast cancer survivors were older than non-exposed participants. Additionally, they generally had completed higher levels of education and more often had diabetes mellitus and a history of myocardial infarction. Lastly, although the numbers of never smokers were similar between the two groups, breast cancer survivors were more frequently former smokers and less often current smokers.

Inflammatory markers

Breast cancer survivors had higher median levels of GLR, PLR, and SII than non-exposed participants. History of breast cancer/cancer treatment was associated with higher inflammatory markers, also after adjustment for age, education, smoking, BMI, diabetes mellitus, history of stroke, history of myocardial infarction, and CES-D sum-score (mean difference for log(GLR) = 0.31, 95% CI 0.24 to 0.37, log(PLR) = 0.14, 95% CI 0.09 to 0.19, log(SII) = 0.31, 95% CI 0.24 to 0.39; Table 2). Inflammatory markers were positively associated with age in both groups [35].

Cognitive performance

Breast cancer survivors had a lower general cognitive factor than non-exposed participants (mean difference = −0.21, 95% CI −0.35 to −0.06, corresponding with an effect of 3.6 years of age given a decline in general cognitive factor of 0.59 points per 10 years; Table 2) [29]. Further adjustment for inflammatory factors changed the estimates slightly, indicating that inflammatory

Table 1 Demographics and characteristics of breast cancer survivors and non-exposed participants

Characteristic	Breast cancer survivors (n = 166)	Non-exposed participants (n = 1344)	P
Age in years, mean (SD)	64.0 (6.7)	57.9 (5.2)	<0.001
Education level, no. (%)			<0.001
Primary	14 (8.4)	158 (11.8)	
Low	59 (35.5)	616 (45.8)	
Intermediate	33 (19.9)	287 (21.4)	
High	60 (36.1)	283 (21.1)	
Body mass index in kg/m^2, mean (SD)	26.9 (4.6)	27.4 (4.8)	0.181
Smoking status, no. (%)			<0.001
Current	16 (9.6)	295 (21.9)	
Former	93 (56.0)	574 (42.7)	
Diabetes mellitus, no. (%)	14 (8.4)	54 (4.0)	0.008
History of stroke, no. (%)	1 (0.6)	19 (1.4)	0.715
History of myocardial infarction, no. (%)	6 (3.6)	11 (0.8)	0.001
CES-D sum-score, mean (SD)	14.5 (3.6)	14.8 (4.4)	0.450
General cognitive factor, mean (SD)	−0.39 (1.14)	0.05 (0.97)	<0.001
Inflammatory markers, median (IQR)			
GLR	2.06 (1.67–2.66)	1.52 (1.20–1.92)	<0.001
PLR	145 (119–176)	124 (102–151)	<0.001
SII	618 (469–796)	443 (328–595)	<0.001
Age at breast cancer diagnosis in years, mean (SD)	42.9 (5.6)		
Time since breast cancer diagnosis, mean (SD)	21.0 (4.5)		

Abbreviations: *CES-D* Center for Epidemiologic Studies Depression Scale, *GLR* granulocyte-to-lymphocyte ratio, *IQR* interquartile range, *PLR* platelet-to-lymphocyte ratio, *SD* standard deviation, *SII* systemic immune-inflammation index

markers explained only a small part of the difference in general cognitive factor in addition to the effect of history of cancer/cancer treatment (mean difference for history of cancer/cancer treatment after adjustment for log(GLR) = −0.18; 95% CI −0.33 to 0.02, log(PLR) = −0.21; 95% CI −0.36 to 0.06, log(SII) = −0.19; 95% CI −0.34 to 0.03).

Association between cognitive performance and inflammatory markers by cancer status

A lower general cognitive factor was associated with higher inflammatory markers in breast cancer survivors (Table 3). In non-exposed participants, higher inflammatory markers tended to be associated with a lower general cognitive factor, albeit not statistically significant.

Table 2 Association between the general cognitive factor and history of cancer and inflammatory markers and history of cancer

Outcome	Model I Mean difference (95% CI)	Model II Mean difference (95% CI)
Inflammatory marker*		
Log GLR	0.30 (0.24 to 0.36)	0.31 (0.24 to 0.37)
Log PLR	0.16 (0.10 to 0.21)	0.14 (0.09 to 0.19)
Log SII	0.30 (0.23 to 0.38)	0.31 (0.24 to 0.39)
Cognition†		
General cognitive factor	−0.18 (−0.34 to −0.03)	−0.21 (−0.35 to −0.06)

Abbreviations: *CI* confidence interval, *GLR* granulocyte-to-lymphocyte ratio, *PLR* platelet-to-lymphocyte ratio, *SII* systemic immune-inflammation index
Model I is a linear regression of the general cognitive factor or log-transformed inflammatory markers on cancer status adjusted for age and education. Model II is as model I plus adjustment for smoking status, body mass index, diabetes mellitus, history of stroke, history of myocardial infarction, and Center for Epidemiologic Studies Depression Scale (CES-D) sum-score
*Mean difference in general cognitive factor between breast cancer survivors and non-exposed participants
†Mean difference in inflammatory markers between breast cancer survivors and non-exposed participants

Table 3 Association between the general cognitive factor and inflammatory markers in breast cancer survivors and in non-exposed participants

Inflammatory marker per SD increase	Breast cancer survivors Mean difference* (95% CI)	Non-exposed participants Mean difference* (95% CI)	P for interaction[†]
Model I			
Log GLR	−0.24 (−0.40 to −0.08)	−0.04 (−0.09 to 0.00)	0.061
Log PLR	−0.13 (−0.29 to 0.03)	0.05 (0.01 to 0.10)	0.003
Log SII	−0.22 (−0.38 to −0.07)	−0.03 (−0.08 to 0.01)	0.053
Model II			
Log GLR	−0.23 (−0.39 to −0.08)	−0.02 (−0.07 to 0.02)	0.038
Log PLR	−0.18 (−0.33 to −0.02)	0.03 (−0.01 to 0.08)	0.003
Log SII	−0.23 (−0.38 to −0.07)	−0.01 (−0.06 to 0.03)	0.033

Abbreviations: *CI* confidence interval, *GLR* granulocyte-to-lymphocyte ratio, *PLR* platelet-to-lymphocyte ratio, *SD* standard deviation, *SII* systemic immune-inflammation index

Model I is a linear regression of the general cognitive factor on each log-transformed inflammatory marker adjusted for age and education. Model II is as model I plus adjustment for smoking status, body mass index, diabetes mellitus, history of stroke, history of myocardial infarction, and Center for Epidemiologic Studies Depression Scale (CES-D) sum-score

*Mean difference in general cognitive factor per standard deviation increase in inflammatory marker

[†]P value for interaction term between history of cancer/cancer treatment and inflammatory marker

The interaction term between inflammatory markers and history of cancer/cancer treatment was significant for each inflammatory marker, indicating that the association between higher inflammation levels and lower general cognitive factor was more pronounced in breast cancer survivors than in non-exposed participants (P for interaction between cancer and standardized log-transformed GLR = 0.038, PLR = 0.003, and SII = 0.033; Fig. 2).

The association between higher inflammatory markers and lower general cognitive factor differed more between breast cancer survivors and non-exposed participants with a higher BMI than in those with a lower BMI. However, stratified analyses for BMI showed that the effect of one–standard deviation increase in inflammatory marker on general cognitive factor was higher among

breast cancer survivors with a BMI below 27.3 kg/m^2 compared with those with a higher BMI (Table 4).

Discussion

This study is the first report investigating the association between blood cell–based inflammatory markers and cognitive performance in breast cancer survivors with an average time since cessation of chemotherapy of more than 20 years. Breast cancer survivors had lower global cognitive performance and higher inflammatory markers compared with women without a history of cancer. The tendency for lower global cognitive performance with higher inflammatory markers was more pronounced in breast cancer survivors, suggesting a potential role for inflammation in the pathophysiology of cognitive problems in cancer

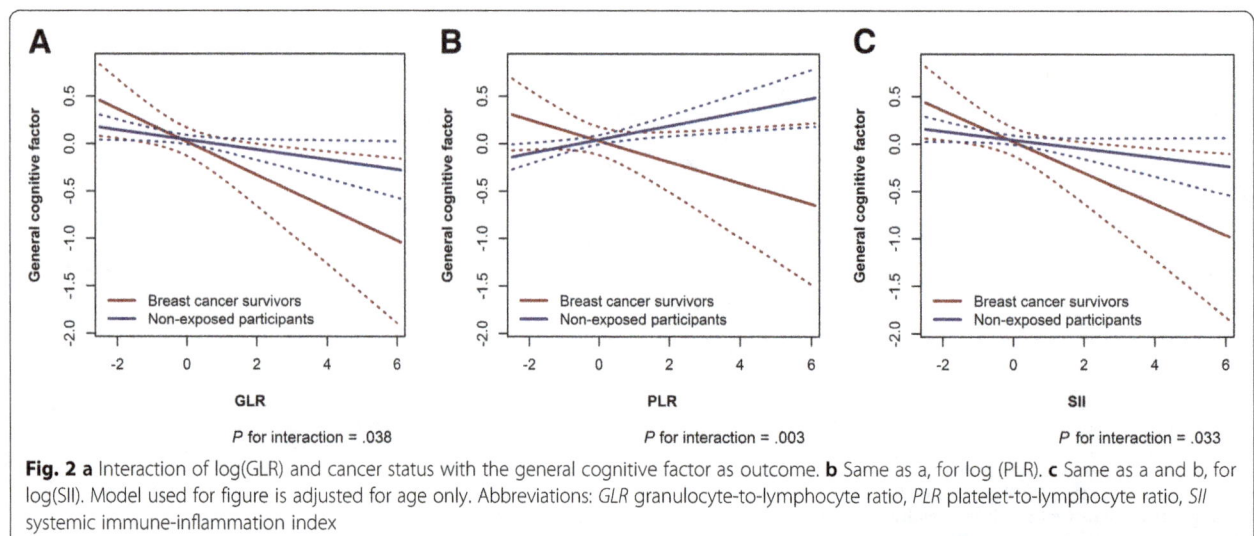

Fig. 2 a Interaction of log(GLR) and cancer status with the general cognitive factor as outcome. **b** Same as a, for log (PLR). **c** Same as a and b, for log(SII). Model used for figure is adjusted for age only. Abbreviations: *GLR* granulocyte-to-lymphocyte ratio, *PLR* platelet-to-lymphocyte ratio, *SII* systemic immune-inflammation index

Table 4 Association between the general cognitive factor and inflammatory markers in breast cancer survivors and in non-exposed participants stratified for mean body mass index

Inflammatory marker per SD increase	Breast cancer survivors		Non-exposed participants		P for interaction[†]
	Mean difference*	95% CI	Mean difference*	95% CI	
BMI < 27.3 kg/m²					
	n = 104		n = 749		
Log GLR	−0.29	−0.49 to −0.10	−0.04	−0.10 to 0.02	0.480
Log PLR	−0.22	−0.42 to −0.02	0.01	−0.05 to 0.08	0.309
Log SII	−0.28	−0.48 to −0.09	−0.04	−0.10 to 0.02	0.564
BMI > 27.3 kg/m²					
	n = 62		n = 595		
Log GLR	−0.16	−0.41 to 0.09	0.01	−0.06 to 0.08	0.013
Log PLR	−0.16	−0.42 to 0.10	0.05	−0.02 to 0.12	<0.001
Log SII	−0.12	−0.38 to 0.14	0.02	−0.05 to 0.09	0.005

Abbreviations: *BMI* body mass index, *CI* confidence interval, *GLR* granulocyte-to-lymphocyte ratio, *PLR* platelet-to-lymphocyte ratio, *SD* standard deviation, *SII* systemic immune-inflammation index

Model I is a linear regression of the general cognitive factor on each log-transformed inflammatory marker adjusted for age and education. Model II is as model I plus adjustment for smoking status, diabetes mellitus, history of stroke, history of myocardial infarction, and Center for Epidemiologic Studies Depression Scale (CES-D) sum-score.

*Mean difference in general cognitive factor per standard deviation increase in inflammatory marker

[†]P value for interaction term between history of cancer/cancer treatment and inflammatory marker

survivors. This effect was not modified by BMI. More insight in mechanisms underlying cognitive problems could help identifying those women who are at an increased risk of cognitive problems and developing prevention strategies.

We previously reported on differences in cognitive performance between breast cancer survivors and non-exposed participants [2]. In this previous study, we tested between-group performance differences of individual cognitive outcome measures that were currently used to construct the general cognitive factor and observed that breast cancer survivors performed worse compared with non-exposed participants within several cognitive domains. This suggested that cognitive problems in cancer survivors can be long-lasting. In the present study, we evaluated global cognitive performance using the general cognitive factor because we did not expect a specific cognitive domain to be affected by inflammation. We chose to use a robust cognitive summary measure, thereby reducing the number of comparisons.

Interestingly, levels of inflammatory markers were higher in breast cancer survivors, compared with non-exposed participants, on average 20 years after cancer treatment. Inflammation plays a critical role in tumorigenesis, tumor progression, and cancer metastasis [36, 37]. Research has shown that chronic inflammation is associated with an increased cancer risk [37]. Moreover, different markers of inflammation, such as cytokines, C-reactive protein, and NLR, are often elevated in patients with cancer and are associated with poor survival [9, 15–17, 24, 38]. One study investigating

inflammation levels after cancer treatment found that C-reactive protein and cytokine levels were elevated up to 5 years after treatment [19]. Our observation that systemic inflammation markers are higher in breast cancer survivors compared with non-exposed participants on average 20 years after cancer treatment suggests deregulation of the immune system. Whether this is a consequence of cancer or cancer treatment (or both) or a pre-existing deregulation before cancer development cannot be determined with the present study.

The found association of blood cell–based inflammatory markers and cognitive performance in breast cancer survivors is in line with previous observations before, during, and shortly after therapy [6, 17, 18]. Two studies investigated the link between inflammation and cognitive performance prior to the start of cancer treatment. The first study showed that elevated levels of interleukin-6 (IL-6) in patients with acute myelogenous leukemia or myelodysplastic syndrome were associated with poorer executive functioning before cancer treatment [14]. The second study showed that high levels of soluble tumor necrosis factor receptor type II (sTNF-RII) were related to reduced verbal memory performance in patients with newly diagnosed breast cancer [5]. More studies in patients with breast cancer have tried to elucidate the role of inflammation in impaired cognitive performance during chemotherapy and two of these studies identified specific cytokines to be involved. Williams et al. focused on sTNR-RII and found that higher levels of this receptor were associated with visual memory performance [10]. Cheung et al. observed an association between increased levels of IL-6 and IL-1β and poorer psychomotor speed performance during chemotherapy [8]. Shortly after cancer treatment, higher levels of sTNF-RII were associated with increased memory complaints [11], and on average 5 years after cancer treatment, elevated IL-6 and TNFα levels were associated with worse verbal memory [13]. Importantly, the association between inflammation and cognitive performance is supported by animal studies. Acute peripheral immune challenges using lipopolysaccharide resulted in cognitive impairments in a spatial working memory task in mice. Cognitive impairments were observed 1.5–2 h after injection in tumor-bearing mice but not in tumor-free mice. These cognitive effects could be prevented when using a technique to enhance innate immune reactivity [39]. Together, these results support the hypothesis that inflammation has a role in the complex pathogenesis of both short-term and longer-term cognitive problems in patients with cancer.

Owing to our study design, we cannot determine whether the association between inflammation and impaired cognitive performance is causal. However, also a causal association could not illuminate the exact underlying mechanisms by which inflammation leads to brain changes and subsequent cognitive problems. Peripheral pro-inflammatory cytokines are able to cross the blood–brain barrier, which may initiate the release of local cytokines [40]. Local cytokine production could result in neurotransmitter deregulation, increased oxidative stress, and decreased neurogenesis and neuroplasticity, which in turn can lead to cognitive dysfunction [41]. It is also possible that inflammation induces epigenetic changes and chromosomal instability, which can be persistent and therefore could be associated with long-term cognitive problems [42].

Our study has several strengths. First, we have a large sample size of breast cancer survivors who have been treated on average more than 20 years ago, enabling us to investigate long-term effects. Moreover, we used non-exposed participants from a population-based cohort study, who underwent the same examinations as the breast cancer survivors. This design provided standardized ascertainments of outcome and covariates. All participants received a neuropsychological test battery, enabling us to investigate global cognitive function by the general cognitive factor. Lastly, we were able to investigate inflammation status using blood cell–based inflammatory markers, which are low-cost and easy to use in the clinic.

Study limitations include the design by which we cannot disentangle the effects of cancer and cancer treatment on cognition and levels of inflammatory markers. Some studies show that patients treated with chemotherapy have higher inflammatory markers during and after treatment compared with chemotherapy-naïve patients [12]. However, because inflammatory markers and cognitive problems can already

occur in patients with newly diagnosed cancer, it is unlikely that inflammation is important only in chemotherapy-treated patients [5]. Owing to the cross-sectional design, we do not have information about cognitive performance and levels of inflammatory markers before cancer diagnosis and treatment. Moreover, patients with breast cancer nowadays receive chemotherapy regimens other than CMF, either with or without adjuvant endocrine therapy, limiting the generalizability to current patients with breast cancer.

However, cyclophosphamide and 5-fluoroacil are still frequently used in other regimens for adjuvant chemotherapy. Furthermore, we were not able to exclude individuals whose systemic inflammatory markers may have been elevated because of acute infections and to control for acute-phase reactants such as C-reactive protein, but we expect that this effect is similar for cancer survivors and non-exposed participants. Lastly, we need to emphasize that by measuring the GLR, PLR, and SII, we cannot identify the exact phenotype of the underlying immune cell populations. Although these markers are proven to be related to chronic systemic inflammation, it is unknown whether they also reflect higher levels of pro-inflammatory cytokines. In other words, we cannot confirm that observed shifts in the granulocytes, lymphocytes, and platelets cause higher cytokine levels and thereby are functional. To elucidate the exact immune cell populations involved in increases of the GLR, PLR, and SII, determination of different cytokines is needed.

Conclusions
We found that breast cancer survivors who had been treated with chemotherapy on average more than 20 years ago have higher blood cell–based inflammatory markers compared with women without a history of cancer. Higher levels of inflammatory markers tended to be associated with poorer cognitive performance in both cancer survivors and cancer-free women, and expression was stronger in breast cancer survivors. This finding suggests that inflammation could have a role in the pathogenesis of long-term cognitive impairment in cancer survivors. Further prospective studies are important to determine the causality of the association and to investigate the effects of lowering inflammation on the development of cognitive problems in cancer patients and survivors, for instance, by exercise or anti-inflammatory drugs.

Abbreviations
15-WLT: 15-Word Learning Test; BMI: Body mass index; CES-D: Center for Epidemiologic Studies Depression Scale; CI: Confidence interval; CMF: Cyclophosphamide, methotrexate, and fluorouracil; GLR: Granulocyte-to-lymphocyte ratio; IL: Interleukin; LDST: Letter-Digit Substitution Test; MRI: Magnetic resonance imaging; NLR: Neutrophil-to-lymphocyte ratio; PLR: Platelet-to-lymphocyte ratio; PPB: Purdue Pegboard Test; RS-III: Third subcohort of the Rotterdam Study; SII: Systemic immune-inflammation index; sTNF-RII : Soluble tumor necrosis factor receptor type II; TNF: Tumor necrosis factor; WFT: Word Fluency Test

Acknowledgments
We gratefully thank all participants and staff for their time and commitment to the study. The authors are grateful for the intellectual contributions that K.E. de Visser, Division of Immunology, Netherlands Cancer Institute, made to this study.

Funding
This work was supported by the Dutch Cancer Society (grant number NKI-20157737). The Rotterdam Study is funded by Erasmus Medical Center and Erasmus University, Rotterdam, Netherlands Organization for the Health Research and Development (ZonMw), the Research Institute for Diseases in the Elderly (RIDE), the Ministry of Education, Culture and Science, the Ministry for Health, Welfare and Sports, the European Commission (DG XII), and the Municipality of Rotterdam. The funders had no role in study design, data collection and analysis, decision to publish, or preparation of the manuscript.

Authors' contributions
KDW, SBS, and MAI contributed to study design. MAI and SBS contributed to funding. VK contributed to data collection. KDW contributed to data analysis. All authors contributed to data interpretation and critical revision and approved the final manuscript.

Competing interests
The authors declare that they have no competing interests.

Author details
[1]Department of Psychosocial Research and Epidemiology, Netherlands Cancer Institute, Plesmanlaan 121, 1066 CX Amsterdam, the Netherlands. [2]Department of Epidemiology, Erasmus MC - University Medical Center Rotterdam, PO Box 2040, 3000 CA Rotterdam, the Netherlands. [3]Department of Psychiatry, The University of Utah, 501 Chipeta Way, Salt Lake City, UT 84108, USA. [4]Department of Neuro-oncology, Netherlands Cancer Institute, Plesmanlaan 121, 1066 CX Amsterdam, the Netherlands. [5]Brain and Cognition, Department of Psychology, University of Amsterdam, Nieuwe Achtergracht 129-B, 1018 WS Amsterdam, the Netherlands.

References
1. Janelsins MC, Kesler SR, Ahles TA, Morrow GR. Prevalence, mechanisms, and management of cancer-related cognitive impairment. Int Rev Psychiatry. 2014;26:102–13.
2. Koppelmans V, Breteler MM, Boogerd W, Seynaeve C, Gundy C, Schagen SB. Neuropsychological performance in survivors of breast cancer more than 20 years after adjuvant chemotherapy. J Clin Oncol. 2012;30:1080–6.
3. Ahles TA, Saykin AJ. Candidate mechanisms for chemotherapy-induced cognitive changes. Nat Rev Cancer. 2007;7:192–201.
4. Ahles TA, Root JC, Ryan EL. Cancer- and cancer treatment-associated cognitive change: an update on the state of the science. J Clin Oncol. 2012;30:3675–86.
5. Patel SK, Wong AL, Wong FL, Breen EC, Hurria A, Smith M, et al. Inflammatory Biomarkers, Comorbidity, and Neurocognition in Women With Newly Diagnosed Breast Cancer. J Natl Cancer Inst. 2015;107.
6. Lyon DE, Cohen R, Chen H, Kelly DL, McCain NL, Starkweather A, et al. Relationship of systemic cytokine concentrations to cognitive function over two years in women with early stage breast cancer. J Neuroimmunol. 2016;301:74–82.
7. Briones TL, Woods J. Dysregulation in myelination mediated by persistent neuroinflammation: possible mechanisms in chemotherapy-related cognitive impairment. Brain Behav Immun. 2014;35:23–32.
8. Cheung YT, Ng T, Shwe M, Ho HK, Foo KM, Cham MT, et al. Association of proinflammatory cytokines and chemotherapy-associated cognitive impairment in breast cancer patients: a multi-centered, prospective, cohort study. Ann Oncol. 2015;26:1446–51.
9. Pusztai L, Mendoza TR, Reuben JM, Martinez MM, Willey JS, Lara J, et al. Changes in plasma levels of inflammatory cytokines in response to paclitaxel chemotherapy. Cytokine 2004;25:94–102.
10. Williams AM, Shah R, Shayne M, Huston AJ, Krebs M, Murray N, et al. Associations between inflammatory markers and cognitive function in breast cancer patients receiving chemotherapy. J Neuroimmunol. 2018;314:17–23.
11. Ganz PA, Bower JE, Kwan L, Castellon SA, Silverman DH, Geist C, et al. Does tumor necrosis factor-alpha (TNF-alpha) play a role in post-chemotherapy cerebral dysfunction? Brain Behav Immun. 2013;30(Suppl):S99–108.
12. Pomykala KL, Ganz PA, Bower JE, Kwan L, Castellon SA, Mallam S, et al. The association between pro-inflammatory cytokines, regional cerebral metabolism, and cognitive complaints following adjuvant chemotherapy for breast cancer. Brain Imaging Behav. 2013;7:511–523.
13. Kesler S, Janelsins M, Koovakkattu D, Palesh O, Mustian K, Morrow G, et al. Reduced hippocampal volume and verbal memory performance associated with interleukin-6 and tumor necrosis factor-alpha levels in chemotherapy-treated breast cancer survivors. Brain Behav Immun. 2013;30(Suppl):S109–16.
14. Meyers CA, Albitar M, Estey E. Cognitive impairment, fatigue, and cytokine levels in patients with acute myelogenous leukemia or myelodysplastic syndrome. Cancer. 2005;104:788–93.
15. Janelsins MC, Mustian KM, Palesh OG, Mohile SG, Peppone LJ, Sprod LK, et al. Differential expression of cytokines in breast cancer patients receiving different chemotherapies: implications for cognitive impairment research. Support Care Cancer. 2012;20:831–9.
16. Lippitz BE. Cytokine patterns in patients with cancer: a systematic review. Lancet Oncol. 2013;14:e218–28.
17. Seruga B, Zhang H, Bernstein LJ, Tannock IF. Cytokines and their relationship to the symptoms and outcome of cancer. Nat Rev Cancer. 2008;8:887–99.
18. Wang XS, Shi Q, Williams LA, Mao L, Cleeland CS, Komaki RR, et al. Inflammatory cytokines are associated with the development of symptom burden in patients with NSCLC undergoing concurrent chemoradiation therapy. Brain Behav Immun. 2010;24:968–74.
19. Vardy JL, Booth C, Pond GR, Zhang H, Galica J, Dhillon H, et al. Cytokine levels in patients (pts) with colorectal cancer and breast cancer and their relationship to fatigue and cognitive function. Suppl J Clin Oncol. 2007;18S:9070.
20. Templeton AJ, McNamara MG, Seruga B, Vera-Badillo FE, Aneja P, Ocana A, et al. Prognostic role of neutrophil-to-lymphocyte ratio in solid tumors: a systematic review and meta-analysis. J Natl Cancer Inst. 2014;106:dju124.
21. Kwon HC, Kim SH, Oh SY, Lee S, Lee JH, Choi HJ, et al. Clinical significance of preoperative neutrophil-lymphocyte versus platelet-lymphocyte ratio in patients with operable colorectal cancer. Biomarkers. 2012;17:216–22.
22. Hu B, Yang XR, Xu Y, Sun YF, Sun C, Guo W, et al. Systemic immune-inflammation index predicts prognosis of patients after curative resection for hepatocellular carcinoma. Clin Cancer Res. 2014;20:6212–22.
23. Ethier JL, Desautels D, Templeton A, Shah PS, Amir E. Prognostic role of neutrophil-to-lymphocyte ratio in breast cancer: a systematic review and meta-analysis. Breast Cancer Res. 2017;19:2.
24. Chen J, Deng Q, Pan Y, He B, Ying H, Sun H, et al. Prognostic value of neutrophil-to-lymphocyte ratio in breast cancer. FEBS Open Bio. 2015;5:502–507.
25. Ikram MA, Brusselle GGO, Murad SD, van Duijn CM, Franco OH, Goedegebure A, et al. The Rotterdam Study: 2018 update on objectives, design and main results. Eur J Epidemiol. 2017;32:807–50.

26. Patton KT, Thibodeau GA. Anatomy and Physiology. 9th ed. St Louis: Elsevier; 2016.
27. Wulaningsih W, Holmberg L, Abeler-Doner L, Ng T, Rohrmann S, Van Hemelrijck M. Associations of C-Reactive Protein, Granulocytes and Granulocyte-to-Lymphocyte Ratio with Mortality from Breast Cancer in Non-Institutionalized American Women. PLoS One. 2016;11:e0157482.
28. He W, Yin C, Guo G, Jiang C, Wang F, Qiu H, et al. Initial neutrophil lymphocyte ratio is superior to platelet lymphocyte ratio as an adverse prognostic and predictive factor in metastatic colorectal cancer. Med Oncol. 2013;30:439.
29. Hoogendam YY, Hofman A, van der Geest JN, van der Lugt A, Ikram MA. Patterns of cognitive function in aging: the Rotterdam Study. Eur J Epidemiol. 2014;29:133–40.
30. Diabetes mellitus. Report of a WHO Study Group. World Health Organ Tech Rep Ser. 1985;727:1–113.
31. Bos MJ, Koudstaal PJ, Hofman A, Ikram MA. Modifiable etiological factors and the burden of stroke from the Rotterdam study: a population-based cohort study. PLoS Med. 2014;11:e1001634.
32. Hak AE, Pols HA, Visser TJ, Drexhage HA, Hofman A, Witteman JC. Subclinical hypothyroidism is an independent risk factor for atherosclerosis and myocardial infarction in elderly women: the Rotterdam Study. Ann Intern Med. 2000;132:270–8.
33. Mirza SS, de Bruijn RF, Direk N, Hofman A, Koudstaal PJ, Ikram MA, et al. Depressive symptoms predict incident dementia during short- but not long-term follow-up period. Alzheimers Dement. 2014;10(5 Suppl):S323–9 e321.
34. Rubin DB. Multiple imputation for nonresponse in surveys. New York: Wiley; 1987.
35. Lin BD, Hottenga JJ, Abdellaoui A, Dolan CV, de Geus EJ, Kluft C, et al. Causes of variation in the neutrophil-lymphocyte and platelet-lymphocyte ratios: a twin-family study. Biomark Med. 2016 [Epub ahead of print].
36. Coussens LM, Werb Z. Inflammation and cancer. Nature. 2002;420:860–7.
37. Shacter E, Weitzman SA. Chronic inflammation and cancer. Oncology (Williston Park). 2002;16:217–26 229; discussion 230–212.
38. Pierce BL, Ballard-Barbash R, Bernstein L, Baumgartner RN, Neuhouser ML, Wener MH, et al. Elevated biomarkers of inflammation are associated with reduced survival among breast cancer patients. J Clin Oncol. 2009;27:3437–44.
39. Bever SR, Liu X, Quan N, Pyter LM. Euflammation Attenuates Central and Peripheral Inflammation and Cognitive Consequences of an Immune Challenge after Tumor Development. Neuroimmunomodulation. 2017;24:74–86.
40. Ren X, St Clair DK, Butterfield DA. Dysregulation of cytokine mediated chemotherapy induced cognitive impairment. Pharmacol Res. 2017;117:267–73.
41. Wang XM, Walitt B, Saligan L, Tiwari AF, Cheung CW, Zhang ZJ. Chemobrain: a critical review and causal hypothesis of link between cytokines and epigenetic reprogramming associated with chemotherapy. Cytokine. 2015;72:86–96.
42. Lyon D, Elmore L, Aboalela N, Merrill-Schools J, McCain N, Starkweather A, et al. Potential epigenetic mechanism(s) associated with the persistence of psychoneurological symptoms in women receiving chemotherapy for breast cancer: a hypothesis. Biol Res Nurs. 2014;16:160–74.

Permissions

The contributors of this book come from diverse backgrounds, making this book a truly international effort. This book will bring forth new frontiers with its revolutionizing research information and detailed analysis of the nascent developments around the world.

We would like to thank all the contributing authors for lending their expertise to make the book truly unique. They have played a crucial role in the development of this book. Without their invaluable contributions this book wouldn't have been possible. They have made vital efforts to compile up to date information on the varied aspects of this subject to make this book a valuable addition to the collection of many professionals and students.

This book was conceptualized with the vision of imparting up-to-date information and advanced data in this field. To ensure the same, a matchless editorial board was set up. Every individual on the board went through rigorous rounds of assessment to prove their worth. After which they invested a large part of their time researching and compiling the most relevant data for our readers.

The editorial board has been involved in producing this book since its inception. They have spent rigorous hours researching and exploring the diverse topics which have resulted in the successful publishing of this book. They have passed on their knowledge of decades through this book. To expedite this challenging task, the publisher supported the team at every step. A small team of assistant editors was also appointed to further simplify the editing procedure and attain best results for the readers.

Apart from the editorial board, the designing team has also invested a significant amount of their time in understanding the subject and creating the most relevant covers. They scrutinized every image to scout for the most suitable representation of the subject and create an appropriate cover for the book.

The publishing team has been an ardent support to the editorial, designing and production team. Their endless efforts to recruit the best for this project, has resulted in the accomplishment of this book. They are a veteran in the field of academics and their pool of knowledge is as vast as their experience in printing. Their expertise and guidance has proved useful at every step. Their uncompromising quality standards have made this book an exceptional effort. Their encouragement from time to time has been an inspiration for everyone.

The publisher and the editorial board hope that this book will prove to be a valuable piece of knowledge for researchers, students, practitioners and scholars across the globe.

Contributors

Aiping Shi, Ye Du, Dong Song, Ming Yang, Sijie Li, Bing Han and Gang Zhao
Department of Breast Surgery, The First Hospital of Jilin University, 71 Xinmin street, Changchun 130021, Jilin Province, China

Pin Gao and Ying Jin
Department of Breast Surgery, The First Hospital of Jilin University, 71 Xinmin street, Changchun 130021, Jilin Province, China
Division of Pediatric Surgery, Department of Surgery, Children's Research Institute, Medical College of Wisconsin, 8701 W Watertown Plank Rd, Milwaukee, WI 53226, USA
Division of Pediatric Pathology, Department of Pathology, Children's Research Institute, Medical College of Wisconsin, 8701 W Watertown Plank Rd, Milwaukee, WI 53226, USA

Zhimin Fan
Department of Breast Surgery, The First Hospital of Jilin University, 71 Xinmin street, Changchun 130021, Jilin Province, China
College of Life Sciences, Nankai University, 94 Weijin Road, Tianjin 300071, China

Wenquan Hu
Division of Pediatric Surgery, Department of Surgery, Children's Research Institute, Medical College of Wisconsin, 8701 W Watertown Plank Rd, Milwaukee, WI 53226, USA
Division of Pediatric Pathology, Department of Pathology, Children's Research Institute, Medical College of Wisconsin, 8701 W Watertown Plank Rd, Milwaukee, WI 53226, USA

Yajun Duan and Xiang Wang
Division of Pediatric Surgery, Department of Surgery, Children's Research Institute, Medical College of Wisconsin, 8701 W Watertown Plank Rd, Milwaukee, WI 53226, USA

Division of Pediatric Pathology, Department of Pathology, Children's Research Institute, Medical College of Wisconsin, 8701 W Watertown Plank Rd, Milwaukee, WI 53226, USA
Department of Human Anatomy, Histology and Embryology, Key Laboratory of Carcinogenesis and Translational Research (Ministry of Education) and State Key Laboratory of Natural and Biomimetic Drugs, Peking University Health Science Center, Beijing 100191, China

Qing Robert Miao
Division of Pediatric Surgery, Department of Surgery, Children's Research Institute, Medical College of Wisconsin, 8701 W Watertown Plank Rd, Milwaukee, WI 53226, USA
Division of Pediatric Pathology, Department of Pathology, Children's Research Institute, Medical College of Wisconsin, 8701 W Watertown Plank Rd, Milwaukee, WI 53226, USA
College of Life Sciences, Nankai University, 94 Weijin Road, Tianjin 300071, China

Hongquan Zhang
Department of Human Anatomy, Histology and Embryology, Key Laboratory of Carcinogenesis and Translational Research (Ministry of Education) and State Key Laboratory of Natural and Biomimetic Drugs, Peking University Health Science Center, Beijing 100191, China
College of Life Sciences, Nankai University, 94 Weijin Road, Tianjin 300071, China

Holly Holliday, Laura A. Baker, Simon R. Junankar and Alexander Swarbrick
The Kinghorn Cancer Centre, Cancer Research Division, Garvan Institute of Medical Research, Darlinghurst, NSW 2010, Australia

St Vincent's Clinical School, Faculty of Medicine, UNSW, Darlinghurst, NSW 2010, Australia

Susan J. Clark
St Vincent's Clinical School, Faculty of Medicine, UNSW, Darlinghurst, NSW 2010, Australia
Epigenetics Research Program, Genomics and Epigenetics Division, Garvan Institute of Medical Research, Darlinghurst, NSW 2010, Australia

Christopher J. Sevinsky, Faiza Khan, Leila Kokabee and Douglas S. Conklin
Cancer Research Center, Department of Biomedical Sciences, State University of New York, University at Albany, CRC 342, One Discovery Drive, Rensselaer, NY 12144-3456, USA

Anza Darehshouri
Electron Microscopy Core Facility, The University of Texas Southwestern Medical Center, 5323 Harry Hines Boulevard, Dallas, TX 75390, USA

Krishna Rao Maddipati
Lipidomics Core Facility, Wayne State University, 435 Chemistry Bldg., Detroit, MI 48202, USA

Vassilena Tsvetkova and Serena Bonaguro
Department of Surgery, Oncology and Gastroenterology, University of Padova, Via Gattamelata 64, 35128 Padova, Italy

Maria Vittoria Dieci, Gaia Griguolo, Federica Miglietta, Grazia Vernaci, Giulia Tasca, Pierfranco Conte and Valentina Guarneri
Department of Surgery, Oncology and Gastroenterology, University of Padova, Via Gattamelata 64, 35128 Padova, Italy

Medical Oncology 2, Istituto Oncologico Veneto IRCCS, Via Gattamelata 64, 35128 Padova, Italy

Tommaso Giarratano, Carlo Alberto Giorgi and Giovanni Faggioni
Medical Oncology 2, Istituto Oncologico Veneto IRCCS, Via Gattamelata 64, 35128 Padova, Italy

Enrico Orvieto
Department of Pathology, Azienda Ospedaliera di Padova, Padova, Italy

Federico Piacentini
Department of Medical and Surgical Sciences of Mother, Child and Adult, University of Modena and Reggio Emilia, Modena, Italy

Guido Ficarra
Division of Pathology, University Hospital of Modena, Modena, Italy

Claudia Omarini
Department of Medical Oncology, University Hospital of Modena, Modena, Italy

Rocco Cappellesso
Surgical Pathology and Cytopathology Unit, Department of Medicine, University of Padova, Padova, Italy

Camillo Aliberti
Radiology, Istituto Oncologico Veneto IRCCS, Padova, Italy

Hans Wildiers
Department of General Medical Oncology, Leuven Cancer Institute, University Hospitals Leuven, Leuven, Belgium

Patrick Schöffski
Department of General Medical Oncology, Leuven Cancer Institute, University Hospitals Leuven, Leuven, Belgium
Department of Oncology, Faculty of Medicine, Laboratory of Experimental Oncology, KU Leuven, Herestraat 49, B-3000 Leuven, Belgium

Sara Cresta and Silvia Damian
Department of Medical Oncology, Fondazione IRCCS Istituto Nazionale dei Tumori, Milan, Italy

Ingrid A. Mayer
Department of Medicine, Vanderbilt University Medical Center, Nashville, TN, USA

Steven Gendreau and Jill M. Spoerke
Oncology Biomarker Development, Genentech Inc, South San Francisco, CA, USA

Isabelle Rooney and Stina M. Singel
Product Development Oncology, Genentech Inc, South San Francisco, CA, USA

Kari M. Morrissey
Clinical Pharmacology, Genentech Inc, South San Francisco, CA, USA

Vivian W. Ng
Biostatistics, Genentech Inc, South San Francisco, CA, USA

Eric Winer
Department of Medical Oncology, Dana-Farber Cancer Institute, Boston, MA, USA

Tanjina Kader
Cancer Genetics Laboratory, Peter MacCallum Cancer Centre, Melbourne, VIC, Australia
The Sir Peter MacCallum Department of Oncology, University of Melbourne, Melbourne, VIC, Australia
Cancer Genomics Program, Peter MacCallum Cancer Centre, Melbourne, VIC, Australia

Ian G. Campbell
Cancer Genetics Laboratory, Peter MacCallum Cancer Centre, Melbourne, VIC, Australia
The Sir Peter MacCallum Department of Oncology, University of Melbourne, Melbourne, VIC, Australia
Department of Pathology, University of Melbourne, Parkville, VIC, Australia

Kylie L. Gorringe
The Sir Peter MacCallum Department of Oncology, University of Melbourne, Melbourne, VIC, Australia
Cancer Genomics Program, Peter MacCallum Cancer Centre, Melbourne, VIC, Australia
Department of Pathology, University of Melbourne, Parkville, VIC, Australia

Prue Hill
Department of Anatomical Pathology, St Vincent's Hospital, Fitzroy, VIC, Australia

Emad A. Rakha
Department of Histopathology, University of Nottingham and Nottingham University Hospitals NHS Trust, City Hospital, Nottingham, UK

Jia Wu and Ruijiang Li
Department of Radiation Oncology, Stanford University School of Medicine, 1070 Arastradero Road, Stanford, CA 94305, USA

Xuejie Li and Xiaodong Teng
Department of Pathology, First Affiliated Hospital of Zhejiang University, Hangzhou 310058, Zhejiang, China

Sandy Napel and Bruce L. Daniel
Department of Radiology, Stanford University School of Medicine, Stanford, CA 94305, USA

Daniel L. Rubin
Department of Radiology, Stanford University School of Medicine, Stanford, CA 94305, USA
Department of Biomedical Data Science, Stanford University School of Medicine, Stanford, CA 94305, USA
Center for Biomedical Informatics Research, Department of Medicine, Stanford University School of Medicine, Stanford, CA 94305, USA

Maider Zabala, Dalong Qian and Michael F. Clarke
Institute for Stem Cell Biology and Regenerative Medicine, School of Medicine, Stanford University, 265 Campus Drive, Stanford, CA 94305, USA

Neethan Amit Lobo
Institute for Stem Cell Biology and Regenerative Medicine, School of Medicine, Stanford University, 265 Campus Drive, Stanford, CA 94305, USA.
Cell and Molecular Biology Program, University of Michigan, Ann Arbor, MI, USA

John A. Reid
Biomedical Engineering Institute, College of Engineering, Old Dominion University, 5115 Hampton Blvd, Norfolk, VA 23529, USA

Peter A. Mollica, Robert D. Bruno and Patrick C. Sachs
School of Medical Diagnostic and Translational Sciences, College of Health Sciences, Old Dominion University, 5115 Hampton Blvd, Norfolk, VA 23529, USA

Sara Donzelli, Elisa Milano, Andrea Sacconi, Giovanni Blandino and Giulia Fontemaggi
Oncogenomics and Epigenetics Unit, IRCCS Regina Elena National Cancer Institute, Via Elio Chianesi 53, 00144 Rome, Italy

Magdalena Pruszko, Maciej Zylicz and Alicja Zylicz
Department of Molecular Biology, International Institute of Molecular and Cell Biology in Warsaw, Księcia Trojdena 4, 02-109 Warsaw, Poland

Silvia Masciarelli, Ilaria Iosue and Francesco Fazi
Department of Anatomical, Histological, Forensic and Ortho-paedic Sciences, Section of Histology and Medical Embryology, Sapienza University of Rome, Via A. Scarpa, 16, 00161 Rome, Italy

Laboratory affiliated with Istituto Pasteur Italia-Fondazione Cenci Bolognetti, Rome, Italy

Elisa Melucci, Enzo Gallo and Marcella Mottolese
Pathology Department, IRCCS Regina Elena National Cancer Institute, Via Elio Chianesi 53, 00144 Rome, Italy

Irene Terrenato
Biostatistics Unit, Scientific Direction, IRCCS Regina Elena National Cancer Institute, Via Elio Chianesi 53, 00144 Rome, Italy

Jeannette T. Bensen, Mariaelisa Graff, Kristin L. Young, Melissa A. Troester and Andrew F. Olshan
Department of Epidemiology, Gillings School of Global Public Health, University of North Carolina at Chapel Hill, Chapel Hill, NC 27599, USA

Praveen Sethupathy
Department of Biomedical Sciences, College of Veterinary Medicine, Cornell University, Ithaca, NY 14853, USA

Joel Parker
Department of Genetics, University of North Carolina at Chapel Hill, Chapel Hill, NC 27599, USA

Kevin Currin
Department of Genetics, University of North Carolina at Chapel Hill, Chapel Hill, NC 27599, USA
Biological and Biomedical Sciences Program, University of North Carolina at Chapel Hill, Chapel Hill, NC 27599, USA

Chad V. Pecot
Department of Medicine, Division of Oncology, School of Medicine, University of North Carolina at Chapel Hill, Chapel Hill, NC 27599, USA

Stephen A. Haddad, Lynn Rosenberg and Julie R. Palmer
Slone Epidemiology Center at Boston University, Boston, MA 02215, USA

Edward A. Ruiz-Narváez
Department of Nutritional Sciences, University of Michigan School of Public Health, Ann Arbor, MI 48109, USA

Christopher A. Haiman
Department of Preventive Medicine, Keck School of Medicine, University of Southern California/Norris Comprehensive Cancer Center, Los Angeles, CA 90033, USA

Christine B. Ambrosone, Chi-Chen Hong, Lara E. Sucheston-Campbell, Qianqian Zhu and Song Liu
Department of Cancer Prevention and Control, Roswell Park Cancer Institute, Buffalo, NY 14263, USA

Song Yao
Department of Biostatistics and Bioinformatics, Roswell Park Cancer Institute, Buffalo, NY 14263, USA

Elisa V. Bandera
Cancer Prevention and Control, Rutgers Cancer Institute of New Jersey, New Brunswick, NJ 08903, USA

Kathryn L. Lunetta
Department of Biostatistics, Boston University School of Public Health, Boston, MA 02118, USA

Aarti Sethuraman, Martin Brown, Raya Krutilina, Zhao-Hui Wu, Tiffany N. Seagroves, Lawrence M. Pfeffer and Meiyun Fan
Department of Pathology and Laboratory Medicine, and the Center for Cancer Research, University of Tennessee Health Science Center, 19 South Manassas Street, Memphis, TN 38163, USA

D. Aggouraki and V. Georgoulias
Laboratory of Tumor Cell Biology, School of Medicine, University of Crete, Heraklion, Greece

G. Kallergi
Laboratory of Tumor Cell Biology, School of Medicine, University of Crete, Heraklion, Greece

Department of Biochemistry, University of Crete, Greece Medical School, Heraklion, Greece

N. Zacharopoulou and C. Stournaras
Department of Biochemistry, University of Crete, Greece Medical School, Heraklion, Greece

S. S. Martin
Department of Physiology, Marlene and Stewart Greenebaum Comprehensive Cancer Center, University of Maryland School of Medicine, 655 W. Baltimore Street, Baltimore, MD, USA

Erin D. Giles
Department of Nutrition and Food Science, Texas A&M University, 373 Olsen Blvd; 2253 TAMU, College Station, TX 77843, USA

Paul S. MacLean
Anschutz Health and Wellness Center, University of Colorado Anschutz Medical Campus, Aurora, CO 80045, USA
Department of Medicine, Divisions of Endocrinology, Metabolism, and Diabetes, University of Colorado Anschutz Medical Campus, Aurora, CO 80045, USA
Department of Pathology, University of Colorado Anschutz Medical Campus, Aurora, CO 80045, USA

Troy Schedin
Department of Medical Oncology, University of Colorado Anschutz Medical Campus, Aurora, CO 80045, USA

Ann D. Thor, Elizabeth A. Wellberg and Steven M. Anderson
Department of Pathology, University of Colorado Anschutz Medical Campus, Aurora, CO 80045, USA

Sonali Jindal
Department of Cell, Developmental and Cancer Biology, Oregon Health and Science University, 3181 S.W. Sam Jackson Park Rd, Mailing Code: L215, Portland, OR 97239, USA

Pepper Schedin
Department of Cell, Developmental and Cancer Biology, Oregon Health and Science University, 3181 S.W. Sam Jackson Park Rd, Mailing Code: L215, Portland, OR 97239, USA
Knight Cancer Institute, Oregon Health and Science University, 1130 NW 22nd Ave #100, Portland, OR 97239, USA

Dean P. Edwards
Departments of Molecular and Cellular Biology and Pathology Immunology, Baylor College of Medicine, Houston, TX 77030, USA

Ann H. Rosendahl
Division of Oncology and Pathology, Clinical Sciences, Lund University, SE-221 85 Lund, Sweden

Signe Borgquist
Division of Oncology and Pathology, Clinical Sciences, Lund University, SE-221 85 Lund, Sweden
Clinical Trial Unit, Skåne University Hospital, Lund, Sweden

Kamila Czene
Department of Medical Epidemiology and Biostatistics, Karolinska Institute, Solna, Sweden

Per Hall
Department of Medical Epidemiology and Biostatistics, Karolinska Institute, Solna, Sweden
Department of Oncology, Södersjukhuset, Stockholm, Sweden

Judith S. Brand
Department of Medical Epidemiology and Biostatistics, Karolinska Institute, Solna, Sweden
Clinical Epidemiology and Biostatistics, School of Medical Sciences, Örebro University, Örebro, Sweden

Nirmala Bhoo-Pathy
Julius Centre University of Malaya (JCUM), Faculty of Medicine, University of Malaya, Kuala Lumpur, Malaysia

Mozhgan Dorkhan
Global Medical Affairs, Novo Nordisk A/S, Søborg, Denmark
Institution for Clinical Sciences, Lund University, Lund, Sweden

Arantzazu Zubeldia-Plazaola, Leire Recalde-Percaz, Núria Moragas, Mireia Alcaraz, Xieng Chen, Mario Mancino, Patricia Fernández-Nogueira, Aleix Noguera-Castells, Anna López-Plana, Estel Enreig, Paloma Bragado and Gemma Fuster
Institut d'Investigacions Biomèdiques August Pi i Sunyer (IDIBAPS), Barcelona, Spain
Department of Medicine, University of Barcelona, Barcelona, Spain

Pedro Gascón
Institut d'Investigacions Biomèdiques August Pi i Sunyer (IDIBAPS), Barcelona, Spain
Department of Medicine, University of Barcelona, Barcelona, Spain
Department of Medical Oncology, Hospital Clínic, Barcelona, Spain

Miquel Prats de Puig
Department of Medicine, University of Barcelona, Barcelona, Spain
Department of Senology, Clínica Planas, Barcelona, Spain

Flavia Guzman
Histopathology-Citology, Anatomical Pathology Service, Centro Médico Teknon, Barcelona, Spain

Neus Carbó
Department of Biochemistry and molecular Biomedicine, University of Barcelona, Barcelona, Spain

Vanessa Almendro
Division of Medical Oncology, Department of Medicine, Harvard Medical School, Dana-Farber Cancer Institute, Brigham and Women's Hospital, Boston, MA, USA

Eleanor Broadberry, James McConnell, Jack Williams, Nan Yang, Egor Zindy, Angela Leek, Rachel Waddington, Leena Joseph, Miles Howe, Qing-Jun Meng and Charles H Streuli
Wellcome Centre for Cell-Matrix Research and Manchester Breast Centre, Faculty of Biology, Medicine and Health, University of Manchester, Manchester M13 9PT, UK

Anja Kathrin Wege, Stefan Buchholz, Simone Diermeier-Daucher, Olaf Ortmann and Gero Brockhoff
Clinic of Gynecology and Obstetrics, University Medical Center Regensburg, Regensburg, Germany

Dominik Chittka
Clinic of Gynecology and Obstetrics, University Medical Center Regensburg, Regensburg, Germany
Department of Nephrology, University Hospital Regensburg, Regensburg, Germany

Monika Klinkhammer-Schalke
Tumor Center Regensburg, University of Regensburg, Regensburg, Germany

Florian Zeman
Center for Clinical Studies, University Hospital Regensburg, Regensburg, Germany

John L. Hopper, Gillian S. Dite and Prue C. Weideman
Centre for Epidemiology and Biostatistics, The University of Melbourne, Parkville, VIC, Australia

Robert J. MacInnis, Roger L. Milne and Graham G. Giles
Centre for Epidemiology and Biostatistics, The University of Melbourne, Parkville, VIC, Australia
Cancer Epidemiology and Intelligence Division, Cancer Council Victoria, Melbourne, VIC, Australia

Kelly Anne Phillips
Centre for Epidemiology and Biostatistics, The University of Melbourne, Parkville, VIC, Australia

Division of Cancer Medicine, Peter MacCallum Cancer Centre, Melbourne, VIC, Australia
Sir Peter MacCallum Department of Oncology, The University of Melbourne, Melbourne, VIC, Australia

Yuyan Liao, Nur Zeinomar and Jeanine M. Genkinger
Department of Epidemiology, Mailman School of Public Health, Columbia University, 722 W 168th St, 7th Floor, New York, NY, USA

Mary Beth Terry
Department of Epidemiology, Mailman School of Public Health, Columbia University, 722 W 168th St, 7th Floor, New York, NY, USA
Herbert Irving Comprehensive Cancer Center, Columbia University Medical Center, New York, NY, USA

Gord Glendon
Lunenfeld-Tanenbaum Research Institute, Sinai Health System, Toronto, ON, Canada

Julia A. Knight
Lunenfeld-Tanenbaum Research Institute, Sinai Health System, Toronto, ON, Canada
Dalla Lana School of Public Health, University of Toronto, Toronto, ON, Canada

Irene L. Andrulis
Lunenfeld-Tanenbaum Research Institute, Sinai Health System, Toronto, ON, Canada
Departments of Molecular Genetics and Laboratory Medicine and Pathobiology, University of Toronto, Toronto, ON, Canada

Melissa C. Southey
Department of Pathology, Genetic Epidemiology Laboratory, The University of Melbourne, Parkville, VIC, Australia
Precision Medicine, School of Clinical Sciences at Monash Health, Monash University, Clayton, CA

VIC 3168, USA

Wendy K. Chung
Herbert Irving Comprehensive Cancer Center, Columbia University Medical Center, New York, NY, USA
Departments of Pediatrics and Medicine, Columbia University, New York, NY, USA

Sue-Anne McLachlan
Department of Medicine, St Vincent's Hospital, The University of Melbourne, Parkville, VIC, Australia
Department of Medical Oncology, St Vincent's Hospital, Fitzroy, VIC, Australia

Michael L. Friedlander
Prince of Wales Clinical School, University of New South Wales, Sydney, NSW, Australia
Department of Medical Oncology, Prince of Wales Hospital, Randwick, NSW, Australia

Antonis C. Antoniou
Department of Public Health and Primary Care, Centre for Cancer Genetic Epidemiology, University of Cambridge, Cambridge, UK

Stephanie Nesci
Division of Cancer Medicine, Peter MacCallum Cancer Centre, Melbourne, VIC, Australia

kConFab Investigators
Sir Peter MacCallum Department of Oncology, The University of Melbourne, Melbourne, VIC, Australia
The Research Department, The Peter MacCallum Cancer Centre, Melbourne, VIC, Australia

Saundra S. Buys
Department of Medicine and Huntsman Cancer Institute, University of Utah Health Sciences Center, Salt Lake City, UT, USA

Mary B. Daly
Department of Clinical Genetics, Fox Chase Cancer Center, Philadelphia, PA, USA

Esther M. John
Department of Medicine and Stanford Cancer Institute, Stanford University School of Medicine, Stanford, CA, USA

Jaroslaw Suchanski
Department of Biochemistry and Molecular Biology, Faculty of Veterinary Medicine, Wroclaw University of Environmental and Life Sciences, C.K. Norwida 31, 50-375 Wroclaw, Poland

Maciej Ugorski
Department of Biochemistry and Molecular Biology, Faculty of Veterinary Medicine, Wroclaw University of Environmental and Life Sciences, C.K. Norwida 31, 50-375 Wroclaw, Poland
Laboratory of Glycobiology, Hirszfeld Institute of Immunology and Experimental Therapy, Polish Academy of Sciences, Wroclaw, Poland

Tomasz Owczarek
Department of Biochemistry and Molecular Biology, Faculty of Veterinary Medicine, Wroclaw University of Environmental and Life Sciences, C.K. Norwida 31, 50-375 Wroclaw, Poland
Present address: Department of Medicine, Herbert Irving Comprehensive Cancer Center, Columbia University Medical Center, New York, NY, USA

Aleksandra Piotrowska, Aleksandra Nowak and Jedrzej Grzegrzolka
Department of Histology and Embryology, Wroclaw Medical University, Wroclaw, Poland

Piotr Dziegiel
Department of Histology and Embryology, Wroclaw Medical University, Wroclaw, Poland
Department of Physiotherapy, Wroclaw University School of Physical Education, Wroclaw, Poland

Pawel Pasikowski
EIT+ Wroclaw Research Center, Wroclaw, Poland

Bartlomiej Kocbach
Laboratory of Glycobiology, Hirszfeld Institute of Immunology and Experimental Therapy, Polish Academy of Sciences, Wroclaw, Poland

Andrzej Wojnar
Lower Silesian Oncology Center, Wroclaw, Poland

Michael Hauptmann
Department of Psychosocial Research and Epidemiology, Netherlands Cancer Institute, Plesmanlaan 121, 1066 CX Amsterdam, the Netherlands.

Kimberly D. van der Willik
Department of Psychosocial Research and Epidemiology, Netherlands Cancer Institute, Plesmanlaan 121, 1066 CX Amsterdam, the Netherlands
Department of Epidemiology, Erasmus MC - University Medical Center Rotterdam, 3000 CA Rotterdam, the Netherlands

Vincent Koppelmans
Department of Psychosocial Research and Epidemiology, Netherlands Cancer Institute, Plesmanlaan 121, 1066 CX Amsterdam, the Netherlands
Department of Epidemiology, Erasmus MC - University Medical Center Rotterdam, 3000 CA Rotterdam, the Netherlands
Department of Psychiatry, The University of Utah, 501 Chipeta Way, Salt Lake City, UT 84108, USA

Sanne B. Schagen
Department of Psychosocial Research and Epidemiology, Netherlands Cancer Institute, Plesmanlaan 121, 1066 CX Amsterdam, the Netherlands
Brain and Cognition, Department of Psychology, University of Amsterdam, Nieuwe Achtergracht 129-B, 1018 WS Amsterdam, the Netherlands

M. Arfan Ikram
Department of Epidemiology, Erasmus MC - University Medical Center Rotterdam, 3000 CA Rotterdam, the Netherlands

Annette Compter
Department of Neuro-oncology, Netherlands Cancer Institute, Plesmanlaan 121, 1066 CX Amsterdam, the Netherlands

Index

www.ingramcontent.com/pod-product-compliance
Lightning Source LLC
Chambersburg PA
CBHW061329190326
41458CB00011B/3945